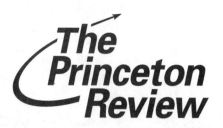

BEST 168
MEDICAL
SCHOOLS

2007 EDITION

Random House, Inc.
New York
www.PrincetonReview.com

Malaika Stoll

The Princeton Review, Inc.
2315 Broadway
New York, NY 10024
E-mail: bookeditor@review.com

ISBN: 0-375-76566-2

Manufactured in the United States of America.

Publisher: Robert Franek
Editors: Adrinda Kelly, Michael Palumbo
Account Manager: David Soto
Production Manager: Scott Harris
Production Editor: Christine LaRubio

9 8 7 6 5 4 3 2 1

2007 Edition

Acknowledgments

Special thanks must go to the hundreds of med students and scores of admissions officers who have supplied information for this book over the years. This year's edition owes a great debt to the efforts of many: to Michael Palumbo, Adrinda Kelly, Christine LaRubio, and Scott Harris for their editorial and design talents; to David Soto for heading the data collection efforts; to Ben Zelevansky for his data-pouring wizardry and sense of humor; and to Robert Franek, Publisher, for his enthusiasm.

Contents

Preface

For over 25 years The Princeton Review has offered preparatory courses and tutoring for standardized tests such as the SAT, MCAT, LSAT, GRE, GMAT, and USMLE. More than 100,000 students took our courses last year, and hundreds of thousands have bought our "Cracking" series test-prep books. At the center of our approach is the desire to help students tear away the anxiety and sense of helplessness that have surrounded these entrance exams for so many years. The Princeton Review has long been an advocate of students' right to be informed consumers, and works to make sure that information on these tests is readily accessible to all.

In addition to being consumers of entrance exams, students are also consumers of education. Before investing in a graduate degree, they have the right and the need to gather as much information as possible. We hope that this publication will provide students with a viable means of achieving this goal. The *Best 168 Medical Schools* contains the essentials students will need to answer both basic and advanced questions regarding their list of prospective medical schools. The 2007 edition is our most complete medical school handbook to date; it contains 126 accredited allopathic schools in the United States, including Puerto Rico (we've retained a separate profile for the University of Minnesota Medical School—Duluth), 16 accredited allopathic schools in Canada, 20 accredited osteopathic schools, and a brand new section profiling 6 accredited naturopathic schools in the U.S. and Canada.

When viewing individual schools listed in this year's guide, you will find the union of painstakingly researched school profiles coupled with school-specific statistical data. Each profile has been sent to the medical school itself for review prior to publication so that we may provide our readers with the most accurate and current information about the programs. The data presented was the most up-to-date available at the time of publication; students should consult the schools' websites for further information.

Two of the Southern schools featured in this book were affected by hurricanes during the past year. Tulane University School of Medicine and Louisiana State University School of Medicine in New Orleans were closed for either all or part of the Fall 2005 semester. As a result, these two schools were unable to participate in our profile review campaign, but each will have the opportunity to update its information for the 2008 edition of the book. We advise prospective students considering schools in the South, particularly those in Louisiana and Eastern Texas, to contact each school for a full update on any changes to the medical school experience that may have occurred as a result of the hurricanes.

We hope this book will serve as an important guide as you research, gather, and consider information before embarking on your medical career, and we wish you the best of luck as you pursue your career in medicine. If you have questions, comments, or suggestions, we welcome them. Please give us your insights:

The Princeton Review
Best 168 Medical Schools
2315 Broadway
New York, NY 10024
bookeditor@review.com

We appreciate your input and want to make our books as useful to you as they can be.

Sincerely,
Adrinda Kelly and Michael Palumbo
Co-editors
Admissions Services
The Princeton Review

1 How to Use This Book

Although some people describe medical school education as somewhat canned—and downplay the differences between schools—real, concrete differences do exist. Some differences, like the fact that a family medicine clerkship lasts two weeks at one school and eight at another, might not seem like a big deal, but such details may help convey a school's priorities. The school profile section of this guide will help you to discern such differences, and in doing so, match your interests with the school that can best fulfill them. But don't just use this book to decide where to apply; use it also as a resource to help you decide when to apply—or if you really want to apply after all. The detailed information about course offerings and facilities will help you prepare for interviews. Examine the profiles for descriptions of each program's fundamental academic approach and resources, the student body, and the school's emphasis as evidenced by the path its graduates take. These are all good points to bring up in an interview and will aid your decision of where to attend.

As you review the school profiles, keep the following in mind:

- *Just as admissions offices rely too heavily on quantitative measures to evaluate candidates (MCAT and GPAs), applicants probably rely too much on school ranking in deciding where to apply and where to go to school. Often, the criteria for determining a school's ranking have little to do with how well a school will train you or how enjoyable your experience will be (NIH research dollars, for example). Thus, you will find no quantitative rankings in this book.*

- *Our goal is to present accurate and complete descriptions of medical schools. Note that the admissions offices of each medical school had the opportunity to read and edit our write-ups. The data presented in this book was the most up-to-date at the time of publication. In deciding where to apply or where to go, you should consult the schools' websites in addition to using this book as part of your research. Take every opportunity to meet with medical students at the schools in which you are interested. Speak with more than just one student—and with students in different years—at each school.*

- *In response to managed care and other trends, many medical schools that traditionally focused on research or specialty medicine now claim to focus on primary care. Whether a school really has changed its focus may be partially gleaned from the percentage of graduates entering primary care fields. Note, however, that definitions of primary care vary (some include ob/gyn for example).*

- *In the Graduates section (under Students), a statistic on what percent of students match within their top one, two, or three residency preferences may appear. Less prestigious schools often have impressive rates. This is due in part because students only rank schools that they have a good chance of getting into (and at which they obtained an invitation to interview). In addition, students at less prestigious schools are less likely to enter highly specialized residency positions that are typically the most competitive. Please note that this stat is often misleading.*

- *For most schools, we list website addresses—they are often helpful and some include candid student opinions. Try to visit these websites before you make a commitment to apply, interview, or attend.*

HOW THIS BOOK IS ORGANIZED

The 2007 edition of this book includes 142 U.S. and Canadian accredited allopathic medical schools. You may notice that we no longer list Puerto Rican schools separate from U.S. schools. The AAMC lists them under one umbrella, and so do we. The profile of each school is broken down into five text sections—Overview, Academics, Students, and Admissions. Three categories of hard stats supplement the general data in the allopathic profiles—Student Body, Admissions, and Cost and Aid—listed in the shaded sidebar column. We also created supplementary chapters of lists—including a general overview and admissions requirements—of the 20 accredited osteopathic schools, and of the 6 accredited naturopathic schools.

Here's what you will find in the various text and statistic sections for each school profile:

PROFILE

ACADEMICS

First, we give you a basic look at the academic program—quarter system or semester, pass/fail or honor, and USMLE requirements. Then we break it down in accordance with how your own studies will be broken down—Basic Sciences and Clinical Training—outlining the academic requirements and path of each. Here you will find out how much time you have to spend hunched over a book versus the fun part—hunched over, say, a cadaver. We will often use the term "selective" to describe certain clinical requirements. It means that students have some choice within a specified area: Selective courses are less "free" than an "elective" (which might also have some restrictions).

STUDENTS

Discover where your potential classmates call home and who they are—percentage-wise. In the Student Life section, we describe what kind of recreation facilities are available, where you might live, where you might go out. We also include information about the graduates. Who are the grads of this school—primary care physicians, surgeons, public health administrators—and in what type of community do they choose to practice?

ADMISSIONS

The Requirements section details what the school is looking for in its prospective students. Pay special attention to the Suggestions section for some hints about how to impress the school. Then whip out your Palm Pilot—the Process section will tell you the dates you need to know and key stats about who gets interviews (and then who the lucky recipients of the fat envelopes are).

SIDEBAR

The shaded column next to each school listing contains the following information:

STUDENT BODY

Type: Is the school private or public? This is important information that is closely tied to the cost of tuition. In addition, public schools are often open only to state residents.

Enrollment: Total number of students enrolled in the medical school.

% male/female: Gender breakdown based on total enrollment.

% underrepresented minorities: Percentage of African Americans, Native Americans, Mexican Americans, and mainland Puerto Ricans in the total enrollment.

 # applied: The number of people who applied to the school in the most recently reported year, presented as the total number, and the number of out-of-state/province residents who applied.

 # accepted: The number of applicants who were accepted at the school in the most recently reported year. Also broken down in terms of total and out-of-state/province.

 # enrolled (out-of-state): The number of out-of-state applicants who were accepted who actually entered the school as first-year medical students in the most recently reported entering class.

Average age: The average age of entering class.

FACULTY

total faculty: The number of faculty employed by the medical school.

% female: Percentage of female faculty members.

% minority: Percentage of underrepresented minorities present on the faculty.

% part-time: Percentage of part-time faculty members.

student-faculty ratio: The ratio of faculty members to enrolled students.

ADMISSIONS
Overall GPA

Average undergraduate grade point average of the students who matriculated in the most recently reported entering class.

MCAT

Average MCAT scores of the students who matriculated in the most recently reported entering class, broken down into the following areas: Biology, Physics, Verbal, and Essay.

Application Information

Outlines all the dates and facts you need to know:

Regular application: The latest date by which the school must receive all application materials for regular admission.

Regular notification: The latest date by which the school will notify prospective students of its decisions concerning regular admission.

Early application: The latest date by which the school must receive all application materials for the early decision plan.

Early notification: The latest date by which the school will notify prospective students of its decisions concerning admission to the early decision plan.

Are transfers accepted? Yes or No.

Admissions may be deferred? Yes or No.

Interview required? Yes or No.

Application fee: How much does it cost to apply?

Admissions Requirements (Required): Required qualifications in order for an applicant to be considered for admission into the school's program.

Admissions Requirements (Optional): Additional suggested qualifications for applicants—not required for admission.

Overlap schools: The other schools to which applicants are most likely to apply.

COSTS AND AID

Tuition & Fees

Most recent yearly tuition figures available for both state residents and nonresidents. The amount of money students can expect to spend on books and fees is listed here as well.

Financial Aid

% students receiving aid: Percentage of medical students at the school receiving some sort of financial aid.

Average grant: The amount of money in grants students receive on average.

Average loan: The amount of money students borrow on average.

Average debt: How much do students owe when they get out?

2 So You Want to Be a Doctor . . .

A GLIMPSE AT MEDICINE IN THE TWENTY-FIRST CENTURY

Do you want to be a doctor? If your answer is yes, use this chapter to prepare yourself for what lies ahead. (This chapter can also prepare you for medical school interviews—you can impress interviewers with your knowledge of current trends in health care!) If you're not yet sure whether medicine is the career for you, this chapter will help you decide. Learn about current issues as well as potential future trends in health care, medicine, and physician practice. The purpose of this chapter is to provide a glimpse of what life will be like for you as a doctor. Although it is impossible to predict the future, research and analysis have allowed us to identify some of the issues that will shape medicine in the coming years.

DECISIONS, DECISIONS . . .

Becoming a doctor requires a real commitment, so your decision to pursue this career path should be an informed one. You should consider information from discussions with medical professionals as well as from books such as this one. Talk to as many doctors as you can. Find out how they spend their days, and what they love and don't love about their profession. Think about whether you could fill their shoes and whether you would thrive in doing so. Always consider your source when gathering information. For example, TV shows with exciting plots and attractive actors glamorize medicine, whereas newspapers sometimes do the opposite by highlighting negative trends and emphasizing scandal.

While you are fortunate to have hundreds of career options to choose from, having so many choices can be confusing and overwhelming. Don't let indecision paralyze you. Consider taking time off after college to work in medical or nonmedical fields, to travel, or to volunteer before applying to medical school. This type of experience serves the dual purpose of allowing you to assess your interest in medicine and giving you something to write about in your medical school application essays (not to mention that it can be fun and meaningful, depending on what you do). The chapter in this book on nontraditional medical school applicants discusses several alternative paths to medical school. In deciding whether medicine is the career for you, you should also reflect on the paths that you won't be taking. Are you deciding between being a teacher or a doctor? Why not teach for a year or two and then reconsider medical school? The skills you learn teaching will help you explain medical issues to patients if you decide to become a physician.

Perhaps you feel that there are too few rather than too many career possibilities from which to choose. Some people consider medicine, law, and other obvious professions because they just don't know what else is out there. In this situation, there is nothing like spending a couple of years in the "real" world. This will expose you to various professions and career options. Even working for a temp agency can be beneficial; it can provide exposure to a number of fields and organizations. Learning about other options might confirm your interest in medicine or could lead you in another direction. Either way, it will be a valuable use of your time.

WHAT IT TAKES TO BE A DOCTOR

In some ways, being a doctor in the United States in the twenty-first century is similar to being a doctor in any number of cultures during just about any time period. There are a few traits that are essential, no matter where you are, or what century you're in. Consider the following questions:

Do you want to spend your life helping others?
Doctors heal people, save lives, and help others—often through direct, face-to-face interactions. According to a recent survey of medical school students, "helping others" is their primary motivation for pursuing an MD.[1] If this is your motivation, you're in good company. However, there are other altruistic careers out there, all of which involve less schooling and less debt than medical school. The desire to help others should be one, but not your only, reason for becoming a doctor.

Do you enjoy working hard?
Medicine is an incredibly challenging field. This was the case a hundred years ago when doctors worked to fight yellow fever, polio, and influenza, and it is the case today as health professionals try to prevent and treat heart disease, cancer, AIDS/HIV, and influenza, while dealing with the constraints of managed care. Consider medicine only if you love challenges and you know you want tremendous challenge in your professional life. As you read through this chapter, think about whether the challenges involved in practicing medicine are the ones that appeal to you. For example, a physician who is 20 years out of medical school is still expected to be familiar with the latest medical developments. One of the challenges of practicing medicine is a commitment to lifelong learning.

---

[1] Princeton Review survey of medical students

Are you interested in science and health issues?

If you enjoyed some aspects of your science courses (few people enjoy all aspects of pre-medical course work) and you find yourself drawn to health issues, there is a good chance that you will enjoy studying and practicing medicine. Although medicine has changed significantly over the years, its roots remain in basic science.

Do you like working with different people?

With the exception of a few fields, medicine involves working with people, many of whom may be very different from you. If science interests you but working with people does not, you may wish to consider a PhD rather than an MD (this choice also involves less debt). You might also look into an MD that allows you to do only research.

WHAT IT'S LIKE TO BE A DOCTOR

What is life like as a doctor in the twenty-first century? Although it varies a great deal depending on specialty, geographic region, employment situation, and so on, we can get a general idea by examining recent data.[2, 3]

PATIENT CARE

Most doctors—90 percent—spend their time seeing patients; in fact, they see 20 to 25 patients per day on average. Doctors generally work in one of three situations: solo, as part of a group practice, or as an employee of a hospital or organization. The most common reason people go to the doctor is for some sort of check-up or test. Other common reasons for doctor visits are respiratory (allergies, the flu), gastrointestinal (heart burn, nausea), and psychological (e.g., depression) complaints. An important responsibility of the primary care physician is to identify potentially serious issues during routine examinations. On the other side of the spectrum, a major challenge for doctors with highly specialized training (e.g., oncologists, cardiologists, and surgeons) is to work intensely to save and improve lives. The most common causes of mortality (death) in the United States are listed below.

Top Ten Causes of Mortality in the United States[4]

1. *Diseases of the heart (heart disease)*

2. *Malignant neoplasms (cancer)*

3. *Cerebrovascular diseases (stroke)*

4. *Chronic lower respiratory diseases (e.g., emphysema, asthma, bronchitis)*

[2] Association of American Medical Colleges. AAMC Data Book. Statistical Information Related to Medical Schools and Teaching Hospitals. January 2003.

[3] The Future of American Medicine. American Medical Association, Council on Long Range Planning and Development, 1994.

[4] National Center for Health Statistics, Deaths: Leading Causes for 2002.

5. *Accidents*

6. *Diabetes mellitus (diabetes type 2)*

7. *Influenza and pneumonia*

8. *Alzheimer's disease*

9. *Nephritis, nephrotic syndrome, and nephrosis (kidney disease)*

10. *Septicemia (blood poisoning)*

Note that all of the above except Alzheimer's are preventable. Preventive medicine and the interdisciplinary approach are important elements of practicing medicine.

WORKLOAD AND COMPENSATION

On average, doctors work 58 hours per week. Obstetricians work longer hours, 62 per week, while the typical psychiatrist works shorter hours, 49 per week. Although their annual incomes have decreased over the past few years, physicians are still the highest paid professionals in the country. The following table presents median annual income for nine areas of practice. Incomes listed are after expenses (such as staff and malpractice insurance) but before taxes.

Medical Field	Annual Income
Anesthesiology	$266,000
General/Family Practice	$142,000
Internal Medicine	$150,000
Ob/Gyn	$238,000
Pathology	$212,000
Pediatrics	$144,000
Psychiatry	$143,000
Radiology	$286,000
Surgery	$261,000
ALL PHYSICIANS	$160,000

The figures listed above do not account for residents, who are notoriously underpaid. The national median salary for a resident is about $35,000. In the interest of patient safety, there have been some efforts—at the state and hospital level, and among residents themselves—to limit the number of hours that residents work each week. These efforts have been somewhat successful. However, despite the rules limiting the workweek to 80 hours, many residents continue to work more than 100 hours per week. Why are residents required to work so hard? In part, it's because hospitals depend on residents as a cheap source of labor, since they are paid much less than other physicians and somewhat less than nurses and other health professionals.

PRESTIGE

Almost universally, being a doctor carries prestige. Doctors are generally thought to be smart, well educated, hard-working, caring, and dedicated. Even in this era of managed care and malpractice lawsuits, doctors are well respected. In a recent Harris poll, Americans ranked "doctor" as the most prestigious profession/occupation.[5] You should consider the degree to which having a prestigious career is important to you. Other health professions, although perhaps less glamorous, also involve healing and helping others.

TRENDS IN MEDICINE IN THE TWENTY-FIRST CENTURY

Several trends in medicine that began during the past few decades are likely to continue well into the twenty-first century. These trends have implications for you, the aspiring doctor. They will impact the nature of your work, the structure of the organization in which you work, your salary, the relationship you have with patients, and above all, the quality of the health care you deliver.

In the sections that follow, we consider some important trends (we call them the Top Ten, with a disclaimer that predicting the future is difficult) affecting medicine in the twenty-first century.

Top Ten List: Trends in Medicine in the Twenty-First Century

1. *Development of new technology*

2. *Increased health care costs*

3. *Evolution of health care delivery and payment systems*

4. *Greater reliance on primary and preventive care*

5. *More guidelines for patient care*

6. *A possible surplus of physicians, at least in certain specialty areas*

[5] Doctors reign, teachers gain, lawyers wane in public esteem. *New York Times.* 11/1/2000.

7. *Improved gender and ethnic diversity among physicians*

8. *An aging patient population*

9. *The emergence of new ethical issues*

10. *Changes in academic medicine and medical education*

Note that the above list is by no means complete. Also, the trends listed are interrelated and are not necessarily in order of importance.

NEW TECHNOLOGY

Medicine and health care has improved during the past few decades largely because of technological advancement; there are probably even more exciting developments on the horizon. The term *technology* is often used broadly. In the health care arena, it means the development of new drugs, procedures, techniques, and means of communication that, if used correctly, have the potential to improve diagnosis, care, and patient outcomes.

- *Medications and Procedures. The increase in life expectancy over the past few decades is partially due to improvements in medications and procedures. For example, the death rate due to heart disease is declining because of better drugs (hypertension, heart, and cholesterol medications) and surgical techniques.*

- *Laboratory Techniques. Often, improvements in laboratory tools or techniques lead to important discoveries. For example, better tools allowed the human genome to be mapped.*

- *The Internet. Patients who are Internet users arrive at their doctor's office well-informed about their illness. On the other hand, the Internet houses a great deal of misinformation. The physician who is Web-savvy can guide patients to informative websites and Web-based support groups. The Internet is an invaluable tool for research.*

- *Telemedicine. Telemedicine is defined by the American Telemedicine Association as "the use of medical information exchanged from one site to another via electronic communication for the health and education of the patient or health care provider and for the purpose of improving care." Sharing of radiographic images and patient information (X-rays, MRIs) via computer between physicians is an important current application. In the future, we may see telemedicine bring the expertise of specialists to rural or other remote areas.*

- *Other Computer Applications. Computerized database systems are used for billing and patient records. Some physicians take advantage of software programs made for hand-held devices. These can be used for note-taking, reference, or even patient management. Not surprisingly, it is often the younger doctors (and medical stu-*

dents) who are the most comfortable with computer technology. Interest in and understanding of relevant computer applications can give you an advantage when it comes to working with older, more experienced doctors; instead of just learning from them, you will have something to contribute. The key is being able to explain, teach, and pass on your knowledge effectively.

HEALTH CARE COSTS

The United States spends more money per capita on health care than any other country in the world. Some believe that the U.S. offers the best medical care in the world, thereby justifying the high cost. Others note that, according to indicators such as life expectancy and infant mortality, the U.S. lags behind other industrialized countries. In 1960, six percent of the U.S. Gross Domestic Product (the sum total of all expenditures, by all people, in a given country) went to health care. In 2000, that figure climbed to 20 percent, meaning that nearly a fifth of the GDP went to health-related goods and services. There are many theories as to what has caused this escalation, two of which are discussed below.

Technology

As discussed above, technological advances usually serve to improve health care and health outcomes. However, technology is often cited as a major cause of rising health care costs. When new tools are developed and advertised, hospitals and physicians may feel pressure to purchase and use them, even if the benefit of the new device is still questionable. Someone ultimately pays for such purchases, and thus we see rising health care costs. The MRI—an imaging device that, for about $2,000, provides pictures of a patient's organs—is often thought to be overused in this country. For example, there are more MRI machines in Orange County, California, than in all of Canada.[7] It is important to remember, however, that technological advances can also serve to reduce costs. By preventing illness and reducing the spread of disease, new vaccines (anti-influenza, for example) lower the cost of treatment for society overall. New surgical instruments and the development of medication in pill form facilitate the use of outpatient procedures instead of expensive hospital stays.

Incentives

Patients are generally far removed from the cost of their care, and therefore have little incentive to keep costs down. Employers and the government—not patients themselves—foot most of the bill for health care, creating a system of "third-party payers."[8] Some believe that since patients don't pay much for their own health care, they "overuse" it, thereby driving government and employer health care expenditures up.

---

[7] "By the Numbers: Health Care Costs." *Scientific American.* April 1999.

[8] The United States relies largely upon an employer-based health care financing system, which means that most people (60 percent) receive health benefits through their work. In other words, employers pay for employees' health care—typically by taking responsibility for paying monthly premiums. Twenty percent of the population receives government health care benefits in the form of Medicare (everyone over 65 is eligible) or Medicaid (eligibility based on financial need).

As a physician, you will undoubtedly feel pressure to keep health care costs down. In many practice settings, doctors are scrutinized on the basis of the cost of the tests and treatments they prescribe. For example, primary care doctors are sometimes encouraged to limit referrals to specialists. All doctors may be monitored for "overuse" of expensive tests and equipment. Physicians face difficult decisions as they attempt to provide excellent care at a lower cost: if a patient has a slim chance of benefiting from an expensive treatment, should that treatment be employed? The physician must balance the cost of treating with the risk of not treating.

HEALTH CARE DELIVERY SYSTEMS

The push for management of health care costs has led to the growth of managed care. One of the most important trends of the past few decades has been the replacement of simple fee-for-service plans by the growth of the managed care industry.

Fee-for-Service

Before managed care, health care was delivered on a "fee-for-service" basis. Medicare (federally funded health insurance for those over 65 years of age) remains a fee-for-service program. Under a fee-for-service system, doctors and hospitals perform a service (a check-up, an operation, etc.) and charge a fee for the service. Typically, the patient's health insurance company pays the fee for whatever medical service the patient wants or needs. The patient pays the health insurance company a monthly premium or, if the patient has health benefits from his employer, the employer pays the monthly premiums. The insurance company calculates monthly premiums based on how much it pays out to hospitals and doctors each year for all people enrolled in the insurance plan.

Managed Care

Managed care was introduced as a response to rising health care costs, and has succeeded in slowing the rate at which health care costs rise. Thus, the trend towards managed care will probably continue. Although managed care is often thought to be synonymous with Health Maintenance Organizations (HMO), an HMO is, in fact, just one of many systems for managing care.[9]

Managed care usually involves set monthly premiums that are lower than those in fee-for-service plans, and this makes those paying the premiums (usually the employers) happy. How do managed care organizations keep their premiums down? By keeping their financial outlays down. Under managed care, expenditures are typically controlled through several mechanisms:

---

[9] HMOs specify the doctors and hospitals that participants must use. Another example of a managed care organization is a Preferred Provider Organization (PPO). PPOs encourage the use of certain providers ("preferred providers") but will also cover part of the cost of doctors and hospitals outside of the preferred provider network.

- *Participants in a managed care plan agree to use doctors and hospitals that are part of the plan, and these providers are either paid yearly salaries or charge reduced fees for services rendered.*
- *Primary care physicians serve as "gatekeepers" in limiting the use of expensive medical specialists.*
- *Guidelines/regulations are implemented that attempt to limit the use of expensive tests and equipment in unnecessary situations.*
- *Inpatient care is reduced and there is more emphasis on outpatient services (care that does not involve an overnight hospital stay). Associated with the movement towards outpatient care, hospitals are filling fewer of their beds and are seeing a decline in length of stay (LOS) for hospital patients.*

Managed care has generated discontent among some patients and providers. In a recent study,[10] over half of those surveyed said that managed care lessens quality of care. Patients are often frustrated by red tape, the inability to choose one's own doctor, short visits, long waits, obstacles to seeing specialists, and limitations on coverage. Many doctors object to managed care because the cost-cutting mechanisms may compromise patient care, and because physician salaries and autonomy are reduced under managed care arrangements.

However, there can be advantages in working for a managed care organization. For one, doctors are often salaried, which means that they earn a specified amount each year, and their income does not depend on finding clients. Doctors also tend to work fewer hours per week, which is probably good both for doctors and for patients. For better or for worse, being a doctor in the twenty-first century is likely to involve practicing in a managed care environment of some form.

The Uninsured

This section on health care delivery and payment would be incomplete without discussing the uninsured. At least 15 percent of people in the United States have no health insurance. The U.S. is unique among industrialized nations in that respect, and it is not exactly something to be proud of. Individuals without health insurance tend to seek medical care—typically through an emergency room—only after a health problem has become really serious. This is obviously bad for the patient, who with early treatment might have avoided serious complications. It is also costly to society, because prevention and early treatment are less expensive than late intervention. Most people—physicians and nonphysicians alike—believe that everyone should have access to health care. However, there is less agreement on how universal access should be achieved and funded. Doctors will need to speak out to assure that this issue is addressed as soon, and as equitably, as possible.

---

[10] Harvard/Harris Poll, analyzing 25 public opinion surveys. 1997.

PRIMARY AND PREVENTIVE CARE

Most observers predict that as managed care grows, primary care physicians will continue to play a very important role, and the demand for primary care doctors will remain relatively high. Primary care physicians may be either MDs, DOs, or NDs (see page 22 for a description of each degree).

Gatekeepers

Before the days of managed care, if a person discovered an odd-looking spot on his skin, he could go directly to a dermatologist and be reimbursed by his insurance company for the visit. An important tenet of managed care has been the requirement that enrollees see a primary care physician prior to visiting a specialist. Family practice, pediatrics, internal medicine, and ob/gyn are typically considered primary care fields. The primary care physician serves as a "gatekeeper," presumably reducing unnecessary visits to expensive specialists.

Without the training of a specialist (a dermatologist in our example above), the primary care physician may not be equipped to judge the seriousness of some conditions. Missing a pre-cancerous skin lesion, for example, may cause hardship for the patient later on. On the other hand, if a primary care doctor refers *all* patients with skin lesions to the dermatologist, the system has failed because each patient required two doctor visits rather than one.

Integrated Approach

A benefit of this emphasis on primary care is that, in theory, patients develop a long-term relationship with their primary care doctor who is better able to understand the social, economic, and community-related issues associated with their health. The primary care doctor presumably has an understanding of all physiologic systems. This comprehensive knowledge facilitates diagnosis or at least allows the physician to make the initial decision about what next steps will lead to diagnosis. Primary care physicians are well-positioned to address behavioral changes, such as exercise programs, that aid in the prevention of disease.

Prevention

Several of the major causes of morbidity (illness) and mortality (death) in the U.S. are preventable. Emphysema, for example, is often the result of heavy smoking. The most common type of diabetes is linked with obesity. We have learned that the spread of HIV can be reduced through educational programs and behavioral interventions. The high death rate in this country due to violent crime is often attributed to the prevalence of handguns, a situation that could be addressed through legislation. Advances in genetics could potentially revolutionize preventative medicine by allowing physicians to identify people who are going to get sick before they show any symptoms of disease.

Prevention is preferable to treatment for the obvious reason that, with prevention, illness is reduced or even eliminated altogether. Whether prevention efforts are cost-effective depends upon the disease, its prevalence, and the technology employed. For example, mammography is helpful in detecting breast cancer at a treatable stage and can potentially prevent mortality and reduce the high costs associated with treating end-stage cancer. It is sensible and cost-effective to offer mammograms to women above a certain age. However, it is probably unreasonable to encourage women in their 20s to have annual mammograms because breast cancer at this age is rare and, furthermore, can be difficult to spot on a mammogram from a woman of this age.

GUIDELINES FOR PATIENT CARE

Fundamental to medicine are the doctor-patient relationship, the belief that each patient must be considered individually, and the principle that doctors should be allowed to use their best judgment when providing care. Do these ideals conflict with the recent trend of using guidelines in clinical medicine?

Evidenced-Based Medicine or Cookbook Medicine?

Doctors vary tremendously in their approach to medicine and disease treatment. This is why, in serious illness, a second opinion is usually recommended. In recent years, there has been increased use of Evidenced-Based Medicine (EBM) in clinical practice. EBM employs *scientific evidence* for the purpose of standardizing and improving patient care. Quantitative indicators such as rate of reduction of disease are typically used to evaluate procedures and treatments. The goal of EBM is to establish guidelines for clinical decision-making based on the results of studies, particularly randomized clinical trials (these are generally considered the most accurate type of study).

Some doctors worry that the trend towards EBM de-emphasizes physician judgment, results in strict guidelines for treatment, and amounts to "cookbook medicine." On the other hand, EBM's supporters say that its population-based approach actually complements the one-on-one tradition of medicine by allowing doctors to defend their decisions with data. However, there are many diseases and clinical situations for which the EBM literature fails to provide clear evidence. In some cases, the risks and benefits of a particular therapy may differ depending on the study examined.

Cost Consciousness

Occasionally, guidelines that dictate clinical care are based on cost-cutting objectives rather than on sound medical evidence. Such "guidelines" may compromise patient care. Going back to our mammogram example, an HMO might encourage physicians to recommend mammograms to all women over 50, when research suggests that mammograms are highly beneficial for women in their 40s as well. It is the physician's ethical responsibility to give his patient honest and up-to-date medical advice (in this case, to recommend mammograms after age 40). At the same time, the physician may want to support the cost-cutting goals of his employer. This is the type of conflict that doctors face in the current era of cost-consciousness. There are no easy answers. However, familiarity with medical evidence and the rules of the organization will at least allow you to make informed decisions.

Physician Surplus or Physician Shortage?

From 1970 to 1990 there was a sharp increase in the number of residency positions in the U.S., largely as a result of government policy encouraging such growth. During the same period, there was a much less dramatic increase in the patient population. Some said that we were training too many doctors and that we would see a surplus. Since 1990, however, the number of residency programs has remained relatively stable, while the patient population has grown (partially as a result of an aging population). The surplus never occured; now some experts predict a shortage.

Whether we have a physician surplus, shortage, or neither, there will always be rural and inner-city areas that are in need of doctors. To combat this problem, federal and state-funded programs offer financial incentives to doctors who agree to work in underserved areas. There is also a shortage of physicians from certain ethnic backgrounds. It is important to have a physician population that represents the population that it serves. Most medical schools attempt to recruit students of ethnic backgrounds that are underrepresented in medicine.

Diversity Among Physicians

Increased diversity among physicians is a positive trend and may result in better patient care.

Women

Approximately 49 percent of entering medical students are women. This is remarkable considering that just 20 years ago, women accounted for about 30 percent of medical students, and in 1960, less than 7 percent of medical students were women. Today, about 25 percent of practicing physicians are women, and this percentage will continue to rise. There are outstanding women physicians in every imaginable medical field. However, women are especially well represented in fields like pediatrics and ob/gyn, and less well represented in other fields like surgical subspecialties. Several theories and generalizations have been put forth to help explain why women are attracted to some fields more than others. One such theory is that once there is a critical mass of women within a field, it becomes a more welcoming environment for other women. Also, people tend to be interested in fields that have personal relevance. Finally, many women tend to avoid fields with the very longest residencies (only 10 percent of neurosurgery residents, for example, are women).

Minorities

The medical profession is slowly becoming more ethnically diverse, as increased numbers of nonwhite medical school graduates enter the work force. This increase in diversity reflects the changing demographics of the U.S. population, better and more widely available educational opportunities, and active minority recruitment on the part of medical schools. If this trend continues, we will someday have a physician work force that is representative of the population at large, including African Americans, Mexican Americans, Puerto Ricans, other Hispanics, Native Americans, and other underrepresented minorities. In 2004, underrepresented minorities made up 16 percent of entering medical school classes[11].

Aging Population

In 2020, the median age in the U.S. will be 40 years, up from 36 in 2000 and 30 in 1960. As the population ages, the demand for medical care increases: the average number of doctor visits per year is three for the population at large, but is six for those over 74 years old. The aging of the American population contributes to rising health care costs. Because 99 percent of individuals over 65 are covered by Medicare, government expenditures on health care are expected to rise. The paperwork involved in treating a patient with Medicare is notoriously time-consuming.

An older population will cause growth within certain fields, such as geriatrics, internal medicine, orthopedics, and cardiovascular medicine. The incidence of chronic disease, meaning disease that is long-lasting and often incurable, will increase. Thus, physicians will often be called upon to provide palliative care that addresses symptoms when the underlying disease cannot be cured. Physician-researchers will be encouraged to find treatments for conditions that afflict the elderly, such as Alzheimer's Disease.

Ethical Issues

Physicians have always dealt with important ethical issues related to life and death. As a physician in the twenty-first century, some of your ethical dilemmas are likely to involve the conflict between saving money and saving lives. Consider the following scenario:

> You are a pediatrician, seeing a patient you have never seen before. The patient is a very ill 6 year old without health insurance. Do you treat her, knowing that you will hear about it later? Or do you send her to the free clinic across town, even though it will entail a long bus ride for the sick girl?

Ethical issues surrounding end-of-life care will become increasingly relevant because of an older patient population. For example:

> Your patient is 80 years old and suffers from terminal lung cancer, which has spread to his brain. There are no cures for this man at this stage, so your care has been focused on keeping him comfortable. He can't breathe on his own, is incoherent, and has been more or less motionless in the hospital for one week. His daughter does not want you to remove life support. What do you do?

[11] Association of American Medical Colleges. AAMC Data Warehouse: Applicant Matriculant File as of Oct 14, 2004.

The rule of doctor-patient confidentiality can also be the basis for ethical issues. Consider this situation:

> You have been treating a young man in the hospital for a lung infection. During his hospital stay, he was tested for HIV and the test results were positive. He is unwilling to discuss the matter, does not want medications that will help his HIV symptoms, and appears to be in denial. Do you have a responsibility to alert the man's wife?

Unfortunately, some medical schools barely address ethics, leaving you on your own to learn about and think through important ethical issues. A mentor, someone whose opinion you respect, can serve as a resource for sorting out ethical questions. If you feel strongly about a particular issue, you should consider getting involved—through writing, attending conferences, or engaging in dialogue.

CHANGES IN ACADEMIC MEDICINE AND MEDICAL EDUCATION

Most medical schools are directly affiliated with teaching hospitals. Three advantages to this arrangement are the following:

- *Medical students have the opportunity for hands-on learning.*
- *Patients are treated by expert physicians and benefit from the latest technology.*
- *The academic environment coupled with the clinical facilities provide an ideal setting for research that ultimately pushes medicine forward and improves care.*

Academic medical centers throughout the country are having a tough time financially, leading some experts to question their future viability. Although medical school tuition seems incredibly high, it does not cover the actual cost of medical education; academic medical centers have historically depended on income from clinical activities to subsidize medical education, research activities, and management of a teaching hospital. As discussed, the shift toward outpatient medicine has resulted in reduced earnings for hospitals. For academic medical centers, this means less revenue to cover their high costs. As more and more academic medical centers face financial crisis, there will be pressure to cut costs and/or raise revenue significantly. We might see academic medical centers restrict their patients to those who can pay higher fees, or perhaps we'll see an increase in government funding and/or medical school tuition.[12]

In response to these changes in medicine and health care, most medical schools are attempting to revise their curriculum. Some of the revisions we see are the following:

- *Less time spent in lecture. Educators recognize that in this age of technology and information, there are simply too many facts to learn. Rather than inundate students with a massive amount of information, some medical schools hope to teach students general concepts that will prepare them for a lifetime of learning.*

[12] Keynotes on Health Care. AAMC. 34 (1) Winter, 2000.

- *More clinical problem-solving during the first two years. With all that we know, and all the treatment options available today, physicians must be thinkers and problem-solvers.*

- *Greater emphasis on health economics, health care management, and public health. Doctors should understand the interdisciplinary nature of health care, and the forces that affect medicine.*

- *Better training in outpatient medicine, with the use of outpatient clinics and doctors' offices for clinical rotations of outpatient facilities.*

With the requirement of at least 11 years of post-high school training, becoming a physician takes longer in the U.S. than anywhere else in the world. This is costly to society. Some people predict that as a result of financial pressures, the amount of schooling required to become a doctor will be reduced. For the time being, however, you have a long (but exciting) road ahead of you.

CONCLUSION: IS MEDICINE YOUR CALLING?

Whether you will be able to work effectively amidst all these changes depends in part on your flexibility. According to the American Medical Association, ". . . The next 10 to 15 years will be a period of substantial change for physicians. Physicians who are flexible, adaptable, and responsive to changing circumstances are likely to prosper during such a period."[13]

Apart from flexibility, what other traits will help you succeed and find job satisfaction as a physician in the twenty-first century?

What It Takes to Be a Doctor in the Twenty-First Century

Compassion—*a critical part of healing*

Advocacy—*for your patients and for those without health care*

Leadership—*in improving health care at the team, hospital, and policy level*

Lifelong learning—*there will always be more to know*

Interpersonal skills—*communication with patients and among providers is key*

Negotiation—*ability to work around bureaucratic constraints*

Grasp—*of increasing amounts of medical knowledge and of a health care system in flux*

Ask yourself: Is medicine your CALLING?

[13] ibid

3 So You Still Want to Be a Doctor . . .

Congratulations! The good news is that you are on your way to entering one of the most rewarding and respected fields, one of the few altruistic careers that pays a livable wage. The bad news is that, even armed with all the information we can give you and the help of a premed advisor, the application process is still tough. The painful reality is that there are about 33,000 applicants for approximately 18,000 spots. The good news, however, is that if you are persistent and have worked hard for the past several years to make yourself a competitive candidate, you have a good chance of obtaining a certified letter and a career that will keep you challenged and fulfilled for the rest of your life.

WHAT MAKES A COMPETITIVE APPLICANT?

Well, that's the $115,218 question (average debt of current medical school graduates). In 2005, the average matriculated (accepted) medical student had an undergraduate science GPA of 3.56, a nonscience GPA of 3.70, and an overall GPA of 3.63; the average matriculated (accepted) medical student had average MCAT scores of 9.7 Verbal Reasoning, 10.1 Physical Science, 10.4 Biological Sciences, and a P on the Writing Sample. But while GPA and MCAT scores will play a large role in the admissions decision, they aren't everything. Solid numbers are a good start, but medical schools are also quite interested in who you are, why you want to be a physician, and whether or not you have a clue about what being a doctor is like. Therefore, in addition to strong grades and scores, you will strengthen your application by having volunteer activities listed, some experience in scientific academic research, demonstrated leadership roles, interesting extracurricular activities, a well-written personal statement, excellent communication skills, and solid recommendation letters. All these application pieces will provide the admissions committee with a fuller picture of who you are than mere numbers can convey.

Also, keep in mind that despite the odds, there are always large numbers of normal, sane people who actually didn't get straight A's or perfect MCATs who still manage to get into medical school. You can be one of them, and this book can help you to package yourself and target schools that are likely to appreciate your unique strengths. If you have a hunch that your set of qualifications is not what traditional medical school admissions committees are looking for, consider a few alternate career paths. This book covers allopathic (MD) programs in the U.S., Puerto Rico, and Canada (many Canadian schools accept only Canadians), osteopathic (DO) programs, and includes a brand new section on naturopathic (ND) programs. Don't rule out programs or schools in other health fields, such as dental school, nursing school, and physician assistant programs.

ALLOPATHIC MEDICINE

Allopathic schools confer the MD on their graduates, and allopathic training is by far the most widely available and recognized type of medical training. There are 142 accredited MD schools in the U.S., Puerto Rico, and Canada. Both the Canadian and Puerto Rican medical schools in this book are part of the American Association of Medical Colleges (AAMC). Teaching methodology varies among schools. The "traditional" model consists of two years of basic science followed by clinical rotations. The "systems-based" program is organized around physiologic systems, such as the lung or kidney. The "case-based" model teaches through clinical vignettes. There are also schools offering hybrids of these approaches. Most schools have made a concerted effort to get students together with patients at a much earlier stage in their education—it used to be that medical students might not come in contact with any patients until they'd already been through two years of school. At most schools, the last two years are spent doing clinical rotations. Even if you're sure that your calling in life is plastic surgery, you're going to have to do a pediatrics rotation. Most medical students really enjoy having a chance to delve into the various specialties, and this structure provides an excellent opportunity to learn about the areas you hope to pursue.

Allopathic training will give you the option to practice in any of the medical specialties, and the MD is universally recognized worldwide as a medical degree. For an abundance of information on all aspects of allopathic training and practice, visit the AAMC website (www.aamc.org).

OSTEOPATHIC MEDICINE

Osteopathic medicine in the United States got its start in the late 1800s. Its founding father was Dr. Andrew Taylor Still, who established the American School of Osteopathy in Kirksville, Missouri, in 1892. The various regulatory bodies (osteopathic versions of AAMC and the AMA) were well underway by the early 1900s, and are now the American Osteopathic Association (AOA) and the American Association of Colleges of Osteopathic Medicine (AACOM). There are currently 20 colleges of osteopathic medicine throughout the United States, and the DO is only issued in the United States. Visit the AOA's website at www.aoa-net.org and the AACOM's website at www.aacom.org to find out more about these organizations.

Osteopathic medicine has an interesting history; until fairly recently, its focus on preventive care, communication with the patient, and a holistic approach to health was considered to be somewhat radical. Now, of course, much of what osteopathic medicine has always espoused is rapidly becoming part of all medical training. In addition to a philosophical difference in approach, an important distinction between osteopathic and allopathic training is that osteopaths are taught an additional modality of treatment called manipulation (not to be confused with chiropractic manipulation, which has an entirely different system of education and is not recognized as a fully licensed medical degree). The osteopathic philosophy posits that there is a unity between a living organism's anatomy and physiology. Osteopathic science includes "the behavioral, chemical, physical, spiritual, and biological knowledge related to the establishment and maintenance of health as well as the prevention and alleviation of disease." Osteopathic concepts emphasize the following principles[1]:

1. *The human being is a dynamic unit of function.*

2. *The body possesses self-regulatory mechanisms that are self-healing in nature.*

3. *Structure and function are interrelated at all levels.*

4. *Rational treatment is based on these principles.*

What this means to the average osteopathic student is that he or she has to learn all of the same science as his or her allopathic counterpart, plus osteopathic diagnosis and treatment, in the same amount of time. Practicing osteopaths have another way of helping their patients that allopaths do not. Osteopaths achieved full-practice rights in 1973, although some states certified osteopaths to practice in all public hospitals as complete physicians and surgeons much earlier.

As you might guess from their philosophy and training, many osteopathic doctors choose to become primary care physicians. Most work in family practice, internal medicine, pediatrics, ob/gyn, and general surgery. In the words of one osteopathic dean, they tend to be generalists first and specialists second. However, there are DOs in just about every area of modern medical practice, from neurological surgery to psychiatry, oncology, and emergency medicine. Although DO was not traditionally considered a research degree, the DO/PhD combination is becoming more common, and the AOA is becoming much more active in encouraging research activities, particularly in primary care.

At most osteopathic schools, matriculates have undergrad GPAs of about a 3.4 and combined MCAT scores of just under 25. In 2005, there were 8,300 applicants for approximately 3,000 seats. However, osteopathic schools do have a reputation for "looking past the numbers" and place a very strong emphasis on the whole picture of the candidate. This often makes osteopathic school an attractive choice for nontraditional, older students whose GPAs from their first trek through undergraduate school prove prohibitive in most allopathic programs. If you have a few blemishes on your academic record but a life that suggests you'll make a dedicated physician, you should consider applying to osteopathic schools.

---

[1] *AOA Yearbook of Osteopathic Physicians 1996*, Chicago: AOA, p. 732.

Most premeds trying to decide whether or not to apply to osteopathic schools worry about what will happen to them after they graduate and apply for a residency. Osteopathic graduates participate along with allopaths and foreign medical graduates (both American and nonresident) in the National Resident Matching Program (NRMP)—the Match. DOs can apply for either osteopathic or allopathic residencies, and for that reason, many take both the USMLE (United State Medical Licensing Examination) and the COMLEX (Comprehensive Osteopathic Medical Licensing Examination, which is a series of exams administered by the National Board of Osteopathic Medical Examiners). Louisiana is the only state that does not recognize the COMLEX and requires DOs to pass the USMLE to be licensed. The best way to decide which path is right for you is to spend time with both MDs and DOs and talk to them at length about their practices.

NATUROPATHIC PROGRAMS

Students enrolled in a school of naturopathic medicine are conferred the doctor of naturopathic medicine (ND) degree upon graduation. The program in naturopathic medicine consists of two years of classroom instruction in standard medical school sciences and two years of clinical training under the supervision of a licensed ND. Graduates of naturopathic medical school programs are licensed as primary care physicians who can use natural therapies such as nutrition, homeopathy, acupuncture, hydrotherapy, and lifestyle modification to treat disease, and combine these therapies with conventional medical treatments when appropriate.

Naturopathic physicians (NDs) take a holistic approach to healing, and aim to cure disease by taking advantage of the body's self-regenerative powers and harnessing the restorative power of nature. Like osteopaths, naturopathic physicians endeavor to treat the whole person by taking into account the emotional, genetic, and environmental factors that have influenced their state of health. Unlike osteopaths, however, naturopathic physicians emphasize natural remedies. NDs also differ from allopaths (MDs); rather than limiting their treatment to synthetic drugs and invasive procedures, NDs predominantly utilize natural medicines and procedures. Naturopathic physicians work to identify and eliminate the *cause* of disease, and are guided by six basic principles:

1. *Do no harm*

2. *Utilize the healing power of nature*

3. *Identify and treat the causes*

4. *Treat the whole person*

5. *Focus on preventive medicine*

6. *Practice doctor-as-teacher*

Naturopathic medicine gained major visibility in the U.S. in the late 1800s, when Dr. Benedict Lust opened the nation's first health food stores and helped put the spotlight on diet and nutrition as the primary means to staying healthy. Naturopathic medicine was hugely popular until WWII when rapid advancements in medicine and technology caused it to lose ground to more high-tech forms of treatment, leading to a near-monopoly in health care practices by the chemical and drug industries. Today, a new crop of scientifically focused proponents of naturopathy largely guided by the principles of EBM, have been able to prove that diet and lifestyle have a significant impact on health, placing naturopathic medicine in the spotlight once more.

Students considering a naturopathic medical program should know that the ND license to practice medicine is only valid in 15 U.S. states and four Canadian provinces, and graduates are subject to passing national licensing exams. However, legal provisions do allow for the practice of naturopathic medicine in several of the unlicensed states. (See *www.aanmc.org* for a list of states and provinces.) NDs may also practice in countries outside of the United States, based on requirements specific to each country. Each of the Association of Accredited Naturopathic Medical Colleges (AANMC) schools is accredited by the Council on Naturopathic Medical Education (CNME), and prepares graduates to sit for board examinations with the North American Board of Naturopathic Examiners (NPLEX). Naturopathic medical schools are looking for applicants who are thoroughly committed to the efficacy of natural therapies and are flexible enough to deal with the challenge of formulating personalized treatment plans. Some opportunities for specialization include dermatology and allergies, women's medicine, pediatrics, diabetes and blood pressure treatment, and cancer treatment and research, to name a few. In order to figure out whether an ND career is right for you, talk to other NDs. Compare their experiences with those of the MDs and DOs you know.

FOREIGN MEDICAL SCHOOLS

If you are seriously considering attending a foreign school but want to practice in the U.S., make sure you take a hard look at the prospective school's USMLE pass rate and residency placement rate. Although foreign schools are much easier to get into, they will put you in just as much debt as U.S. schools, without the same assurance of a career after graduation that will enable you to pay it off.

THE NUMBERS GAME

Because of the sheer volume of applications they have to wade through, admissions officers have to make some initial screening decisions based largely on GPA and MCAT scores—deceptively simple acronyms for the arcane processes they represent.

Your GPA, for the purposes of applying to medical school, consists of your science GPA (biology, chemistry, physics, and math), your nonscience GPA (every other class you ever suffered through), and your cumulative GPA. These are calculated for your undergraduate career, any nondegree-seeking postsecondary work, and any degree-seeking postsecondary programs. In other words, you could conceivably have nine GPAs. Each medical school has its own policies for deciding which GPA means the most to them when they're choosing which applicants to interview and/or matriculate. The average GPA of all applicants (not necessarily accepted) in 2005 was a 3.37 science, a 3.60 nonscience, and a 3.48 overall. It is extremely difficult to get into medical school with a cumulative GPA below 3.0. Your GPA is the single most important element of your application because it is the best predictor of your academic readiness.

Although community college classes may count as part of your GPA, they may not always be acceptable as prerequisite premedical course work. If you are planning to take some of your core premed courses (biology, chemistry, physics) at a community college, it's an extremely good idea to do some advance planning and call some of the schools that you're interested in to make sure that they have no qualms about community college credit. Similarly, if you took an AP class in high school and then tested out of a core class, such as physics, you may run into trouble when you apply unless you've taken upper-division course work in that subject. Again, it is very much to your advantage to check with a few medical schools and your pre-health advisor to make sure that your academic record doesn't have any holes in it.

Your GPA and MCAT score are interrelated. The MCAT is an immensely important part of your application, but not as important as your GPA. As a standardized test, it provides only a snapshot of your academic readiness. Your MCAT score is made up of four separate marks: verbal reasoning, physical sciences, biological sciences, and the writing sample. Verbal reasoning and the science sections are scored from 1 to 15. The writing portion of the MCAT requires that you write two essays, which generate a single score. This score is reported as a letter J–T, where J is low and T is high. The average score for all applicants on each section in 2005 was 8.9 verbal, 9.1 physical sciences, 9.5 biological sciences, and a P on the writing sample.

The writing sample, added to the MCAT a few years ago in an attempt to ensure the applicant's ability to communicate, is largely ignored by admissions committees. Virtually the only time the writing sample is looked at very carefully is in the case of a disconnected application—a beautifully written personal statement with low verbal scores and/or a low writing sample score. Some schools will also consider the writing score if they are evaluating the English ability of English as a Second Language applicants. This does not mean that you can take a nap during the writing sample. You should make every effort to answer the questions in a coherent and focused way on the off-chance that the committee decides to closely examine your score.

THE SUM OF YOUR EXPERIENCE

Although your GPA and MCAT score play a large role in your application, admissions committees are also looking for several other attributes. They are quite interested in who you are, why you want to be a physician, and whether or not you have a clue about what being a doctor is really like.

Exposure to the Health Care Field

Although students with no discernible exposure to health care still matriculate, the vast majority of successful premeds have some experience, usually volunteer work, in a hospital, clinic, hospice, or other health care setting. Some premeds are qualified enough to find part-time paying positions as emergency medical technicians (EMTs), nurse's aids, or organ and blood bank workers, while other "nontraditional" applicants may have had full-time careers in health care. Your goal should be to hold a volunteer or paid position for at least six months. Many premedical programs have specific classes you can take that include organized volunteer time as part of their course work—even if you are a returning adult student and not officially registered as premed. You can often get college credit for community service work in the medical field. Although it may seem difficult to find the time to volunteer, it will make a huge difference as you work on your personal statement and get through your interviews. You will have stories to tell, and will be able to speak far more effectively about the reasons that you want to become a physician.

Leadership Experience and Community Service

Leadership can mean many things, and being a leader, say, within your family, can be as important as being class president. One of the simpler ways to prove your abilities is to join a club or campus organization and get elected to office. You can also lead youth- or religiously-affiliated organizations, or participate in a variety of community service organizations such as food banks, literacy programs, and mentoring. The key is to demonstrate sincere commitment and have some longevity with whatever cause you decide to embrace, so that you can achieve a measure of responsibility. If you are serious about practicing primary care medicine, for example, this is your chance to build your resume and to start proving yourself. Find a clinic that needs a dedicated volunteer and get your feet wet.

Research

Academic research is quite a bit easier to get involved with than you might think. Research labs are always looking for drones—read "undergrads"—to help with the unlovely business of test-tube cleaning and organism counting. With any luck, however, you should be able to find a program in which you will actually be able to conduct experiments and write about the results. If you are considering a career in academic medicine, you should try to get involved in research projects as early in your undergraduate career as you can convince someone to take you. One way to find out about cool research projects is to sit down with a teaching and research assistant over a cup of coffee and ask about the various projects going on in their departments. Alternatively, check out the science department websites at your university for information on current research.

HUMANITY

Medical schools are interested in training bright, empathic, communicative people who have a strong interest in science and a wide-ranging intellect. They are not interested in students with perfect grades who have clearly never done anything else with their lives than try to break the curve in chemistry class. The schools want to graduate physicians who will listen to their patients and be able to effectively use the myriad tools available to heal them. What this means is that there is no magic system that will create an unbroken path into medical school. You can major in art history, modern dance, or biochemistry—it doesn't matter, as long as you take the classes you need to fulfill medical school requirements. You can take a few years off and join the Peace Corps or go straight to med school upon college graduation. Admissions committees will be trying to discern what you have learned from your experiences and how the things you have seen and done nurtured the values that have led you to pursue a medical career.

THE "Z" FACTOR IN MEDICAL SCHOOL ADMISSIONS

Although many medical schools will claim not to use a formula when it comes to evaluating an applicant, in actuality, almost all employ an initial screening process that weeds out applicants based on a cut-off score. While the formula used to arrive at this score varies from institution to institution, it's sure to involve the following three elements: GPA, MCAT score, and a "Z" factor. The "Z" factor represents the bonus points an institution will award based on an applicant's ethnicity, participation in varsity athletics, and any other extraordinary activity and/or circumstance that the applicant may have experienced. Keep in mind that each medical school has its own target score. In order to maximize your rating, focus on improving your GPA and MCAT numbers so that you don't have to rely on bonus points awarded for the "Z" factor to achieve the school's cut-off score.

THE APPLICATION PROCESS

There are many factors to consider when applying to medical schools. The first rule of thumb is to apply broadly and include "safety" schools where you will most likely be accepted. Besides the obvious clinical and scholastic goals, it is important to look for a school in a location that suits you. Although you may think that you won't see the light of day for four years, you should apply to schools that are in geographic areas that appeal to you and will provide outlets for your hobbies and interests.

APPLYING TO ALLOPATHIC MEDICAL SCHOOLS

Most allopathic medical schools use AMCAS®, the American Medical Colleges Application Service, which is a centralized and standardized application that is handled by the AAMC, the Association of American Medical Colleges. In the spring of 2001, the AAMC switched to an entirely Web-based AMCAS application. The online application is available directly from www.aamc.org. The AMCAS application costs $160 for the first school; the fee is $30 for each additional school. If you have significant financial hardship, you can apply directly to AMCAS for a fee waiver on their services. You will also need to prepare transcript requests for every postsecondary school you ever attended, even if you only took one class there or the credits transferred elsewhere. Undergraduate colleges will send your transcripts to AMCAS, who forwards them to all medical schools to which you are applying. AMCAS begins accepting transcripts on March 15 each year and completed applications on June 1. It will take a couple of weeks for AAMC to process everything, at which point you'll receive a "transmittal notification." You can call and use AAMC's voicemail to check your status (you can reach AAMC on the Web at www.aamc.org or by phone at 202-828-0600). At most universities and colleges, your pre-health advisor will help you navigate the AMCAS application, which can be fairly baffling. One of the toughest parts of the application is the "Personal Comments" page, where you have exactly one typewritten, single-spaced page to explain your life and convince them that you should be one of the chosen few. Needless to say, this part of the application takes time and patience—be sure to read through the suggestions and advice for working on it that are included later in this chapter. Please note that the seven public medical schools in Texas have their own application service called TMDSAS (Texas Medical Dental Schools Application Service). In addition, two U.S. allopathic medical schools do not participate in any application service at all. Those schools are: Columbia University College of Physicians and Surgeons and the University of North Dakota School of Medicine and Health Sciences. If you're interested in attending these schools, or any of the 17 accredited Canadian medical schools, you'll need to contact each school directly to obtain an application.

When you are choosing which schools to apply to, make sure that you check their in-state residency requirements. Although many allopathic schools are private, there are quite a few public schools that receive free money every year from out-of-state applicants they are prohibited from accepting into their programs. It doesn't matter how qualified you are; if you aren't a state resident, you can't get in.

APPLYING TO OSTEOPATHIC SCHOOLS

Osteopathic schools use their own internal system, called AACOMAS®, which in many ways works exactly the same way as AMCAS. Both paper and online applications are available from AACOM. You can request an application from their website at www.aacom.org, or call 301-968-4100. Like the AMCAS application, AACOMAS takes some time to fill out, so make sure you get started early. It also includes a personal statement, but it's even shorter than AMCAS's—you only have half of a page to explain why you want to be an osteopathic physician. You will also need to get a recommendation from a DO, a fact that takes some applicants by surprise. If you are serious about osteopathic school, search for a mentor DO as early as possible. One of the nice things about AACOMAS is that all osteopathic schools use it—you don't have to worry about tracking down additional applications. Because osteopathic schools are private institutions, they don't have residency requirements (although some may have tuition breaks for residents of particular states). If you are interested in going to an osteopathic school, investigate all of your options and choose one based on your interest in the program and living conditions in the area.

APPLYING TO NATUROPATHIC SCHOOLS

The admission process varies slightly at each of the six AANMC schools. In general, naturopathic medical schools require a bachelor's degree and a base of undergraduate science courses that include physics, biology, and general and organic chemistry for an applicant to be considered. Math and psychology courses may also be specified. Admission into most of the naturopathic medicine programs requires students to have completed three years of premedical training. The duration of an ND program is the same as that of an MD program, with residency period optional. Check with each school you are considering in order to make sure that you've met all prerequisites and that you fully understand their application procedures. It is worth noting that the MCAT is not required, but is optional for admission into a naturopathic medical school.

WHEN TO APPLY TO MEDICAL SCHOOL

Whether you're applying to osteopathic, allopathic, or naturopathic medical schools, you need to apply as early as you can in the process. In general, premedical students begin the application process in the spring semester of their junior year, or approximately a year and a half before they want to enter medical school. The vast majority of medical schools engage in some type of rolling admissions, which means that they read and evaluate applications as the folders arrive. Admissions officers are only human. Even though they make every effort to give the same consideration to applicant number 6,005 as they give to applicant number 1, the sheer volume of applications takes its toll on their patience and enthusiasm. In practical terms, this means that if you take the April MCAT (Medical College Admission Test) and get your applications in by late June, you will have a distinct advantage over someone taking the August test. Even if you turn in your AMCAS or AACOMAS application early, many medical schools will not look closely at your application until they have a copy of your MCAT scores. Each year, students are accepted with August test scores and applications that arrived late in the process. Unfortunately, there are also large numbers of students who are not accepted but would have had a decent chance had they applied earlier. Basically, you should try for every possible advantage. Turning in your application early can certainly help to give you an edge. Also, procrastinators take note: AMCAS is serious about its deadlines. If an application or transcript is late, you'll get it back.

INFORMATION ABOUT THE MCAT TEST

The MCAT (Medical College Admissions Test) is administered by the AAMC and is an admissions requirement for most allopathic and osteopathic medical school programs. More than 60,000 students take the test each year. The test is broken up into four sections: physical sciences, biological sciences, verbal reasoning, and a writing sample. All of the questions (with the exception of the writing sample) are multiple-choice.

Recently, the AAMC announced that in 2007, the MCAT will become a computer-based test (CBT) and paper-and-pencil exams will be eliminated. Here's a breakdown of changes to the test format that will occur when the MCAT becomes a CBT:

- *MCAT CBT will have 33 percent fewer questions.*
- *MCAT CBT will be shorter (approximately 5 and a half hours vs. the current testing time of 8 hours).*
- *Students will receive their MCAT scores more quickly (30 days vs. 60 days).*
- *MCAT will be offered more frequently throughout the year (19 testing dates).*
- *Students will have optional breaks instead of mandatory breaks.*
- *Test will be given in smaller, climate-controlled rooms.*
- *Students will have their identities verified using electronic fingerprint verification technology.*

Students who are taking the MCAT in 2006 shouldn't be affected by the format change since the paper-and-pencil exam will be administered through August 2006. If you're taking the MCAT in 2007 or later, you can see that the new test has its advantages: it's shorter, has fewer questions, and you'll receive your score report faster. However, if AAMC gives you the option to take the MCAT CBT while they are testing the new format this year, we strongly recommend you take the standard paper-and-pencil version. The MCAT CBT being tested by AAMC will be the same exact exam as the paper-and-pencil version, but it will be given on a computer. You've practiced and prepared for the paper-and-pencil exam, and that's how you should take the real thing.

When to Take the MCAT

According to the "AMCAS Survival Guide" (an official publication of the AAMC) you should, "if possible, take the Medical College Admissions Test (MCAT) on the April test date." As evidence, they cite the admissions cycle—earlier is better. Of course, not all applicants' academic schedules realistically allow them to take the April test. The new MCAT to be rolled out in 2007 will enable greater flexibility in scheduling by providing students with 19 test dates to choose from throughout the year. To register for the MCAT online, visit the AAMC website.

If you have not finished most of the prerequisites for the test—two semesters each of biology, physics, general chemistry, and organic chemistry—you probably should not sit for the exam. If you are determined to try the test without being fully prepared, take advantage of the fact that you can take a practice test at any Princeton Review office. It is much, much better to find out precisely what your current scoring levels are on a practice exam than to have to explain a woefully low score on a later medical school application.

It is possible, although it's certainly not the best idea, to take the last semester of one of the required science courses concurrently with studying for the MCAT. If you find yourself in this situation, it is vitally important to lighten your course load so that you will be able to adequately study for the exam while maintaining good grades in your courses. Thoroughly studying for the MCAT is not a small task.

How to Study for the MCAT

You are correct in assuming that since you're reading a book published by The Princeton Review, we're a little biased as to how we think you should study for the MCAT. The short answer here is that for most people, taking a course to prepare for the MCAT is worth the investment in both time and money. This is simply because MCAT scores are as important as your GPA in terms of admissions criteria. The MCAT is a tedious and wretched business, and having a class full of fellow sufferers at least makes you feel less alone in your pain. A class also forces you to study in a reasonable way, cover the material effectively, get plenty of practice, and gives you the resources to shore up any gaps in your academic preparation.

There are some people who do not need much preparation for the MCAT, and you'll meet them in medical school. They'll be getting honors designations in all of their classes while maintaining their world rankings as premier ice climbers/Sanskrit poets/master chefs. Unless you're pretty sure you're one of them (you might qualify if you're reading this while skydiving), you'll need some help with the test.

First, assume that you will be spending about 20 hours a week for several months studying for the MCAT. Although it doesn't test everything you've learned in school, it will feel that way. And, if you're rusty or haven't studied one of the subjects in awhile—physics, general chemistry, organic chemistry, and biology—you're going to have to do some in-depth review. At the same time, you have to keep in mind that this is a standardized test, and even though it's one of the better ones available, it still suffers from the same flaws as all other standardized tests—a fact that you can use to your advantage.

The key to doing well on the exam is to know the material, and then to know the test. The MCAT consists of four timed sections administered over a period of more than five hours.

The MCAT tests basic sciences—but don't assume that the exam is a science test similar to the kind you have learned to take as an undergraduate. Fundamentally, the MCAT is a verbal test, which is why on average, humanities majors tend to get slightly better scores in all of the sections than any other major. They are seeing a test format that they are used to: passages and questions. Science majors, on the other hand, are generally used to manipulating formulas and answering questions that may have a setup, but are not embedded in a long series of paragraphs.

In practice, it is much easier to raise your score if you start with low science numbers but a high verbal score. Unfortunately, most examinees are in exactly the opposite position. This is of real concern because more and more medical schools have come to regard scores that are out of balance as undesirable. They will often look more favorably on a candidate with three tens than someone with an eight verbal and two twelves. In order to change your verbal score, you will have to practice the type of causal, linear logic that it tests. AAMC releases five previous MCATs, including one that is free, and a couple of books of practice items (any formal test preparation course should give you reams of additional practice material). If you don't have access to test preparation courses, you will probably find yourself rapidly running out of verbal practice material, although most college bookstores are reasonably well stocked with practice materials relating to the science portions of the MCAT. You can use reading comprehension sections from other graduate-level standardized tests such as the GRE or LSAT to supplement your verbal study, but keep in mind that the passages in these tests were not written to be read under the same time constraints as were the MCAT passages. In addition, you may want to consider using online training materials.

MCAT SCORE REPORTING—FULL DISCLOSURE

Gone are the days when prospective med students could choose whether or not to release their MCAT scores to schools before seeing them. The MCAT is, in fact, moving toward a "full disclosure" policy, whereby scores from any MCAT taken in 2003 or later will automatically be reported as part of the examinee's test history. AMCAS and the medical schools you're applying to will always receive your MCAT Testing History Report, or THx Report (previously known as the Additional Score Report). If you took the MCAT between 1991 and 2002, those scores won't be released unless you request it. Still, the dates of those tests will appear on the THx Report.

Although you'll no longer have the option to withhold MCAT scores except in the case of older test dates, this isn't necessarily a bad thing. In the past, schools knew when you withheld your scores, and as you might imagine, they could interpret this in many different ways. Although some schools told us that they did not hold it against you if you withheld your scores, other said they were inclined to look negatively on withheld scores and would rather see your entire test history. Problem solved! Seriously though, these issues may still come into play if you choose to withhold test scores from 2002 or earlier.

There are a few perks to the new THx Report online system too: the reports are free and you can check out your score online much earlier—as soon as it's available to the AAMC.

Check out www.PrincetonReview.com for more information on the MCAT, including a detailed discussion of changes to the test.

YOUR BUDDING CAREER AS A NOVELIST

If you've ever harbored any fantasies of becoming a writer, now is your chance. If you've ever harbored fantasies of wiping the art of composition from human memory in retaliation for the suffering you endured in your freshman English class, you're going to have to find a way to cope. The personal comments section of the ACOMAS and AMCAS application is your chance to convince the committee that you are more than the sum of your numbers and that you deserve a chance at an interview.

Idea Generators

It is extremely difficult to write about anything important in a page or less, so assume that you will be spending some quality time with your computer. To get started, you can try a couple of different approaches to get your fingers moving:

Clustering

You may remember this from Freshman composition. You probably thought it was silly back then, but it just might save you now. Get a large blank piece of paper and write down a few words to describe some of the experiences that have led you to pursue medical school. Or jot down some interesting, sad, or memorable experiences and later link them to your interest in medicine. You don't have to write them down in any particular order, just scatter your thoughts across the page. After you have several topics to work with, see if you can spot any patterns. Some of them will probably be interrelated. Next, generate longer descriptions of the words you wrote. For example, try to explain what you mean by "intellectual challenge." Was there a particular class you took? A paper you wrote? After you have some ideas on paper, try pulling them together based on the patterns of relationships you see between the topics. For example, telling a story about helping to clean a wound while volunteering in the ER might be a good way of letting the reader know that compassion is one of your qualities. It is often more effective to let the reader draw conclusions rather than spelling them out. For example, relate how you felt while treating a patient and let the reader see that you are compassionate. Don't write, "That experience demonstrates my compassion."

Free Writing

This is particularly helpful if you find that you are having trouble figuring out where to start. All you have to do is sit down and force yourself to write about anything that comes into your mind. Don't worry about punctuation or grammar—just write for several pages. Take a break and look back at what you wrote. Most of the time, you'll be surprised to discover the beginnings of an idea. Keep a notepad with you and by your bed. Jot down ideas as they come to you.

Talk, Talk, Talk

One way to avoid writer's block and get started is to talk into a tape recorder, or bribe a friend to write as you speak. Sometimes, an empty screen or page can be intimidating in and of itself. You can get started on your essay by telling your story to a tape recorder, or by having a friend write down what he or she thinks is interesting or important as you explain why you want to go to medical school. Don't expect to have suddenly generated your essay in this way. However, you can generate some material with which to start writing.

Three Basic Approaches

There are many different ways to structure the personal essay, but there are three basic approaches that can be used alone or in combination.

"My History in School"

This essay focuses on college experiences. It works well for people whose grades are fairly high and who want to emphasize their growth during the college years. The essay should be about your development, specialties, and strengths. The best essays usually have specific examples. It helps to have a specific class, professor, paper, or experience that crystallizes your experiences and ties into your goals. One of the benefits of this essay is a built-in chronology and organizational structure.

"My Life History"

In this essay, focus on a few events or main ideas that illustrate the qualities you can bring to medicine. If your whole life clearly leads up to being a physician (even if it might not have seemed that way at the time), this can be a good choice. One of the pitfalls of this structure is that it can let you ramble and lose coherency. Although you need to give a brief overview of your life, you also need focus your paragraphs around individual ideas.

"The Story"

This is often the most effective essay if it's done correctly. Focus on one or two stories that illustrate some of the points listed above. The story essay is the most fun for admissions officers to read, and is the most likely to be coherent and cohesive. You don't have to go overboard with adjectives and turns of phrase to write effective narrative. Just pick a few moments that most clearly define why you want to be a physician.

Key Bragging Points

No matter the subject you plan to focus on, the following are points that you should consider incorporating into the finished essay:

Academic Strength

You can discuss this generally, or with a specific example of a class, an assignment, or a moment in which you enjoyed an intellectual challenge. Medical school will require a lot of hard work. What demonstrates your love of hard work?

Commitment to Ideals

No one expects you to be Mother Teresa, but most good physicians have a streak of empathy and altruism.

Balance

What makes you whole? What balances the hardworking academic powerhouse that you are?

Careful, Complex Thinking

It is very difficult to explain something as complicated as your motivation to be a physician. Most people, when writing about a defining moment in their lives, assume that the audience is right there with them. This is not the case. You have to explain what you think and feel after you describe the event. Don't assume that the admissions committee is going to fill in the blanks for you.

Why You Want to Be a Doctor

The question you should ask yourself is why—when many other people who've had similar life/career/academic experiences take one look at the horrendous hours involved in medical training and decide that teaching or counseling are perfectly good alternatives—you want to be a doctor. For instance, although many physicians decide to be doctors because of an early experience with the illness of a family member, there are far greater numbers of people with the same background who never consider medicine—but would still describe themselves as compassionate and moved to help people. You have to force yourself to ascertain what odd mixture of qualities—intellectual and emotional—have convinced you that going more than $100,000 in debt in the era of HMOs is a good idea.

Reasons, Not Excuses, for Weakness

Do not attempt to cover up or gloss over any deficiency, academic or otherwise. You will earn yourself points by honestly and openly dealing with your less-than-sterling qualities. If you have a couple of low grades or if you had a bad semester, briefly explain what happened, discuss what the experience taught you, and move on.

Good, Clever, Interesting Writing

Translation: Lots and lots and lots of drafts. Everybody has a distinct voice, and you're not going to survive medical school without a sense of humor. Find a way to get both qualities across without resorting to clichés. Prohibited phrases include: Lifelong learning, challenge of a lifetime, healing the mind as well as the body, childlike wonder, frail hands, quiet desperation, and any variations on these overused terms.

Overall Conservative Tone

Shock value doesn't work, despite the tales you might have heard about cartoons and poems. Admissions committees expect you to take the exercise seriously, and to treat the process with respect. Humor is fine, but it needs to be subtle.

Show, Don't Tell

One of the traps of the personal statement is to rewrite your resume in prose. Instead of listing your accomplishments, explain what they mean to you and show how they have affected your life. For example, if you really want to practice primary care, it is far more effective for you to explain in detail what motivates you than to simply state your goal.

The Evolution of the Essay

Good essays tend to evolve and often bear very little resemblance to rough drafts. Don't be afraid to start over, or to let the essay build on itself. If you write something that doesn't use any of the forms described above but that you feel gets across the points you want to make, then that is the essay you should stick with. Don't force yourself into a mold.

No matter what your essay looks like, however, there are a few general issues that you should think about.

Focus

Your essay must communicate specific points clearly and effectively. This means that every time you write a sentence that could be used in any other essay, you need to cross it out and start over. For example, "I truly enjoy working with people" could be the opening line in an application for Fry Guy at McDonald's just as easily as it could be a statement about the profound impact you want to have on your patients' health.

Editing

No mistakes. If you are not one of those people who goes around making a pest of themselves by correcting everyone else's grammatical errors, you need to find one. Most colleges and universities have writing centers with free editorial assistance, or you can check the local college paper for teaching assistants who are willing to edit for food. No matter what, make sure someone else reads your essay.

Interest

Everyone has a compelling style, and you need to write until you find yours. You are who you are for a reason; you have to write until that reason becomes apparent to anyone reading the essay.

Relevance

At some point, the reader will have to have a very clear sense of just why they should let you into their medical school. Don't get so caught up in explaining your inner child that you forget to mention your desire to become a doctor.

Coherence

Make sure your essay fits together. You shouldn't be able to move a paragraph or a sentence when you're finished.

Remember that your entire personality is not going to be reflected in this essay, nor can you entirely offset an otherwise weak application. But this is your big chance to talk to the committee, so make the most of it. Spend the necessary time to draft and rework your essay until it is the best measure of your writing ability and candidacy for medical school.

SECONDARIES AND LETTERS OF RECOMMENDATION

After medical schools receive your application, they will send you what's called a "secondary." Some schools send all of their applicants a secondary, while others go through an initial cut (usually based totally on GPA and MCAT scores). One of the reasons that schools like to send out secondaries is that they usually charge you about $50 for the privilege of filling them out. Secondaries usually include a variety of essay topics that are slightly more directed than the "personal comments" in either the ACOMAS or AMCAS. The following are some typical secondary questions:

- *What is your favorite novel?*

- *What are your hobbies?*

- *Where do you see yourself in ten years?*

- *Name a leadership role that you've taken and what it taught you about yourself.*

- *What has been your greatest academic achievement? What has been your greatest academic failure?*

- *What type of medicine do you think you might want to practice?*

As you can see, most of these essays seem fairly simple, but that doesn't mean you shouldn't spend time thoughtfully filling them out. Many secondaries are quite lengthy, so it's a good idea to fill them out as you get them, unless you've decided for some reason not to continue with your application to the school. If you find that the cost of sending back secondaries rapidly becomes prohibitive, you can call the individual schools and request a fee waiver. If you were eligible for a waiver from AMCAS, for example, you will probably be able to have most of your secondary fees waived.

You should also take care of your letters of recommendation at the secondary stage. If you are a student who is still in school and you have access to pre-health advising, your letters will probably be handled by that office, and at least one of your letters will probably be from the pre-health advisor. Usually, your recommenders will write one letter that the advising office will copy and send to your list of schools. If you are a returning adult, you may have to take care of all the requests and letters yourself.

Letters of recommendation for medical school work in much the same way as any other such letters; you will have much better luck if you approach your potential recommender with a copy of your resume, transcript, and personal statement. Try to make an appointment to speak to the person to discuss with them the various schools to which you are applying—and to make your case. Even if you have been out of school for awhile, you should try to get at least one letter from a former professor. Medical schools are interested in your character, your desire to be a physician, your academic preparedness, and your intellectual ability. Although most employers could attest to some of those qualities, you will probably need a letter from a professor that discusses your academic abilities. As an undergrad or in your post-bacc program, try to build relationships with faculty members so they can write something meaningful about you. Don't ask for a letter from someone famous unless they know you pretty well. Name-dropping is not considered to be particularly attractive in a prospective medical student.

Although many returning adults feel awkward approaching professors they might not have spoken with in several years, most are pleasantly surprised to discover that for the most part, professors do tend to remember their students, and most are happy to write them letters of recommendation. Both current and former students should also consider asking for letters from doctors with whom they have worked or volunteered— and remember that if you're applying to an osteopathic school, you have to have a letter from a DO.

Once you discover how painless it really is to get a letter of recommendation, you may be tempted to go into overdrive on the theory that inundating the committee with reams of stationary will force them to recognize your worthiness. Resist this! Do not send more letters than the school asks for. The committee will not read them, and you will not have done yourself any favors. The only time you might consider sending extra letters is if you are placed on hold after an interview, and have in the meantime been working with someone who you feel would be able to contribute some additional information about your abilities.

MINORITY RECRUITMENT

Minority status refers to ethnicities that are *underrepresented* in medicine, such as Native Americans, African Americans, Latinos, Native Hawaiians, and some other specific groups. If you are not sure whether you qualify as a minority in this sense, you should contact AMCAS. Many public and private medical schools recognize the value of educating physicians who may choose to work in underserved areas and communities. Some committees look favorably on a candidate with a background that suggests he or she will fill this need. In some cases, this amounts to a preference for candidates with specific ethnic backgrounds—but it is a preference that occurs after a field of equally qualified applicants is generated from the initial pool. Medical schools are simply too competitive to accept candidates who are not up to the intellectual challenge of medicine. This selectivity advantage often extends to people of any ethnicity who come from underserved rural areas and seem inclined to return there to practice medicine.

There is also a type of minority status that AMCAS recognizes that deals only with economic factors and does not take into account ethnicity or country of origin. To be considered a "financially disadvantaged" minority, you need to have been under financial strain for a long period of time, and to have been the recipient of federal aid in the form of AFDC, welfare, food stamps, or other such programs. Your financial situation needs to have had an ongoing and persistent negative effect on your ability to procure education, housing, food, etc. In other words, the average two-job-struggling-to-make-ends-meet college student does not qualify. This minority status is reserved for those who have struggled uphill their entire lives, and have somehow managed to make it through undergraduate school. The basic rule of thumb here is: If you are a financially disadvantaged minority, you probably know it. If you're in doubt, you probably aren't.

Medical schools are faced with a problem that is actually a boon for the quality of health care in the U.S.: They literally have more good applicants than they can take. This means that medical schools can easily fill their classes with students who are academically qualified. Medical schools have the opportunity to select from this pool those students who are most likely to improve underserved communities and help those with the most need. The AAMC has sought to increase enrollment of underrepresented minorities in recent years. AOA has recently instituted a minority scholarship, the Sherry R. Arnstein Minority Student Award, to boost minority recruitment at osteopathic schools.

WHAT HAPPENS AFTER YOU'VE BEEN ACCEPTED

So you've achieved the impossible, the best-case scenario: multiple acceptances. First, congratulations. Second, it's probably not a good idea to share your good fortune with too many of your premed friends, unless you don't particularly want to keep them and you've first removed all the sharp objects from the room.

BACK TO REALITY

After the giddiness wears off, you will have to deal with the best problem you will ever have: choosing which school to attend. Remember that you have lots of time to choose the medical school that best fits your goals and lifestyle. You can hang on to your acceptances until May 15, at which point schools will begin dropping your name off of their acceptance lists if you have not committed. Remember, however, that most of your fellow premeds do not share your enviable position. If you are accepted by a school that you know you will not attend, notify them before the deadline so that they can offer the seat to someone else. If you are on the waitlist for a school you really want, don't hesitate to write a short note letting the committee know that their school is your first choice.

Factors to Consider

So while you are basking in your acceptance, think seriously about the following factors, but don't selfishly hold onto too many acceptances while you are deliberating.

How much does the school emphasize and reward teaching?

This is a huge concern and often overlooked. Look into how much the school values teaching versus how much they emphasize research. This can be the difference between being taught and being forced to teach yourself. The best way to determine teaching quality is to ask current students for their opinions.

What are community, social life, and support systems like?

Talk to current students to determine the overall community of the school. You'll be there for four years, and you certainly won't be studying all—okay, most, but not all—of the time. Are the students accepting the rigors of med school with a positive attitude or do they waste all of their extra energy complaining? What is the quality of life in general like at this school? Do students study together? Is it a community or commuter lifestyle?

What's the quality of the residents?

The residents are the ones who will be teaching you when you're a med student, so of course you want them to be good. You should presumably be able to approximate the quality of the residents based on the quality of postgraduate training programs (residency programs) at the hospitals affiliated with the school.

How family-friendly are the school and its surroundings?

If you're a returning adult student with a family, look into the spouse/partner support services available at the schools you're considering. Getting through medical school will be hard on you and your family, and many places have begun programs that allow spouses/partners to attend special seminars and support groups that acclimate you to the pressures of your chosen educational and career path. Will your partner be able to find work/activities he or she enjoys?

Where will you be living?

Believe it or not, you will occasionally escape to the outside world. Make sure that the activities and hobbies you enjoy are available somewhere in the general vicinity. If you come from one climate and are moving to another, consider how that will affect you. Also, find out how close the clinical facilities are to the school and housing. The closer, the better.

What kind of research opportunities are available?

Some schools are much better equipped than others, and it's not always the "name" schools that are doing the most cutting-edge research. Different schools have different specialties, and some benefit from affiliated schools of public health, business, or law. Other schools offer paid research opportunities.

Traditional or systems-based?

Teaching methodologies include traditional (two years of science plus two years of rotations), organ-based (learn everything about the liver), case-based (learn science by delving into patient histories), and everything in between. Which method will be best for you? It is difficult to know. It is also likely that other issues are more important for you to consider, such as the school's regard for education, commitment to teaching, and responsiveness to student input and overall academic climate. These issues may prove more important than the curricular grid (i.e., when you take anatomy), in terms of how much you learn and how much you enjoy learning.

What kind of financial aid offer are they making?

Is the offer good for all four years? In comparing offers between schools, consider cost of living differences and variation in the terms of loans.

How much will you owe?

This is the most important financial aid statistic a school can offer because it encompasses tuition, expenses, and financial aid. No matter what kind of financial package you get, you will most likely owe a staggering sum when you graduate, and it all eventually has to be paid back. As an intern and resident, you won't be making much in the way of a salary ($38,000 in 2002). Although most physicians eventually achieve a comfortable living (average of $160,000 annual salary in 2002), the practice of medicine is in such a state of flux that it is impossible to predict what kinds of jobs and compensation will be available 10 years from now. A public university education, while perhaps not carrying quite the cachet as a private school, may save you tens of thousands of dollars and relieve some of the stress associated with gargantuan debt.

BEHIND DOOR NUMBER 1 . . . MORE STANDARDIZED TESTS!

Most medical students take the USMLE Step 1 (and/or the first COMLEX—the COMLEX exams go in the same order as the USMLEs) at the end of the second year of medical school. Osteopathic students must pass the USMLE to obtain allopathic residency spots. Step 1 is often used to determine whether or not a student has "passed" their pre-clinical course work and can continue into their third and fourth years of training. Step 2 is usually taken during the third or fourth year of school during clerkships. At this point, the vast majority of senior U.S. medical students go through the Match in order to obtain residency positions. Very few contract privately for their first year of graduate medical training. Most programs in the Match now use ERAS (Electronic Residency Application Service), which is administered by AAMC, rather than a traditional paper application. Step 3 is usually taken after at least one year of residency (most physicians do at least three years of residency, but still take the test after the first year). The USMLE is written and scored by the National Board of Medical Examiners, which administers Steps 1 and 2. Step 3 is administered by the state. The state confers the license; the USMLE is a prerequisite.

INTERNATIONAL MEDICAL GRADUATES

International medical graduates (IMG) go through a special process to be granted licensure in the U.S. Before you can start a residency program, you need to be certified by the Education Commission for Foreign Medical Graduates (ECFMG). To be certified, an IMG must complete the following five steps:

- *Take USMLE Steps 1 and 2.*

- *Send medical credentials and fill out the paperwork necessary to show proof of medical education.*

- *Take the English test administered by the ECFMG.*

- *If you don't pass the English test, you can take the Test of English as a Foreign Language instead.*

- *Take the Clinical Skills Assessment, which is a live "standardized patient" exam.*

After this, contact the board of the state in which you want to practice for the Step 3 requirements (each state determines its own passing score). You can get a residency either through the NRMP Match or through a private contract. After passing Step 3 and following any other state guidelines, you are granted a temporary license to practice in that state.

If you are currently in a medical program abroad and thinking about transferring to a U.S. medical school, you need to contact the school and ask about its transfer policies. In general, it is extremely difficult to transfer into a U.S. medical school.

ANOTHER PRINCETON REVIEW RESOURCE FOR PROSPECTIVE MED STUDENTS

If you're a premed student and want an in-depth, holistic guide to becoming the best possible applicant to med school, check out The Princeton Review's *Planning a Life in Medicine*, available in our online bookstore: www.princetonreview.com/college/bookstore.asp.

HIGH SCHOOL STUDENTS

If you've picked up this book and you're still in high school, you're very much ahead of the game. You can get started on the road to medical school by participating in volunteer activities and researching potential college choices to learn about their premedical training. Remember, you can major in any subject that interests you as long as you complete your premedical courses. Choose a subject you enjoy, and you are more likely to earn good grades and get into medical school. A few schools have special programs that funnel students through their undergraduate education directly into medical school. If you are interested in these programs, you should contact the following schools directly for more information:

Boston University

Brown University

Case Western University

East Tennessee State University

George Washington University

Howard University

Louisiana State University—New Orleans

Louisiana State University—Shreveport

Michigan State University

New York University

Northwestern University

University of Alabama

University of Miami

University of Michigan

University of Missouri—Kansas City

University of Rochester

University of South Alabama

University of Southern California

University of Wisconsin

IMPORTANT CONTACT ORGANIZATIONS

AMERICAN ASSOCIATION OF COLLEGES OF OSTEOPATHIC MEDICINE (AACOM)
5550 Friendship Boulevard
Suite 310
Chevy Chase, MD 20815-7231
301-968-4100
301-968-4101 (fax)
www.aacom.org

AMERICAN ASSOCIATION OF MEDICAL COLLEGES (AAMC)
2450 N Street, NW
Washington, DC 20037-1126
202-828-0400
202-828-1125 (fax)
www.aamc.org

ASSOCIATION OF ACCREDITED NATUROPATHIC MEDICAL COLLEGES
4435 Wisconsin Avenue, NW Suite 403
Washington, DC 20016
202-237-8150 or 866-538-2267 (toll-free)
202-237-8152 (fax)
www.aanmc.org

AMERICAN OSTEOPATHIC ASSOCIATION (AOA)
142 East Ontario Street
Chicago, IL 60611-2864
800-621-1773
312-202-8200 (fax)
www.osteopathic.org, www.do-online.org

EDUCATIONAL COMMISSION FOR FOREIGN MEDICAL GRADUATES
3624 Market Street
Philadelphia, PA 19104-2685
215-386-5900
215-386-9196 (fax)
www.ecfmg.org

FEDERATION OF STATE MEDICAL BOARDS
400 Fuller Wiser Road
Suite 300
Euless, TX 76039-3855
817-868-4000
817-868-4099 (fax)
www.fsmb.org

NATIONAL BOARD OF MEDICAL EXAMINERS

3750 Market Street
Philadelphia, PA 19104-3102
215-590-9500
215-590-9457 (fax)
www.nbme.org

TEXAS MEDICAL AND DENTAL SCHOOLS APPLICATION SERVICE

702 Colorado, Suite 6400
Austin, TX 78701
512-499-4785
512-499-4786
www.utsystem.edu/tmdsas
(Texas public schools do not use AMCAS)

4 Advice for the "Nontraditional" Applicant

Forty years ago, most medical school applicants shared certain traits. The "traditional" medical school applicant was white, male, and just older than 20. Most likely, he majored in biology or chemistry while in college. Although he knew that medical school would be difficult and that his career would be challenging, he looked forward to choosing from a wide range of medical specialties and being financially secure. As a trained professional, he would possess real skills and expertise and, as a result, could expect to enjoy authority and autonomy.

The past few decades have seen substantial changes both in the composition of the medical school applicant pool and in the professional opportunities available to medical school graduates. Based on the previous idea of the traditional medical student, women and minority applicants could be considered "nontraditional," but the term is currently used to describe applicants who are older than most med students. The average age of applicants is between 23 and 26, but a significant and increasing proportion of applicants are several years older.

Some of these older applicants, always intending to apply to medical school, completed premedical requirements during their years as undergraduates, and simply postponed medical school to work, travel, or start a family. Others were unsuccessful at gaining admission directly out of college and are attempting a second or third time. Another group considered medical school in college, but did not complete requirements or the application process. Some older applicants never seriously considered medicine until after they graduated college and were involved in another occupation. Whatever the reason for postponing, older applicants now represent a significant proportion of the medical school candidate pool.

Aspiring doctors who did not take the prerequisite science courses in college or did not excel in them face a formidable challenge. These individuals have a minimum of seven years of medical school and residency on the horizon and, in addition, must complete (and do well in) one to two years of basic science courses before even applying to medical school. Nonetheless, thousands of adults, despite the arduous path ahead of them, decide to tackle this challenge. This chapter is intended as a source of information and support for nontraditional applicants at all stages of the application process. It is written by a nontraditional applicant and includes input from others who are or were in the same category. Follow eight nontraditional applicants through the entire process—from decision-making, to post-bacc training, to MCAT preparation, and acceptance. The group is composed of real individuals[1] coming from a wide range of backgrounds, some elements of which will hopefully resemble aspects of your own situation. When these people decided that medical school was their goal, this is who they were and what they were doing:

- *Becky, a 28-year-old who completed two years of college and had worked as a medical assistant for 10 years.*

- *Pete, a 28-year-old with a law degree who was unhappy in his field.*

- *Tina, a 27-year-old art history major who was working in a gallery and dating a medical student.*

- *Bob, a 35-year-old chemistry professor at a small college.*

- *Mitch, a 30-year-old former Peace Corps volunteer who was working in international development.*

- *Jacob, a 24-year-old volunteer firefighter. A car accident and subsequent hospitalization kept him from completing organic chemistry while in college. Discouraged, he dropped out of the premedical track.*

- *Eve, a 42-year-old wife and mother of three who graduated college 20 years ago, and had little experience working outside of the home.*

- *Donald, an engineering graduate student who decided that he needed more human contact in his work.*

DECIDING THAT MEDICINE—AND MEDICAL SCHOOL—IS WHAT YOU WANT

Some of these people were absolutely sure about going to medical school. Jacob, for example, had always known. Tina, who was fascinated by what her boyfriend studied in medical school, had a strong hunch. Donald imagined that being a physician would give him what he felt was missing from his career, but he had limited contact with the medical field and had not fully considered other options that would give him more personal interaction.

---

[1] Names have been changed.

Being reasonably sure about medicine is important because you will invest time, money, and energy into the medical school preparation and application process. It is also important because admissions officers will look for indications of your commitment. If you are sure of it, your commitment is more likely to come through in your personal statement and your interview.

If you have never worked or volunteered in a medical setting, you should explore opportunities to do so. You might arrange to informally shadow a physician or to volunteer in a hospital that has a formal program. Some volunteers find that they are given more responsibility at a small clinic than they are in a large hospital, so look into clinic programs as well. Explore opportunities to volunteer in overseas medical projects. Of our eight subjects, those who had more than one medically related experience felt that it was beneficial because they were exposed to the variation that exists within the field. Not only are volunteer activities helpful in your decision-making process, but they will become significant resume builders should you decide to apply to medical school. In addition, they are likely to be valuable and, hopefully, enjoyable experiences.

One way to help determine if medicine is the right career for you is to talk to others who have made the choice. Interview as many people as you can. Talk to practicing physicians, residents, medical students, and those involved in academic medicine such as researchers. Find out what they love and hate about their work. Ask questions that will help you put their comments about medicine in perspective. For example, if you come across someone who positively hated medical school and dislikes being a physician, ask him what part of medical school he hated the least. If his favorite part of the experience was the relaxing cruise-ship vacation he took after his first year, he probably could have made a better career choice for himself. His views of medical school may not be an indication of what the experience will be like for you.

If possible, talk to medical students, practicing physicians, and resident physicians who are or were nontraditional. Find out whether they feel that they made the right decision. What were the biggest sacrifices they had to make? Visit the premedical and medical student discussion pages online where many nontraditional applicants and students share their thoughts. Although we are unaware of books documenting the experiences of nontraditional medical students, at least one book does give accounts of nontraditional applicants.[2] A commonly held view is that nontraditional medical students have more difficulty with the pre-clinical medical curriculum, but excel during the clinical years.[3] Based on our own discussions, however, nontraditional medical students express fewer doubts about their decision to go to medical school than those

[2] Goss, Bryan. *Applying to Medical School for the Nontraditional Student*. 1997: Lakeshore-Pearson Publications. Contact Mountain Books, Albuquerque, NM.

[3] Some studies indicate that nontraditional students do less well in basic science courses. See Blacklow HM et al. *Postbaccalaureate Preparation and Performance in Medical School*. Academic Medicine 1990 June; 65 (6). Other studies refute the claim. See Hall ML, Stocks MD. *Relationship Between Quantity of Undergraduate Science Preparation and Preclinical Performance in Medical School*. Academic Medicine 1995 March; 70: (3).

who went directly from college. Perhaps this is because they appreciate having a second "chance" at a career, or perhaps it is because they gave the decision more thought.

Bob's decision to apply to medical school was influenced by his sister-in-law. She works in medical equipment sales and is five years older than Bob. She encouraged him to follow his dream, saying that she, too, had entertained the idea of becoming a physician when she was 30. She decided against it and at 40 still dreams about doing it today. But with two young children, she feels that it would be too difficult. Bob decided that it would be more painful to spend his life wondering if he should have gone to medical school than to go and—in the worst-case scenario—drop out and return to teaching.

Mitch also found it helpful to talk to people working in totally unrelated fields. He had worked for two years in a clinic in rural Africa and thought that he wanted to become a pediatrician. However, he became discouraged while talking to his friends who were medical students, residents, or newly graduated practicing physicians because it seemed that few people loved everything about what they were doing. Many of his friends warned him of the burden of debt and the prospect of having little free time. One friend told him that in comparison to Mitch's current job, which involved traveling around the world, he would be *bored* in medicine. Mitch then took an informal poll of all his friends who included teachers, writers, business owners, software designers, lawyers, and full-time parents. He found that people in all occupations both love *and* hate certain things about their work.

Although medical students and physicians complain about debt, teachers complain about low salaries, and business owners complain about financial insecurity. All of Mitch's friends in their early 30s complain about working too hard, and about the difficulty of balancing their personal and family lives with their careers. Mitch concluded that despite the initial discouragement he got from friends in the medical profession, people in medicine are among the *most* professionally fulfilled. Although medical students and physicians had complaints, they were engaged in their work and most couldn't imagine a better career. He also noticed that a significant number of nonphysicians he spoke to, although unhappy with their own jobs, still discouraged him from going into medicine. He realized that some of these people had, at one point in their lives, entertained the idea of becoming a doctor. They had successfully talked themselves out of medical school and were sold on all the reasons why *not* to go into medicine. As far as his friend's comment about being bored, Mitch realized that others tended to glamorize his current work because it involved travel. He knew that being a pediatrician would, on a day-to-day basis, be more interesting than the paperwork he dealt with in his current job. Furthermore, he could probably work overseas as a physician if he found himself yearning for travel.

After you follow Mitch's example and grill everyone you know, ask yourself some serious questions. What jobs and experiences have you loved most in your life? Do you foresee medicine providing similar satisfaction? Have you enjoyed some aspects of your medically related work? Do you have the skills it takes to become a physician? To be fulfilled as one? Whether or not to pursue a career in medicine is an important decision that will affect many years of your life. Give yourself time, both for information gathering and personal reflection. Write down your thoughts on what is influencing your decision. Whether or not you decide to go for it, if you carefully weigh the decision now, you will be less likely to doubt it later on.

Resist feeling that because you are "older," you should make your decision to enter medical school as quickly as possible. Medical school, internship, and residency require at least seven years to complete. Moreover, medicine is a career of lifelong learning. Start finding things to enjoy about the process of becoming a doctor now. Deciding to go to medical school is part of the process. Try not to stress too much about the decision, and find some satisfaction in your information gathering and self-reflection.

GETTING INTO MEDICAL SCHOOL AS A NONTRADITIONAL APPLICANT

If you are reading this, you have probably decided to move forward with your plan to become an MD, DO, or ND. Hopefully, your level of maturity and your life experience have allowed you to make a well-informed decision that a student just out of college may not be in a position to make. Between 20 percent and 30 percent of applicants in the 24- to 37-year-old age range are admitted to medical school, while approximately 45 percent of 21 to 23 year olds are admitted. Although these statistics suggest that the odds are against older applicants, age itself is not regarded as a disadvantage, and may in some cases be a plus. The smaller percentage of older applicants admitted may be partially due to lower GPAs[4] and test scores. Even the most exciting and unique older applicant must have a competitive GPA and MCAT score.

The timing of the admissions process is often an issue for nontraditional applicants. Donald started thinking about medical school midway through his first year of graduate school. We will call this January of Year 1. He realized that he had prerequisites to fulfill and that he wouldn't be eligible to enter medical school the following fall, but thought he would be able to matriculate in the fall of Year 3. Donald quit his graduate program and entered an intensive premedical curriculum, completing his requirements by January, Year 2. He took the MCAT in April, Year 2. If Donald had taken premedical courses part-time rather than full-time, he could not have adhered to this schedule. Had he done poorly on the MCAT the first time, he could have been delayed an entire year

---

[4] Smith, SR. *A Two-Year Experience with Premedical Postbaccalaureate Students Admitted to Medical School.* Academic Medicine; 1991: 66:1.

and postponed entrance until Year 4. As a result of the timing of the admissions process, it takes two to four years to matriculate after deciding to pursue medical school. The following are the important dates to remember as you think about timeframe and requirements:

- *April: MCAT is given. You should have completed all prerequisite science courses by this date. (Please note that more MCAT test dates will be added in 2007.)*

- *June: AMCAS (preliminary) applications are accepted. Filling out the AMCAS application requires all undergraduate, graduate, and post-bacc transcripts (they accept transcripts beginning on March 15, but the completed application isn't accepted until June 1). You will need your own copies, and you will need to have copies sent directly to AMCAS. It is important to submit AMCAS applications as soon as possible because most schools offer rolling admissions.*

- *August: MCAT is given. Use this test date only if you need to improve your scores from the April test. You will indicate on your AMCAS application whether you intend to take (or retake) the test on this date. If so, many schools will not look at your application until August scores are available (some time in October). The penalty for this delay may very well outweigh your score improvement. Thus, unless you anticipate significant score improvement, the August MCAT is not advised. (Please note that more MCAT test dates will be added in 2007.)*

- *August: Medical schools to which AMCAS applications have been submitted begin sending secondary applications. Some schools will review AMCAS applications closely, and send secondary ones to a limited number of applicants. Others send them to everyone who applies through AMCAS. There is almost always an additional fee. In some cases, secondary applications require essays or short-answer questions that focus on motivation, personal characteristics, values, and experiences. In other cases, the application is very simple and similar to the AMCAS application. Thus, receiving a secondary application may be an indication that a school is interested in you. When you return the application and fee, you demonstrate your interest in the school. Schools often want these back within two to four weeks. You will also need to submit recommendations at this time. Some schools ask for a photo.*

- *August–May: Based on AMCAS and secondary applications and recommendations, applicants are invited to interview during this period. Some schools conduct all their interviews during one or two months, while others spread them out. Most schools accept 25–50-plus percent of interviewed candidates. Thus, getting an interview is an excellent sign. Most admissions decisions are also made during this period, with the exception of applicants who fall into a "hold" or "wait list" category.*

- *June–August: Wait listed candidates may be accepted.*

ACADEMIC REQUIREMENTS

Most medical schools require or strongly prefer that applicants have a BA or BS degree from a four-year accredited college or university. All medical schools require a minimum level of science preparation that includes approximately one year each of biology, chemistry, organic chemistry, and physics. Some nontraditional candidates meet these requirements by taking night courses while simultaneously working part- or full-time. Others enroll full-time at private or public undergraduate institutions. Some choose to enroll in special "post-baccalaureate premedical" programs (we call them post-bacc programs) offered by a surprisingly large number of colleges and universities (see Chapter 10 for a comprehensive listing of post-bacc programs). Post-bacc programs vary widely in terms of cost, rigor of course work, grading system, percentage of graduates admitted to medical school, structure and flexibility of curriculum, duration, size, and class composition. Unlike medical schools, post-bacc programs are neither accredited as such, nor ranked.

Becky needed to complete her BA in addition to fulfilling science prerequisites. When she decided it was time to take a shot at fulfilling her long-time dream of becoming a physician, she lived and worked in California, which has some of the most selective state-affiliated medical schools in the country. Becky decided to move to another state and complete her BA there so that she would be qualified for admission to the state's medical school. Becky enrolled full-time for three years to complete her BA—not all of her previous college credits transferred—and fulfill all her science requirements.

Becky's strategy is interesting and may be advisable for others in similar situations who are prepared to relocate. Before moving across the country, be sure that you understand your new state's criteria for determining residency. In some states, being a full-time student does not ensure resident status. Becky might have saved herself a year of schooling had she looked at more colleges and possibly uncovered schools willing to award her credit for all her previous college work.

Tina graduated from a prestigious college but had taken neither science nor math classes while in school. She was also concerned about her undergraduate GPA, which was 2.9. To make herself a more competitive applicant, she wanted to demonstrate both competence in the sciences and overall improved study skills. Some post-baccalaureate premedical programs are quite structured and involve only the minimum science prerequisites; Tina felt that she needed more than this to make up for her undergrad GPA. One of Tina's options was to apply to a post-bacc program that allows participants to take additional courses beyond those in the required scientific disciplines. This type of program tends to be somewhat flexible, allowing students to spend as much time as needed to fulfill requirements and take any additional courses. Students get the opportunity to learn foreign languages, improve writing or math skills, or take courses often recommended—but not required—by medical schools such as biochemistry or statistics. Other post-bacc programs apply students' course work toward a master's degree.

Tina decided not to enter an organized post-bacc program. Instead, she enrolled full-time as a nondegree candidate at a local, private university. This gave her access to larger course offerings. One of the advantages of post-bacc programs is that they are compact, scheduling courses and labs so students may complete all requirements within a year. Tina was less worried about speed and more interested in earning excellent grades. Another important consideration for Tina was letters of recommendation. Medical schools usually prefer that applicants submit a composite letter from their premedical advisor who is typically an administrator or dean, a department head, a specified faculty member, or some type of counselor. The letter discusses the student's qualifications and incorporates comments from his or her premedical professors. Because Tina chose a small school, she had the opportunity to get to know her professors and, presumably, to secure meaningful comments from them. At some colleges, only degree-earning students have full access to premedical and other advisors, but Tina was able to identify one who agreed to write a letter for her. One advantage to true post-bacc programs is that the premedical advisors are able to write appropriate letters of recommendation for nontraditional applicants.

Some premedical candidates are highly concerned with getting through the application process quickly and have no interest in prolonging premedical course work. Pete had a 3.7 GPA in college and an excellent record in law school. He had no need to prove himself scholastically, but just wanted to "get the sciences out of the way." He was a good candidate for a highly selective post-bacc program. To be admitted to one of these programs, applicants must submit detailed information including personal statements, prior standardized test scores, and several recommendations. Interviews are often required. These programs seek to admit students who will not only complete the course work, but who are likely to be accepted to medical school. Often, the brochures for these programs boast the percentage of graduates who have been admitted into medical school. Although a high acceptance rate is partially a reflection of the quality and resources of the program itself, it also indicates that they accept well-qualified students. In one year, Pete was able to complete all his sciences and study for and take the MCAT.

Pete took advantage of an arrangement between his post-bacc program and a medical school, allowing him to enter medical school in the fall following completion of premedical course work. Thus, he avoided an "in between" year generally devoted to the medical school application process. Several selective post-bacc programs offer this type of arrangement, affiliation, or linkage with a number of medical schools. In some cases, the medical school and the post-bacc program are part of the same university. Many nontraditional candidates are disappointed to discover that top medical schools such as Harvard, University of Pennsylvania, and Columbia do not offer these arrangements with their own university's post-bacc program.

Pete took the shortest path possible to medical school. In the fall of 1996, he left the law firm where he was working, and in the fall of 1997, he was beginning medical school. He was happy to skip the long and stressful medical school application process, having been through a similar experience with law school. While ideal for some, Pete's path is neither available nor advisable for everyone. The short, intensive post-bacc programs are grueling and may be too fast-paced for some people. Graduates of these programs often claim their post-bacc work was more demanding than medical school itself. Although these programs can serve as excellent preparation for medical school, they may discourage people who could have succeeded had they enrolled in a more relaxed program.

Earning acceptance to a post-bacc program with affiliated medical schools does not assure your acceptance to medical schools. Post-bacc students in these programs usually apply to the affiliated schools, but acceptances are only provisional, and conditional upon securing a minimum GPA and MCAT score. Only a handful of medical schools participate in these linkages, and each school limits the number of positions available through the direct admissions route. Pete chose his post-bacc program in part because one of the linked medical schools interested him. If none of the medical schools that allow admission through this route appeal to you, saving one year now is probably not worth spending four years someplace you don't want to be. Generally, medical schools agree to these arrangements as a means of enrolling students who they would otherwise not attract. Thus, if you are accepted as a post-bacc student to one of these schools, you are not likely to be accepted to other schools if you apply through the regular admissions process. Another disadvantage to these arrangements is that they are usually binding: if you get in, you must go. If you earn a perfect score on the MCAT, you cannot withdraw and apply to your dream school for the following year. Additionally, you have no opportunity to compare financial aid packages.

While Donald, Tina, Pete, and Becky quit their jobs to enter premedical studies full time, Mitch, Jacob, and Eve opted for part-time schooling. Eve wanted to ease into school, and decided to take one course at a time. She enrolled in a general chemistry class through the extension office of a local public university. Her children spent summers at camp and with relatives, allowing her to take a compact organic chemistry course during the summer. The following school year, she enrolled in a two-semester biology course, and she took an intensive physics course the next summer. Eve was concerned that her age would hurt her chances of being accepted to medical school. Some premedical advisors believe that being older than 40 may be a slight disadvantage.[5] However, had she crammed all of the required science courses into just one year, she would have only been one year younger when she applied to med school, but a whole lot more frustrated and perhaps not as appealing a candidate because her grades could have suffered. In retrospect, Eve's only regret about taking courses "on her own" is that she missed the camaraderie and support that she might have had in a post-bacc program. An advantage to post-bacc programs is that you will meet people facing challenges similar to your own.

[5] See the article, "Is It Too Late For Me To Go To Medical School?" by Leon C. Dorosz, Professor and Chair, Department of Biological Sciences, San Jose State University.

Most medical schools advise nontraditional applicants to demonstrate success in *recent* course work. Bob had fulfilled all the prerequisites in college about 15 years earlier. Since Bob had a graduate degree in science and remained active in an academic environment, the fact that he completed his prerequisite courses years earlier did not hurt him. His hurdle was the MCAT, for which he reviewed intensely.

The grading systems vary tremendously among undergraduate institutions and post-bacc programs. Some material that you learn as a premed, such as the basic biochemical processes, will serve you in medical school. Other topics, like whether your rowboat sinks or rises if you fall into the water, might not. As a premedical student, your goals should be to figure out whether you enjoy studying science, to learn the material for the MCAT, and to get good grades.

Some colleges and universities with post-bacc programs assign nontraditional students to regular, undergraduate science courses. You attend lectures, labs, and exams alongside undergraduates and may or may not be graded on the same curve as your younger classmates. Most likely, the mean score of post-bacc students is somewhat higher than that of the rest of the class. Undergraduates shouldn't be penalized by your presence since, after all, you already have your BA. Thus, schools with significant numbers of post-bacc students are likely to separate them from the undergraduates for grading purposes. Unfortunately, this practice could hurt you because you may be competing with your undergraduate classmates for positions in medical schools. Your cumulative test score of 90 percent put you in the middle of the post-bacc curve and earned you a C, while your classmate's 90 percent put him at the front end of the undergraduate curve and earned him an A. Although a letter of recommendation could explain that you did in fact maintain a 90 percent average, a C is still a C.

Some post-bacc programs address this issue by setting the post-bacc curve higher. The mean score will represent a B grade rather than a C grade. Highly selective post-bacc programs usually recognize that all their students were strong in college, and will set the mean somewhere in the A– or B+ range. If a college that does not have a formal post-bacc program allows you to enroll in science courses, your GPA might be slightly higher because you will be graded with your classmates, many of whom are probably less focused and less serious than you about maintaining excellent grades. Note, however, that many medical schools consider the caliber of undergraduate institutions when evaluating GPAs. This applies to traditional and nontraditional applicants alike.

THE MCAT

The MCAT is a day-long exam that is currently offered twice yearly at locations throughout the country. It is composed of four sections. An individual's raw score (number wrong out of number possible) on each section is compared with those of test-takers nationwide and is converted to a scaled score. Because most MCAT takers have never sat through an all-day exam, many find the experience a test of endurance and concentration as much as a test of knowledge (see page 30 for more information on the MCAT).

Virtually all medical schools require the MCAT. Schools evaluate MCAT scores in different ways. Some have devised formulas that incorporate MCAT results and GPAs and produce numerical scores to assign to candidates. In some cases, if an applicant's score falls above a cutoff, he will receive a secondary application or perhaps be invited to interview. Although certain sections of the MCAT may be weighted more heavily than others by some admissions offices, most schools regard all sections except the essay as equally important. In some formulas, the MCAT and GPA carry roughly equal weight, while in others one is weighted more heavily. A number of schools claim that GPA is more important than MCAT. Although this may be true, consider such statements in light of the recent outcry against standardized tests. A school that admits to using test scores as its primary means of weeding out applicants could be regarded as lazy and discriminatory.

Most schools claim not to use specified formulas or cutoff points and indicate that they might consider an applicant with a very low MCAT score if other aspects of his application are extraordinary. But generally, admissions committees rely heavily on MCAT scores because they are considered a strong indicator of success in the first two years of medical school, and because they are the easiest part of an application to judge. Examining the average MCAT scores of accepted students at a school gives you a rough idea of what score you will need to gain admission there.

The MCAT is important for all applicants, but may be especially so for nontraditional applicants. Eve's college grades were 20 years old. Over the years, colleges and universities have made changes and adjustments to grading scales and curricular requirements. Thus, her GPA might not be comparable to that of someone who graduated from the same school in 2005. Furthermore, how she performed in college 20 years ago is probably not a great indicator of how she will fare in medical school today. Grades in post-bacc courses are important, but as mentioned earlier, there is wide variation in grading policies among post-bacc programs and between regular undergraduate courses and the same courses within post-bacc programs. The benefit of the MCAT is that it is standardized, supposedly allowing admissions committees to compare the aptitude of people with different backgrounds.

When preparing for the MCAT, consider that the results of that one day of work are nearly as important as all your other academic achievements. Beyond striving for a sound academic background, most medical school applicants—both traditional and nontraditional—take some sort of MCAT preparation course like the ones offered by The Princeton Review. For some, a test-prep course teaches material never learned, or never absorbed, in class. For others, it relieves some anxiety associated with standardized tests, and thereby allows for an improved performance. For those lacking self-motivation, taking a course is a good way to encourage studying.

Some post-bacc programs offer an MCAT review along with premedical courses. Usually, such a review will be much less intensive than a course offered by an outside organization. In Pete's post-bacc program, most students enrolled in a private course that met twice weekly for three months prior to the April MCAT. Since the post-bacc program itself was so intensive and required many hours per day of studying, the students needed to be pushed to devote time to MCAT preparation. Pete did not take the course because he felt confident that he would enter medical school the following fall through the arrangement he had made with an affiliated medical school. The medical school required Pete to take the MCAT and to score at least a nine in all subjects. By January of his post-bacc year, Pete was scoring eights or higher in all sections, and reasoned that, by finishing his premedical courses and studying for the MCAT on his own, he could score nines.

Formal MCAT courses typically include three or four practice, full-length MCATs. The exams are scored, giving students an idea of their strengths, weaknesses, and overall progress throughout the course. Pete obtained practice MCATs through the Association of American Medical Colleges (AAMC), and set aside three Saturdays prior to the April exam to take them. For those who do not take a course, it is important to order these practice exams and to be disciplined about taking them.[6] The exams come with tables that allow you to convert your raw score to the scaled score that gives you an accurate idea of how you'll score on an actual MCAT. There are a number of books available that review important MCAT topics and offer tips for taking the exam.

Review books and courses are a good idea for both nontraditional and traditional students, although nontraditional students who have been out of the standardized test scene for many years may particularly need the help. For example, when Becky took her first practice exam, she was discouraged because she was barely able to complete half of the questions in the science sections. MCAT questions are not arranged in order of difficulty, and Becky was spending too much time on really tough passages that appeared early in the sections. She improved her score significantly on the science sections just by training herself to skip and go back to difficult passages.

Some nontraditional applicants have an advantage on the verbal section. By just being older, you may have had more time than a college student to read a wide variety of books. Eve loves reading, and found the verbal section to be a confidence builder. Becky, who did not read extensively for work or pleasure, found the verbal section very difficult. Donald, who learned English as his second language, studied more for the verbal section than for both science sections combined. Becky improved her verbal score by focusing on concentration skills. One way to do this is to read slightly complicated or technical magazine and journal articles every day for several months before the MCAT. Force yourself to concentrate for an extended period of time each day.

---

[6] Practice exams are real MCATs from years past. Visit www.aamc.org/students/mcat/start.htm.

Health care has changed dramatically in the United States, and some experts argue that physicians in the twenty-first century (see Chapter 2) will have to possess a wider range of skills than was previously considered adequate. Not only must physicians be experts in their respective fields, but it is advantageous to understand the financial, legal, ethical, and political issues surrounding health care provision. Medical schools recognize the need for well-rounded physicians. The schools now offer revised curriculums that include nonscience courses, and they admit more and more nonscience majors.

As a nontraditional applicant, you have unique experiences and skills. These will help differentiate you from other applicants and can be an important strength. The AMCAS personal statement, essays for secondary applications, and the interview are opportunities for you to shine. Although you are probably tired of being asked why you want to become a doctor, you will have to figure out how to answer the question with sincerity and enthusiasm. As a nontraditional applicant, your motivation for pursuing a career in medicine is an extremely important consideration for admissions committees.

Despite recognizing the value of nontraditional students, admissions committees may be skeptical of applicants who are embarking on their second or third career. Essays and interviews are also opportunities for you to address their concerns and doubts about your motivation. In interviews, Donald was often asked what made him so sure he wouldn't drop out of medical school as he had engineering school. The school's concern is that poor judgment with respect to your first career choice may suggest the possibility of poor judgment in your decision to apply to medical school. Or perhaps the worry is that some people are eternally unfulfilled and will therefore be unfulfilled by a career in medicine. Many people believe that if you are good at something, you enjoy it. Thus, not liking your previous job suggests to some that you were bad at it and that you may possess some hidden faults.

All medical school applicants—both traditional and nontraditional—must figure out how to package themselves. Like wrapping a present that is oddly sized, some nontraditional applicants have to be creative in their packaging. Donald's strategy was to maintain a positive attitude. He told interviewers that some of the things that attracted him to engineering, such as the analytic thinking required, also applies to medicine. He asked interviewers whether some of the principles in engineering would translate to physiological issues. He emphasized his excellent academic record, his success in science courses, and his demonstrated willingness to work hard in school. He also stressed how much he enjoyed volunteering at a clinic. He did his best to be personable and talkative, thereby showing off his "people skills" rather than restating what was written in his essay—that he was switching fields because he wanted to work directly with people.

Tina's story—that she was bored working in an art gallery and envious of her boyfriend's career—would not get her into medical school without clarification. Tina enjoyed certain aspects of her job, such as interacting with artists and clients. She loved much of the art with which she worked, particularly the pieces that were highly expressive and revealed human emotion. On the other hand, she missed a sense of social purpose in her gallery work, and she felt that she wasn't being intellectually challenged. Tina packaged herself as passionate, people-oriented, and interested in helping others. She was good at her job but knew that it would not engage her for life. Through her work, she came to know what she liked and disliked, what fulfilled her and what did not. Unlike children of physicians who are likely to consider medicine as a potential career from an early age, Tina never thought about it as a realistic pursuit until her 20s when her boyfriend entered medical school. Now that she had an idea of what medical school and medicine were like, and now that she knew herself better, she was ready to commit to the career. Because she enjoyed working with people, she envisioned a career in primary care. She believed that as a result of her studies and work in the art world, she had good insight into the mental capacity and emotions of people. She wondered if psychiatry was the field for her.

Packaging Jacob was relatively straightforward. He had a reasonably consistent interest in medicine, demonstrated by earlier premedical courses and more recent firefighting work that involved some emergency medical skills. In Jacob's personal statement, he needed to address the reasons he dropped out of the premedical track in college. Jacob had been hospitalized, and this experience was emotionally difficult for him. Being in a hospital and being around sick and dying people was enough to make him question whether he really could be a physician. When he returned to school, he was less committed to going to medical school and decided to focus on completing his major and general requirements with good grades. After graduation, he fully recovered and had regained his interest in medicine. He took several first aid courses, volunteered in an emergency room, trained to become a fireman, and looked around for post-bacc programs. In his essay, Jacob brought up the doubts that he had about becoming a physician, and discussed how he overcame them. Had he glossed over his hospital experience and the fact that he only took one semester of organic chemistry in college, admissions committees may have concluded that he "just couldn't cut it" as a premed. By addressing the situation, he presented himself as someone who matured and grew from a difficult experience.

Some medical schools read the essays and personal statements of all applicants and use them, along with grades and scores, for initial screening. Others only read essays after some applications have been weeded out. If you are filling out applications, you are at the point where you can't do much about your grades or scores. However, you can write an excellent personal statement. Enlist a friend, relative, advisor, or coworker who is well-read and writes well to review your statement and make suggestions. Have someone who really knows you read it to be sure that you have conveyed your strengths. On the AMCAS application, exactly one page is provided for an applicant's personal statement. The resume of a nontraditional applicant is probably longer than that of a college senior, and limiting your statement to one page may seem difficult. However, you need not mention all of your accomplishments, experiences, or reasons for pursuing medicine. Choose your most impressive accomplishments, your most meaningful experiences, and your most compelling reasons for pursuing medicine (see page 31 for more advice on how to compose a good essay).

There are countless approaches to writing a personal statement. Becky wrote about learning. By focusing on a concept, she subtly brought up her relevant accomplishments and experiences and explained her motivation for wanting to go to medical school. During her career as a nurse, she learned a tremendous amount from doctors, other nurses, patients, and families. She loved applying her knowledge to her daily work and seeing her work pay off in the people she helped. However, she felt that her formal education did not enable her to really understand disease, treatments, and the healing process. Having worked closely with physicians, she understood that they didn't always know everything. She felt, however, that they had the tools to ask the right questions. Asking and answering questions, addressing problems and solving them, and observing others and analyzing their techniques are among the activities Becky looked forward to in medical school.

Eve concentrated on the doctor-patient relationship, discussing vivid memories of her own pediatrician and comparing the relationship she had with him to that of her children and their current pediatrician. She was able to elaborate on her accomplishment of raising three well-adjusted children, a feat that involved serving as caretaker, healer, friend, manager, teacher, advisor, and so on. Mitch described a few of his work experiences in Africa and Latin America, focusing on the ones that were most directly related to health care issues. He wrote that although he enjoyed working overseas, he felt that he would be able to contribute more as a physician than as a project manager. Jacob's prose included personal accounts of saving peoples' lives as a firefighter, and how fulfilling he found that aspect of his work.

The secondary application may have general questions that allow you to elaborate on topics mentioned in the AMCAS essay. Some secondaries contain questions about particular experiences that you may have had, such as research, community service, or employment. Some questions focus on your values and personal experiences. Chapter 7 of this book includes a profile of each allopathic medical school. In the "Application Process" section of each description, we give the percentage of AMCAS applicants who generally receive secondaries. Some schools send secondary applications to a very limited number of applicants, and receiving a secondary from these schools means that you made it through a significant screening.

All schools limit the number of applicants that they interview. If you have been invited to interview, it is a sign that you are a "competitive" applicant and you should be pleased. If you receive several interview invitations, the odds are that you will get into medical school. Nontraditional applicants who have interesting life experiences have an advantage in interviews because there is more to talk about than college courses or summer jobs. In addition, you may have had more experience interviewing for jobs and other educational programs than a college student. Hopefully, this will allow you to be more relaxed during the interview process.

In writing a personal statement, you are able to edit, rewrite, rethink, and start over. In an interview, you don't have this luxury. Being relaxed is important, but so is being prepared. Interviewers may ask about courses you have taken. Before going into an interview, review your academic transcripts. Which courses were your favorites? Your least favorite? Why? How do your preferences relate to your desire to go to medical school? If there are any particularly low or high grades, be prepared to discuss what went on in those classes. Review your AMCAS and secondary applications. Be sure that you can discuss every experience you have listed or discussed. Think of some sort of interesting, impressive, (tastefully) funny, or meaningful comment for each experience. Be prepared to answer questions about your childhood. What aspect of yourself do you really hate talking about? Be ready to talk about it, or figure out a good way to divert the conversation from it. What (of relevance) do you know about and enjoy talking about? Think about ways to introduce this subject into your interview.

Although most interviews are one-on-one, some schools use panels of more than one interviewer. Some schools offer group interviews where you interview alongside other applicants. Interviewers may be faculty members, administrators, medical students, or members of the community. Older applicants may find that interviewing with current students, who could be somewhat younger, is challenging. An important part of being a physician is the ability to communicate and to get along with all types of people in all types of positions. The interview is an opportunity to demonstrate your skills in this area.

There are predictable interview questions, such as, "Why do you want to go to medical school?" Others are much less predictable, and may even be surprising or shocking. You may be asked about your strategy for balancing personal/family life and medical school, or whether you intend to have children. These questions might seem to be inappropriate, particularly to women. However you choose to answer such questions, it is probably best *not* to get defensive. It is reasonable to have concerns about these issues. Tina found that she got a good response when she turned the questions around and asked the interviewer whether *he* felt being a medical student/resident/physician was stressful on a marriage and what *he* felt about having children while in medical school. For more advice on interviewing techniques, turn to Chapter 6.

CHOOSING YOUR MEDICAL SCHOOL

Due to the intense competition in medical school admissions, most premedical advisors recommend that applicants apply to at least 10 schools. Some applicants, particularly those from states with competitive state-affiliated medical schools and whose grades and test scores are below average, should apply to 30 or more schools. In deciding which and how many schools to apply to, it is valuable to talk to a premedical advisor. They will help you determine how strong your application is.

The average MCAT scores of students at a particular school are an indicator of how difficult it is to get in. Be sure to apply to a few "safety" schools to which you have a better chance of being admitted. Medical school admission and rejection decisions don't always make sense. Donald was accepted to some of the most prestigious schools in the country, but not to his own state school. This element of chance is one reason it's better to apply to a number of schools and not to set your hopes on a single school.

For legal reasons, most schools claim that "age is not a factor in admissions." One way to evaluate a school's attitude toward nontraditional students is to look at its student body. Are there a significant number of nontraditional students? What is the average age of incoming students, and what is the age range? Typically, a school's student body reflects its applicant pool, and some schools with fewer nontraditional students simply have fewer nontraditional applicants. If a school that interests you has few nontraditional students, you may want to ask why. It is possible that the school is looking to diversify its student population and will be particularly interested in your application. Medical schools that have arrangements with post-bacc programs are clearly interested in nontraditional students. You should explore them carefully.

Some people argue that all the medical schools in the United States are very good and that there is no particular reason to aspire toward a "top" school. An important difference between medical school and many other graduate or professional degree programs is that medical training does not end at graduation. Rather, a physician's formal education continues during internship, residency, and possibly into fellowship experiences. In terms of job opportunities, where you do your residency could be more important than where you go to school. While attending a well-reputed school will help in residency placement, doing well at a lesser-known school will also allow you to secure a desirable residency. On the other hand, an advantage to attending a well-reputed school is the comfort of knowing that you don't necessarily have to graduate at the top of the class in order to be competitive after graduation.

For those who want to practice strictly clinical medicine, there are factors to consider that may be as important as, if not more important, than a school's general reputation, which is often based largely on the research associated with the institution. When evaluating the training you will receive, some of the issues to consider are the school's location, the patient population to which students are exposed, the extent to which first and second year students learn clinical medicine, the format of the basic science curriculum,[7] interdisciplinary aspects of the curriculum,[8] the learning resources available to students, the school's role in the community and as a health care provider, the emphasis on primary care, the grading system, and the accessibility of faculty. Even if you are uninterested in a career in medical research, there are educational benefits to becoming involved in research efforts while in medical school, and you may be interested in schools that facilitate faculty/student collaboration and encourage student participation in research.

Rather than focusing on prestige or a published ranking,[9] concentrate on what you want from a school. Among other features, Mitch wanted access to a school of public health so that he could continue working in public and international health issues. Eve looked for schools that devoted significant resources to primary care. Donald looked for more structured programs, while Becky was interested in programs that allowed flexibility. Jacob applied primarily to schools with strong reputations for emergency medicine. Bob hoped to continue teaching part-time or during summers while in school. He looked for schools that would allow this.

Beyond academic features, there are lifestyle issues to consider that may be quite different from those faced by recent college graduates. In college, Mitch enjoyed being part of a cohesive student body at a small, remote, private school. As a 30-year-old who had spent significant time overseas, he wanted to live in a more multicultural environment. He hoped to have a social life that, to some degree, involved people other than his medical school classmates. Most of the schools he applied to were either in urban areas or were closely associated with a larger university. Tina wanted to remain near her boyfriend and decided to limit her applications to schools in the region of the country where he was studying. Because of her family, Eve had location issues as well. As a nontraditional student, you are likely to have more responsibilities and complexities in your life than a recent college graduate. As a result, you may find that lifestyle issues play a more important role in determining where you apply and where you go to school.

The day of your interview affords a rare opportunity to hear firsthand what it is like to be a student at a particular medical school. During the course of the day, you will probably speak with current students, either formally or informally. Ask the students you meet for the names of nontraditional students within the class. If you have a spouse and/or children, ask for the names of students in similar situations. While interviewing, you will be focused on making a good impression and getting in. Later, however, you

---

[7] Some schools use lectures and labs while others have an entirely case-based approach. A number of schools fall somewhere in the middle, incorporating some of each educational methodology. There is no evidence that a particular curriculum is "best." You need to consider your own learning style.

[8] Presumably, nontraditional students bring an interdisciplinary perspective and benefit from this approach.

[9] There is no definitive ranking. *U.S. News & World Report* publishes a yearly report ranking graduate schools. Be sure to understand the methodology used when reading their findings.

might have some choices to make and you may be desperately trying to differentiate one school from the next. Input from current students, particularly those with backgrounds similar to your own, will be invaluable (for more advice on how to choose a school, turn to page 40).

FINANCIAL ISSUES

The cost of a medical education is daunting for traditional and nontraditional students alike. With the exception of those who have accrued savings in former careers, financing medical school as a nontraditional student involves challenges. Nontraditional students often have higher living expenses associated with off-campus housing, dependents, debt, and other financial responsibilities. With few exceptions, financial aid offices will look at your parents' income and assets in determining assistance packages. This applies to all students, regardless of their age and whether they themselves are parents. If you are married, medical schools will expect your spouse to contribute to the extent that he or she can. If your parents and/or spouse are less than thrilled about supporting you in this endeavor, financial questions can translate to personal/emotional issues. Older medical students will have less time in the workforce to pay off educational debt, and it is unclear whether financial aid offices consider this in making awards (for more information on financial issues, turn to Chapter 5).

You should carefully consider the financial implications of going to medical school, and try to come up with a strategy for dealing with them. If your heart is set on going, financial issues alone should probably not stop you. When deciding where to apply, add to your list of considerations the average debt of graduating students. Even if this figure is not published, financial aid offices will probably provide it if you ask. Look very closely at your state-affiliated medical school because in-state tuition is typically much less than private school costs. Ask financial aid offices about loan repayment programs. Think about ways to trim your budget, such as living with relatives or giving up your car. The material possessions you forego now, and the loan payments you make in the future, should be weighed against the value of having a truly fulfilling career.

5 Financing Medical School

HOW MUCH IS ALL OF THIS GOING TO COST?

There's no doubt that med school is expensive. The average first-year tuition for a U.S. private medical school is upwards of $32,000, and the average tuition at public schools is upwards of $14,000 for in-state residents. When planning for the cost of attending medical school, however, tuition is only part of the picture. You must also pay for books, equipment, housing, utilities, food, insurance, transportation, and miscellaneous costs. All of these expenses add up quickly; depending on where you attend school, they may equal or exceed the price of tuition. Note that tuition is 30 percent higher during second and third years to cover the cost of year-round education.

The cost of a medical education is daunting, but once in practice, physicians are among the most highly paid professionals. In recent years, the difference in pay across specialties has made it difficult to assess physician pay as an overall average. The many options available to current doctors in the way they practice have further complicated this analysis. While all doctors may look forward to earning a comfortable salary, some will be better compensated than others. For example, in 2003 a typical family practitioner made $152,478, while the average for all specialists was $296,464. Although it will be years before today's first-year students make that kind of money, they can assume the financial burden of their education with the confidence that they will one day make enough money to justify the investment.

AND HOW CAN I PAY FOR IT?

Since the medical student of today will be the well-paid physician of tomorrow, medical schools expect the students and their families to be responsible for the cost of their education. Except in cases in which a student has exceptional financial resources, it is essential to rely on outside sources of financial assistance to pay the bill.

FINANCIAL AID PROGRAMS

There are two general types of financial assistance available: loans and scholarships/grants. Loans must be repaid, and have varying interest rates, deferment options, and repayment periods. Many subsidized loans will be available to you only if you have documented need, while other funds are available regardless of your financial situation. Most medical students borrow heavily, relying on the prospect of a generous salary once they begin practice. For 2005 med school graduates, the average debt was $138,093 for students from private schools and $110,460 for students from public schools, and by all indications, these amounts will continue to increase. Scholarships and grants are gifts that need not be repaid. They can be awarded on the basis of several factors—financial need, outstanding academic merit, specific criteria such as gender, or a promise of future service—or a combination of those factors. Note that the financial aid offices of the schools you are accepted to should provide you with a package that covers all costs somehow. The question is how much of the package comes from you or your parents or from high-interest loans.

Loans

Anyone with good credit can borrow enough money to finance a medical education. Borrowing is simplified if you take advantage of federal lending programs. Qualifications are as follows:

- *American citizenship or permanent U.S. resident status*

- *If you are a male 18 years of age or older, you are registered for Selective Service, or you have documentation proving that you are not required to register*

- *You have a good credit history, including good standing on prior student loans*

- *You are an active, enrolled student in good academic standing*

If you have financial resources that disqualify you for some types of need-based aid, but you meet the above requirements, you are still eligible for federal loans (unsubsidized and private loans). The loans for which you qualify may have higher interest rates and offer less favorable repayment schedules than the subsidized loans that are aimed at those with financial need.

Following is a description of five basic types of loans: federal, state, private, charitable, and institutional.

Federal

Federal loan programs are funded by the federal government or are funded by banks and guaranteed by the federal government. Federal loans, particularly the Stafford Loan, are usually the "first resort" for medical student borrowers. Some federal loans such as Perkins or Stafford subsidized loans are need-based, but some higher-interest loans are available to students or their families regardless of financial circumstance.

State

Students who are residents of the state in which they attend medical school may be eligible for state loan programs. Eligibility is often based on need and may be further tied to specific segments of the population (e.g., minority or disadvantaged students, or students who are interested in practicing family medicine in underserved areas of the state). Individual schools can provide you with information about state loan programs.

Private

Privately funded, commercial loans are available from banks and other financial institutions. Interest rates are high! The banks benefit as much from the loan as you do.

Charitable

Charity loans are funded by contributions from foundations, corporations, and associations. A number of private loans are targeted to aid particular segments of the population (e.g., minority or disadvantaged students, women, or students who are interested in practicing family medicine in underserved areas of the state). You may have to investigate to identify all of the charitable loans for which you qualify. The best place to begin your search is in public, undergraduate, and med school libraries. There are also a number of commercial financial aid search services available, but beware—financial aid officers warn that search services sometimes charge hefty fees for information that, in the majority of cases, students can obtain themselves. Private financial aid resources are also available online. Visit the Financial Center at www.PrincetonReview.com to get information on many of them.

Institutional

The amount of loan money available, and the method by which it is disbursed, varies greatly from one school to another. As part of the shift toward emphasizing primary care, some schools offer assistance to students who are committed to providing primary care after graduation. To find out about the resources available at a particular school, refer to its catalog or contact its financial aid office.

In the chart on pages 70 and 71, we have compiled a table of the most commonly used loan programs. Included in this table is information about the characteristics of each loan. The following characteristics are discussed:

Name: The full name of the loan and the acronym, if applicable, by which it is most commonly known.

Source: Information about the organization that funds and administers each loan.

Eligibility: Some loans are need-based. Others are open to people regardless of their financial situation. A few federal and private schools require that a student fit a specific demographic profile. Note that regardless of your age or how long you have been independent of your parents, their income is considered in calculating your need in almost all cases.

TABLE OF LOANS

NAME OF LOAN	SOURCE	ELIGIBILITY	MAXIMUM ALLOCATION
Federal Stafford (Subsidized) Student Loan http://studentaid.ed.gov/ students/publications/ student_guide/index.html	Federal, administered by participating lender	Demonstrated financial need	$8,500/year. The maximum aggregate total for subsidized loans is $65,500. The maximum aggregate total includes any Stafford loans received for undergraduate study.
Unsubsidized Stafford Student Loan http://studentaid.ed.gov/ students/publications/ student_guide/index.html	Federal, administered by participating lender	Not need-based	The total Stafford loan limit is $18,500, including Unsubsidized loans and Subsidized loans not to exceed $8,500. The maximum aggregate total of Stafford loans is $138,500, including Unsubsidized loans and Subsidized loans not to exceed $65,500.*
Health Professions Student Loan/Primary Care Loan (HPSL) Contact school for more information	Federal, administered by school	Exceptional financial need; commitment to primary care	For first- and second-year students, the maximum allocation is the cost of attendance (including tuition, educational expenses, and reasonable living expenses). Third- and fourth-year students may receive allocations beyond this amount.
Perkins Loan (formerly NDSL) Contact school for more information	Federal, administered by school	Demonstrated financial need	$6,000/year, with aggregate of $40,000. Aggregate amount includes undergraduate loans.
Alternative Loan Program (ALP) www.aamc.org/students/ medloans/loanstates/0607/ start.htm	AAMC, administered under MEDLOANS division of AAMC	Not need-based	Cost of attendance minus other aid received. Aggregate: $220,000 (total educational indebtedness from all sources).

*Students pursuing certain health professions and enrolled in programs accredited by the appropriate approved accreditation agency are eligible to receive increased amounts of Unsubsidized Stafford loans. If a student is granted the maximum additional allocation, the maximum aggregate total will be $189,125. This number includes all undergraduate and graduate Subsidized and Unsubsidized Stafford loans. See "Increased Eligibility for Health Professions Students" in the Federal Student Aid Handbook for details and updates.

REPAYMENT AND DEFERRAL OPTIONS	INTEREST RATE	PROS	CONS
10–30 years to repay. Begin repayment 6 months after graduation. Forbearance possible for up to 3 years of residency training.	Variable 4% loan disbursement fee. Capped at *8.25%.	Most common medical school loan. Interest is paid by the government during school. Once you get a loan, later loans are at the same rate.	None
10–30 years to repay. Interest begins to accrue from day loan is disbursed; you can pay the interest or have it capitalized (added to principal). Begin repayment 6 months after graduation. Forbearance possible for up to 3 years of residency training.	Variable 4% loan disbursement fee. Capped at *8.25%.	Not need-based.	Interest is not paid by the government while you're in school.
10 years to repay, beginning 1 year after graduation. Deferrable during residency and under special circumstances.	Fixed, 5%.	Fixed, relatively low interest rate.	Very limited availability.
10 years to repay. Begin repayment 9 months after graduation. Can be deferred for 2 years during residency.	Fixed, 5%.	Fixed, relatively low interest rate.	Low maximum allocation.
Standard: 20 years of interest and principal payments. Alternative: 3 years of interest only and 17 years of interest and principal. Repayment generally begins 3–4 years after graduation, depending on length of residency.	Prime rate plus 1.25%; variable, adjusted monthly. (While in school, prime rate plus 0%. Variable, adjusted monthly.)	High maximum allocation; not need-based.	"Loan of last resort." High interest rate.

*Check http://studentaid.ed.gov/students/publications/student_guide/index.html

Maximum Allocation: There is a maximum amount of money you can borrow from any one program, so many medical students find it necessary to borrow from more than one source. Most loans have both maximum yearly and aggregate loan amounts. Amounts you borrowed from the same loan program for your college education are deducted, in some cases, from the aggregate amount you can borrow in medical school.

Repayment and Deferral Options: Important considerations in structuring your educational debt are how long you have to pay back loans and whether principal and/or interest may be deferred until you have completed your education. This column provides information about the repayment period and deferral options for each loan. It is important to remember that, no matter what the source of a loan, the responsibility for keeping track of loan activity is yours.

Interest Rate: This column provides information about the current interest rate of the loan. Fixed-rate loans use the same interest rate throughout the life of the loan. Variable-rate loans base their interest rate on established financial values, usually 91-day Treasury Bills (T-Bills) or the prime lending rate. Since these rates fluctuate greatly, you should check with a bank to find out the exact interest rate.

Pros: Listed in this category are factors that make this an attractive loan source. Attractive features include long repayment terms, deferral policies that waive both interest and principal throughout medical school and all or part of residency training, and low, fixed-rate interest.

Cons: Listed in this category are factors that make a particular loan unattractive. Such features include short repayment times, limited deferral options, or variable, high-interest rates.

Scholarships/Grants

Some grant, or gift money, comes with no strings attached; these are nonobligatory scholarships. Although such scholarships may be available on the basis of outstanding academic merit alone, others are based on a combination of merit and need. In fact, all federal, nonobligatory scholarships are based on need and may also require that you fit a particular demographic profile. Scholarship amounts vary, and they are administered by the same groups as loans: federal and state governments, private foundations, and institutions. For more information about private, state, and institutional scholarships, contact the financial aid offices at some of the schools to which you are going to apply, or visit the Financial Center at www.PrincetonReview.com.

Obligatory Scholarships

Some federal scholarships are available to students who agree to practice at the Public Health Service, at the Veterans Administration, or in the Armed Forces. These scholarships provide full tuition, some or all expenses, and a monthly stipend. Service-based scholarships, which are not based on need, all carry an obligation to serve at least one

TABLE OF GRANTS

NAME OF GRANT	SOURCE	ELIGIBILITY	SERVICE OF OBLIGATION	AMOUNT OF GRANT
National Health Service Corps (NHSC)	Federal	Need-based; former EFN recipients and students with interest in primary care are preferred.	Two- to four-year contract. Years spent in residency do not count toward fulfilling obligation.	Maximum amount is full tuition and fees plus stipend.
National Medical Fellowship Scholarship (NMF)	Private	First- or second-year underrepresented minority, female, rural, or disadvantaged background with documented financial need.	None	Varies. Awards have ranged from $500–$10,000.
Scholarships for Disadvantaged Students (SDS)	Federal, administered through school	Full-time, financially needy students from disadvantaged backgrounds, enrolled in health professions and nursing programs. U.S. citizens only.	None	Varies; tuition and other educational expenses.
Armed Forces Health Professions Scholarship Program (HPSP)	U.S. Army, U.S. Navy, and U.S. Air Force	Able to serve in military; age restrictions; U.S. citizens only.	One year for every year of support. Years spent in residency do not count toward fulfilling obligation.	Full tuition, "reasonable" fees, and stipend. Student becomes officer in service branch upon matriculation and receives all benefits of rank.

year for every year of support. The advantage—a "free" medical education—is obvious, but this is not an option to take lightly. Time spent in residency—which is often restricted to only military residencies—does not count toward your service debt, so you may be out of medical school for seven to twelve years before you're free of your obligation. Some states and counties also offer service-based scholarship programs or tuition remission programs. Despite their lengthy obligations, service-based scholarships are in high demand. To increase your chances of obtaining one, apply as early as possible. Ask the financial aid offices of schools in which you are interested whom to contact locally for more information. There are also loan repayment programs available to which you apply after you have accrued debt and when you are ready to start working in an underserved area.

THE FINANCIAL AID PROCESS

PREPARING TO APPLY

Many students miss out on potential assistance by making some basic, avoidable mistakes. Top financial aid officers supplied the following common errors and their remedies.

Missing Deadlines and Keeping Poor Records

Like your applications for admission, your financial aid applications should be submitted as early as possible. File your income tax forms early and encourage your parents (all med students are considered dependent by med schools, even if they have been independent for years) to do the same. Photocopy all forms that you submit and note the date you send them. File these forms along with any material related to the decisions of the financial aid committees of the schools to which you apply. Keep careful track of deadlines, which are strongly enforced.

Submitting Information to the Wrong Needs Analysis Service

There are several third-party organizations that assist medical schools in determining the financial need of entering and continuing students. Many applicants assume that because they have submitted information to one of the services for one school, they have done everything they need to do for all the schools they are considering. Making this assumption can have serious repercussions. Until the proper service completes the needs analysis, the financial aid office cannot package your financial aid. To avoid making this mistake, check with the financial aid offices of all the schools to which you are applying to see which service they use. Submit the proper materials to the appropriate service. More detailed information on the needs analysis services and their function can be found under "Calculating Your Contribution."

Having a Poor Credit History

People are often unpleasantly surprised when they see their credit histories. Even relatively minor financial problems, like making a couple of late payments on loans or credit cards, can lower your credit rating. Also, credit bureaus sometimes make mistakes, causing negative, but false, information to show up on your record. Since a bad credit history will make you ineligible for many, if not all, loan programs, it is a good idea to check your credit history before you apply for financial aid. Recent federal legislation has made it possible to get a copy of your credit report free of charge once a year from any of the major credit bureaus. You can visit them online at www.equifax.com, www.experian.com, or www.transunion.com to obtain a copy of your free report.

Defaulting on Undergraduate Student Loans

If you have not kept up with your student loan payments, you will have a very hard time qualifying for loans, especially those funded by the federal government. Clear up any problems with prior student loans well before applying for additional assistance. If you are still in school and have not yet begun repaying your loans, talk to your undergraduate financial aid officer to clarify repayment and deferral options on your loans. Remember that the burden of keeping track of your loan activity is on you, and that once you start medical school, you must keep the lenders apprised of your whereabouts.

APPLYING FOR AID

Schools' policies may vary somewhat, but they all follow the same general lines. To determine whether you qualify and for how much, schools must first determine how much it will cost for you to attend, and then how much of that cost you and your family can absorb.

HOW SCHOOLS DETERMINE THEIR COST

Each medical school prepares a student budget that reflects the expenses associated with being a first-year medical student. Included in this budget are items such as tuition and fees, books, equipment, housing, utilities, food, insurance, transportation, and personal expenses. To some degree, schools customize expenses if a student has particular needs. For example, projected costs may increase if you live off campus.

CALCULATING YOUR CONTRIBUTION

To determine how much you and your family can contribute, medical schools use a needs analysis service. Refer to the financial aid guidelines of the schools you are considering attending. Some schools use more than one service to calculate need, and many ultimately use their own formulas to determine institutional assistance. To make sure you have all the information required to fill out the forms completely, file your previous year's income tax returns early. Because some federal loan programs and some institutions require parental information even from independent or married students, your parents should also file their income tax forms as early as possible.

On the basis of the information you give them, the needs analysis calculates your financial need by subtracting your expected personal and family contribution from the total student budget furnished by the school. If expenses are higher than the estimated contribution, you show financial need.

YOUR TENTATIVE FINANCIAL AID PACKAGE

Most schools will only prepare a financial aid package for accepted students. Once you have been accepted to a school, be on the lookout for a financial aid package. The package can include loans, scholarships, grants, or a combination of these elements. If financial aid is an important consideration in deciding between schools, be sure that you have estimates from all schools by the applicant decision deadline.

ACCEPTING YOUR FINANCIAL AID PACKAGE

Once you matriculate at a school, the financial aid office will put together your actual financial aid package. In most cases, loans will make up a portion of the package. Remember, loans must be repaid—with interest—and the amount of this debt will affect your lifestyle far beyond medical school and residency. For instance, if you borrow a large sum of money for medical school, you may have trouble later obtaining a loan for a large purchase like a car or a house. You are not required to accept all the aid you are offered, so it is in your best interest to borrow only what you need to meet your expenses.

CUTTING COSTS

Medical schools formulate their student budgets by using average expenses for everything except tuition. By making some adjustments to your lifestyle, it is usually possible to undercut this budget and therefore decrease the amount of money you borrow. Following are some strategies recommended by financial aid professionals to reduce debt.

BOOKS AND EQUIPMENT

Buy good-quality used textbooks and equipment whenever possible. Selling books and equipment you no longer need is a good way to earn extra cash.

TRANSPORTATION

Automobile loan payments, insurance premiums, licensing fees, fuel, and maintenance really add up. Evaluate your need for a car before taking one to medical school. If you attend school in a place where public transportation is available or where you can bike or walk to school, leave the car behind. If you must have a car, you can save by raising insurance deductibles and carpooling with fellow students.

INSURANCE

Most medical schools require you to carry medical and, in some cases, disability insurance. Before you buy into the school's plan, check your existing coverage. If your parents still claim you as a dependent, or if you have a spouse whose medical benefits extend to you, you may already have adequate coverage.

OTHER EXPENSES

Millions of Americans find themselves in dire financial straits each year because of revolving credit. Medical students are no exception. If you find that you have trouble avoiding the temptation to pull out the plastic for purchases you can't afford, cut up your cards. Remember, if you can't afford to pay for something with cash or a check, you probably can't afford to charge it either. To keep discretionary expenses from getting out of hand, set up a detailed budget and stick to it. If you've never used a budget before and need help, there are many computer programs that will help you set up a budget, track expenses, and give you reports on how you're doing.

A FINAL WORD

YOUR FINANCIAL AID RIGHTS

- *You have the right to expect that the financial aid office will assist you in obtaining financial aid and information about financial aid opportunities.*

- *Financial aid officers to whom you give information about your/your family's financial profile cannot publicize this information.*

- *You have the right to accept or decline all or part of the aid offered.*

- *You have the right to appeal your financial aid package if your financial aid picture changes for the worse. (This does not necessarily mean, however, that the amount of aid will increase.)*

- *You have the right to examine your financial aid file at any time.*

- *You are entitled to treatment that does not discriminate on the basis of race, creed, age, handicap, gender, or national origin.*

YOUR FINANCIAL AID RESPONSIBILITIES

- *You are responsible for meeting the expenses related to attending medical school.*

- *You are responsible for reading and understanding the conditions and terms of all of the elements in your financial aid package.*

- *You are responsible for submitting financial aid applications on time.*

- *You are responsible for obtaining and filling out financial aid forms and supplying accurate and complete information on these forms.*

- *You are responsible for reporting to your financial aid office any outside scholarships or loans that may affect your amount of need.*

- *You are responsible for using loan funds to pay tuition.*

- *You are responsible for repaying all loans.*

- *You are responsible for notifying all lenders of all changes of address during and after medical school.*

- *You are responsible for keeping accurate and complete records of all financial aid applications and transactions.*

6 The Interview:
Separating the Merely Qualified from the Truly Worthy

Be proud if you're invited to an interview. You've made it through two initial screenings, one before and one after the supplemental application. Usually, this means that the Admissions Committee thinks you're qualified to attend their school. Unfortunately, they also invite a lot of other qualified people, and they don't have space to admit all of you. Therefore, your objective is to convince everyone who interviews you that the school would be a better place with you in it. Easy to say, a little harder to do. It is important to realize that the weight of the interview varies from school to school. At some schools it is the key to admission, while at others it is mainly a formality—more for you than for them.

Because almost everyone has heard horror stories about someone else's interview, most people start to worry about the interview before they even submit their applications. Try to relax. A good interview begins with good preparation. You can start by becoming familiar with the interview process.

WHO CONDUCTS INTERVIEWS?

Different schools have different policies about who conducts the actual interview. In general, schools have a Medical Selection Committee made up of professional admissions or student affairs people and faculty members. Often, especially in more progressive schools, upper-level med students also participate. At some schools, you'll have a couple of separate, one-on-one interviews; at others, you'll be interviewed by a panel. You may be the only applicant in front of a panel (this really seems more like an inquisition), or you may be joined by other candidates.

At many schools, the person or people you speak with become your advocates in the final selection process. When all the interviews in a certain time period are finished and the Selection Committee meets, these people share their observations about you and sometimes recommend a particular action. The final decision, of course, is up to the entire committee.

WHAT CAN I EXPECT?

Expect some interviews to go well and others to go poorly. In the vast majority of cases, the interviewers are trying to build an honest picture of you beyond the numbers, and most try to reduce stress during the interviews. Despite this, you will probably experience one or two "bad" interviews with interviewers who have not read your file and therefore seem disinterested, are insecure or awkward themselves, or are simply having a bad day. Keep this in mind as your interview dates approach.

HOW SHOULD I ACT?

The golden rule for interviews is "Be Yourself." Interviewers have been through all of this before, and they're pretty good at spotting people who are putting on an act or reading from a mental script. What they're trying to find out from this interview is what kind of person you are and how you relate to others. Up until now, you've been only a few sheets of paper, a bunch of numbers, and a (probably horrible) photograph. Now's the time to show them your stuff. But remember: no lying and no BS.

BE PREPARED

You should be ready to answer questions about your motivation to become a physician, your academic background, your extracurricular and leisure activities, your job or research experience, and your views on medical problems and ethical issues. Later in this chapter is a sample of questions that current medical students were asked in their interviews. Some of them are typical; others are truly strange. As you get ready to interview, try to answer some of these questions on your own, and then ask a friend, parent, or professor to grill you. In addition, you may want to audiotape or videotape mock interviews to see how you sound and look. When you choose a guinea pig to be your surrogate interviewer, select someone who will be honest with you about the strengths and weaknesses of your responses. Don't try to memorize answers word for word; canned responses, no matter how valid, are stiff and unconvincing (just look at a video of a presidential debate). It is a good idea, however, to enter an interview with several "stories" or points in mind. Questions are often openended, giving you the chance to direct the conversation toward your strengths and away from your weaknesses.

APPROACH WITH CONFIDENCE

Like dogs, interviewers seem to smell fear. The tone of your interview is often set in the first few seconds, so approach with confidence. Greet your interviewer with a firm handshake and look him or her in the eye. During the interview, be positive. Think of it as a pleasant conversation with someone you'd like to get to know better. A good interview is a dialogue, where there is considerable give and take. Unless your interviewer brings them up, avoid controversial or emotionally charged subjects like abortion. If you're asked your views, state them and move on.

TAKE YOUR TIME

In the course of your interviews, you may be asked scores of questions, some on issues to which you haven't given a great deal of thought. Your interviewers don't expect you to have a ready answer for every one of these questions, but they do expect you to come up with a coherent, well-thought-out response. Many applicants are afraid that if they hesitate, it will seem that they are unprepared. Not so. Good physicians don't rush to a conclusion without considering the facts; rather, they think through a problem before they decide how to act. If a question catches you off guard, take a second to think it through. If it seems ambiguous, don't be afraid to ask for clarification. If you don't know, admit it and ask the interviewer to share the answer. By taking the time to make sure that your response is well conceived and well spoken, you will impress the interviewers as thoughtful and articulate—two characteristics essential in a good doctor.

ASK QUESTIONS

Although the interview is the time for medical schools to find out about you, it is also an excellent opportunity for you to find out more about the school. Before you go to an interview, make sure you've studied the school's information packet and are ready to ask intelligent questions about the program. Search the archives at your undergraduate or public library to see if the school has been in the news and, if so, for what. Remember that most people love to talk about themselves. Ask the interviewer about his work or impressions of the curriculum.

BE ON TIME

Make sure that you get detailed directions before you make the trip and arrive with enough time to park and find the office. If you are invited to interview at several schools in the same geographic region, you might save on travel costs and time by making an interview circuit, visiting several schools on the same trip. This can mean that you have several interviews in the same week or even the same day. Give yourself as much time as possible at each, so that you have time to make the transition, both physically and mentally, from one school to the next. If you can, try to get to each campus early enough to walk around, talk to students, and formulate questions that are specific to the school.

DRESS FOR SUCCESS

Like it or not, looks count. No matter what your usual mode of dress, you should dress conservatively and professionally for your interviews. For men, this means a suit, or a blazer and nice pants (and, of course, a tie); for women, a suit, blazer and skirt or dress pants, or a business-style dress is appropriate. Regardless of your gender, pay attention to detail; even the most beautiful suit looks shabby if your shoes are scuffed and worn, and the effect of a great-looking blazer is ruined by a ragged backpack. Polish your shoes, invest in a nice portfolio or case for your papers, and by all means, iron your clothes. If you are generally somewhat less than conservative in your dress, you may want to tone it down: men, replace the big hoop earring with a stud; women, take off the gold glitter polish and paint on clear. After all, you don't want to be asked, as one of the respondents to our survey was, "Why are you dressed the way you are? Why did you come here looking the way you do?"

CONDUCT YOURSELF PROFESSIONALLY

Admissions committees can see from your application that you are smart, accomplished, and highly regarded by your professors. The interview is an opportunity for them to gauge things that are not so easily conveyed on paper. Medical schools are looking for students with maturity, empathy, and superior interpersonal skills. All of these things come through in the interview. In a group setting, where the committee talks with more than one candidate at a time, you will be observed not only when you answer a question, but also when your fellow applicants are speaking. Keep alert, and show interest. After all, you never know what you may learn that you can use in your next interview.

HOW AND WHEN TO FOLLOW UP ON YOUR INTERVIEWS

First, don't forget to send a thank you note after each set of interviews. You can write several different notes to each of your interviewers, or send just one addressed generally to the interview committee. Don't write a novella in your thank you note. It's fine to mention a particular question or topic you found interesting during your interview, but you should limit yourself to only a few lines. As you might have guessed, it's a good idea to take a few brief notes, such as the interviewer's names and some of the topics they covered, right after you leave the interview. For the thank you notes themselves, you can use any nice stationery paper.

If the school is not entirely certain of the strength of your application relative to other candidates after your interviews, you may be placed on a hold list. Don't despair. You made it as far as the interview process, which (except in the case of some public schools who interview every candidate) means that you have survived some of the initial cuts. Sometimes being put on hold simply means that the school has already accepted enough students that month. You can, however, send supplementary information to further support your application. For example, if you have been doing research, volunteer work, or taking classes that didn't appear on your initial application, and if you didn't get a chance to talk about your new activities during the interview, you can write a short—less than one page—letter outlining your recent accomplishments and send it to the school. This shows that you are still working hard to better your chances of acceptance into medical school.

WHAT ARE THEY GOING TO ASK?

Over the past several years, The Princeton Review has surveyed current medical students about their schools and the medical school application process. The sample interview questions in this section come from those surveys. Although the following list of questions is by no means exhaustive, it is a good sampling of questions that were asked in real interviews in the recent past. When we first decided to ask current med students what they were asked in their interviews, we had no idea how strange—and in some cases disturbing—some of their responses were going to be. Get ready, because while some of the questions are pretty standard, others are truly bizarre.

So You Want to Be a Doctor?

Some of the students we surveyed were unprepared for questions like those that follow, thinking them so mundane that they wouldn't be asked. From our research, however, we can say with confidence that if you're granted even one interview, you're almost sure to be asked several questions about your motivation and suitability for medical school.

- *Why do you want to be a doctor?*
- *The future of medicine looks bleak. Why do you want to go into it?*
- *What articles have you read recently that relate to the reasons you want to become a doctor?*
- *What do you see yourself doing with a medical degree?*
- *Were you influenced by relatives to pursue a career in medicine?*
- *Why do you want to attend [name of school]?*
- *Why should we accept you?*
- *How are your accomplishments better than those of the other candidates in this interview?*
- *Evaluate yourself based on the required evaluation of the interviewer.*
- *Do you think you are motivated enough for medical school?*
- *When you don't get into medical school, what will you do?*
- *What career path would you follow if all the medical schools closed today?*
- *You've taken an odd, nontraditional path to get here. Why are you interested in medicine?*
- *What disadvantages do you see in being an older student?*
- *Can you afford to come here?*

- *How will you finance your medical education?*

- *Describe what you believe to be the financial rewards of medicine.*

- *If doctors were paid as much as teachers, would you still want to be a doctor?*

TELL ME A LITTLE BIT ABOUT YOURSELF . . .

Selection committees use the interview as an opportunity to find out what makes you tick. Prepare yourself for personal questions about your character traits, your coping mechanisms, and your life experiences. You may also be asked to comment on your interpersonal relationships. Always be honest.

- *What is your worst quality?*

- *If you could change anything about yourself, what would it be?*

- *Are you aggressive?*

- *What makes you a fun person?*

- *What makes you angry?*

- *What makes you sad?*

- *What scares you?*

- *Do you like sick people?*

- *Are you afraid of death?*

- *What are you the most proud of?*

- *One of the people who wrote a letter of recommendation for you described you as [adjective]. Do you agree with that description?*

- *Was there a time in your life when you had tremendous responsibility?*

- *What is the wackiest thing you've ever done?*

- *What was the biggest mistake you ever made?*

- *What is the worst thing that has happened to you in the past four years?*

- *Tell me something you wanted to achieve but did not, or something you've failed at. How did you cope with failure?*

- *What role has stress played in your life?*

- *How could you prove to me that you can perform well under stress?*

- *What do you do to alleviate stress?*

- *Tell me about your family.*

- *What role do you play in your family dynamic?*

- *How is your relationship with your parents?*

- *What is the physical health of your parents, and how would you handle an illness of theirs while attending school?*

- *Who is the person in the world to whom you are closest?*

- *Describe your best friend.*

- *What does your closest friend think about your relationship with him or her?*

- *Give one word that a friend would use to describe you.*

IT'S ALL ACADEMIC

Grades, MCAT scores, and courses are fair game for the inquisitive interviewer. You may be asked to explain your performance in a course or to tell what you learned. A hint: To be better prepared for questions of this type, get a copy of your transcript and take a look at it. Look for things that might cause an interviewer to ask a question. Lower than normal grades stick out, as do courses with funny names (like Rocks for Jocks). Then again, be honest.

- *What do you think of the GPA as a valid method of categorizing students?*

- *Why were your first-year grades so bad?*

- *Why do you have so many C grades on your transcript?*

- *Explain your low math grade.*

- *Why are your grades high compared to your MCAT scores?*

- *Do you realize that your MCAT scores aren't anything special?*

- *Tell me about your research.*

- *Have you taken any humanities classes, and what papers did you write in them?*

- *What did you learn in [name of course]? (It's worth noting that some people were asked about normal courses like "Philosophy 101" and others were asked about bizarre courses like "The Art of Murder," "Fairy Tales," and "Play, Games, Toys, and Sports.")*

- *Who was the author of your biochemistry textbook?*

EXTRA, EXTRA, READ ALL ABOUT IT!

Whatever your extracurricular activities and work experiences, you will most likely be asked how they relate to your commitment to and preparedness for studying medicine. Think about your extracurricular experiences and what you learned about yourself, the medical field, and/or working with people as a result of participating in these activities. If you've been out of school for a while and have worked extensively in another field, be ready for questions about why you decided to change fields. Scientific or medical research experience is a plus, but it can be a real liability if you're not able to discuss it in detail.

- *What are your hobbies?*
- *How does your hobby relate to being a doctor?*
- *Have you taught yourself to do anything, and if so, what?*
- *How has working as a [name of job] made you a better candidate for medical school?*
- *What volunteer work contributed to your commitment to become a doctor?*
- *What did you do with your job earnings?*

MEDICAL ISSUES AND ETHICS: WHERE DO YOU STAND?

Interviewers love to ask students about a medical issue or about an ethical dilemma related to medicine. In general, there are no wrong answers to these questions. You should know the terminology (for example, what is the difference between euthanasia and euthenics?), and be aware of some pros and cons for each of these issues. Since the health care crisis and attendant problems in reforming the health care delivery system have been grabbing headlines, you should be prepared to discuss the issues intelligently. No one expects you to be an expert on this or any other issue, but you should do some research before your interviews (read the chapter on medicine in the twenty-first century in this book for a review). Don't be surprised if an interviewer challenges your view on an issue; usually, he or she is trying to see how well you support your argument.

- *What is the greatest problem facing medicine today?*
- *What do you consider the most important thing medicine has done for humanity?*
- *What do you think will be the most significant scientific breakthrough in the next ten years?*
- *If you could find a cure for AIDS or for cancer, which would you choose and why?*
- *If you were Surgeon General, what is the first thing you would do?*
- *If you were the health commissioner of [a large city], what would you do?*
- *What is preventive medicine?*
- *What is the biggest problem family practitioners face?*
- *What are your views on euthanasia?*
- *What do you think about euthenics (not euthanasia)?*
- *What would you do about the alcoholism problem in this country?*

- *What do you think about condoms being distributed in high schools?*

- *What are your views on mandatory HIV testing for doctors and patients?*

- *Current AIDS education programs aren't working; what should we do?*

- *Why will organ rationing be the problem of the future in medicine?*

- *Should people have the right to sell their own organs?*

- *Do you think it's ethical to take the life of a fetus for a cell line to save the life of a sibling with cancer?*

- *Should we spend so much time and effort trying to keep premature infants alive?*

- *If a cure were invented for aging, what repercussions would it have on society in general and the medical profession in particular?*

- *How do you feel about animal research?*

- *What role should politics play in medicine?*

- *Is health care a right or a privilege?*

- *What is your opinion of socialized medicine?*

- *How would you organize health care in an ideal world?*

- *Discuss the health care system of Australia.*

- *What do you think should be done about patients who can't pay for treatment?*

- *What is the difference between Medicare and Medicaid?*

- *What is your opinion of HMOs and PPOs?*

- *How will you react to the death of your first patient?*

- *Who would you go to if your mom needed surgery: a surgeon with good hands and a bland personality or a surgeon with not as good hands with a great personality?*

- *How would you tell your best friend's wife (who is your patient) that she has cancer? What would you do if she then refused to tell her family?*

- *You have to amputate one of the legs of an eight-year-old child. How would you tell him?*

- *Would you give a transfusion to a child whose parents were Jehovah's Witnesses?*

- *If a Hindu, for example, comes in and refuses surgery on the basis of religion, and the surgery is his only hope, what would you do? What if the patient was this man or woman's child?*

- *If you diagnosed a patient with a terminal illness as having only two months to live and the family and the patient wanted to end the turmoil ("pull the plug"), would you allow it or strongly disagree?*

- *What would you do if you saw a bleeding child on the side of the road?*

- *What would you do if you had a female patient who was trying to conceive, and your colleague had that patient's husband, and the husband was HIV positive?*

- *If one of your colleagues refused to treat a patient with AIDS, how would you address that colleague?*

- *How would you react if a fellow medical student had AIDS and entered surgery with you?*

- *Would you let a surgeon with AIDS operate on you?*

- *Would you treat a white supremacist, and should physicians be forced to treat such a patient?*

- *If you made a mistake as a physician, how would you handle it?*

TO CHOOSE OR NOT TO CHOOSE

Abortion is not only a hot political topic, it also seems to be a hot topic for interviews. Some schools are affiliated with hospitals where abortions are performed; some are not. Don't try to guess if the interviewer is hoping you will espouse a particular position; honesty seems the best policy on this issue. If you are asked about your willingness to perform an abortion (as a large number of those we surveyed were), you may want to mention that it is not only your beliefs but also the rules of the hospital or laws of the land that you must consider.

- *What should a physician's role be in the politics of abortion?*

- *What would you do as a physician if you were asked to do something contrary to your stand on abortion?*

- *Would you perform an abortion for a teenager, and would you tell her parents?*

- *How would you justify being a Catholic and going to an institution that allows abortion?*

HAVE YOU HEARD THE NEWS?

Good doctors are aware of, and involved in, the world around them. You may be asked about current events, even things completely unrelated to medicine. The questions that follow are only examples; in most cases, these events are no longer current. To prepare for questions like these, keep up with what's happening. If you get most of your news from the TV or radio, start reading newspapers and news magazines for more in-depth coverage.

- *Who is the U.S. Secretary of State?*
- *What do you think about the political situation in Iraq and surrounding countries?*
- *Do you think the Israelis beat up on the Palestinians?*

PHILOSOPHY 101

From the serious to the silly, questions interviewers ask can make you stop and think. (And for some of these questions, one of the things you might think is, "What does this have to do with med school?")

- *What are the top five priorities of society?*
- *Do you see any parallels between medicine and the priesthood?*
- *What is Zen Buddhism?*
- *Explain Hinduism.*
- *Are you a racist?*
- *Do you believe that racism still exists?*
- *How do you feel about affirmative action?*
- *Would you move to Canada to avoid serving active duty during a military conflict abroad?*
- *What is your view on censorship in the arts?*
- *What would you do if you saw a classmate cheating on a test?*
- *Do you believe in drug legalization?*
- *Do you believe that volunteerism could help eliminate greed from society's social structure?*
- *Is altruism ever pure, without some kind of motive?*
- *Do you believe in life after death?*
- *What is your opinion about natural law ethics?*
- *Explain the mind-body problem.*

- *Are you a vertical or horizontal thinker?*

- *If you could be any cell in the human body, what would you be?*

- *If you were to build a human being, what would you include and exclude?*

- *Define hope.*

TRIED AND TRUE

Some questions sound more like pickup lines than med school interview questions. Although none of those surveyed was asked, "What's your sign?" there were plenty of old favorites that you may as well be prepared for.

- *Are you a person who thinks a glass is half empty or half full?*

- *If you could go back in history and meet anyone, who would it be and why?*

- *If you could talk to someone from the future, what would you ask him or her?*

- *If a genie were able to grant you three wishes, what would they be?*

- *If you were stranded on a desert island, what five books would you want?*

- *If your house was burning down and you could save only one thing, what would it be?*

- *If you could be any vegetable, what would you be?*

- *If you could be any kind of fruit, what would you be?*

- *If you could be any kind of animal, what would you be?*

- *What is your favorite color?*

- *What was the last book you read, and how did it influence your life?*

- *What was the last good movie you saw?*

- *Tell me what you see when you look in the mirror.*

- *What was the most embarrassing moment in your life?*

- *Who is your hero?*

- *If you could invite three role models to dinner, who would they be and why, and what would you serve them?*

- *When you die, what would you like your tombstone to read?*

I'll Take Potpourri for $500, Alex

The students we surveyed were asked some trivia worthy of "Final Jeopardy." The bad news is that because of the very nature of these questions, you can't prepare for them. The good news is that a simple "I don't know" seemed to satisfy the interviewers. For bonus points, ask for the answer or, as one student did, tell them you'll check and get back to them. He did, and subsequently, he got in.

- What is the largest lobbyist group in the U.S.?

- Which state first had women's suffrage?

- What language did Abraham (of the Bible) speak?

- When did Iraq become an independent nation?

- How many numbers that contain 9 are there between 1 and 100?

- What is the capital of Vietnam?

- When and how was Pakistan formed?

- Who won the 1969 World Series?

- What is the difference between European and American eighteenth-century poetry?

- Why was the Civil War fought?

- What is the origin of the name "Cincinnati"?

- What do the e's in e.e. cummings' name stand for?

- When and why was the March of Dimes founded?

- When did Istanbul become Istanbul?

- Name the four non-Arabic-speaking countries in the Middle East.

- What was Thomas Aquinas famous for?

- Who was the architect who built the Great Wall of China?

- Where was Millard Filmore born?

- Give a brief history of the Jesuit order.

- Define the Apollonian and the Dionysian as they figure in the philosophy of Nietzsche.

- Who was the head of NATO during World War II?

- What size tippets do you use on your fly lines with a 14X fly?

A Corollary: I'll Take Science & Medicine for $1,000, Alex

A few interviewees were asked trivia questions that actually related to science and medicine. For the most part, they knew the answers. When they didn't, and the question was obscure, it didn't seem to hurt their chances of getting in. Your undergraduate course work and MCAT review should be preparation enough for a lot of these questions.

- *What was the first industrialized country to practice socialized medicine? The second?*

- *How much does the U.S. spend each year on medical care?*

- *How does a lightbulb work?*

- *Why don't fish die in winter?*

- *Why does ice float on the top of water?*

- *How do you make a protein?*

- *So what is Alzheimer's disease, anyway?*

- *Where is your hamstring region?*

- *Tell me what you know about DNA.*

- *What is the Grignard Reaction?*

- *What is Poisson's equation?*

- *Describe protein structure.*

- *What is PKU?*

Can You Say Inappropriate?

Despite the media attention that issues of gender discrimination and sexual harassment receive, medical school interviewers are still asking questions that, if they were asked in a job interview, would be deemed inappropriate or illegal. These kinds of questions are more common than you would expect. The students who told us they'd been asked these questions (and there were lots of them, mostly female) expressed emotions from confusion to outrage. Still, most admitted to being afraid that they would be rejected if they did anything but reply calmly, and therefore they answered honestly and without additional comment. How you handle a question like this is up to you. At this point, you too might feel that there is too much at stake to make waves, but on the other hand, it is certainly within your rights to ask how the question is relevant or even to politely decline to answer.

- *How did you get such a high score in math? I've never seen such a high score from a woman!*

- *Do you know that you have extraordinarily good looks?*

- *Why do you want to be a doctor rather than a nurse?*

- *Will you faint if I take you into surgery?*

- *Would you feel uncomfortable being alone with a male patient?*

- *How did taking a nude art class make you feel?*

- *What would your ideal date be?*

- *Do you find it hard to find educated black men to date?*

- *Why don't you like men?*

- *How does your boyfriend feel about your going to medical school?*

- *Would having a boyfriend affect your decision in choosing a medical school and career?*

- *Are you prepared to handle possibly losing your boyfriend/girlfriend over the stress and distance?*

- *Are you married?*

- *What kind of person would you like to marry?*

- *Do you plan to marry while in medical school?*

- *Why aren't you married?*

- *How will you deal with being married while in medical school?*

- *What does your husband do?*

- *Why did you get divorced?*

- *Do you plan to remarry?*

- *Do you expect to have a family? If so, why are you applying to medical school?*

- *If you become pregnant, what will you do?*

- *How do you plan to manage a family and a career? After all, you are a woman.*

- *How would you raise your children if you were a doctor?*

- *What would you do if you were sexually harassed at any time during school, residency, or your career?*

- *Are you prepared for the sexual discrimination you will most likely face as a student, resident, intern, and so on?*

EXPECT THE UNEXPECTED

Although most of the questions fall into one of the previous categories, some of the questions are just plain off the wall. Some of the following questions were logical from the perspective of the candidates' background, so be prepared to answer questions about the leisure activities you listed on your application or the experiences you related in your essays. Other questions came straight out of left field. These are unlikely to be repeated, but they give you an idea of the kind of things interviewers ask to catch you off balance. If you're asked a question like this, take your time and think it through. If all else fails, remember, it's better to say "I don't know" than to try to baffle 'em with bull. As one of those surveyed said after an unsuccessful attempt at bluffing, "It doesn't work—they've heard it all before."

- *What would you do if I dropped unconscious right now?*

- *What would you say if you smashed your finger with a hammer?*

- *How tall are you?*

- *How did you get your hair to do that?*

- *Is that your natural hair color?*

- *Why are you dressed the way you are? Why did you come here looking the way you do?*

- *Do you think that anyone can become a singer?*

- *Do you know how to play an instrument?*

- *Who is your favorite classical music composer?*

- *What's your favorite Beatles album?*

- *What is your favorite college football team?*

- *What do you think the chances are that the [team name] will make the playoffs?*

- *Why are the majority of NBA players black?*

- *How much can you bench press?*

- *If you're accepted, will you play on our softball team?*

- *What was your opinion of the rich, yuppie Greek students on your undergraduate campus?*

- *How much do you drink?*

- *Have you ever cheated?*

- *Have you ever tried an illegal substance?*

- *Have you ever stolen a car?*
- *What kind of car do you drive?*
- *What is your opinion of Charlie Brown?*
- *Do you prefer the old* **Star Trek** *or the new one?*
- *Why didn't you take Latin?*
- *Do you dream in Chinese or English?*
- *Do you know how to surf?*
- *Are you most like Madonna, Margaret Thatcher, or Mother Teresa, and why?*
- *What is your favorite card game?*
- *Do you play bingo?*
- *Does your mother know where you are?*

7 Allopathic Profiles

ALBANY MEDICAL COLLEGE

ALBANY MEDICAL COLLEGE

47 NEW SCOTLAND AVENUE, MAIL CODE 3, ALBANY, NY 12208 • ADMISSION: 518-262-5521
FAX: 518-262-5887 • E-MAIL: ADMISSIONS@MAIL.AMC.EDU • WEBSITE: WWW.AMC.EDU

STUDENT BODY

Type	Private
Enrollment	538
% male/female	45/55
% underrepresented minorities	8
# applied (total/out)	6,833/5,369
# accepted (total/out)	313/215
# enrolled (total/out)	94/65
Average age	26

FACULTY

Total faculty (number)	1,522
% female	24
% minority	7
% part-time	64
Student-faculty ratio	3:1

ADMISSIONS

Average GPA and MCAT Scores

Overall GPA	3.5
MCAT Bio	10.1
MCAT Phys	9.8
MCAT Verbal	9.5
MCAT Essay	P

Application Information

Regular application	11/15
Regular notification	12/1
Are transfers accepted?	no
Admissions may be deferred?	yes
Interview required?	yes
Application fee	$100

Academics

Albany Medical College responded to the changing health care needs in the United States by restructuring its curriculum to better address contemporary issues in health care, while simultaneously providing a solid clinical and scientific education. The curriculum focuses specifically on the principles and practices of comprehensive care—health care that addresses the full spectrum of patient needs from medical and preventive to palliative and psychosocial. Grades of honors, excellent, good, marginal, and unsatisfactory are used to evaluate student performance. In the clinical years, narrative assessments of performance are also used as an important evaluation tool. Graduation requirements include passing Step 1 of the USMLE and taking Step 2, including the clinical skills exam.

BASIC SCIENCES: Basic science education is coordinated and integrated in a manner that spans all four years of medical school, systematically increasing basic science knowledge within the context of clinical medicine. By teaching within a clinical context, the college offers a learning environment that focuses on developing problem-solving skills. Basic science concepts are divided into themes or modules that are most often organ-based. Taught in conjunction with clinical case experience, these modules come together to form the foundation for the clinical education. In the first year, students combine basic science instruction with clinical cases to focus on normal function. In the second year, students further expand their knowledge and focus primarily on abnormal function and the disease state. Students learn clinical skills beginning in their firstyear by working within small groups and interacting with standardized patients who are trained to simulate actual illness. Students explore legal, ethical, and humanistic concerns in a 4 year module called Health Care and Society. Systems of health care, epidemiology, biostatistics, and the principles of evidence based medicine are concurrently studied in a 4 year module called Evidence Based Health Care. Fundamental knowledge of nutrition also begins in year one and is integrated in all four years of the curriculum. Managing information is a key component throughout all thematic modules. The Schaffer Library of Health Sciences houses more than 144,000 volumes, 974 journals in print and 8,500 available online, contains 3,900 multimedia programs and has 40 computer stations in the independent learning center. Throughout their medical education, students rely on these resources as well as the support of the library faculty.

CLINICAL TRAINING

An innovative experience, Orientation Clerkship, transitions students from the first two years of the curriculum to the clinical and rotation requirements of the final two years. This two-week clerkship occurs during the summer prior to year 3. These learning opportunities on standardized patients enable medical students to develop, practice, and enhance their clinical skills and abilities. Students participate in mock preceptor rounds, assess their own clinical skills, and perform basic medical procedures. The third-year required clinical clerkships are a combination of hospital-based experiences to hospital- and ambulatory-based experiences. The third-year required clerkships are medicine (12 weeks), surgery (8 weeks), pediatrics (8 weeks), ob/gyn (6 weeks), family practice (6 weeks), and psychiatry (6 weeks). Fourth-year rotation requirements are emergency medicine (4 weeks), neuro/opthomology (4 weeks), critical care (4 weeks), and an elective in either family practice, medicine, surgery, or pediatrics (4 weeks). Required rotations take place primarily at Albany Medical Center Hospital, as well as other regional and local community hospitals, community health centers, psychiatric inpatient units, nursing homes, adult homes, and patients' homes. The remainder of fourth year includes electives chosen by the students.

Students

Of students in the 2005 entering class, 11 percent were underrepresented minorities. Geographic representation was as follows: northeast (66 percent), south (6 percent), midwest (4 percent), west (22 percent), foreign countries (2 percent). There is usually a wide range of ages within the student body. Average class size is 130.

STUDENT LIFE

The student community is very active both on and off campus. There are about 30 campus clubs and organizations, including a student newspaper, outdoor and athletic clubs, support groups for students with similar backgrounds or situations, and groups focused on community activities. For example, one student organization arranges activities for the medical center's pediatric cancer patients, while another brings AIDS education programs to local schools.

GRADUATES

Graduates gain acceptance into some of the top institutions in the nation. Forty percent of the 2004 graduates entered residency programs in primary care.

Admissions

REQUIREMENTS

Requirements are six semester hours each or nine quarter hours of biology, general chemistry, organic chemistry, and physics each of which must include associated labs. When assessing GPAs, the Admissions Committee considers the intensity of each student's course load as well as his or her undergraduate institution. The MCAT is required of all applicants. For those who have retaken the exam, the best set of scores is considered most important, though all scores should be submitted.

SUGGESTIONS

Community service and medically related activities are valued. College courses should be varied and demonstrate breadth and depth. There is no preference for New York State residents.

PROCESS

All AMCAS applicants are sent secondary applications. About 25 percent of those completing secondaries are interviewed. Interviews take place from September through April and are conducted by faculty, students, administrators, and local physicians. The interview day also features a group orientation and the opportunity to meet with deans, faculty, and students. Candidates are notified on a rolling basis and are either accepted, rejected, or under consideration. Albany Medical College offers combined degree programs with Siena College, Union College, and Rensselaer Polytechnic Institute with a special focus on community service, business management, or research, respectively. Interested students should apply during their senior year in high school. The MCAT is waived for students admitted through these joint programs. Students admitted to the programs earn both degrees in seven or eight years, depending on the undergraduate institution.

Admissions Requirements (Required)

MCAT scores, science GPA, nonscience GPA, letters of recommendation, interview, essays/personal statement.

Admissions Requirements (Optional)

State residency, extracurricular activities, exposure to medical profession.

COSTS AND AID

Tuition & Fees

Tuition	$39,637
Room and board (off campus)	$8,500
Cost of books	$1,835
Fees	$30

Financial Aid

% students receiving aid	88
Average grant	$5,942
Average loan	$42,382
Average debt	$161,051

AMERICAN UNIVERSITY OF THE CARIBBEAN
SCHOOL OF MEDICINE

MEDICAL EDUCATION ADMINISTRATIVE SERVICES, 901 PONCE DE LEON BLVD., SUITE 401 CORAL GABLES, FL 33134 ADMISSION: (866)DR2B-AUC (372-2282) • FAX: 786-433-0974 • E-MAIL: ADMISSIONS@AUCMED.EDU • WEBSITE: WWW.AUCMED.EDU

STUDENT BODY

Type	Private
Enrollment	828
% male/female	58/42
# applied	1,420
# accepted	667
# enrolled	299
Average age	25

FACULTY

Total faculty (number)	30
% female	43

ADMISSIONS

Average GPA and MCAT Scores

Overall GPA	3.1
Science GPA	2.9
MCAT Bio	7.8
MCAT Phys	7.5
MCAT Verbal	7.3
MCAT Essay	0

Application Information

Regular application	rolling
Regular notification	rolling
Are transfers accepted?	yes
Admissions may be deferred?	yes
Interview required?	no
Application fee	$75

Academics

American University of the Caribbean (AUC) School of Medicine has provided students with quality medical education since 1978. AUC is fully accredited by the Accreditation Commission on Colleges of Medicine (ACCM), and is recognized by the U.S. Department of Education as having standards comparable to the LCME. AUC students are eligible to sit for the USMLE, obtain U.S. Federal Financial Aid, become active members of AMSA and, upon graduation, obtain residency and licensure throughout the United States. The curriculum is modeled after U.S. medical schools, and classes are taught in English using U.S. textbooks. Students are required to pass the same licensing exams as those taken by U.S. medical students. Faculty members generally hold an MD or PhD and are trained primarily in the United States. The medical school curriculum is comprised of nine and a half semesters. Five semesters of Basic Sciences are taught at the St. Maarten campus, followed by four and a half semesters of Clinical Sciences taught at affiliated hospitals in the United States, England, or Ireland.

BASIC SCIENCES: The first five semesters involve concentrated study of the Basic Medical Sciences on the medical school campus in St. Maarten. Anatomy, biochemistry, and histology are the main focus during the first semester. A logical sequence emphasizing physiology, microbiology, pathology and cell biology during the next two semesters is followed by courses in medical psychology and pharmacology. During the last semester, students experience clinical application of the medical sciences curriculum. Coursework is intended to provide students with the opportunity to familiarize themselves with the USMLE Step 1. Shelf exams are used to assess a student's readiness to be certified to take the medical boards. The fifth semester course, "Biological Basis of Clinical Medicine," encompasses a 15-week board examination review. Students are required to pass the USMLE Step 1 prior to proceeding to clinical rotations.

CLINICAL TRAINING

AUC's Office of Clinical Student Affairs (OCSA) assists students with the USMLE and other certifications. After reporting a passing USMLE Step 1 score, students are scheduled for clinical clerkships in an affiliated teaching hospital in the United States, England, or Ireland. Students are able to submit a preference for a specific geographical area where they would like to rotate. During their 72 weeks of clinical clerkships, OCSA continues to advise students on clerkship options, assist them in obtaining rotations in their chosen area of specialty, and to liaise with hospital administrators to facilitate the students' clerkship experience.

Students

Students are selected from a wide variety of backgrounds. Many entering students have recently completed premedical undergraduate coursework, however, AUC also has non-traditional students who have been practicing as allied health professionals. While over 85 percent of AUC students are U.S. residents, only two-thirds of these are native citizens. This international orientation assures AUC of a richly diverse student body with the opportunity for students to become familiar with the increasing mix of cultures that they will likely encounter throughout their professional career.

STUDENT LIFE

AUC's medical school campus is located in the reputable world-class tourist destination of St. Maarten, where English is commonly spoken, U.S. currency is accepted throughout, and the standard of living is unsurpassed in the Caribbean. A new on-campus dormitory offers entering students fully furnished units with kitchens, ocean views and recreational amenities. Student resources consist of a student government association, medical fraternity, medical honor society, local AMSA chapter, a medical research society, and a spouses organization serving the families and significant others of students. At AUC, students are encouraged to engage in extracurricular activities such as volunteer projects through the community services department.

GRADUATES

AUC alumni secure residencies and are licensed throughout the United States. Along with graduates from U.S. medical schools, AUC graduates utilize the NRMP and ERAS for residency placement. For several years, AUC has ranked higher in NRMP placement than the average for foreign medical school graduate placement. The majority of AUC alumni enter primary care residencies including family medicine, internal medicine, pediatrics and emergency medicine. Popular states for residency training are California, New York, Michigan and Pennsylvania. The Office of Alumni Relations and the AUC Alumni Association help maintain the most up to date records for 4,000 graduates and foster involvement by sponsoring academic and social programs, as well as alumni events.

Admissions

REQUIREMENTS

Students are able to enroll in AUC during September, January, or May. There is no deadline to apply to AUC due to its rolling admissions policy; however, prospective students should plan on completing their application four to five months prior to the semester they are seeking enrollment. The Admissions Committee considers many factors as relevant predictors of a good medical clinician. However, as medical school is a rigorous academic challenge, the Committee must be satisfied that a prospective student has the ability to successfully assimilate the curriculum. For detailed information on application procedures and admissions, see the AUC Web site or contact the admissions office.

Admissions Requirements (Required)

MCAT scores, science GPA, cumulative GPA, letters of recommendation, essays/personal statement, chronological listing of education and work experience.

Admissions Requirements (Optional)

Interview, state residency, extracurricular activities, exposure to medical profession.

COSTS AND AID

Tuition & Fees

Tuition	$22,000
Room and board (on campus)	$16,200
Cost of books	$1,400

Financial Aid

Average Federal Stafford loan	$18,500

* INTERNATIONAL MEDICAL SCHOOL

NOT ACCREDITED BY AAMC

BAYLOR COLLEGE OF MEDICINE

OFFICE OF ADMISSIONS INFORMATION, 1 BAYLOR PLAZA HOUSTON, TX 77030 • ADMISSION: 713-798-4842
FAX: 713-798-5563 • E-MAIL: ADMISSIONS@BCM.EDU • WEBSITE: WWW.BCM.EDU

STUDENT BODY

Type	Private
Enrollment	673
% male/female	52/48
% underrepresented minorities	19
# applied (total/out)	4,285/2,909
# accepted	285
# enrolled (total/out)	168/39
Average age	23

FACULTY

Total faculty (number)	2,111
% part-time	18
Student-faculty ratio	3:1

ADMISSIONS

Average GPA and MCAT Scores

Overall GPA	3.8

Application Information

Regular application	11/1
Regular notification	rolling
Early application	6/1
Early notification	10/1
Are transfers accepted?	yes
Admissions may be deferred?	yes
Interview required?	yes
Application fee	$70

Academics

Students enjoy a flexible and balanced curriculum that helps them prepare for whatever career in medicine they choose. This flexibility is enhanced by the opportunity to create individualized schedules in the clinical curriculum, which, due to a one and a half-year preclinical curriculum, is two and a half years. Throughout all four years, grading is honors, high pass, pass, marginal pass, and fail. Students must take the USMLE Steps 1 and 2 prior to graduation (but performance does not affect graduation). Most students opt to take Step 1 midway through their third year and Step 2 late in their fourth year. About 10 percent of students each year enter one of several combined degree programs offered in conjunction with the University of Houston and Rice University. These programs include the MD/PhD, MD/MBA, and MD/JD degrees. Many of the MD/PhD students are funded annually by the NIH MSTP training grant. Other students are supported by private or institutional sources.

PRECLINICAL CURRICULUM: The preclinical curriculum starts early in August with an integrated course called core concepts. This is followed by a series of interdisciplinary, organ-based modules (e.g., cardiology, respiratory, endocrinology) which are sequenced in order to build on language, vocabulary, and skills. Throughout the 18-month preclinical curriculum, students attend lectures and labs in the morning. Most lectures are available online via streaming video for review. Two afternoons a week, students meet in small groups of 8-10 students with a faculty facilitator or in a preceptor's office, leaving the remaining afternoons open for studying. Complementing the basic science focus of the organ-based modules are courses which emphasize problem solving, early clinical experiences, social and behavioral sciences, and ethics. For example, the two afternoon courses, integrated problem solving and patient, physician, and society, help students develop skills in lifelong learning, use of modern informational technologies, and the basics of patient care. Both faculty and student tutors are available for additional instruction outside of the classroom. State-of-the-art learning resources (print and digital) are available via the Internet, in the Educational Resource Center in the DeBakey Building, or across the street in the Houston Academy of Medicine-Texas Medical Center Library, one of the largest medical libraries in the country. Students also have the opportunity to choose from a wide array of basic science elective experiences (e.g., compassion and the art of medicine, international health care, etc.).

CLINICAL TRAINING

Clinical rotations begin in January of the second year. Required clerkships include the following: medicine (12 weeks), surgery (12 weeks), ob/gyn (8 weeks), pediatrics (8 weeks), psychiatry (8 weeks), neurology (4 weeks), family and community medicine (4 weeks), and surgical subspecialties (4 weeks). Other requirements include four weeks of electives and 20 weeks of electives. Throughout the clinical curriculum, students leave their clinical rotation one afternoon a week to engage in one of three unique courses: clinical applications of the biomedical science (year 1), longitudinal ambulatory care experience (year 3), and mechanisms and management of disease (year 4). As part of the third-year longitudinal ambulatory care experience, students visit community agencies that provide important health-related services to families and patients (e.g., hospice, homeless shelters, etc). At the end of the fourth year, students may elect to take a 2-week course in integrated clinical experiences (ICE), which serves as a transition to residency training. Students train in the Baylor Affiliated Teaching Hospitals (with over 5,000 beds total) in the Texas Medical Center complex and at other sites around the city. Elective credits may be earned at institutions throughout the United States as well as overseas. Students with special interest in care of the under-served, geriatrics, international health, medical ethics, or research can complete elective requirements within a "track" organized around the topic. These students receive a special certificate at graduation. In 2005, Baylor adopted a set of core competency graduation goals and began implementation of a competency-based curriculum in which students will have increased opportunity to receive feedback about specific strengths and weaknesses in their knowledge, skills, and attitudes expected by the competency-based residency training programs they will seek to enter after graduation.

Students

Approximately 70 to 80 percent of students are Texas residents. Students in the class that entered in 2005 came from 54 undergraduate institutions around the country. About 23 percent of students are underrepresented minorities, and a wide age range is seen within the student body. The entering class size is 168.

STUDENT LIFE

A five-day orientation introduces entering students to the school's academic and nonacademic resources and promotes a supportive atmosphere from the beginning. First-year students also benefit from peer counseling groups and professional advising. Numerous organizations promote extracurricular, professional, community service, and religious interests, or offer support for minority or other groups of medical students. Some examples include the Family Practice Club, the Texas Medical Association Medical Student Section, and the Baylor Association of Minority Medical Students. An athletic center with exercise equipment and weights, basketball, racquetball, aerobics, and volleyball is available to medical students. Houston is home to almost two million people and is a center for commerce, industry, arts, and recreation. A dormitory operated by the Texas Medical Center is located near Baylor, although most medical students opt to live off-campus in nearby residential areas.

GRADUATES

Graduates are successful in securing residencies in all generalist and specialty areas. Baylor also administers postgraduate programs.

Admissions

REQUIREMENTS

Prerequisites are one year in each of the following: biology, general chemistry, English, and organic chemistry. Science courses must include associated labs. The MCAT is required and must be from within the past five years. For applicants who have taken the exam on more than one occasion, the most recent set of scores is weighted heavily.

SUGGESTIONS

Approximately 70–75 percent of the positions in each class are reserved for Texas residents, making nonresident positions highly competitive. The April, rather than August, MCAT is recommended. Beyond intellectual ability, Baylor is interested in personal integrity and demonstrated interest in medicine, human compassion, and leadership skills.

PROCESS

Baylor participates in AMCAS. The AMCAS Web-enabled application is available in May preceding the year of anticipated entrance. Approximately 15 percent of applicants are interviewed between September and February. Interviews usually consist of two sessions that are 30 minutes each with a faculty member or medical student. The interview day features a group orientation session, a campus tour, and the opportunity to meet informally with students and faculty members. Of interviewed candidates, about 45 percent are accepted on a rolling basis.

Admissions Requirements (Required)

MCAT scores, science GPA, non-science GPA, letters of recommendation, interview, essays/personal statement.

Admissions Requirements (Optional)

State residency, extracurricular activities, exposure to medical profession.

COSTS AND AID

Tuition & Fees

Tuition	$19,650
Room and board (off campus)	$13,365
Cost of books	$6,298
Fees	$5,198

Financial Aid

% students receiving aid	81
Average grant	$8,823
Average loan	$21,557
Average debt	$67,679

BOSTON UNIVERSITY
SCHOOL OF MEDICINE

715 ALBANY STREET BOSTON, MA 02118 • ADMISSION: 617-638-4630
FAX: 617-638-4718 • E-MAIL: MEDADMS@BU.EDU • WEBSITE: WWW.BUMC.BU.EDU

STUDENT BODY

Type	Private
Enrollment	632
% male/female	47/53
% underrepresented minorities	16
# applied (total/out)	9,589/8,936
# accepted (total/out)	454/372
# enrolled (total/out)	155/132
Average age	22

FACULTY

Total faculty (number)	1,193
% female	37
% minority	8
Student-faculty ratio	1:1

ADMISSIONS

Average GPA and MCAT Scores

Overall GPA	3.65
MCAT Bio	11.03
MCAT Phys	10.91
MCAT Verbal	10.12
MCAT Essay	Q

Application Information

Regular application	11/1
Regular notification	rolling
Early application	8/1
Early notification	10/1
Are transfers accepted?	no
Admissions may be deferred?	no
Interview required?	yes
Application fee	$100

Academics

Several combined degree programs are offered, including the MD/MPH and MD/MBA in which all students accepted into the medical school may apply. Qualified students may pursue a joint MD/PhD program, earning a doctorate degree in anatomy, biochemistry, biomedical engineering, biophysics, behavioral neuroscience, cell biology, genetics, immunology, microbiology, molecular biology, pathology, pharmacology, or physiology. Most students take part in a 4 year curriculum of basic and clinical science, leading to the MD. However, up to 10 students each year enter an alternative curriculum, which spreads out the first year of study into two years to free up time for academic or personal interests. Evaluation uses honors, pass, and fail in addition to narrative reports when possible. Passing the USMLE Step 1 is a requirement for promotion to the third year.

BASIC SCIENCES: An integrated problems course supplements the traditional lecture/lab format of first- and second-year courses. Integrated problems meets in small groups and uses an interdisciplinary approach to tackle case studies that relate to subjects discussed in other courses. First-year courses are biochemistry, endocrinology, essentials of public health, genetics, gross anatomy, histology, immunology, introduction to clinical medicine I (ICM I), neuroscience, physiology, and principles of psychiatry in medicine. ICM I develops an understanding of the doctor-patient relationship and discusses sociocultural issues related to it. Second-year courses are biology of disease I, biology of disease II, ICM II, integrated problems, microbiology and infectious diseases, pathology, pharmacology, psychiatry. In ICM II, students learn to conduct patient interviews and physical examinations. A benefit of the ICM continuum is that instruction involves mentorships with practicing physicians, often in primary care settings. Most basic science instruction takes place in the instructional building, which has classrooms, administrative offices, and a library with 117,000 volumes and 1,300 periodicals. This building connects to the Housman Research Building, which offers a learning center and a computer room.

CLINICAL TRAINING

Required third-year clerkships include the following: Medicine (11 weeks), surgery (11 weeks), family medicine (6 weeks), ob/gyn (6 weeks), pediatrics (6 weeks), and psychiatry (6 weeks). More than half of the fourth year is reserved for electives and many of our students do one or more blocks in international health. Required fourth-year clerkships include the following: Home medicine/geriatrics (4 weeks), neurology (4 weeks), primary care (4 weeks), radiology (4 weeks), and a sub internship (4 weeks). Clinical training takes place at the Boston Medical Center (633 beds), the Veterans Affairs Administration Medical Center (535 beds), and at least 18 other affiliated hospitals and health care facilities. Several research centers are part of the medical center and also serve as educational facilities for medical students.

Students

Underrepresented minorities account for about 18 percent of the student body. The average age of entering students is 22, with a very broad range. Although a large number of states and colleges are represented, a significant proportion of students have completed their undergraduate education on the east or west coast.

STUDENT LIFE

Students are involved in a large number of student organizations, both professional and nonprofessional. These activities range from the Creative Arts Society to volunteer efforts like the Domestic Violence Awareness Project or the Outreach Van that provides medical care to the poor and homeless, to interest groups in the various specialties. Housing is convenient to instructional facilities and promotes cohesion among students. Medical students have access to the academic and athletic facilities of the medical campus as well as those on the Charles River Campus, including the student union and several athletic facilities that offer swimming pools, an ice skating rink, dance, and sailing or rowing on the Charles River. As part of the Introduction to Clinical Medicine courses and clinical rotations, medical students travel in and around Boston, giving them a chance to explore diverse neighborhoods and communities.

GRADUATES

In the 2003 graduating class, the most prevalent specialties were internal medicine (17 percent), pediatrics (16 percent), emergency medicine (8 percent), general surgery (8 percent), family practice (7 percent), anesthesiology (5 percent), diagnostic radiology (5 percent), obstetrics/gynecology (4 percent), and urology (4 percent). In recent years 85–92 percent of graduating students have placed in one of their top three choices in the intern match.

Admissions

REQUIREMENTS

Prerequisites include one year in each of the following: Biology with lab and physics, English, general chemistry with lab, humanities, organic chemistry with lab. In evaluating GPA, factors such as in the intensity of the undergraduate work load are considered. The MCAT is required and must be taken within three years of the date of matriculation. For applicants who have taken the exam more than once, the committee looks at the best set of scores. Advanced placement courses and community or junior college courses are not accepted to fulfill prerequisites.

SUGGESTIONS

In addition to requirements, calculus, genetics, and statistics are recommended as is a broad background in the humanities and social sciences. Applicants are encouraged to take the April MCAT. For applicants who have been out of college for a period of time some recent course work in the biological or physical sciences is advised.

PROCESS

BUSM uses a very limited secondary application, but applicants are invited to provide any additional materials that they believe might be helpful to the Admissions Committee. About 10 percent of the approximately 10,000 AMCAS applicants are invited to interview, with interviews held between October and February. The interview day consists of an introductory session with the associate dean for admissions, a session with staff from the offices of student affairs, minority affairs, registrar, and financial services, lunch with first- and second-year students, and a tour of the facilities with third- and fourth-year students. The interview consists of a one hour session with a faculty member who is on the Admissions Committee. With only 100 positions available for applicants to the four-year program, admission is very competitive. There are several alternate paths to gaining admission. A seven-year program, leading to a BA/MD degree, is offered in conjunction with BU's undergraduate college. The MMEDIC program at BU offers an integrated curriculum composed of liberal arts and medical school courses, enabling pre-selected students to fulfill portions of the requirements of the medical school curriculum. The ENGMEDIC program at BU offers a joint, early selection program for the training of biomedical engineers interested in becoming physicians. The Early Medical School Selection Program was developed with a consortium of historically black undergraduate institutions and colleges with large Hispanic populations to provide an early and more gradual transition into the medical school curriculum beginning with the summer after the second year of undergraduate study.

Admissions Requirements (Required)

MCAT scores, science GPA, non-science GPA, letters of recommendation, interview, essays/personal statement, extracurricular activities, exposure to medical profession.

COSTS AND AID

Tuition & Fees

Tuition	$39,510
Room and board (on campus)	$11,381
Cost of books	$2,153
Fees	$450

Financial Aid

% students receiving aid	79
Average grant	$5,250
Average loan	$46,922
Average debt	$134,089

BROWN UNIVERSITY
BROWN MEDICAL SCHOOL

97 WATERMAN STREET, BOX G-A213, PROVIDENCE, RI 02912 • ADMISSION: 401-863-2149
FAX: 401-863-3801 • E-MAIL: MEDSCHOOL_ADMISSIONS@BROWN.EDU • WEBSITE: BMS.BROWN.EDU/MED/

STUDENT BODY

Type	Private
Enrollment	345
% male/female	42/58
% underrepresented minorities	44
# applied (total/out)	4,324/3,877
# accepted (total/out)	184/173
# enrolled (total/out)	73/64
Average age	24

FACULTY

Total faculty (number)	2,290
% female	34
% minority	14
% part-time	65
Student-faculty ratio	7:1

ADMISSIONS

Average GPA and MCAT Scores

Overall GPA	3.62
MCAT Bio	11.5
MCAT Phys	11.5
MCAT Verbal	10.4
MCAT Essay	Q

Application Information

Regular application	11/1
Regular notification	rolling
Are transfers accepted?	yes
Admissions may be deferred?	yes
Interview required?	yes
Application fee	$85

Academics

Brown was one of the first medical schools to implement a competency-based curriculum, which defines the outcomes of medical education in terms of a core knowledge base and nine abilities. Currently undergoing renewal and redesign, the curriculum will maintain the high level of flexibility that allows students to pursue scholarly goals both within and beyond the traditional areas of medical education. Students are encouraged to develop independent study options either at Brown or sites in the United States or overseas. The school admits about half of its medical students through the Program in Liberal Medical Education (PLME), an 8-year baccalaureate/MD combined degree program. Applicants may be considered for MD/PhD programs in conjunction with Brown graduate departments in the following fields: Artificial organs, biomaterials and cellular technology, biomedical engineering, cell biology and biochemistry, ecology and evolutionary biology, epidemiology and biostatistics, molecular biology, molecular pharmacology and physiology, neuroscience, pathobiology.

BASIC SCIENCES: Principles of patient care and the social and behavioral aspects of medicine are integrated into the basic science curriculum. The first two years are organized into semesters. During the fall semester of the first year, students take physiology, anatomy, histology, and doctoring. During the spring semester of the first year, students take biochemistry, microbiology, pathology, brain and behavior, neurobiology, and doctoring. The basic science courses are not only taught primarily through lectures and labs but also utilize small-group teaching and clinical correlations. Pathophysiology provides a structure for year 2, which is organized around organ systems or concepts such as cardiovascular, renal, hematology, pulmonary, human reproduction, gastroenterology, infectious diseases, supporting structures, and endocrine. Pharmacology, pathology, doctoring, and neurologic pathophysiology and epidemiology are also part of the second-year curriculum. Pre-clinical instruction takes place primarily in the Biomedical Building on the main Brown campus. The Science Library is fully computerized, with online database systems. Medical students have access to all of Brown's academic facilities, including the main library, which houses 2 million volumes. Grading is honors, pass, and fail. Passing Step 1 of the USMLE is not a requirement for promotion.

CLINICAL TRAINING

Patient contact begins in the first year with doctoring, a 2-year clinical skills course. In each semester of doctoring, students spend one half day per week at a community site with a physician-mentor in which theoretical concepts are applied to a real-world setting. Formal clinical training, consisting of required core rotations and electives, occupies the third and fourth years. In total, 50 weeks are devoted to core clerkships and 30 weeks to electives. Requirements include the following: medicine (12 weeks); surgery (8 weeks); pediatrics (6 weeks); ob/gyn (6 weeks); family medicine (6 weeks); psychiatry (6 weeks); community health (6 weeks); medicine, pediatrics, or surgery sub internship (4 weeks); and longitudinal ambulatory (one half day per week for 26 weeks). Clinical training takes place at eight affiliated teaching hospitals in the Providence area including Bradley Hospital, Butler Hospital, The Miriam Hospital, Memorial Hospital of Rhode Island, Rhode Island Hospital, Hasbro Children's Hospital, V.A. Medical Center, and Women and Infants' Hospital. The hospitals attract an ethnically and socioeconomically diverse, urban population. Noteworthy areas of clinical care and research include child/adolescent medicine, psychiatric care, international health, cancer, AIDS/HIV, artificial organs, and diabetes treatment and management. Evaluation of clinical performance uses an honors/pass/fail scale supplemented by narratives. Students are required to take the USMLE Steps 1 and 2 (CK and CS) prior to graduation.

Students

The medical student body is a heterogenous group admitted through several routes. The range of matriculants' ages is 19–47 years, resulting in a class with a diverse set of life experiences. About 75 percent of medical students participate in a community-based activity before graduation, while at least 60 percent of the graduates collaborate on a research project with a faculty sponsor. The American Medical Student Association (AMSA) chapter has a long tradition of service and advocacy; three Brown students have served as president of the national organization during the past 25 years.

STUDENT LIFE

Medical students have full access to the school's recreational activities and facilities. Brown has more than 200 student clubs and organizations that unite students. Although most students choose to live off campus, residence halls and housing co-ops are available.

GRADUATES

In recent years, approximately 17 percent of graduates entered residency programs at hospitals affiliated with Brown. About 45 percent of each class enters primary care residencies.

Admissions

REQUIREMENTS

Students admitted to Brown Medical School must attain competence in the sciences basic to medicine and sufficient to provide adequate preparation for medical school. Applicants are expected to demonstrate competence by successfully completing courses in the following areas of study: Biology (at least one course); chemistry (two courses in general inorganic chemistry and one course in organic chemistry); physics (a two-course sequence for coverage of topics in mechanics, heat, electricity, optics, and radiation physics); and social and behavioral sciences (at least two courses, preferably in anthropology, sociology, psychology, economics, or political science). The MCAT is required for students applying via the standard route of admission. All applicants are selected on the basis of academic achievement, faculty evaluations, evidence of maturity, motivation, leadership, integrity, and compassion. Applicants to the MD/PhD program also are evaluated on the basis of their research accomplishment and potential. Generally, to be eligible for consideration, candidates must present a minimum cumulative grade point average of 3.00 (on a 4.00 scale) in courses taken as a matriculated student at an undergraduate college. Applicants who have attended graduate school must achieve a cumulative grade point average of 3.00 (on a 4.00 scale) in courses taken in graduate school. In addition, applicants must have completed the requirements for a baccalaureate degree prior to matriculation into medical school.

SUGGESTIONS

Admission to Brown Medical School is now available to a greater number of applicants through the standard admissions process and the MD/PhD program.

PROCESS

Brown Medical School accepts applications from qualified graduates of any college or university as part of the standard admissions route. Students are also admitted through the PLME (combined BA-BS/MD program), postbaccalaureate pathway, and the Early Identification Program (EIP). Those interested in applying for the standard route of admission must file an application with the American Medical College Application Service (AMCAS) by 11/1 and submit a secondary application with required documents before 12/31. The PLME application is part of the undergraduate application package. Students enrolled in premedical, postbaccalaureate programs at Bryn Mawr College, Columbia University, and Goucher College apply through the Postbaccalaureate pathway. Students attending schools that are part of the EIP program in Rhode Island should contact their premedical advisors for application procedures. Those interested in applying to the MD/PhD Program must submit an AMCAS application before 10/15 and the Brown secondary application before 11/15; notification of admissions decisions are made before 2/15. Interviews are required of most applicant groups.

Admissions Requirements (Required)

MCAT scores, science GPA, non-science GPA, letters of recommendation, interview, essays/personal statement, exposure to medical profession.

Admissions Requirements (Optional)

State residency, extracurricular activities.

Overlap Schools

Boston University, Columbia University, Cornell University, Dartmouth College, New York University, University of Massachusetts, Tufts University, Yale University.

COSTS AND AID

Tuition & Fees

Tuition	$34,472
Room and board (on campus)	$15,559
Cost of books	$1,705
Fees	$2,981

Financial Aid

% students receiving aid	77
Average grant	$20,127
Average loan	$30,231
Average debt	$88,316

CASE WESTERN RESERVE UNIVERSITY
SCHOOL OF MEDICINE

ASSOCIATE DEAN OF ADMISSIONS, 10900 EUCLID AVENUE CLEVELAND, OH 44106 • ADMISSION: 216-368-2000
FAX: 216-368-4621 • E-MAIL: AXH65@CASE.EDU • WEBSITE: HTTP://CASEMED.CASE.EDU

STUDENT BODY	
Type	Private
Enrollment	587
% male/female	50/50
% underrepresented minorities	46
# applied (total/out)	4,940
# accepted	368
# enrolled	132

Application Information	
Early application	11/15
Early notification	1/15
Are transfers accepted?	yes
Interview required?	yes
Application fee	$60

Academics

The curriculum is decidedly nontraditional, combining several approaches to learning and two distinct paths, each of which provides flexibility. All students participate in the Core Academic Program (CAP), which incorporates the Core Physician Development Program (CPDP), a case-based system. Patient Based Learning (PBL) is introduced in year 1, required clerkships in year 3, and the Flexible Program allows students to participate in pre-clinical and clinical electives throughout the four years. Students who elect the Primary Care Tract (PCT) have enhanced clinical opportunities early in the program and direct contact with primary care providers throughout medical school. Joint MD/PhD programs are offered in physiology, engineering, and biophysics and in 13 divisions of biomedical sciences including nutritional sciences and environmental health. Approximately 10 students in each class are admitted as MD/PhD candidates. A BA/MD is offered in conjunction with the undergraduate college, and approximately 10 students matriculate as part of this yearly program.

BASIC SCIENCES: During the first year, students are presented cellular and developmental biology, integrated human physiology, and the cellular basis of disease by faculty teaching teams representing both basic science and clinical departments. Each course lasts 2 months and is followed by an exam. For the remainder of the first year and for the duration of year 2, students cover basic sciences through study of the individual organ systems, and students retain the information with the help the case-study approach. With this integrated approach to learning, students attend class, and student note-taking collectives are not emphasized. Afternoons are generally free from scheduled courses, allowing for elective study or research. Computer facilities support classroom learning, and computers loaded with first- and second-year course material are available in the MicroComputer Lab. The Health Center Library houses 150,000 volumes. Grading is pass/fail. Students choose their own academic advisors and have a great deal of control over their own courses of study. The USMLE Steps 1 and 2 are required for graduation.

CLINICAL TRAINING
Students have ample opportunity for clinical training outside of traditional clerkships. Most students begin their clinical responsibilities during the first year when they are assigned to either a pregnant woman in the Family Clinic or a patient in the geriatric care program. For two years the student follows the patient and his or her development. Second-year students learn physical diagnosis and history-taking under the supervision of physician preceptors. In the third year, required rotations include family medicine, medicine, neuroscience, ob/gyn, pediatrics, psychiatry, and surgery. Fourth year is devoted to clinical electives. Training takes place at affiliated teaching hospitals including the University Hospitals of Cleveland, Metro-Health Medical Center, Saint Luke's, VA Cleveland, Mount Sinai Medical Center, and the Henry Ford Health System. Some training takes place in clinics rather than in a traditional hospital setting. The patient population represents urban Cleveland and rural Ohio. The Primary Care Tract is a relatively new mechanism for encouraging and training primary care physicians that promotes ongoing student-physician mentorships and intensive primary-care clinical training. Grading during years 3 and 4 is pass/fail/honors.

Students

Case Western is partially supported by the State of Ohio and gives preference to in-state residents, which is reflected in its matriculates. Sixty percent of students are Ohio residents. The student body is slightly more mature than average and is particularly diverse in terms of experience and background. Class size is about 135.

STUDENT LIFE

Although campus residence halls are available, most students choose to live off campus and most rely on cars for transportation to and from school. University-sponsored, married-student housing is unavailable. Student groups are involved in both community and social activities. The structure of the academic program allows time for extracurricular activities, and students participate in both university and community events.

GRADUATES

Of the 140 graduates of a recent class, 52 went on to residency programs in Cleveland; 5 remained in Ohio. The rest went to Pennsylvania (8), Washington (8), and other states (13), New York (7), California (7), Michigan (6), Illinois (5), Maryland (5), Georgia (4), and Texas (4). Specialties were family medicine (22), surgery (17), pediatrics (13), radiology (7), ob/gyn (9), orthopedic surgery (5), psychiatry (5), emergency medicine (4), anesthesiology (3), neurology (3), Ophthalmology (3), pathology (3), urology (2), transitional (2), neurosurgery (2), physical medicine (1), and plastic surgery (1).

Admissions

REQUIREMENTS

Requirements include one year of biology; one year of physics; and two years of chemistry, which should include cover both organic and inorganic. In addition, students should demonstrate writing ability through course work. Recent academic performance is more heavily weighted, and although many older students are admitted, most have taken some relevant courses within the past two years. The MCAT is required, and the most recent set of scores is considered. Due to the rolling admissions process, applicants are encouraged to submit materials as soon as possible.

SUGGESTIONS

Case offers no further recommendations for college courses and accepts students of all undergraduate majors.

PROCESS

About half of those submitting AMCAS applications receive a secondary. Secondaries should be completed promptly and are due by 12/15 at the latest. Less than one-third of those completing secondaries are interviewed, with interviews held from September to March. Students have a one-on-one interview with a faculty member that generally lasts one hour. Those interviewed are notified shortly afterward of their status (accept, reject, or wait list). The wait list is not ranked. About half of the students who are accepted decline the offer, freeing up spaces for wait listed applicants. Wait listed candidates may submit additional material and should indicate if Case Western is their top choice. All Case Western undergraduates are invited to interview at the medical school.

Admissions Requirements (Required)

MCAT scores, science GPA, non-science GPA, letters of recommendation, interview, state residency, extracurricular activities, exposure to medical profession.

Admissions Requirements (Optional)

Essays/personal statement.

COSTS AND AID

Tuition & Fees

Tuition	$37,944
Room and board (on campus)	$7,260
Fees	$530

COLUMBIA UNIVERSITY
COLLEGE OF PHYSICIANS AND SURGEONS

ADMISSIONS OFFICE, 630 WEST 168TH STREET, PO BOX 41, NEW YORK, NY 10032 • ADMISSION: 212-305-3595
FAX: 212-305-3601 • E-MAIL: PSADMISSIONS@COLUMBIA.EDU • WEBSITE: CUMC.COLUMBIA.EDU/DEPT/PS/

STUDENT BODY

Type	Private
% underrepresented minorities	12
# applied (total/out)	4,213/2,069
# accepted (total/out)	302/51
# enrolled (total/out)	149/117
Average age	24

ADMISSIONS

Average GPA and MCAT Scores

Overall GPA	3.7
MCAT Bio	12.0
MCAT Phys	12.2
MCAT Verbal	11.2
MCAT Essay	Q

Application Information

Regular application	11/15
Regular notification	3/1
Are transfers accepted?	yes
Admissions may be deferred?	yes
Interview required?	yes
Application fee	$75

Academics

The Columbia curriculum is multidisciplinary and integrated. It focuses on not only understanding the science, skills, and techniques of medicine, but also appreciating the art and ethics involved. Several joint-degree programs such as the MD/MPH and MD/MBA are offered in conjunction with other schools and departments at Columbia. Qualified students interested in careers in scientific research may pursue a combined MD/PhD, earning the doctorate in fields such as anatomy, biochemistry, biophysics, cell biology, genetics, immunology, microbiology, molecular biology, neuroscience, pathology, pharmacology, and physiology. Medical students are evaluated with an honors/pass/fail system. Successful completion of Steps 1 and 2 of the USMLE are required for graduation.

BASIC SCIENCES: The first two years provides information and experiences essential for all physicians. The majority of instruction is conducted in lectures and lab, but small-group teaching is increasingly emphasized. Students spend approximately 25 hours per week in scheduled activity. The first year (42 weeks) includes clinical practice, gross anatomy, neural science, and an integrated course that covers biochemistry, cell biology, genetics, human development, and physiology. The majority of the second year (40 weeks) is devoted to a multidisciplinary course that examines the basic concepts of immunology, microbiology, pathology, and pharmacology. Physical diagnosis, basic psychiatry, and clinical practice are also taught. Columbia has extensive laboratory, informational, and computer facilities that enhance classroom learning. The Augustus C. Long Health Sciences Library houses nearly 450,000 volumes and is one of the largest medical center libraries in the nation.

CLINICAL TRAINING

In the third year, students complete required rotations in the following: Medicine (10 weeks), surgery (5 weeks), pediatrics (5 weeks), ob/gyn (5 weeks), primary care (5 weeks), psychiatry (5 weeks), neurology (5 weeks), anesthesiology (2 weeks), orthopedics (2 weeks), urology (2 weeks), otolaryngology (1 week), and ophthalmology (1 week). The fourth year consists of 1- and 2-month-long electives drawn from a large number of offerings and student-designed experiences. There are extensive opportunities for clinical electives abroad. Each student is also required to complete a back-to-basic science elective. These include 1-month seminars in advanced pathophysiology, clinical pharmacology, or clinical pathology. Rotations are conducted at various medical centers and hospitals throughout the metropolitan area. Columbia-Presbyterian Medical Center, Harlem Hospital Center, Roosevelt Hospital, St. Luke's Hospital, and other institutions combine for a comprehensive clinical experience.

Students

Columbia attracts an extremely diverse, nationally represented student body. About 10 percent of students are underrepresented minorities. There is a wide age range among incoming students, with significant numbers of students in their late 20s and 30s.

STUDENT LIFE

Despite the rigorous schedule, student life abounds at Columbia. Medical students have access to the recreational and athletic facilities of Columbia University and to university-sponsored cultural events. The P&S Club, the oldest student organization of its kind at any medical school in America, provides a variety of extracurricular activities. Students have opportunities in the fine arts, athletics, and service-oriented projects. In addition, Manhattan offers unparalleled access to museums, concerts, and every imaginable type of dining. Most students live in on-campus housing, which helps make New York affordable. Both residential halls and apartments buildings are available. Newly accepted married students are guaranteed married-student housing.

GRADUATES

Graduates gain acceptance to the most competitive residency programs in the nation. A Columbia education allows students to emphasize academic medicine, research, or primary care.

Admissions

REQUIREMENTS

One year each of biology, English, chemistry, organic chemistry, and physics are required for admission along with the MCAT. For those students who have taken the MCAT more than once, the most recent scores are weighed most heavily. Thus, there is no advantage in withholding scores. Columbia does not admit students on a rolling basis. Therefore, submitting MCAT scores from the fall of the admission year does not place applicants at a disadvantage.

SUGGESTIONS

The Admissions Committee is interested in the depth and breadth of an applicant's extracurricular experiences. Community service, artistic activities, athletics, and medically related experiences are all valuable. It is valuable to denote that Columbia is an applicant's first choice for medical school, particularly for those who have been placed on the wait list.

PROCESS

Columbia is a participant in the AMCAS application. All applicants are invited to fill out the P&S secondary application, which can be accessed through the Columbia website. Between Labor Day and early March, approximately 25 percent of applicants are invited for an interview. The interview day consists of one session with a faculty member who is a member of the Admissions Committee. Applicants also have lunch and tour the facilities with a current medical student. About 15 percent of interviewed applicants are accepted, with notification occurring in early March. A wait list is also created at this time. Wait listed applicants may send additional information to update their files.

Admissions Requirements (Required)

MCAT scores, science GPA, non-science GPA, letters of recommendation, interview, essays/personal statement, extracurricular activities, exposure to medical profession.

Admissions Requirements (Optional)

State residency.

Overlap Schools

Harvard University.

COSTS AND AID

Tuition & Fees

Tuition	$36,876
Room and board (on campus)	$14,969
Cost of books	$1,750
Fees	$3,055

CORNELL UNIVERSITY
JOAN & SANFORD I. WEILL MEDICAL COLLEGE

OFFICE OF ADMISSIONS, 445 EAST 69TH STREET, NEW YORK, NY 10021 • ADMISSION: 212-746-1067
FAX: 212-746-8052 • E-MAIL: CUMC-ADMISSIONS@MED.CORNELL.EDU • WEBSITE: WWW.MED.CORNELL.EDU

STUDENT BODY

Type	Private
Enrollment	412
% male/female	50/50
# applied 5,177	
# accepted 262	
# enrolled (total/out)	101/65
Average age	24

FACULTY

Total faculty (number)	2,340

ADMISSIONS

Average GPA and MCAT Scores

Overall GPA	3.72
MCAT Bio	11.9
MCAT Phys	11.9
MCAT Verbal	10.8
MCAT Essay	P

Application Information

Regular application	10/15
Regular notification	3/10
Early application	8/1
Early notification	10/1
Are transfers accepted?	yes
Admissions may be deferred?	yes
Interview required?	yes
Application fee	$75

Academics

A revised curriculum strives to limit the time students spend in lectures, thereby promoting independent and interactive learning and research. The curriculum integrates basic and clinical sciences, utilizes problem-based learning, includes principles of public health, and encourages student research efforts. Joint MD/PhD programs can be pursued in conjunction with the Weill Graduate School of Medical Sciences, Rockefeller University, and the Sloan-Kettering Institute in the following fields: biochemistry, cell biology, immunology, molecular biology and genetics, molecular pharmacology, neuroscience, physiology, and microbiology. Fifteen students per year may enter joint programs.

BASIC SCIENCES: The curriculum was completely revised and has been both highly successful and widely emulated. The first and second years of study consist of five basic science courses and medicine, patients, and society. In the first year, the basic science courses are molecules to cells and genetics, human structure and function, and host defenses. In the second year, they are brain and mind and basis of disease. The core basic science courses are sequential, integrated, interdisciplinary block courses that employ problem-based learning (PBL) in small groups. PBL emphasizes active learning and requires the student first to identify issues needed to solve a medical problem, then to seek out the information needed to solve the problem, and then to reconvene in small groups with the faculty to apply the information learned. Lectures are few and emphasize the conceptual framework of a field. Anatomic dissection and experimental laboratories complete the learning experience. The course medicine, patients, and society approaches the doctor-patient relationship from both the conceptual and practical perspectives. For one day each week throughout each year, students spend the morning in seminar and the afternoon in physicians' offices. Areas treated include medical interviewing, physical diagnosis, human behavior in illness, medical ethics, public health, biostatistics, clinical epidemiology, and others. Thus, students learn these vital topics in a patient-centered context. The evaluation system uses an honor/pass/fail scale.

CLINICAL TRAINING

Upon completion of the second year, students take three introductory clinical courses: clinical pharmacology, anesthesia, and the introductory clerkship. The third year is dedicated to clinical learning and emphasizes the core clerkships, including medicine, surgery, pediatrics, obstetrics-gynecology, psychiatry, neurology, and primary care. In these courses, students are assigned to clinical inpatient and outpatient services at New York-Presbyterian Medical Center and throughout the network of clinical affiliates. Clinical affiliates include the Hospital for Special Surgery, a leader in the fields of orthopedics, rheumatology, and sports medicine; Memorial Sloan-Kettering Cancer Center, one of the premier facilities in the world devoted to the study and treatment of cancer; The New York Methodist Hospital; and others throughout the city. Students are integral members of the health care team and actively care for patients under the supervision of the faculty. The fourth year focuses on completion of clinical requirements, a sub internship, and electives. While electives can be taken at any time in the third or fourth years, most students focus on three major types of electives in the fourth year: Clinical electives, often in subspecialty areas; research; and international electives. Each year up to half of the fourth-year class spends time abroad, typically in Cornell-funded programs that combine clinical care and research in the third world: South America, the Caribbean, Africa, and Asia. In the month before graduation, eight weeks of advanced basic science allow students to study leading-edge biomedical science in depth.

Students

In a typical class, students graduated from over 40 different undergraduate institutions and came from over 25 different states. Class size is 101.

STUDENT LIFE

Despite the urban environment, students are cohesive and student life is apparent around the Medical College. Ninety-five percent of students live within three blocks of campus, generally in college-owned dorms or apartments. The rent is subsidized and competitive for New York. In the residence halls, there are athletic facilities for student use. Student organizations, including those that support women and minority students, are active. Parks, including Central Park, are accessible, as are an abundance of museums, theaters, shops, and restaurants. Students do not own cars.

GRADUATES

Graduates gain acceptance to the nation's top residency programs. Many stay in New York City for postgraduate training.

Admissions

REQUIREMENTS

Weill/Cornell requires 24 semester credit hours in science courses, including two semesters each of biology, general chemistry, organic chemistry, and physics. In addition, six semester hours of English are required. The science GPA is given considerable weight. The MCAT is required and is used to assist the Admissions Committee in assessing the GPAs of applicants who typically come from a wide range of undergraduate backgrounds. If an applicant has repeated the MCAT, the both scores are considered.

SUGGESTIONS

Beyond required courses, Weill/Cornell recommends one to two additional upper division biology courses for nonscience majors. For students who graduated college several years ago, recent science course work is suggested. The Medical College is interested in the extracurricular activities of applicants, particularly if they demonstrate commitment and dedication. Some exposure to the field of medicine is also desirable. Biomedical research is recommended.

PROCESS

All AMCAS applicants receive secondary applications. About 13 percent of applicants who complete secondaries are invited to interview, and about 30 percent of those who interview are offered a place in the first-year class. Interviews are held from October through February and consist of two sessions that are 30 minutes each, each with a member of the Admissions Committee. Decisions are announced by 3/15. For a wait listed candidate, submitting supplemental material can serve to strengthen his or her application and is also helpful in that it indicates interest in attending Weill/Cornell.

Admissions Requirements (Required)

MCAT scores, science GPA, non-science GPA, letters of recommendation, interview, essays/personal statement, extracurricular activities, exposure to medical profession, secondary application.

Admissions Requirements (Optional)

State residency.

COSTS AND AID

Tuition & Fees

Tuition	$32,320
Room and board (on campus)	$9,977
Cost of books	$1,800
Fees	$1,325

Financial Aid

% students receiving aid	83

CREIGHTON UNIVERSITY
SCHOOL OF MEDICINE

OFFICE OF ADMISSIONS, 2500 CALIFORNIA PLAZA, OMAHA, NE 68178 • ADMISSION: 402-280-2799
FAX: 402-280-1241 • E-MAIL: MEDSCHADM@CREIGHTON.EDU • WEBSITE: MEDICINE.CREIGHTON.EDU

STUDENT BODY

Type	Private
Enrollment	460
% male/female	54/46
% underrepresented minorities	8
# applied (total/out)	3,948/3,759
# accepted (total/out)	315/285
# enrolled (total/out)	120/106
Average age	23

FACULTY

Total faculty (number)	295
% female	23
% part-time	7
Student-faculty ratio	1:1

ADMISSIONS

Average GPA and MCAT Scores

Overall GPA	3.7
MCAT Bio	10.0
MCAT Phys	9.9
MCAT Verbal	9.5
MCAT Essay	P

Application Information

Regular application	12/1
Regular notification	rolling
Early application	6/1–8/1
Early notification	10/1
Are transfers accepted?	yes
Admissions may be deferred?	yes
Interview required?	yes
Application fee	$75

Academics

The educational program is divided into four years based on: (1) biomedical fundamentals; (2) organ- and disease-based concepts; (3) clinical clerkships; and (4) elective clinical experiences. Students may apply to PhD programs in several areas of biomedical science, medical microbiology, or pharmacology and pursue the degree jointly with the MD. The grading system at Creighton uses honors/pass/fail supplemented with written, narrative evaluations. Students are not ranked against their peers.

BASIC SCIENCES: In some cases, basic sciences are taught using the traditional lecture/lab format and in others, small groups and case-based learning are used. First- and second-year students are in scheduled sessions of some sort for about 25 hours per week. First-year courses, comprising the first unit, are anatomy, ethics in medicine, evidence based medicine, host defense, molecular and cell biology, microbiology, neuroscience, human development in medicine, interviewing and physical exam, and pharmacology. Many students use the summer between years 1 and 2 for funded research projects. The second component, organized by organ-and disease-based concepts, occurs during the second year. Concepts or systems include cardiovascular, endocrinology, reproductive, gastrointestinal, infectious disease, muscular/skeletal, multi-systems courses, respiratory, renal-urinary, hematology/oncology, and psychiatry. Throughout year 2, students take psychological and social dimensions of medical practice, in which they are exposed to health policy, public health, medical ethics, and behavioral science issues. During years 1 and 2, students also participate in clinical activities related to the patient physical and examination. Tutoring and review sessions for the USMLE Step 1 are provided. Creighton's Bio-Information Center houses 200,000 books and maintains extensive multimedia resources, computer teaching laboratories, and computerized literature search facilities. Passing the USMLE Step 1 is a requirement for progression to third year. Students at Creighton benefit from the new onsite computer testing facility for administration of their exams, which is one of eight in the nation.

CLINICAL TRAINING

Second-year students take part in a longitudinal care clerkship, which demands one-half day per week. This allows students to develop longer-term relationships with mentors and patients. Third-year, core clerkships are primary care (8 weeks, encompassing internal medicine and family medicine); inpatient general medicine (8 weeks); psychiatry (8 weeks); surgery (8 weeks); pediatrics (8 weeks); and ob/gyn (8 weeks). Fourth-year guidelines require that students select one surgery elective, one critical care elective, one primary care sub internship, one neurology clerkship, and participate in senior colloquium. The remaining 28 weeks are reserved for residency interviewing and electives. CUMC (404 beds) is the primary teaching hospital. Other sites for clinical training include Omaha Children's Hospital, Omaha Veterans Medical Center, and Bergen Mercy Medical Center. During the summer, Creighton students have the opportunity to gain clinical experience through volunteer efforts in medical settings in the Dominican Republic or in communities closer to home.

Students

Among the 115 students in a recent class, California, Minnesota, and Nebraska accounted for 37 percent of the students' home states, though 28 states and 3 foreign countries were represented. Sixty-four colleges were represented, with about 30 percent of the class having graduated from Creighton—either with an undergraduate or a graduate degree. About 84 percent of the students were science majors. The age range was 21 to 37, with an average age of 23. Of the entire class, 50 percent are women, 6 percent are members of underrepresented minority groups (mostly Hispanic and African American), 10 percent are married, and 6 percent have at least one parent who is an MD alumnus/alumna of Creighton.

STUDENT LIFE

The student body is cohesive and supportive, as evidenced by a student-published *Wellness Chronicle* that offers tips and shares experiences on issues such as exercise, nutrition, mental health, relationships, and spirituality. Through clubs, organizations, and extensive volunteer opportunities, students associate with one another outside of an academic setting. The School of Medicine is part of the main campus of Creighton, allowing medical students to take advantage of programs and facilities of the greater university and to integrate with students from other programs. The physical fitness center, the student center, and graduate student housing are all convenient to the School of Medicine. Omaha is a comfortable, friendly, and inexpensive city, allowing students to meet their own lifestyle needs. Affordable off-campus housing is widely available.

GRADUATES

Our students have gained entrance into virtually all available specialty areas and prestigious programs throughout the United States. During the last three years an average of 52 percent of the graduates enter primary care specialties, defined as internal medicine, family practice, or pediatrics. This is well above the national average of 48 percent. Creighton alumni are found in every state but are more numerous in the Midwest and Western regions.

Admissions

REQUIREMENTS

Requirements are biology (8 semester hours), chemistry (8 hours), organic chemistry (8 hours), physics (8 hours), and English (6 hours). The MCAT is required, and scores must be from within the past three years. For applicants who have retaken the exam, the best set of scores is considered.

SUGGESTIONS

No particular courses or majors are recommended beyond requirements, but advanced courses including biochemistry and/or molecular biology are a plus. Studying overseas is encouraged, as are volunteer and community activities that demonstrate motivation and character.

PROCESS

All AMCAS applicants receive a secondary application, and about 15 percent of those returning secondaries are invited to interview. Interviews are held from September through the spring and consist of one 30-minute session with a faculty or alumnus member of the Admissions Committee, and one session with a medical student who is usually a committee member. A tour of the campus and lunch with current medical students are also provided. About half the interviewed candidates are initially offered a place in the class, with notification occurring on a rolling basis. Wait listed candidates may send supplementary information, such as grades and updates on extracurricular activities.

Admissions Requirements (Required)

MCAT scores, science GPA, non-science GPA, letters of recommendation, interview, essays/personal statement, extracurricular activities, exposure to medical profession, volunteer service.

Admissions Requirements (Optional)

State residency.

Overlap Schools

Georgetown University, Loyola University Chicago, Medical College of Wisconsin, Saint Louis University, The University of Iowa, University of Minnesota, University of Nebraska at Omaha.

COSTS AND AID

Tuition & Fees

Tuition	$37,519
Room and board (on campus)	$16,680
Cost of books	$2,955
Fees	$806

Financial Aid

% students receiving aid	94
Average grant	$20,000
Average loan	$53,599
Average debt	$142,000

DALHOUSIE UNIVERSITY
FACULTY OF MEDICINE

5849 UNIVERSITY AVENUE, HALIFAX, NOVA SCOTIA, CANADA B3H 4H7 • **ADMISSION:** 902-494-1874
FAX: 902-494-6369 • **E-MAIL:** MEDICINE.ADMISSIONS@DAL.CA • **WEBSITE:** WWW.ADMISSIONS.MEDICINE.DAL.CA

STUDENT BODY

Type	Public
Enrollment	91
% male/female	37/63
% underrepresented minorities	37
# applied 581	
# accepted 91	
# enrolled 91	

FACULTY

Total faculty (number)	1,311
% female	30
% part-time	32

ADMISSIONS

Average GPA and MCAT Scores

Overall GPA	3.5
MCAT Bio	10.0
MCAT Phys	10.0
MCAT Verbal	9.0
MCAT Essay	0

Application Information

Regular application	10/31
Regular notification	3/1
Are transfers accepted?	no
Admissions may be deferred?	no
Interview required?	yes
Application fee	$70

Academics

The progressive Case-Oriented Problem-Stimulated (COPS) curriculum prepares students for the pressures and problems facing physicians today. The COPS curriculum uses real-life patient cases and is based on a tutorial system that emphasizes group learning, contextual learning, communication skills, and clinical interaction with patients. In addition to the MD curriculum, programs leading to master's and PhD degrees are offered. Some students opt for a combined degree program, earning both an MD and a graduate degree in a biomedical or related field.

BASIC SCIENCES: In their first two years, students are organized into small groups and build their basic science knowledge by examining matter relevant to patient cases. Faculty/staff tutors guide the group's learning process. Students also choose specific areas of medicine for an elective period and begin to acquire clinical skills in the first month of school. The first academic period lasts 40 weeks and covers the following subjects: Embryology and reproduction; human body; metabolism and function; pathology, immunology, and microbiology; genetics; pharmacology; and clinical epidemiology and critical thinking. During the second academic period, students learn brain and behavior; skin, glands, and blood; respiratory and cardiovascular; genitourinary, gastrointestinal, and musculoskeletal; and population health, community service, and critical thinking. Throughout the first and second years, students have ongoing patient contact through the patient-doctor unit and have the opportunity to take elective courses. Teaching, research, and administration take place within two buildings, the Sir Charles Tupper Medical Building and the Clinical Research Center. The patient-doctor sessions are organized within the hospitals and pair the students with a clinical preceptor each week. Additionally, students attend the Learning Resource Centre weekly where they participate in small groups in hands-on skills and procedures such as casting, blood gases, tubes and wires. Each student also completes case practice sessions that support each unit and use simulated patients. The students gain exposure to pediatrics, psychiatry, and various disciplines of medicine. The Kellogg Health Sciences Library houses more than 150,000 books and journals. The library is fully computerized and provides links to other libraries on campus.

CLINICAL TRAINING

The clerkship is organized into two phases, each of which has a central theme. All clerks will begin in an introduction to clerkship unit for 1 month in which clinical skills, procedures, history-taking, and physical-taking skills will be reviewed for all students. Phase 1 includes medicine, surgery, obstetrics and gynecology, pediatrics, family medicine, emergency medicine and psychiatry. Each unit will be accountable for integrating objectives from other disciplines and ambulatory and community experiences will be expected. Phase 2 begins with elective rotations offering the clerks maximum choice or remediation depending on their performance. In the final unit, continuing and preventive care, clerks are required to complete 3-week rotations in long term care and care of the elderly and again have an opportunity for a choice of rotations. Clerks will be evaluated frequently to receive feedback on their progress to guide self-directed learning. The major teaching hospitals are within walking distance of the school. They include a 202-bed pediatric hospital, a 254-bed obstetrics hospital, a psychiatric hospital, a rehabilitation center, and two large tertiary care adult hospitals. Other affiliated hospitals, clinics, and outpatient facilities also provide important training sites for medical students.

Students

Each entering class has 90 students. In a recent class, 81 students were from the maritime provinces and 9 were from non-maritime regions. At least 50 percent of students are women.

STUDENT LIFE

Although the academic workload is heavy, students are encouraged to pursue nonacademic interests. All students belong to the Dalhousie Medical School Society (DMSS), which promotes the interests of medical undergraduates. The DMSS organizes social and sporting events and raises money to support various nonprofit organizations. Through the student advisory, students have access to informal counseling, activities, and organized discussions that are coordinated and sponsored by other students. Dalhousie offers a variety of housing options on campus, including residencies, singles rooms, and shared apartments. Outside of the campus, the city of Halifax offers a wide variety of entertainment, leisure, and shopping activities.

GRADUATES

Many graduates choose to enter postgraduate training at Dalhousie. Areas of training include family practice, numerous surgical and medical specialties, and laboratory medicine.

Admissions

REQUIREMENTS

The MCAT is required, and scores cannot be more than five years old. A baccalaureate degree is required for entrance to Dalhousie medicine. There are no absolute prerequisite courses, though a minimal science background is advisable for success on the MCAT. Maritime applicants (those from Nova Scotia, New Brunswick, and Prince Edward Island) should have a minimum academic average of a B+, while nonmaritime applicants should have at least an A average.

SUGGESTIONS

Applicants from nonmaritime provinces and countries other than Canada should be exceptionally qualified. In addition to place of residence and academic credentials, the Admissions Committee reviews recommendations, results of personal interviews, and the applicant's extracurricular interests and activities.

PROCESS

For applications and details on the admissions cycle, view the website at www.admissions.medicine.dal.ca or contact the Admissions Office at the phone number and/or address above. Applications are available online only, beginning 9/1 of each year.

Admissions Requirements (Required)

MCAT scores, nonscience GPA, letters of recommendation, interview, essays/personal statement, extracurricular activities, exposure to medical profession, official school transcripts.

Admissions Requirements (Optional)

Science GPA, state residency.

Overlap Schools

Memorial University Newfoundland.

COSTS AND AID

Tuition & Fees

In-state Tuition	$12,806
Out-of-state Tuition	$18,446
Cost of books	$2,000
Fees	$674

Financial Aid

Average grant	$4,000
Average loan	$12,000

DARTMOUTH COLLEGE
DARTMOUTH MEDICAL SCHOOL

3 ROPE FERRY ROAD, HANOVER, NH 03755-1404 • ADMISSION: 603-650-1505
FAX: 603-650-1560 • E-MAIL: DMSADMISSIONS@DARTMOUTH.EDU • WEBSITE: WWW.DMS.DARTMOUTH.EDU

STUDENT BODY	
Type	Private
Enrollment	298
% male/female	50/50
# applied (total/out)	4,537/4,484
# accepted (total/out)	259/248
# enrolled (total/out)	82/76
Average age	24

FACULTY	
Total faculty (number)	2,078

ADMISSIONS

Average GPA and MCAT Scores

Overall GPA	3.7
MCAT Bio	10.7
MCAT Phys	10.7
MCAT Verbal	10.9

Application Information

Regular application	11/1
Regular notification	rolling
Are transfers accepted?	yes
Admissions may be deferred?	yes
Interview required?	yes
Application fee	$75

Academics

Dartmouth Medical School (DMS), founded in 1797, is the nation's fourth oldest. Well-known for its commitment to teaching, excellence in clinical care, and a strong sense of collegiality, DMS is also an important research institution. In the past decade, annual research grants and contracts awarded to DMS increased by more than 100 percent. Annual grant support today totals over $131 million. The innovative New Directions curriculum integrates study of the basic and clinical sciences throughout the four years of medical school. Dartmouth's New Directions combines small-group discussions, problem-based learning, independent study, and traditional classroom presentations in a unique mix to supply focus and support without hindering individual learning and creativity. DMS is a small school, with a national student body, where opportunities for collaboration with the faculty abound. The medical school is located on the campus of Dartmouth College in Hanover, NH, one of the nation's classic college towns. DMS students are well-traveled, with the opportunity to participate in clinical clerkships and electives around the country and throughout the world.

BASIC SCIENCES: Structured class time in both years 1 and 2 totals approximately 20 hours per week. During the three terms of year 1, which last 13 weeks, students focus on the human organism's physical and psychosocial functioning. They gain a strong basic science grounding through course work in human gross anatomy and embryology, microscopic anatomy, microbiology, immunology, neuroscience, pathology, and physiology. The year also includes an integrated course called the biochemical and genetic basis of medicine. Topics in biostatistics and epidemiology are introduced, as well as biochemistry and metabolism. The major component of year 2 is an interdisciplinary pathophysiology course called the scientific basis of medicine. Principles of medical pharmacology is another important second-year course.

CLINICAL TRAINING

Clinical training begins at the start of the first year when students are paired with a faculty preceptor in the on doctoring course. On doctoring continues through the second year. The Dartmouth-Hitchcock Medical Center was recently identified by Solucient, a leading health care data company, as one of America's top 16 major teaching hospitals. A second major training facility, the White River Junction VA hospital, was awarded the Robert W. Carey Quality Achievement Award, the Department of Veteran's Affairs' highest quality award, two years in a row. Systemwide, the Dartmouth-Hitchcock Clinic conducted almost 1.5 million patient visits last year. In addition to other teaching sites in New England, students can complete clinical clerkships in Dartmouth-affiliated teaching hospitals in Alaska, Arizona, California, Connecticut, Florida, New Mexico, and New Zealand. Fellowships from the Dartmouth International Health Group have made it possible for DMS students to explore health care opportunities throughout the world.

Students

DMS is located on the campus of Dartmouth College, an Ivy-League institution with an international student body and reputation. DMS students participate fully in the life of the institution and have access to the facilities, events, activities, and society that are part of the academic community. Students may enjoy national performing arts groups, professional theater, and high-quality films at Dartmouth's Hopkins Center. The Hood Museum of Art, the Berry Sports Center, Thompson Arena, and Alumni Gymnasium are other focal points of interest. Dartmouth's athletic facilities include a ski area, golf course, horse farm, boathouses, and approximately 5,000 acres on Mount Moosilauke. Many medical students volunteer in the community through such organizations as Planned Parenthood, the Good Neighbor Health Clinic, HEART (Health Education, and Rescue Training), and the DMS Dermatones, a singing ensemble. There are several medical interest groups at the medical school. On-campus housing is available, though the majority of students live off-campus.

STUDENT LIFE

Student life at DMS is marked by a strong sense of community and collaborative spirit. In an entering class of approximately 70 individuals, approximately 60 different undergraduate institutions are represented along with every region of the country and several foreign countries. Students of color and international students comprise approximately 30 percent of the student body. Though medical education is demanding, DMS students do not typically view medical school as four years set aside. The environment is rich in opportunities for intellectual and personal growth.

GRADUATES

Graduates are successful in securing residencies in all fields at locations across the country. The Dartmouth-Hitchcock Medical Center sponsors 41 ACGME accredited residency and fellowship training programs.

Admissions

REQUIREMENTS

One year (8 semester hours) each of general biology, general chemistry, organic chemistry, and physics, along with one-half year of calculus, are required. Facility in written and spoken English is also required. MCAT results are strongly recommended and must be no more than three years old.

SUGGESTIONS

Biochemistry is a recommended course, although it is not required. In addition to scientific acumen, applicants should demonstrate motivation and interest in their chosen major, which need not be science. Relevant research, medical experience, social service, and other co-curricular activities are important evidence of commitment.

PROCESS

All AMCAS applicants to DMS receive a secondary application, which must be completed by 12/31. Approximately 650 applicants are invited to interview from a pool of roughly 5,000 candidates. Interviews occur from September to April and take place on the Dartmouth campus. Dual degree applicants (MD/PhD, MD/MBA, MD/MPh) also interview at Dartmouth. About 30 percent of those interviewed are admitted. A small number are placed on the waiting list.

Admissions Requirements (Required)

Science GPA, nonscience GPA, letters of recommendation, interview, essays/personal statement.

Admissions Requirements (Optional)

MCAT scores, state residency, extracurricular activities, exposure to medical profession.

COSTS AND AID

Tuition & Fees

Tuition	$34,500
Room and board (on campus)	$8,750
Cost of books	$2,500
Fees	$775

Financial Aid

% students receiving aid	85
Average grant	$18,730
Average loan	$29,850
Average debt	$112,600

DREXEL UNIVERSITY
COLLEGE OF MEDICINE

2900 QUEEN LANE, PHILADELPHIA, PA 19129 • ADMISSION: 215-991-8202
FAX: 215-843-1766 • E-MAIL: MEDADMIS@DREXEL.EDU • WEBSITE: WWW.DREXELMED.EDU

STUDENT BODY

Type	Private
Enrollment	1,016
% male/female	50/50
% underrepresented minorities	15
# applied (total/out)	6,475/5,795
# accepted (total/out)	846/686
# enrolled (total/out)	231/218
Average age	24

FACULTY

Total faculty (number)	577
% female	38
% minority	6
% part-time	11

ADMISSIONS

Average GPA and MCAT Scores

Overall GPA	3.5
MCAT Bio	11.0
MCAT Phys	10.0
MCAT Verbal	10.0
MCAT Essay	0

Application Information

Regular application	12/1
Regular notification	10/15
Early application	8/1
Early notification	10/5
Are transfers accepted?	yes
Admissions may be deferred?	yes
Interview required?	yes
Application fee	$75

Academics

With its dedication to academic and clinical excellence and a historic commitment to diversity, the College of Medicine has earned national recognition as an institution that provides innovation in medical education. Medical students are trained to consider each patient's case and needs in a comprehensive, integrated manner, taking into account more factors than the presenting physiological condition. Most students follow a four-year curriculum, leading to the MD. Students can gain research experience through the Summer Research Fellowship Program, which provides a stipend in exchange for full-time research in the laboratory of a participating mentor. The combined MD/MPH program is available, as are MD/MBA and MD/PhD programs, through which students may earn graduate degrees in bioengineering, microbiology and immunology, molecular and cell biology and genetics, molecular pathobiology, neuroscience, pharmacology and physiology, and biochemistry. The Medical Humanities Scholars Program allows students who are particularly interested in the humanistic elements of medicine to graduate with the designation of Humanities Scholar. The Women's Health Education Program incorporates women's health into all aspects of medical education. Medical students are evaluated using the grades of Honors/Highly Satisfactory/Satisfactory/Unsatisfactory. Passing Step 1 of the USMLE is required for promotion to year 3, and passing Step 2 of the USMLE is required for graduation.

BASIC SCIENCES: College of Medicine students choose between two innovative academic curricula for their first two years of study. IFM, Interdisciplinary Foundations of Medicine, integrates the basic science courses and presents them through clinical symptom-based modules. Students learn in lectures, labs, and small group settings. The Program for Integrated Learning (PIL), a problem-based curriculum, takes place primarily in small groups, and is supervised and facilitated by faculty. Laboratories and resource sessions complement the case studies. In both curricula, first-year students are introduced within their first few weeks to clinical experience and community service. Standardized patients and model examination rooms are some of the facilities used to enhance clinical instruction in the courses. Students also spend time in offices of primary care physicians, thereby gaining firsthand experience with patient care. Both curricula teach students to think like physicians from their first days on campus.

CLINICAL TRAINING

Required rotations, most of which are completed in the third year, are medicine (12 weeks), surgery (12 weeks), pediatrics (6 weeks), ob/gyn (6 weeks), psychiatry (6 weeks), neurology (4 weeks), an internal medicine sub internship (4 weeks), and family medicine (6 weeks). The College of Medicine has many affiliated hospitals to accommodate students who wish to work in large tertiary care hospitals and those who prefer small community hospitals. Our academic campuses include leading hospitals in Pennsylvania, New Jersey, and Delaware. A sampling of our clinical sites includes: Hahnemann University Hospital, St. Christopher's Hospital for Children, Allegheny General Hospital, Saint Peter's University Hospital, Friends Hospital, Lehigh Valley Hospital, York Hospital, Abington Memorial Hospital, Monmouth Medical Center, and Pinnacle Health.

Students

About 50 percent are women, at least 25 percent of students are nontraditional, having pursued other interests or careers in between college and medical school, and 15 percent of students are underrepresented minorities.

STUDENT LIFE

Despite the relatively large class size, students are cohesive and supportive. The College of Medicine offers a variety of clubs and activities that are both academically and socially oriented. Many students are involved in community outreach activities in local public schools, health clinics, and rehabilitation centers. Students have access to a new onsite fitness center at the College of Medicine. Philadelphia, a diverse and interesting city with a large student population, is replete with history, culture, sports, clubs, and restaurants. For additional attractions, New York and other urban areas can be easily reached by train or car. Affordable and attractive housing surrounds the Queen Lane campus.

GRADUATES

Drexel graduates do very well in the residency matching program, both in primary care and in more specialized fields. Matches for the last two years can be viewed on the school's website.

Admissions

REQUIREMENTS

Requirements are two semesters each of biology, English, general chemistry, organic chemistry, and physics. Science courses should include associated labs. The MCAT is required, and scores should be from within the past two years. For applicants who have retaken the exam, the most recent set of scores is weighted most heavily.

SUGGESTIONS

Beyond prerequisites, recommended courses include ethics, history, philosophy, psychology, and other social science and humanities courses. An advanced course in molecular biology or genetics is strongly encouraged. The College of Medicine seeks highly qualified and motivated students who demonstrate the desire, intelligence, integrity, and emotional maturity to become excellent physicians. Drexel medical students have the opportunity to utilize advanced technology to aid their learning with extensive access to educational materials online. The college encourages applications from those who have demonstrated a commitment to the service of others and who appreciate the significance of both technology and humanity in clinical care. Students who are interested in careers as generalist physicians, those who come from Pennsylvania, and those who come from populations that are underrepresented in medicine are particularly encouraged to apply. Applicants must be U.S. citizens or permanent residents.

PROCESS

All AMCAS applicants receive secondary applications. About 20 percent of those that submit secondary applications are interviewed between September and April. The interview typically consists of two sessions: An open file session with a faculty member or administrator, and a closed file session with a student. Of interviewed candidates, about half are accepted on a rolling basis. Wait listed candidates may send transcripts or other material to update their files. An alternate route to admissions is through BA/MD and BS/MD (3+4) programs organized in conjunction with Drexel, Lehigh, and Villanova Universities, and Rosemont College. We also have early assurance programs with Allegheny College, Monmouth University, Muhlenberg College, Ursinus College, West Chester University, and Wilkes University for students interested in 4+4 programs. For highly qualified post-baccalaureate students at participating institutions, a provisional acceptance to the College of Medicine may be granted, contingent on successful completion of the pre-medical curriculum. Post-baccalaureate programs through which this type of arrangement is possible are found at Bryn Mawr College, Columbia University, Goucher College, Scripps College, University of Pennsylvania, and West Chester University.

Admissions Requirements (Required)

MCAT scores, science GPA, non-science GPA, letters of recommendation, interview, essays/personal statement.

Admissions Requirements (Optional)

State residency, extracurricular activities, exposure to medical profession, research.

Overlap Schools

Eastern Virginia Medical School, New York Medical College, Penn State University MBA, Rush Medical College of Rush University, Temple University, Thomas Jefferson University, UMDNJ.

COSTS AND AID

Tuition & Fees

Tuition	$36,770
Room and board (on campus)	$9,500
Cost of books	$12,155
Fees	$1,120

Financial Aid

% students receiving aid	85
Average grant	$47,641
Average loan	$49,707
Average debt	$174,343

DUKE UNIVERSITY
SCHOOL OF MEDICINE

COMMITTEE ON ADMISSIONS, PO BOX 3710, DUMC, DURHAM, NC 27710 • ADMISSION: 919-684-2985
FAX: 919-684-8893 • E-MAIL: MEDADM@MC.DUKE.EDU • WEBSITE: HTTP://MEDSCHOOL.DUKE.EDU

STUDENT BODY

Type	Private
Enrollment	402
% male/female	53/47
% underrepresented minorities	18
# applied (total/out)	5,023
# accepted (total/out)	183/161
# enrolled (total/out)	101

ADMISSIONS

Average GPA and MCAT Scores

Overall GPA	3.8
MCAT Bio	12.0
MCAT Phys	12.0
MCAT Verbal	11.0
MCAT Essay	Q

Application Information

Regular application	11/1
Regular notification	3/1
Are transfers accepted?	no
Admissions may be deferred?	yes
Interview required?	yes
Application fee	$80

Academics

By condensing the basic sciences into the first year and scheduling required clinical clerkships for the second year, Duke allows medical students additional opportunities for research, clinical, or other enriching experiences during their third year. Those who are particularly interested in research may apply for joint MD/PhD programs in fields such as anatomy, biochemistry, biomedical engineering, cell biology, genetics, immunology, microbiology, molecular biology, neuroscience, pathology, pharmacology, and physiology. Other joint degree programs are the MD/JD, MD/MBA, MD/MPH, MD/MPP, and the Medical Historian Program, which leads to an MD and either an MA or PhD in history. In most courses, medical students are evaluated by the grades pass with honors, pass, incomplete, or fail. The USMLE is not required for graduation, though most students opt to take it, and virtually all pass each section with scores in the 90th percentile or higher.

BASIC SCIENCES: A new introduction to critical care course meets weekly during the first and second years and integrates clinical and basic science concepts. Each week during the first year, practice alternates between the classroom, where students meet in small groups, and the clinics, so that shortly after lessons are learned, they are applied. Computers are issued to all students to be used in the practice course for informational and instructional purposes. Also, part of the course is an intensive 3-week preparation for year II segment, which prepares students for clinical rotations. Other first-year courses, taught primarily in a lecture/lab format, are organized into five blocks, so that no more than three subjects are tackled at a time. Courses are biochemistry, cell biology, genetics, gross anatomy, microanatomy, physiology, neurobiology, microbiology, immunology, pathology I, pharmacology, and pathology II. In total, first-year students are in class or scheduled sessions for approximately 30 hours per week. Classes are held in buildings central to the medical complex. The Medical Center Library houses 276,000 books, including a renowned medical history collection. The Medical Library Education Center has electronic classroom and multimedia areas. Basic science concepts are reinforced during clinical rotations in the second year.

CLINICAL TRAINING

Preparation for and exposure to clinical medicine begins during the first year, as part of the introduction to critical care course. The year-long preparation for clinical clerkships provides students with significant experience in clinical settings before the beginning of their formal clerkships in year 2. Clerkship requirements are fulfilled in the second year. They are: medicine (8 weeks), ob/gyn (8 weeks), pediatrics (8 weeks), psychiatry (6 weeks), cost-effective care (2 weeks), surgery (8 weeks), and family medicine (8 weeks), or neurology and family medicine (4 weeks each). Clinical training takes place at Duke Hospital (1,124 beds), Durham Veterans Affairs Medical Center (455 beds), Lenox Baker Children's Hospital, Durham Regional Hospital (451 beds), and at multiple affiliated hospitals and clinics. The third year is spent in research as part of an independent scholarship project, which may be in behavioral neuroscience, biomedical engineering, biometry, biophysics, cancer biology, cardiovascular studies, cell and regulatory biology, epidemiology health services and health policy, immunology, infectious diseases, neurobiology, ophthalmology and visual studies, and pathology. Third-year students may design a year of mentored research at Duke or at approved extramural sites (e.g., NIH) or students may begin the dual degree curricula. During their fourth year, students complete clinical training through elective clerkships. There are more than 150 electives offered at Duke. In addition, students may spend up to 2 months in rotations at other institutions.

Students

In the most recent class, 22 percent of the students are underrepresented minorities, most of whom are African American. Women account for 49 percent of the class, and the average age is 22, with an age range of 19–42. Forty-three undergraduate institutions are represented, the top six being Duke, Harvard, North Carolina State, Johns Hopkins, UNC at Chapel Hill, and Yale. Twenty-eight states are represented, and the top five are North Carolina, California, New York, Ohio, and Virginia. Class size is 100.

STUDENT LIFE

Students, faculty, and administrators come together for events that promote a sense of community, congeniality, and friendship within the medical school. For example, the Dean hosts five Dean's Desserts for medical students to interact with teaching, research, and clinical faculty during the year. Organizations based on volunteer work, professional goals, or extracurricular interests are numerous. Medical students have access to all of Duke's athletic and recreational facilities. Durham is popular with students, offering parks, shopping districts, restaurants, and museums. Mountains and beaches are just a few hours away. Convenient campus-owned apartments, some of which have athletic facilities, are available on a limited basis. Social events sponsored by various medical school-based organizations provide opportunities for students to interact together. A fitness facility located with the major hospital complex for medical students and house staff only has recently opened.

GRADUATES

Graduates enter top residency programs, in primary and specialty fields. Most students get their top choice for residency appointment.

Admissions

REQUIREMENTS

Prerequisites are one year each of English, inorganic chemistry, organic chemistry, physics, biology, and calculus. The MCAT is required, and scores must be from within the past four years. If the exam has been taken on multiple occasions, the most recent set of scores is generally considered. For those who have taken time off after college, science work must have been completed not more than seven years before matriculation at Duke.

SUGGESTIONS

An introductory course in biochemistry is recommended. The character, motivation, and dedication of applicants is considered along with academic merits. Extracurricular activities, particularly those that are medically related, community service, volunteer experience, research exposure, and work experience are all considered in admission.

PROCESS

About 60 percent of AMCAS applicants receive secondary applications. Of those returning secondaries, about 30 percent are interviewed. Interviews are conducted from September through February, and consist of two half-hour sessions with members of the Admissions Committee. On interview day, students also receive a campus tour, and have the opportunity to eat lunch and speak with students. About one-third of interviewees will be considered for admission.

Admissions Requirements (Required)

MCAT scores, science GPA, non-science GPA, letters of recommendation, interview, essays/personal statement, extracurricular activities, exposure to medical profession.

Admissions Requirements (Optional)

State residency.

Overlap Schools

Harvard University, Johns Hopkins University, Stanford University, University of Pennsylvania, Washington University.

COSTS AND AID

Tuition & Fees

Tuition	$32,916
Room and board (off campus)	$15,240
Cost of books	$2,480
Fees	$6,684

Financial Aid

% students receiving aid	85
Average grant	$21,110
Average loan	$24,500
Average debt	$68,848

EAST CAROLINA UNIVERSITY
BRODY SCHOOL OF MEDICINE

OFFICE OF ADMISSIONS, 600 MOYE BOULEVARD, GREENVILLE, NC 27834 • ADMISSION: 252-744-2202
FAX: 252-744-1926 • E-MAIL: SOMADMISSIONS@MAIL.ECU.EDU • WEBSITE: WWW.ECU.EDU/BSOMADMISSIONS

STUDENT BODY	
Type	Public
Enrollment	288
% male/female	50/50
% underrepresented minorities	34
# applied (total/out)	873/128
# accepted (total/out)	72/0
# enrolled (total/out)	72/0
Average age	24

ADMISSIONS

Average GPA and MCAT Scores

Overall GPA	3.5
MCAT Bio	9.0
MCAT Phys	9.0
MCAT Verbal	9.0
MCAT Essay	P

Application Information

Regular application	11/15
Regular notification	rolling
Early application	6/1–8/1
Early notification	10/1
Are transfers accepted?	yes
Admissions may be deferred?	no
Interview required?	yes
Application fee	$60

Academics

All first- and second-year students are paired with community physician mentors and have the opportunity for ongoing patient contact and exposure to primary health care settings. Grading uses are A, B, C, and F. In addition, honors may be awarded in some instances. Passing the USMLE Step 1 is a requirement for promotion to year 3, and passing the USMLE Step 2 is a requirement for graduation. Joint PhD/MD programs can be arranged on a case-by-case basis.

BASIC SCIENCES: During the first two years, students spend about 28 hours per week in classes, most of which are taught in a lecture/lab format. Small group discussions, problem-based learning, and an introduction to clinical medicine are also part of the basic science curriculum. First-year courses are behavioral science, biochemistry, clinical skills I, embryology, ethical and social issues in medicine, genetics, gross anatomy, histology, neurobiology, microbiology and immunology, primary care preceptorship, and physiology. Second-year courses are clinical skills II and clinical aspects of lifestyle abuse, ethical social issues in medicine, introduction to child development, introduction to medicine, pathology, pathogenic microbiology, pharmacology, primary care preceptorship, and psychopathology and human sexuality. Clinical skills II and clinical aspects of lifestyle abuse addresses behavioral aspects of health maintenance both for patients and physicians. The Academic Support and Counseling Center assists students in a variety of ways, including enrichment sessions and tutorials. Most classes take place in the Brody Medical Sciences Building, a modern facility that has classrooms with computer and video technology, large laboratories, auditoriums, and a clinical outpatient center. The presence of a clinical facility in this classroom structure suggests the importance of integrating basic and clinical sciences at East Carolina. Another building used frequently by first- and second-year students is the W.E. Laupus Health Sciences Library, which has 52,900 volumes and 1,550 subscriptions in addition to computer and audiovisual learning aids.

CLINICAL TRAINING

Required clerkships are family medicine (8 weeks), internal medicine (8 weeks), ob/gyn (8 weeks), pediatrics (8 weeks), psychiatry (8 weeks), and surgery (8 weeks). At least 10 of these 48 weeks are spent in an ambulatory setting. Fourth-year students make selections from specified categories including primary care experiences (2 months), surgical selectives (1 month), medicine selectives (1 month), transition to residency (1 month), and electives (4 months). Clinical training takes place at sites throughout Eastern North Carolina, with the cooperation of the school's extended faculty members, some of whom practice in remote, rural areas. Training also takes place at the Developmental Evaluation Clinic, Eastern Carolina Family Practice Center, Pitt County Memorial Hospital (731 beds), specialized research institutes, and at rural affiliated hospitals throughout the state.

Students

Virtually all students are North Carolina residents, many of whom attended college outside of the state. More than 20 percent of students are underrepresented minorities, mostly African Americans. Almost half of entering students have taken some time off between undergraduate and medical school. In a recent entering class, the mean age at matriculation was 26. Class size is 72.

STUDENT LIFE

The university has an active student union and facilities such as student lounges, theaters, concert halls, museums, and an athletic center. Medical students are not only integrated into the greater campus community but also have a cohesive social life among themselves. Medical student groups are organized around volunteer efforts, professional interests, support groups, and religious affiliations, among other themes. Examples are the Generalist Physicians in Training Interest Group, the Medical Student Council, Peer Counseling, the Christian Medical/Dental Fellowship, and the Greenville Community Shelter Clinic. Greenville is known for its gentle climate and low cost of living, both assets for medical students. There are plenty of housing options, both on and off campus, for married or single students.

GRADUATES

The goal of the Generalist Physician Initiative is that at least half of medical school graduates enter primary care fields. There are at least 12 residency programs and several fellowship programs offered at Pitt County Memorial Hospital, with the majority of positions in internal medicine, family medicine, and emergency medicine.

Admissions

REQUIREMENTS

One year each of biology, English, general chemistry, organic chemistry, and physics are all required. Laboratories are required with all science courses. The MCAT is required and must be no more than three years old. For those who have retaken the exam, the most recent set of scores is generally considered. State residency, or close affiliation with the state, is a requirement for admission.

SUGGESTIONS

Beyond required courses, students are advised to take humanities and social science courses and an additional year of English. Taking classes that are part of the medical school curriculum is not recommended. Extracurricular activities that involve exposure to the medical practice are important. The Admissions Committee looks for applicants who are likely to contribute to meeting the health care needs of North Carolina.

PROCESS

All AMCAS applicants who are state residents (or who demonstrate strong ties to the state) are sent secondary applications. About 60 percent of those returning secondaries are interviewed, with interviews taking place between August and April. The interview consists of two sessions with faculty or student members of the committee, which last between 30–60 minutes. On interview day, applicants have an opportunity to meet with students and tour the campus. About 15 percent of interviewed candidates are accepted, while others are rejected or wait listed. Candidates awaiting a decision may send additional information to enhance their files.

Admissions Requirements (Required)

MCAT scores, science GPA, non-science GPA, letters of recommendation, interview, state residency, essays/personal statement, extracurricular activities, exposure to medical profession.

COSTS AND AID

Tuition & Fees

In-state Tuition	$6,034
Out-of-state Tuition	$30,724
Cost of books	$1,153
Fees	$1,644

Financial Aid

Average grant	$8,259
Average loan	$12,720
Average debt	$43,714

EAST TENNESSEE STATE UNIVERSITY
JAMES H. QUILLEN COLLEGE OF MEDICINE

JAMES H. QUILLEN COLLEGE OF MEDICINE, PO BOX 70580, JOHNSON CITY, TN 37614-1708 • **ADMISSION:** 423-439-2033
FAX: 423-439-2110 • **E-MAIL:** SACOM@ETSU.EDU • **WEBSITE:** COM.ETSU.EDU

STUDENT BODY	
Type	Public

FACULTY	
Student-faculty ratio	1:1

ADMISSIONS

Application Information

Regular application	11/15
Regular notification	7/1
Early application	6/1–8/1
Early notification	10/1
Are transfers accepted?	yes
Admissions may be deferred?	yes
Interview required?	yes
Application fee	$50

Academics

Quillen College of Medicine offers the following degrees of study: Doctor of medicine, master of science, and doctor of philosophy. Most students earn an MD in four years, through either the traditional track or the rural primary care track (RPCT). Quillen admits a medical class of 60 each fall. Quillen's major educational emphasis is primary care and rural medicine. The Biomedical Science Graduate Program offers study leading to the doctor of philosophy and master of science in biomedical science. The purpose of the program is to prepare students for careers in research and education in the life sciences. Students receive their degrees in biomedical science with a concentration in one of the following five areas of basic science: Anatomy and cell biology, biochemistry and molecular biology, microbiology, pharmacology, and physiology.

BASIC SCIENCES: With the exception of clinical work, basic science courses are taught primarily in a lecture/lab format. Students are in scheduled sessions for about 24 hours per week. First-year courses for all students are anatomy, biochemistry, biostatistics and epidemiology, communication skills for health professionals, cell and tissue biology, physiology, geriatrics, behavorial science and lifespan development, and human development biology and genetics. Traditional students also take case-oriented learning, while RPCT students take introduction to rural health, rural and community health, and health assessment/examination. Patient contact begins in case-oriented learning for traditional track students and as part of weekly visits to rural health providers for RPCT students. The second-year curriculum for all students is geriatrics, neuroscience, microbiology, immunology, pathology, pharmacology, practicing medicine, and psychiatry. Traditional track students take clinical skills and clinical preceptorship while RPCT students take rural health needs, health assessment, and patient/client assessment. Instructional facilities are located in a newly constructed, multimillion dollar basic sciences building on the grounds of the Mountain Home Veterans Affairs facility. The medical library, also located on the same databases, has almost 100,000 volumes, several online medical databases, educational software programs, computerized access to the university library system, computers for student use, and rooms for audiovisual study, reading, and conferences. Evaluation uses an A–F grading system. Students must pass Step 1 of the USMLE for promotion to the third year.

CLINICAL TRAINING

Third-year required rotations for traditional track students are family medicine (8 weeks), ob/gyn (8 weeks), pediatrics (8 weeks), psychiatry (8 weeks), internal medicine (8 weeks), and surgery (8 weeks). RPCT students take part in shorter rotations in the same specialties, and are required to complete a 16-week primary care clerkship in a rural area. During the fourth year, all students complete a minimum of 16 weeks of electives. RPCT students have additional rural, primary care requirements, and traditional tract students must take internal medicine and senior surgery. Clinical training takes place in the following three cities: Bristol, Kingsport, and Johnson City, and in neighboring rural towns. Affiliated hospitals are The Johnson City Medical Center, VA Medical Center, Woodridge Psychiatric Hospital, Johnson City Specialty Hospital, Northside Hospital, The Holston Valley Hospital, Indian Path Medical Center, Bristol Regional Medical Center, and Hawkins County Hospital. In total, these hospitals provide 3,000 patient beds. Evaluation uses an A–F grading system, and the USMLE Step 2 is required for graduation.

Students

Almost all students are from Tennessee or the immediately surrounding areas. Most students went to college in Tennessee, although undergraduate institutions from around the country are represented in the medical student body. About 15 percent of students are underrepresented minorities, most of them African American. Class size is 60.

STUDENT LIFE

Medical students take advantage of the extracurricular opportunities at ETSU, such as its theater, films, intramural sports, and athletic and recreational facilities. They are active in a wide variety of special interest and service organizations. Housing options include campus housing as well as a selection of apartments, townhouses, condominiums, and houses for rent or sale. As an urban area, Johnson City offers many services and attractions.

GRADUATES

More than 60 percent of Quillen graduates pursue careers in primary care medicine and 22 percent practice in rural settings. Quillen provides a strong background in both the art and science of medicine, and graduates who wish to pursue advanced training in specialty areas have a high degree of success getting into residency programs of their choice.

Admissions

REQUIREMENTS

Applicants must complete chemistry (8 semester hours), organic chemistry (8 hours), physics (8 hours), biology (8 hours), and communication skills (9 hours). An additional 49 hours of course work is required. The MCAT is required and should be no more than two years old. The April MCAT is advised as the August exam will delay application processing.

SUGGESTIONS

Other recommended courses are comparative vertebrate anatomy, histology, mammalian anatomy, advanced mathematics, statistics, biochemistry, microbiology, public speaking, history, economics, philosophy, psychology, social science, and foreign languages. For those who have been out of school for a significant period of time, recent course work is helpful. The Admissions Committee looks for traits and experiences that are consistent with primary care practice. Admissions is particularly competitive for out-of-state residents, and with the exception of applicants from the contiguous Appalachian region who are interested in primary care, out-of-state applicants must have extremely strong qualifications to be considered.

PROCESS

About one-third of AMCAS applicants are sent secondary applications. Of those submitting secondaries, the majority of Tennessee residents and about 10 percent of out-of-state residents are invited to interview between September and March. Applicants receive two interviews with faculty, medical students, administrators, or community members, which last one hour. Of interviewed candidates, about 40 percent of Tennessee residents and 15 percent of out-of-state residents are accepted on a rolling basis. Others are either rejected or wait listed. Generally, only a few students are accepted from the wait list.

Admissions Requirements (Required)

MCAT scores, science GPA, non-science GPA, letters of recommendation, interview, state residency, essays/personal statement, extracurricular activities, exposure to medical profession.

COSTS AND AID

Tuition & Fees

In-state Tuition	$14,390
Out-of-state Tuition	$29,332
Room and board (off campus)	$12,000
Cost of books	$1,360
Fees	$553

Financial Aid

% students receiving aid	91
Average grant	$8,000
Average loan	$28,000
Average debt	$94,000

EASTERN VIRGINIA MEDICAL SCHOOL

OFFICE OF ADMISSIONS, 700 WEST OLNEY ROAD, NORFOLK, VA 23507-1607• ADMISSION: 757-446-5812
FAX: 757-446-5896 • E-MAIL: NANEZKF@EVMS.EDU • WEBSITE: WWW.EVMS.EDU

STUDENT BODY

Type	Private
Enrollment	432
% male/female	47/53
% underrepresented minorities	12
# applied (total/out)	2,565/1,846
# accepted (total/out)	335/197
# enrolled (total/out)	110/50

ADMISSIONS

Average GPA and MCAT Scores

Overall GPA	3.5
MCAT Bio	10.0
MCAT Phys	9.8
MCAT Verbal	9.5

Application Information

Regular application	11/15
Early application	6/1–8/1
Early notification	10/1
Are transfers accepted?	yes
Admissions may be deferred?	yes
Interview required?	yes
Application fee	$90

Academics

The curriculum is designed to help students master both the science of medicine and the art of clinical problem solving. A combined MD/PhD program is available for qualified students, leading to the doctorate degree in one of the biomedical science fields. For medical students interested in medical research, summer research projects are available. Medical students are evaluated with honors, high pass, pass, and fail.

BASIC SCIENCES: The first two years are devoted to basic sciences that are fundamental to the practice of medicine. Students also learn the clinical skills of physical diagnosis and interviewing. Throughout the first two years, students are in class or other scheduled sessions for about 25 hours per week. Lectures, labs, and small-group discussions are the instructional modalities used. First-year courses are the following: Biochemistry, gross anatomy, histology, human development, introduction to the patient/longitudinal generalist mentorship, medical ethics, medical molecular and cellular biology, neuroscience, physiology, the doctor, and the patient. Second-year courses are the following: Biostatistics, epidemiology, introduction to the patient/longitudinal mentorship, medical ethics, microbiology/immunology, pathology, pathophysiology, pharmacology, and psychopathology.

CLINICAL TRAINING

Required third-year clerkships are family medicine (6 weeks), internal medicine (12 weeks), ob/gyn (8 weeks), pediatrics (8 weeks), psychiatry (6 weeks), and surgery (8 weeks). Fourth-year required clerkships include 4 weeks of surgical specialties, 2 weeks of geriatrics, 1 week of substance abuse, and 25 weeks of electives, which may be selected from basic science and clinical offerings. For clinical training, students have access to a wide range of facilities including the East Coast's largest naval hospital, full-service community hospitals, interdisciplinary primary care centers, one of the largest Level I shock trauma centers in the state, private hospitals, a prestigious children's hospital, and clinics built for the medically underserved.

Students

At least 70 percent of students are Virginia residents. The student body has a number of older or nontraditional students, and the average age of incoming students is often around 26. Underrepresented minorities account for approximately 7 percent of the student body. Class size is 105.

STUDENT LIFE

EVMS supports students' nonacademic lives and puts significant resources into the well-being of its students. Each fall, students and faculty members convene at a nearby resort for the orientation retreat sponsored by the school's Human Values in Medicine Program. The retreat provides a relaxed and informal atmosphere and allows incoming students the chance to interact before classes begin. Throughout the year, students are involved in a number of organizations and events, including ongoing community-service projects and a monthly Friday-night social hour. In general, the school's location in the Hampton Roads area is ideal for medical students, offering urban conveniences, the friendliness of a small town, and the attractions of a beach community. Most medical students live in the section of Norfolk near the medical school known as Ghent, a beautiful neighborhood of tree-lined streets and Victorian houses. EVMS also owns and operates an apartment complex near the school that offers housing for both married and single students. Washington, DC, with its many attractions and recreational opportunities, is only a 4-hour drive.

GRADUATES

From 20 percent to 25 percent of graduates are accepted into one of the many residency programs sponsored by the Eastern Virginia Graduate School. Other graduating students are successful in securing residency positions at institutions throughout the state and at locations around the country.

Admissions

REQUIREMENTS

Required courses are one year each of biology, chemistry, organic chemistry, and physics, all with associated labs. Applicants are expected to have a B or better in these courses. The MCAT is required, and scores should be from no more than two years prior to the date of application. For applicants who have retaken the exam, the best set of scores is weighed most heavily. Thus, there is no advantage in withholding scores.

SUGGESTIONS

In addition to academic transcripts, an applicant's experiences and background are examined. Personal characteristics are evaluated during the interviews, and honesty and spontaneity are considered essential qualities. Interviewers are interested in an applicant's concept of a physician's role, motivation, sensitivity to the needs of others, and communication skills.

PROCESS

After an initial screening of academic credentials, state residency, and other factors, about 50 percent of AMCAS applicants are sent secondary applications. A slightly larger percentage of state-resident applicants are asked to submit secondaries. Of those returning secondaries, about one-third are interviewed between September and March. Interviews consist of one session with a small panel of faculty members and medical students. On interview day, candidates also have the opportunity to meet with current students, tour the campus, and attend group information presentations. About one-third of interviewed candidates are accepted on a rolling basis. Alternate paths to admission are possible for students at schools that have special arrangements with EVMS. These are Old Dominion University, The College of William and Mary, Norfolk State University, Hampton University, and Hampden-Sydney College.

Admissions Requirements (Required)

MCAT scores, science GPA, non-science GPA, letters of recommendation, interview, extracurricular activities, exposure to medical profession.

Admissions Requirements (Optional)

State residency, essays/personal statement.

COSTS AND AID

Tuition & Fees

Tuition	$18,975
Cost of books	$1,000
Fees	$2,966

Financial Aid

% students receiving aid	90

EMORY UNIVERSITY
SCHOOL OF MEDICINE

1440 CLIFTON ROAD NE, SUITE 115, ATLANTA, GA 30322-4510 • ADMISSION: 404-727-5660
FAX: 404-727-5456 • E-MAIL: MEDADMISS@EMORY.EDU • WEBSITE: WWW.MED.EMORY.EDU

STUDENT BODY

Type	Private
Enrollment	462
% male/female	51/49
% underrepresented minorities	28
# applied (total/out)	3,759/3,233
# accepted (total/out)	308/244
# enrolled (total/out)	114/77
Average age	23

FACULTY

Total faculty (number)	1,952
% female	35
% minority	12
% part-time	9
Student-faculty ratio	4:1

ADMISSIONS

Average GPA and MCAT Scores

Overall GPA	3.64
MCAT Bio	11.4
MCAT Phys	11.2
MCAT Verbal	10.7
MCAT Essay	P

Application Information

Regular application	10/15
Regular notification	rolling
Are transfers accepted?	yes
Admissions may be deferred?	yes
Interview required?	yes
Application fee	$80

Academics

The 4 year medical curriculum begins with basic science courses combined with medical problem-based learning, medical decision making, pre-clinical experiences, and patient-doctor course work that provides outstanding preparation for the clinical experiences, which make up the third and fourth years. Emory offers joint-degree programs that allow qualified students to explore interdisciplinary aspects of medicine. Students may enter a combined MD/MPH program organized with the School of Public Health. In conjunction with the Graduate School of Arts and Sciences, medical students may earn the PhD degree concurrently with the MD.

BASIC SCIENCES: The basic science portion of the curriculum is comprehensive and engaging, with an instructional methodology that relies on lectures, small-group problem-based learning sessions, and labs. Introductory clinical experiences, discussions about the doctor-patient relationship, medical decision making, and the behavioral aspects of medicine are integrated with basic science concepts during the first and second years. First-year (9 months) courses are anatomy, embryology, biochemistry, neuroscience, physiology, cell biology and histology, and genetics. There is also an opportunity between the first and second years to take a clinical preceptorship or to engage in summer research projects within the 10-week block. The second year (9 months) includes courses in microbiology/immunology, pathology, human behavior/psychopathology, clinical methods, pharmacology, pathophysiology, and medical problem solving.

CLINICAL TRAINING

The third and fourth years consist of 21 months of required clerkships that also include 2 months that may be taken for vacation or residency interviewing; only 19 months of actual course work are required for graduation. Required clerkships include the following: Clinical medicine (junior year, 12 weeks taught with dermatology); clinical surgery (8 weeks with a clinical anesthesiology component within it); clinical gynecology/obstetrics (6 weeks); clinical pediatrics (6 weeks); clinical psychiatry (6 weeks); advanced clinical medicine (senior year, 4 weeks); clinical family medicine (4 weeks); clinical neurology (4 weeks); clinical medical ethics and professionalism stressed throughout the curriculum; emergency medicine (4 weeks); clinical radiology (2 weeks); surgery selectives and elective courses offered in a wide variety of areas. These clerkships take place within the wide scope of Emory-owned hospitals, facilities, and affiliated institutions such as Emory University Hospital, Emory Crawford Long Hospital, Grady Memorial Hospital, Children's Health Care of Atlanta at Egleston, Wesley Woods Center for Geriatrics, and Atlanta Veterans Administration Medical Center. These institutions offer a diverse patient community and clinical diagnosis.

Students

Students at Emory are encouraged to find time to pursue outside interests while balancing the school schedule.

STUDENT LIFE

Students have access to the organizations, events, and facilities of both the medical and undergraduate schools. As a release from studying, students use the athletic center, which is modern and comprehensive. Students also participate in intramural sports. Medical students organize community service projects and participate in local and national medical student organizations, which serve to integrate students into the greater community and often provide additional clinical exposure. Atlanta is an excellent city for students as it is affordable and offers many cultural, recreational, and entertainment opportunities. While many choose to live off campus, where apartments and houses are plentiful and affordable, many choose to live in the new Clairmont campus residential community. Located within walking distance to the main campus, it includes modern luxury apartments, recreational areas, a student center, dining facilities, and much more. In addition, Georgia's climate is conducive to many outdoor recreational amenities, offering both urban and rural opportunities year-round.

GRADUATES

Graduates and undergraduates intermingle at the dining facilities, athletic center, and campus wide activities.

Admissions

REQUIREMENTS

In addition to the traditional requirements of 1 year each of biology, chemistry, physics, and organic chemistry, Emory also requires 6 semester hours of English and 18 semester hours of humanities and behavioral/social science course work. The MCAT is required. For applicants who have retaken the exam, the best set of scores is typically weighted most heavily. Emory operates a rolling admissions process, making it beneficial to submit MCAT scores and application material early in the summer.

SUGGESTIONS

In addition to required courses, genetics and biochemistry are both strongly recommended. It is also important that students have patient contact in a clinical setting and show interests outside of medicine. Research experiences, volunteerism, and evidence of professionalism are also highly valued.

PROCESS

All verified AMCAS applicants are sent a supplemental application. Of the supplemental applications received, approximately 750 are invited to interview between October and February. Emory conducts group interviews that involve three applicants, two faculty members, and a current medical student. An additional one-on-one interview is conducted with a faculty member. On interview day, candidates meet the Dean of Admissions, tour the campus and affiliated clinical locations, and meet Emory medical students and faculty. Following the interview, accepted students are notified on a monthly basis. Students placed on the alternate list are encouraged to submit new information to update their files.

Admissions Requirements (Required)

MCAT scores, science GPA, non-science GPA, letters of recommendation, interview, essays/personal statement, extracurricular activities, exposure to medical profession, Emory Supplemental Application.

Admissions Requirements (Optional)

State residency.

Overlap Schools

Duke University, Johns Hopkins University, Medical College of Georgia, University of Pennsylvania, Vanderbilt University, Washington University, Yale University.

COSTS AND AID

Tuition & Fees

Tuition	$36,000
Room and board (off campus)	$17,568
Cost of books	$2,108
Fees	$534

Financial Aid

% students receiving aid	80
Average grant	$19,877
Average loan	$36,141
Average debt	$114,078

FLORIDA STATE UNIVERSITY
COLLEGE OF MEDICINE

ADMISSIONS OFFICE, 1115 WEST CALL STREET, TALLAHASSEE, FL 32306-4300 • ADMISSION: 850-644-7904
FAX: 850-645-1420 • E-MAIL: MEDINFORMATION@MED.FSU.EDU • WEBSITE: WWW.MED.FSU.EDU/

STUDENT BODY

Type	Public
Enrollment	115
% male/female	61/39
% underrepresented minorities	31
# applied (total/out)	272/5
# accepted (total/out)	57/1
# enrolled (total/out)	46/0
Average age	23

FACULTY

Total faculty (number)	194
% female	26
% minority	13
% part-time	64
Student-faculty ratio	1:1

ADMISSIONS

Average GPA and MCAT Scores

Overall GPA	3.6
MCAT Bio	9.4
MCAT Phys	8.9
MCAT Verbal	8.3
MCAT Essay	0

Application Information

Regular application	12/1
Regular notification	4/15
Early application	8/1
Early notification	9/3
Are transfers accepted?	no
Admissions may be deferred?	yes
Interview required?	yes

Academics

The FSU College of Medicine is truly a 21st century medical school. Created in June of 2000 by the Florida legislature, it is the first new medical school the country has seen in a generation and, as such, it is charting a new course for medical education.

BASIC SCIENCES: The basic science component of the training program takes place on the FSU campus and is integrated into the culture and value system of the liberal arts university. The curriculum is based on a biopsychosocial foundation that balances biomedicine, medical humanities, and social sciences. Clinical training will take place on the front lines of the health care delivery system in the North Florida region and throughout the state. The emphasis will be on ambulatory care settings such as physicians' clinics, HMOs, and chronic care facilities in rural, urban, and suburban areas. Because the FSU medical school will partner with existing medical facilities and practitioners throughout the state rather than operate a teaching hospital, students will have the opportunity to learn on the front lines of the health care system. Community campuses are being developed in Tallahassee, Pensacola, and Orlando and are planned for Jacksonville, Sarasota, and Fort Myers in partnership with local hospitals and practices. Nonprofit community corporations in each location will provide community representation and input into the medical education program, as well as planning and coordination of student clinical experiences. A campus dean chairs each community corporation, which also is responsible for community education, fundraising, and advocacy on issues related to medical education.

Students

In partnership with Florida communities, the FSU College of Medicine is creating a new model of medical education and research that uses interdisciplinary teams and emerging technologies. Building upon the FSU Program in Medical Sciences, a first-year medical school program begun in 1971, the college's educational program is designed to produce compassionate physicians who will practice patient-centered medicine and who are prepared to practice in a rapidly changing health care environment. FSU trains the physicians of tomorrow in such a way that they will become lifelong learners equipped to teach themselves what they need to know in an era of tremendous innovation in knowledge management and information technology.

STUDENT LIFE

The Florida State University College of Medicine carefully selects students who are outstanding academically and are committed to the college's mission of service to Florida's medically underserved populations. FSU medical students come from all over Florida and are culturally diverse. Many come from small towns and rural areas, but the state's major metropolitan areas are also well represented. A number of students are older than average for medical school and bring a broad range of professional and life experiences, while others come straight out of undergraduate programs. Most are active in student organizations, community service projects, and medical outreach programs.

Admissions

REQUIREMENTS

The College of Medicine is searching for students who have demonstrated through their lifestyle a commitment of service to others. The college encourages applications from traditional students, nontraditional students, and students from rural, inner city, or other medically underserved areas of the state of Florida. FSU College of Medicine is an Early Start

Program. Classes begin on June 1. Students apply through the AMCAS. Some are invited to submit a secondary application. FSU COM accepts approximately 50 students each year. An applicant should be a legal resident of Florida and should have completed the following required prerequisite courses: Biochemistry, biology, chemistry, English, organic chemistry, and physics. An applicant should meet academic standards predictive of success in medical school including academic grade point average and MCAT (Medical College Aptitude Test) score. An applicant's MCAT score should be dated no more than three years prior to the beginning of the year of the application cycle. A bachelor's degree is required by the time of matriculation to medical school. If an applicant is currently enrolled in a degree program, the program must be completed and final transcripts provided to the College of Medicine Admissions Office prior to the beginning of classes in May. An applicant should be a legal resident of Florida. Non-U.S. citizens must possess a permanent resident Visa.

The first-year class had a cumulative GPA of 3.62, an overall BCPM of 3.53, and the following MCAT mean scaled scores: VR/8.4; PS/8.9; WS/0; BS/9.3. While these statistics serve as guidelines, the College of Medicine considers applicants as individuals. Applicants are assessed on their qualifications without discrimination in regard to gender, sexual orientation, color, age, disability, race, religion, veteran status, or national origin. It is not possible to provide places for all acceptable applicants to the College of Medicine; consequently, failure to be accepted is not necessarily an indication that a student is considered unsuitable for a medical career. The College of Medicine is searching for students who have demonstrated through their lifestyle a commitment of service to others.

ELIGIBILITY

An applicant should have completed the following required prerequisite courses: Biochemistry, biology, chemistry, English, organic chemistry, and physics. Undergraduate degree credit that has been granted to the student on the basis of the College-Level Examination Program (CLEP), an International Baccalaureate Program (IB), an Advanced Placement Program (AP), or participation in dual enrollment will be accepted provided the credit appears on the official transcript.

An applicant must apply through the American Medical College Application Service (AMCAS) and submit the required supplemental application form. Information regarding applying through AMCAS can be obtained at the College of Medicine Pre-health Advising Office at 850-644-7678. If an applicant is invited, he or she will interview with two members of the Admissions Committee. Not all applicants are invited for interview, and such interviews are conducted only on the FSU College of Medicine campus at a prescribed time. An applicant who has been away from academic work for a prolonged period may require additional college work in order to be competitive. All applicants must apply online at the AAMC's website, www.aamc.org/students/start.htm. Applicants may begin to certify and submit their AMCAS application beginning June 1. The deadline for submitting applications to AMCAS is December 1.

PROCESS

The regular admission process begins in September and continues until late March. Interviews are scheduled between September and March and applicants are discussed and voted upon by the Admissions Committee. Typically about 150 applicants are interviewed each admission cycle. Those candidates who are accepted outright are sent acceptance letters. All others are held until the final meeting at the end of March, when all candidates for whom a decision has not been made are reviewed again and high alternate, alternate, and hold lists are compiled. Letters are sent informing applicants of their status.

The Admissions Committee utilizes all appropriate information including academic, personal, experiential, and demographic data in the selection process. Personal qualities such as motivation, sensitivity to the needs of others, excellent oral communication skills, and maturity receive particular attention along with strong academic credentials. In addition, personal attributes such as compassion and altruism that are, in the view of the committee, essential to the art of good medical practice are of special interest in the selection process.

Admissions Requirements (Required)

MCAT scores, science GPA, non-science GPA, letters of recommendation, interview, state residency, essays/personal statement, extracurricular activities, exposure to medical profession.

Overlap Schools

University of Florida, University of Miami, University of South Florida.

COSTS AND AID

Tuition & Fees

In-state Tuition	$13,349
Room and board (on campus)	$6,274
Room and board (off campus)	$13,461
Cost of books	$7,601
Fees	$1,400

Financial Aid

% students receiving aid	90
Average grant	$1,200
Average loan	$22,962

THE GEORGE WASHINGTON UNIVERSITY
SCHOOL OF MEDICINE AND HEALTH SCIENCES

OFFICE OF ADMISSIONS, 2300 I STREET, NW, ROSS HALL 716, WASHINGTON, DC 20037 • ADMISSION: 202-994-3506
FAX: 202-994-1753 • E-MAIL: MEDADMIT@GWU.EDU • WEBSITE: WWW.GWUMC.EDU/EDU/ADMIS

STUDENT BODY

Type	Private
Enrollment	675
% male/female	45/55
% underrepresented minorities	16
# applied (total/out)	7,776
# accepted (total/out)	358
# enrolled (total/out)	177
Average age	24

FACULTY

Total faculty (number)	2,419
% female	34
% minority	24
% part-time	74
Student-faculty ratio	1:1

ADMISSIONS

Average GPA and MCAT Scores

Overall GPA	3.55
MCAT Bio	9.82
MCAT Phys	9.52
MCAT Verbal	9.41
MCAT Essay	P

Application Information

Regular application	12/1
Regular notification	rolling
Early application	6/1–8/1
Early notification	10/1
Are transfers accepted?	yes
Admissions may be deferred?	yes
Interview required?	yes
Application fee	$105

Academics

The George Washington University School of Medicine and Health Sciences is located in the heart of Washington, DC. Within the larger mission of the university, the vision of The George Washington University Medical Center is to be a preeminent academic health institution, dedicated to improving the health and well-being of our local community, our country, and beyond. The Medical Center works to achieve this goal through commitment to excellence and innovation in education and to research that expands the frontiers of science and knowledge.

BASIC SCIENCES: The George Washington University MD curriculum prepares well-trained physicians to complete residencies in primary care or specialized areas of concentration. Our medical school also stresses education through cooperation and collaboration rather than competition and emphasizes working with groups of colleagues and coworkers. Courses in anatomy, biochemistry, immunology, microbiology, neurobiology, and physiology constitute the first-year study. The second-year curriculum focuses on abnormal human biology through courses in pathology, pharmacology, and an interdisciplinary, organ-system course titled introduction to clinical medicine (ICM).

CLINICAL TRAINING

The School of Medicine curriculum contains a unique course titled the practice of medicine (POM). This revolutionary course, spanning all four years, allows students to begin clinical training during their first year of medical school while at the same time learning the traditional basic sciences. During POM, students learn about the doctor-patient relationship, essential communication skills, basic clinical assessment skills of interviewing and physical examination, professionalism, ethics, and many issues of the medicine-society interface.

The GW Clinical Learning and Simulation Skills (CLASS) Center is housed on the sixth floor of the GW Hospital. Dedicated to education and research, the center features cutting-edge technology in a setting that is among the most innovative in the nation. It is in this setting that students gain the comprehensive clinical exposure, feedback, and evaluation they need to become both technically adept and humane caregivers for their patients. This hands-on experience proves invaluable in preparation for the USMLE Step II, Clinical Skills.

Students

The Fall 2005 entering class hailed from 32 different states, spanning the United States from Oregon to Florida and matriculating from 82 different undergraduate institutions. Forty percent of incoming students were nonscience majors and 17 percent held various graduate degrees. Last year's entering class ranged in age from 20–47 years old.

STUDENT LIFE

The GW campus is nestled in the Foggy Bottom area of Washington, DC, and is within walking distance of the White House and many other governmental, historical, and cultural landmarks. The campus is subway-accessible; the Foggy Bottom/GWU metro stop sits immediately outside of the School of Medicine. A new Student Opporutunity Office provides a wealth of resources and coordinates the new track programs. A state-of-the-art Health and Wellness Center, one block from Ross Hall, is an 188,000-square-foot facility that hosts a wide variety of fitness and instructional classes; walk-in recreation; and sport club, intramural, and wellness programs and services.

GRADUATES

The GW SMHS maintains a national reputation for placing qualified graduates into quality residency programs. Many students choose to continue their postgraduate work at GW and be a part of our new state-of-the-art hospital. In fact, of the graduating class of 2006, 19 members remained at GW to complete their residencies. Some of the other institutions at which members of the class of 2006 were placed include Yale University, Mt. Sinai Hospital, and the Mayo Clinic. The following list indicates some of the specialties and/or programs that were most highly matched by GW graduates: Anesthesia, emergency medicine, family practice, ob/gyn, medicine, pediatrics, psychiatry, radiology, surgery, and urology.

Admissions

REQUIREMENTS

Applicants must have completed 90 semester hours at an accredited American or Canadian college or university prior to matriculation. Applicants must be United States or Canadian citizens or United States permanent residents.

Applicants must have completed 6 credits of English as well as 6 credits of lecture and 2 credits of lab in each of the following sciences at an accredited American or Canadian college or university prior to matriculation: Biology (botany or biochemistry courses do not fulfill this requirement), general chemistry, organic chemistry, and physics. Last year's entering class averaged an overall GPA of 3.56 and a science GPA of 3.46.

The MCAT is required and should be taken no more than three years prior to the year of medical school matriculation.

SUGGESTIONS

We strongly urge you to complete your file as early as possible.

PROCESS

Once the Admissions Office receives an AMCAS application, the secondary application is sent to the applicant. GW requires three letters of recommendation (two from science faculty and one from someone who is familiar with your personal traits), and a premedical advisor letter or committee advisory letter. It will take 4–5 weeks to process your application and letters of recommendation after we have received them. The application process is very competitive, as there are over 9,000 applicants for approximately 175 seats. Interviews and acceptances are offered on a rolling admissions basis. Please note the following deadlines:

* AMCAS: 12/1

* GW Secondary Application: January 1 (postmarked)

* Letters of recommendation: January 1 (postmarked)

* Each year the Admissions Office offers approximately 1,000 interviews to selected applicants. These interviews are blind (the interviewers do not read the applicant's file prior to the interview). Although we only offer interviews from September to March, acceptances into the class may be offered any time after 10/15 until early August. All final decisions will be mailed to applicants.

Admissions Requirements (Required)

MCAT scores, science GPA, non-science GPA, letters of recommendation, interview, essays/personal statement, extracurricular activities, exposure to medical profession.

Admissions Requirements (Optional)

State residency.

COSTS AND AID

Tuition & Fees

Tuition	$41,193
Room and board (off campus)	$13,950
Cost of books	$4,697
Fees	$360

Financial Aid

% students receiving aid	80
Average grant	$9,550
Average loan	$38,500
Average debt	$136,000

GEORGETOWN UNIVERSITY
SCHOOL OF MEDICINE

OFFICE OF ADMISSIONS, 3900 RESERVOIR ROAD, NW, WASHINGTON, DC 20007 • ADMISSION: 202-687-1154 •
E-MAIL: MEDICALADMISSIONS@GEORGETOWN.EDU • WEBSITE: HTTP://SOM.GEORGETOWN.EDU/

STUDENT BODY

Type	Private
Enrollment	699
% male/female	56/44
% underrepresented minorities	26
# applied	8,832

ADMISSIONS

Average GPA and MCAT Scores

Overall GPA	3.6

Application Information

Regular application	10/20
Regular notification	10/15
Are transfers accepted?	yes
Interview required?	yes
Application fee	$130

Academics

While most students earn their MD through a 4 year program, some extend their studies more than five years to take part in year-long research projects between their second and third years. Others participate in combined degree programs leading to the MD and the PhD in biochemistry, bioethics, biophysics, cell biology, molecular biology, microbiology and immunology, pathology, pharmacology, physiology, neuroscience, tumor biology, or other disciplines. The proximity of the National Institute of Health facilitates student involvement in important research projects, either during summers or year-long periods. Medical students are evaluated with grades of honors, high pass, pass, and fail, with the exception of elective courses, which are usually taken as satisfactory/unsatisfactory. Passing Step 1 of the USMLE is a requirement for promotion to year 3, and passing Step 2 is a graduation requirement.

BASIC SCIENCES: The first two years focus on basic science instruction but incorporate interdisciplinary courses; principles of patient care; problem-based learning modules; and ethical, social, economic, and religious aspects of health care as well. Lectures, labs, and small-group discussions are the teaching methods used, with students in scheduled sessions for about 22 hours per week. A student-run note taking service assists with the volume of material presented during the first two years. First-year courses are ambulatory care, biochemistry, biostatistics and epidemiology, embryology, endocrinology, gross anatomy, introduction to health care, introduction to the patient, medical data and reasoning, microscopic anatomy, neurobiology, and physiology. Second-year courses are ambulatory care, clinical problem solving, microbiology and immunology, pathology, pharmacology, physical diagnosis, and psychiatry. Also during the second year, 2 hours each week are reserved for elective courses, some of which may be taken at Georgetown's main campus. Basic science instruction takes place in several science/research buildings that are part of the medical center complex. The Dahlgren Memorial Library houses over 177,000 volumes and subscribes to over 1,800 journals. Within the library is the Biomedical Academic Computer Center (BACC), with a variety of audiovisual, computer, and educational services. Students have access to the Internet, e-mail, medical software, and databases.

CLINICAL TRAINING

Third-year required rotations are medicine (12 weeks), surgery (12 weeks), pediatrics (6 weeks), ob/gyn (6 weeks), neurology (4 weeks), psychiatry (4 weeks), and family medicine (4 weeks). Fourth-year requirements are medicine (6 weeks), surgery (6 weeks), emergency medicine (4 weeks), selectives (20 weeks), and electives (20 weeks). Medical students train at the Georgetown University Hospital (407 beds) and at nine other affiliated federal and community hospitals in the Washington, DC, metropolitan area. Electives may be taken abroad through Georgetown's International Programs or through individually arranged clerkships. Examples of possible training sites are the Bahamas, Colombia, and the Dominican Republic.

Students

Virtually all states are represented in the student body. Among students in the entering class, 49 percent majored in biological sciences, 24 percent in physical sciences, 18 percent in social sciences, and 9 percent in various humanities or other disciplines. Approximately 11 percent of students are underrepresented minorities. Class size is 165.

STUDENT LIFE

Though Georgetown is a Jesuit institution, the school encourages students of all denominations to express their spirituality. In addition to religious organizations, student groups focused on professional interests and community service are active. Outside of the classroom, students socialize at organized events and informally in common areas such as the new Student Lounge in the Pre-clinical Science Building. Medical students take advantage of the Yates Memorial Field House, which is conveniently located behind the library. It has a pool, track, squash and tennis courts, a fitness center, and other athletic facilities. At the Leavey Center, students enjoy performing arts, shops, services, and restaurants. Washington, DC has vast cultural and recreational opportunities. Admission to the Smithsonian museums is free, restaurants abound, Rock Creek Park offers running and biking trails, and the city's attractions are all accessible on the metro system. A free shuttle between the medical center and nearby metro stations is provided. Baltimore, Philadelphia, and New York are easily reached by train, and the Appalachian Mountains and the Atlantic coast are within a few hours drive. All students live off campus, within walking or biking distance of campus.

GRADUATES

Graduates are successful in securing residency positions at institutions throughout the country.

Admissions

REQUIREMENTS

Prerequisites are 1 year each of biology, chemistry, English, math, organic chemistry, and physics. One semester of biochemistry may be substituted for 1 semester of organic chemistry. Science courses should include associated labs. The MCAT is required, and scores should be from within the past three years. All sets of scores are considered.

SUGGESTIONS

Recommended courses include biochemistry, computer science, cellular physiology, genetics, embryology, biostatistics, physical chemistry, and quantitative analysis. Applications are not processed until MCAT scores are received. Thus, the April MCAT is preferable to the August exam. The Admissions Committee considers character, maturity, and motivation along with academic achievement.

PROCESS

All AMCAS applicants are sent secondary applications. Of those returning secondaries, about 15 percent are interviewed between September and May. Interviews consist of one session with a faculty member or senior medical student. Also on interview day, candidates have lunch with medical students, tour the campus, and attend informational meetings. About 20 percent of interviewees are accepted. Notification begins after 10/15 and continues on a rolling basis. A few highly qualified Georgetown undergraduates may be accepted to the School of Medicine during their sophomore year without MCAT scores.

Admissions Requirements (Required)

MCAT scores, science GPA, non-science GPA, letters of recommendation, interview, state residency, extracurricular activities, exposure to medical profession.

Admissions Requirements (Optional)

Essays/personal statement.

COSTS AND AID

Tuition & Fees

Tuition	$33,670
Room and board (on campus)	$10,560
Cost of books	$1,759
Fees	$1,330

Financial Aid

% students receiving aid	75

HARVARD UNIVERSITY
HARVARD MEDICAL SCHOOL

OFFICE OF ADMISSIONS, 210 GORDON HALL, 25 SHATTUCK STREET, BOSTON, MA 02115 • **ADMISSION:** 617-432-1550
FAX: 617-432-3307 • **E-MAIL:** ADMISSIONS_OFFICE@HMS.HARVARD.EDU • **WEBSITE:** WWW.HMS.HARVARD.EDU

STUDENT BODY

Type	Private
Enrollment	735
% male/female	43/57
% underrepresented minorities	22
# applied	5,396
# accepted	250
# enrolled	165
Average age	23

FACULTY

Total faculty (number)	9,352

ADMISSIONS

Average GPA and MCAT Scores

Overall GPA	3.79
MCAT Bio	12.04
MCAT Phys	12
MCAT Verbal	11.01
MCAT Essay	Q

Application Information

Regular application	10/15
Regular notification	3/7
Are transfers accepted?	no
Admissions may be deferred?	yes
Interview required?	yes
Application fee	$85

Academics

Two distinct programs are available at Harvard—the New Pathway and the Health Science and Technology (HST) Program. All entering students are assigned to one of five societies, organizational units used both to structure academic activities and to facilitate interaction among students and between faculty and students. Joint-degree opportunities include the MSTP, other MD/PhD programs designed in collaboration with science and nonscience graduate departments, the combined MD/MPH, and an MD/MPP with the Kennedy School of Government. More than half of the students take at least five years to complete their education to take full advantage of scholastic and research opportunities, some of which are actually off campus and perhaps overseas.

BASIC SCIENCES: Students in the first year of the New Pathway concentrate on biomedical and social sciences. The year is divided into six sections: Chemistry and biology of the cell, genetics, the human body, immunology, physiology, and pharmacology. Students are also introduced to clinical medicine in their first year. Year 2 has four segments: Human nervous system, human systems I, human systems II, and pathology. Concepts of behavioral and community health are integrated into the basic science studies. During the first two years, lectures are scheduled for only one hour out of each day. Lectures are enhanced with tutorials and labs, but most learning takes place outside of the classroom environment. Students are responsible for addressing specific clinical challenges through independent and small-group research and analysis. Participants in HST also manage their own learning but pose questions to answer through research rather than answering questions that arise through case presentations. During the fall semester of year 1, HST students take the following: Cellular and molecular immunology, functional human anatomy, genetics, human pathology, and molecular biology. During the spring semester, students take endocrinology; cardiovascular, renal, and respiratory pathophysiology; and research. Electives in social and clinical medicine are taken throughout the year. During year 2, students take gastroenterology, microbial pathogenesis, neuroscience, reproductive biology, and research during the first semester and clinical medicine, hematology, pharmacology, and psychopathology during the second semester. HST students complete a thesis as part of their requirements. Computers, loaded with curriculum-related software and linked with online data sources, are considered an important information management tool and are accessible in the Educational Center, the library, and the residence hall. The Countway Library of Medicine has one of the largest biomedical collections in the country. Grading is Satisfactory/Unsatisfactory for all courses. Passing Step 1 of the USMLE is required prior to graduation.

CLINICAL TRAINING

Patient contact begins in year 1, when students learn to take histories and become familiar with basic elements of the physical exam. Formal clinical instruction begins in year 3, when HST and New Pathway students join for required clerkships. These are medicine (4 months), women's and children's health (3 months), surgery (3 months), neurology (1 month), psychiatry (1 month), and radiology (1 month). Throughout years 3 and 4, students take part in ongoing, part-time primary care training. Year 4 is composed mostly of electives, which can be clinical and/or research oriented. Elective credit may be earned from several departments at Harvard University or from MIT. Clinical training takes place at Harvard-affiliated hospitals, which are Beth Israel Medical Center, Brigham and Women's Hospital, Cambridge Hospital, The Center for Blood Research, The Children's Hospital, The Dana-Farber Cancer Institute, DVA Medical Center, Harvard Pilgrim Health Care, Joslin Diabetes Center, Judge Baker Children's Center, Massachusetts Eye and Ear, Massachusetts General, Massachusetts Mental Health Center, McLean Hospital, Mount Auburn Hospital, Schepens Eye Research, and Spaulding Rehab Hospital. Evaluation of student performance in clinical settings uses a high honors/honors/satisfactory/unsatisfactory scale. Narrative comments accompany these marks. In addition to formal rotations, students can gain experience in clinical environments through volunteer activities such as the Urban Health Project, which provides preventive and curative care to community health centers and underserved populations. Students must pass the USMLE Step 2 to graduate.

Students

About 75 percent of students were science majors in college. About 20 percent of the members of a typical class are underrepresented minorities, and about 30 percent took significant time off between college and medical school. Students are from all around the country. Class size is 165, of which 30 are HST and 135 are New Pathway participants.

STUDENT LIFE

The compact class schedule allows students to take part in activities of the medical school, the greater university, and the city of Boston. About 50 percent of medical students live in Vanderbilt Hall, a renovated building adjacent to the medical school. Married students live either off campus or in university-owned apartments. Students are active in organizations focused on topics ranging from support for various minority groups, to abortion rights, to soccer.

GRADUATES

Approximately half of each graduating class remains at Harvard for their residencies. The University of California at San Francisco also appears to be a popular choice. Of the graduating class, the most common specialty choices were internal medicine (34 percent), pediatrics (13 percent), general surgery (9 percent), and orthopedic surgery (7 percent).

Admissions

REQUIREMENTS

Requirements include one year of biology with lab, college-level calculus, expository writing, and physics with lab. Two years of chemistry are required, both of which should involve laboratory experience. For New Pathway applicants, at least 16 additional credit hours in nonscience courses are required. For HST applicants, calculus through differential equations and calculus-based physics are required. The quality of an applicant's undergraduate institution is assessed in evaluating his or her GPA. The MCAT is required, and all scores are considered.

SUGGESTIONS

Unlike many schools with rolling admissions, decisions at Harvard are made after all interviews are complete. Thus, applicants submitting scores from the August MCAT are not penalized. There is no preference for particular undergraduate majors, but demonstration of academic excellence is expected. In addition, most successful applicants have impressive professional, volunteer, community service, or other extracurricular achievements.

PROCESS

Harvard participates in AMCAS, and in the past, about 14 percent of applicants were interviewed. Interviews take place from September through January and consist of two sessions that last one hour each with a member of the Admissions Committee. Decisions are made in late February, and all applicants are notified at once. A wait list is established at that time, but usually only a few candidates are ultimately accepted from the list.

Admissions Requirements (Required)

MCAT scores, science GPA, nonscience GPA, letters of recommendation, interview, essays/personal statement, extracurricular activities.

Admissions Requirements (Optional)

State residency, exposure to medical profession.

COSTS AND AID

Tuition & Fees

Tuition	$35,800
Room and board (on campus)	$10,180
Room and board (off campus)	$11,525
Cost of books	$2,064
Fees	$2,976

Financial Aid

% students receiving aid	74
Average grant	$21,500
Average loan	$25,000
Average debt	$97,390

HOWARD UNIVERSITY
COLLEGE OF MEDICINE

ADMISSIONS OFFICE, 520 WEST STREET, NW, WASHINGTON, DC 20059 • ADMISSION: 202-806-6270
FAX: 202-806-7934 • E-MAIL: SHUMPHREY@HOWARD.EDU • WEBSITE: WWW.MED.HOWARD.EDU

STUDENT BODY

Type	Private
Enrollment	454
% male/female	51/49
% underrepresented minorities	59
# applied (total/out)	4,940/4,592
# accepted (total/out)	368/283
# enrolled (total/out-of-state)	138/118

ADMISSIONS

Application Information

Regular application	12/15
Regular notification	10/15
	until filled
Are transfers accepted?	no
Admissions may be deferred?	yes
Interview required?	yes
Application fee	$45

Academics

Although most students earn their MD in four years, some are given permission to complete requirements over a five-year period. The College of Medicine and the Graduate School of Arts and Sciences offer a joint MD/PhD program. The departments that award the PhD are the following: Anatomy, biochemistry, biology, chemistry, genetics, microbiology, pharmacology, and physiology.

BASIC SCIENCES: Basic sciences are presented primarily in a lecture/lab format. Students are in scheduled classes from 25 to 30 hours per week. First-year courses are anatomy; biochemistry; histology; microbiology; immunology; neuroscience; physiology; psychiatry; introduction to patient care, in which students visit clinics and interact with physicians; and introduction to psychodynamic thinking, which discusses healthy and pathological mental mechanisms. Second-year courses are the following: Genetics, epidemiology, immunology, microbiology, pathology, pathophysiology, pharmacology, physical diagnosis, physiology, and psychopathology. Grading is honors/satisfactory and unsatisfactory, and academic support services such as workshops, tutorials, and summer sessions are available. The USMLE Step 1 is required for promotion to the third year. Instruction takes place in the Seeley G. Mudd Building, which features auditoriums, laboratories, audiovisual, and computer-assisted study areas. The Health Sciences Library has 260,000 volumes and journals, video equipment, and a computer linkage with the National Library of Medicine.

CLINICAL TRAINING

Patient contact begins in the first year in introduction to patient care. Throughout medical school, students have the opportunity to gain clinical experience by volunteering and participating in community outreach programs. Others gain research experience through work at NIH or other prominent institutions. Formal clinical training begins in year 3 (or year 4 for those in a 5-year course of study), with the following required clerkships: Medicine (12 weeks), surgery (8 weeks), ob/gyn (8 weeks), pediatrics (8 weeks), psychiatry (6 weeks), rehabilitation and neurological disease (4 weeks), and family practice (4 weeks). For 2 hours per week, during one semester, third-year students attend lectures on ethical and legal issues in health care. Senior-year requirements are medicine (4 weeks) and surgery (4 weeks). In addition, students take 20–24 weeks of electives in 4-week blocks. Evaluation of clinical performance uses honors/satisfactory/unsatisfactory, and the USMLE Step 2 is required for graduation. Clinical training takes place largely at Howard University Hospital (300 beds). Other sites used are Howard University Cancer Center, Center for Sickle Cell Disease, Walter Reed Army and National Naval Medical Centers, DC General Hospital, St. Elizabeth's Hospital, VA Medical Center, Providence Hospital, Greater Southeast Community Hospital, Prince George's Hospital Center, Washington Hospital Center, and National Rehabilitation Hospital.

Students

About 60 percent of the students are African American, and about 10 percent are from African or Caribbean countries. An average of 30 states and several foreign countries are usually represented. From 10 percent to 20 percent of the students in each entering class attended Howard for undergraduate premedical studies. About 20 percent of entrants are considered nontraditional, having taken time off between college and medical school and participated in some sort of post-baccalaureate premedical program. Class size is 110.

STUDENT LIFE

Medical students enjoy both an active campus life and involvement in the greater community. They may participate in Howard University activities, such as its radio and television stations, intramural athletic teams and events, conferences, and social or special-interest clubs. Washington, DC is a center for cultural, academic, recreational, and obviously, political activities. In addition to being an international city, DC has a strong local, predominantly African American community that is highly diverse. The College of Medicine is part of Howard's downtown campus, which is metro accessible and convenient to lively neighborhoods and interesting parts of the city such as the White House and Smithsonian Museums. Housing for graduate students is available in modern, university-owned apartments. However, most students live off campus and either walk or take public transportation to school.

GRADUATES

About 25 percent of African American physicians practicing in the United States are Howard alumni. Howard graduates secure postgraduate positions at institutions all over the country. Significant numbers enter one of the 16 residency programs at Howard University Hospital or at DC General Hospital, where they are also supervised by Howard faculty.

Admissions

REQUIREMENTS

Requirements are the following: biology (8 hours), chemistry (8 hours), organic chemistry (8 hours), physics (8 hours), college math (6 hours), and English (6 hours). The MCAT is required and must have been taken within the past three years.

SUGGESTIONS

Beyond required courses, biochemistry, cell biology, and developmental biology or embryology are recommended. For students who have taken time off after college, recent course work is helpful. The Admissions Committee values activities that demonstrate an interest in working with underserved communities.

PROCESS

All AMCAS applicants receive secondary applications. Of those submitting secondaries, about 10 percent are interviewed with faculty or administrators. Others are rejected, advised to retake the MCAT, or put in a hold category and considered for interview later in the year. Of those interviewed, 70 percent are accepted on a rolling basis, and the rest are either rejected or wait listed. Wait listed candidates may submit supplementary information and grades. A limited number of high school seniors are accepted into a combined BS/MD program organized with Howard's College of Arts and Sciences that allows students to earn both degrees in a 6-year period. Through an early entrance program, a few students nationwide may be admitted to the College of Medicine after their college junior year.

Admissions Requirements (Required)

MCAT scores, science GPA, non-science GPA, letters of recommendation, interview, state residency, extracurricular activities, exposure to medical profession.

Admissions Requirements (Optional)

Essays/personal statement.

COSTS AND AID

Tuition & Fees

Tuition	$15,980
Fees	$903

Financial Aid

% students receiving aid	85
Average debt	$63,000

INDIANA UNIVERSITY
SCHOOL OF MEDICINE

ADMISSIONS OFFICE, 1120 SOUTH DRIVE, FESLER HALL 213, INDIANAPOLIS, IN 46202 • ADMISSION: 317-274-3772
FAX: 317-278-0211 • E-MAIL: INMEDADM@IUPUI.EDU • WEBSITE: WWW.MEDICINE.IU.EDU/

STUDENT BODY

Type	Public
Enrollment	1,159
% male/female	55/45
% underrepresented minorities	11
# applied (total/out)	2,760/2,104
# accepted (total/out)	409/100
# enrolled (total/out)	280/38
Average age	26

FACULTY

Total faculty (number)	1,291
% female	48
% minority	2

ADMISSIONS

Average GPA and MCAT Scores

Overall GPA	3.68
MCAT Bio	10.3
MCAT Phys	9.9
MCAT Verbal	9.8
MCAT Essay	P

Application Information

Regular application	12/15
Regular notification	10/15
Early application	6/1–8/1
Early notification	10/1
Are transfers accepted?	yes
Admissions may be deferred?	yes
Interview required?	yes
Application fee	$50

Academics

The School of Medicine in Indianapolis is part of the Indiana University (IU) Medical Center, which includes schools of nursing, dentistry, and allied health sciences. The Medical Center complex occupies 85 acres and is situated one mile from downtown Indianapolis. In conjunction with the University Graduate School, The School of Medicine offers selected students an opportunity to pursue MS or PhD degrees along with an MD. Through this program, degrees may be earned in anatomy, biochemistry, biophysics, genetics, humanities, microbiology, neurobiology, pathology, pharmacology, physiology, toxicology, and social studies disciplines.

BASIC SCIENCES: First-year students select one of the following nine locations for their pre-clinical studies: IU Bloomington, IU Indianapolis, Lafayette Center at Purdue, University of Notre Dame, Ball State University, Indiana State University, University of Evansville, Indiana University Northwest, or Fort Wayne Center for Medical Education at Purdue. While the curriculum is essentially the same at each campus, the methods of instruction may differ, with some programs relying more or less on case-based learning. At all schools, the core basic science courses are complemented by early clinical correlations. Throughout the first two years, scheduled classes account for 26–28 hours per week. At the Indianapolis campus, 80 percent of class time is devoted to lectures and labs, and 20 percent is used for small-group discussions. First-year courses are the following: Anatomy, biochemistry, evidence-based medicine, histology, microbiology, physiology, immunology, patient/doctor relationship, and concepts of health and disease, which teaches students how to apply basic science concepts to clinical problems. Year 2 courses include biostatistics, clinical medicine, medical genetics, neurobiology, pathology, and pharmacology. With the exception of clinical medicine, during which students join medical teams in hospitals, second-year courses use lectures and labs as instructional techniques. The Medical Center offers all modern learning tools, including computers and audiovisual equipment. The Ruth Lilly Medical Library (200,000 volumes) is located in the Medical Research Building in Indianapolis and serves the Schools of Medicine and Nursing. All campuses have affiliated library systems, and all libraries are electronically linked. The libraries have access to 400 databases and online informational resources. Evaluation uses an honors/high pass/pass/fail system. Passing the USMLE Step 1 is a requirement for promotion to third year.

CLINICAL TRAINING

All students spend their third year on the Indianapolis campus, rotating through 11 hospitals in the local area. The patient population is drawn from both urban and rural areas. Year 3 is largely composed of required rotations which include the following: medicine (8 weeks), surgery (9 weeks), pediatrics (8 weeks), ob/gyn (5 weeks), psychiatry (4 weeks), neurology (4 weeks), anesthesia (2 weeks), and family medicine (4 weeks). The required fourth-year clerkships are a sub-internship in medicine (4 weeks), emergency medicine (4 weeks), and radiology (4 weeks). Year 4 is mostly dedicated to elective study, which may be pursued off campus, around the country, or overseas. Students are required to achieve an intermediate level in all nine competencies and an advanced level in three competencies, pass both the USMLE Step 2 Clinical Knowledge and Clinical Skills examinations, and pass an OSCE in the fourth year to be eligible for graduation. Evaluation of clinical performance uses an Honors/High Pass/Pass/Fail system, augmented by narratives.

Students

Typically, 86 percent of the students in each entering class are Indiana residents. About 11 percent are underrepresented minorities, most of whom are African Americans. Approximately 4 percent of students are older than 30 at the time of matriculation.

STUDENT LIFE

Students are given a voice in school administration and curriculum development through an elected student government. Though student life differs from one campus to another, in general medical students benefit from the social and cultural offerings of a large university system. There is a wide range of lifestyles among students, with some living on campus in residence halls or apartments and others living off campus. Medical students have access to all campus recreational facilities and events.

GRADUATES

Slightly less than half of the 2006 graduating class entered residency programs in Indiana. Other popular locations for postgraduate training were Michigan, Illinois, and Ohio. The most common specialty choices were internal medicine (15 percent of the class), family medicine (13 percent), anesthesia (11 percent), pediatrics (10 percent), surgery (6 percent), and diagnostic radiology and emergency medicine (5 percent each). Approximately 44 percent of the graduating class entered fields considered to be primary care.

Admissions

REQUIREMENTS

The following undergraduate courses are required (one year each): Biology, chemistry, organic chemistry, and physics. All courses must include labs. Beyond GPA, the quality of an applicant's undergraduate course load is considered rather than the quantity of extra course hours. The MCAT is required and must be no more than four years old. If an applicant has retaken the MCAT, the most recent score is considered.

Invitations to join our community are based on scholarship, character, references, academic performance, and personal interview. IUSM gives preference to Indiana residents and nonresidents with significant ties to the state of Indiana; however, each year we also invite nonresidents to join our community. We uphold and honor equal opportunity guidelines.

SUGGESTIONS

Undergraduate course work in social sciences and humanities is important. For applicants who have taken significant time off after college, some recent course work is useful. The April, rather than August MCAT, is strongly recommended. Among out-of-state applicants, those with strong qualifications and some sort of ties to the state are the most likely to be admitted. The school aims to admit candidates who are likely to choose careers in primary care.

PROCESS

Almost all Indiana residents receive a secondary application, and about 93 percent of those returning secondaries are interviewed. Among out-of-state applicants, only highly qualified candidates are sent secondary applications and about 10 percent are invited to interview. Interviews take place on Wednesdays from September through February and are scheduled in the order in which completed applications are received. Interviews consist of a one-hour session with a team of faculty members. Notification occurs on a monthly basis, beginning in October. Applicants are accepted, rejected, or deferred and reevaluated later in the year. In the spring, a wait list is established. Wait-listed candidates may submit supplementary material if it adds new information to their files.

Admissions Requirements (Required)

MCAT scores, science GPA, non-science GPA, letters of recommendation, interview, state residency, essays/personal statement, extracurricular activities, exposure to medical profession.

Overlap Schools

Michigan State University, University of Illinois at Chicago, Washington University.

COSTS AND AID

Tuition & Fees

In-state Tuition	$23,276
Out-of-state Tuition	$42,130
Room and board (on campus)	$8,284
Room and board (off campus)	$9,968
Cost of books	$4,100
Fees	$755

Financial Aid

% students receiving aid	93
Average grant	$2,800
Average loan	$35,500
Average debt	$142,000

JOHNS HOPKINS UNIVERSITY
SCHOOL OF MEDICINE

733 NORTH BROADWAY, SUITE G-49, BALTIMORE, MD 21205 • ADMISSION: 410-955-3182
FAX: 410-955-7494 • E-MAIL: SOMADMISS@JHMI.EDU • WEBSITE: WWW.HOPKINSMEDICINE.ORG

STUDENT BODY

Type	Private
Enrollment	464
% male/female	55/45
% underrepresented minorities	14
# applied (total/out)	4,289/3,648
# accepted (total/out)	255/232
# enrolled (total/out)	121/109
Average age	23

ADMISSIONS

Average GPA and MCAT Scores

Overall GPA	3.84
MCAT Bio	11.9
MCAT Phys	11.7
MCAT Verbal	10.88
MCAT Essay	Q

Application Information

Regular application	10/15
Regular notification	rolling
Early application	7/1–8/15
Early notification	10/1
Are transfers accepted?	no
Admissions may be deferred?	yes
Interview required?	yes
Application fee	$75

Academics

In 1992 Hopkins implemented a revised curriculum that introduced case-based learning, exposure to clinical settings during the first year, and a physicians and society (P&S) course, which integrates social, economic, and ethical perspectives into the 4 year basic and clinical science curriculum. Studies leading to both an MD and a PhD or MA/MS in the following fields are possible: Biochemistry, cellular and molecular biology, biological chemistry, biomedical engineering, biophysics, biophysics/molecular biophysics, cell biology and anatomy, cellular and molecular medicine, genetics, history of medicine, history of science, medicine and technology, human genetics and molecular biology, immunology, medical and biological illustration, neuroscience, pharmacology, molecular sciences, physiology, and public health. The combined MD/MPH is particularly popular, which is not surprising given the excellent reputation of the School of Public Health.

BASIC SCIENCES: The first year is organized into the following four blocks, all 10 weeks in length: Molecules and cells (block 1), anatomy and developmental biology (block 2), neuroscience and clinical epidemiology (block 3), and organ systems (block 4). The P&S course is year-long as is introduction to clinical medicine, in which students spend two days a month working with a private physician. During the first year, classes end at 1:00 P.M. 4 days a week, giving students ample time to study. Many students take on research projects during the summer between their first and second years. Second-year students study pathology, pathophysiology, and pharmacology, which are offered as yearlong courses. All three courses are integrated and are organized around organ systems. Lectures, discussion, case-study, and labs are all important components of the basic science curriculum. With relatively few hours of scheduled lectures, students generally attend classes and do not rely on student note-taking cooperatives. Grading is honors/high pass/pass/fail. Faculty members, assigned to incoming students, both advise and monitor their progress. The Welch Medical Library and its three affiliated sites own over 380,000 books and subscribe to about 3,000 journals. It provides resources that support instruction, such as extensive database and Internet tools. The USMLE is not used for grading or promotional purposes.

CLINICAL TRAINING

Facilities for clinical training include the Johns Hopkins Hospital complex, which is comprised of numerous affiliates, is housed in 37 buildings, and contains over 1,100 beds. In addition to serving the urban population of Baltimore and the surrounding areas, Johns Hopkins Hospitals attract patients from around the country and the world. Students are exposed to patient care at renowned institutions such as the Wilmer Eye Institute, Adolf Meyer Center for Psychiatry, Brady Urological Institute, Clayton Heart Center, Meyerhoff Center for Digestive Diseases, the Children's Center, Oncology Center, Halsted Surgical Service, and Osler Medical Service. Students are also encouraged to pursue clinical experiences away from Hopkins and a significant number do so overseas. With faculty input, students determine the order of their required clerkships and electives. Requirements are the following: Medicine (9 weeks), surgery (9 weeks), pediatrics (9 weeks), psychiatry (4 weeks), neurology (4 weeks), ob/gyn (6 weeks), emergency medicine (4 weeks), ambulatory internal medicine (3 weeks), and opthalmology (1 week). Clinical instruction is generally carried out in small groups, and individual initiative is encouraged. Grading is honors/high pass/pass/fail for both required and elective courses. Through its subsidiaries, the Johns Hopkins Health Systems provides statewide health care services to individuals and health-plan participants. This integration into managed care operations, coupled with large federal research grants, suggest that the institution is financially stable.

Students

The diversity of the student body reflects the school's national reputation. A typical class has students from 35 different states and 70 or more colleges. As is the case with most top schools, half the entrants are women. Efforts are made to recruit ethnic minorities, and approximately 15 percent of the student body are from underrepresented minorities groups. Class size is limited to 120.

STUDENT LIFE

For some, social life revolves around school, where students spend a great deal of time. Others, particularly those from the area or with families, have lives outside of the medical school. Housing is available for single students or for married students living alone, in Reed Hall dorms adjacent to campus. However, most choose to live in apartments off campus. For those accustomed to New York or Washington, DC, the housing situation in Baltimore is good. The Housing Office assists students in their apartment searches. Recreational facilities, including a full-size gym, are free to medical students and are located next to Reed Hall. Several medical societies exist, including a Women's Medical Alumni Association, which provides support for women students and physicians. There is also a Student National Medical Association, which is active in both campus and community minority affairs.

GRADUATES

Graduates of Hopkins have their pick of residency programs, even those graduating with GPAs that are at the lower end of their class. About 50 percent of graduates enter primary care specialties; 20 percent ultimately enter academic medicine or work primarily in research.

Admissions

REQUIREMENTS

In addition to the typical requirement of 1 year each of biology, chemistry, organic chemistry, physics, and 1 year of calculus (or 1 semester of calculus and 1 semester of statistics), 24 semester hours of humanities and social sciences combined are required. Advanced placement credits accepted by the applicant's undergraduate institution may be submitted in lieu of taking the required courses for calculus, chemistry, and physics. Johns Hopkins does participate in AMCAS. The online secondary application may be accessed at any time after June 1, once the applicant has received an AAMC ID number but before the December 1 deadline.

SUGGESTIONS

Hopkins is concerned with both the academic and personal records of applicants and notes that intellectual progress through college is important. Extracurricular activities need not be medically related but should demonstrate humanistic values and perseverance.

PROCESS

About 15 percent of applicants are invited for interviews, which occur between September and March, and about 29 percent of those interviewed are accepted on a rolling basis. Applicants are interviewed by Admissions Committee members, and regional interviews may be arranged for applicants living a distance from Baltimore. At Admissions Committee meetings, decisions are made to admit, reject, or wait list applicants. In April, wait-listed candidates are notified of their position on the list.

Admissions Requirements (Required)

MCAT scores, science GPA, non-science GPA, letters of recommendation, interview, essays/personal statement.

Admissions Requirements (Optional)

State residency, extracurricular activities, exposure to medical profession.

Overlap Schools

Columbia University, Cornell University, Duke University, Harvard University, Stanford University, University of Pennsylvania, Yale University.

COSTS AND AID

Tuition & Fees

Tuition	$33,000
Room and board (on campus)	$9,080
Room and board (off campus)	$10,770
Cost of books	$1,890
Fees	$2,965

Financial Aid

% students receiving aid	80
Average grant	$15,836
Average loan	$20,000
Average debt	$95,919

LOMA LINDA UNIVERSITY
SCHOOL OF MEDICINE

LOMA LINDA UNIVERSITY SCHOOL OF MEDICINE LOMA LINDA, CA 92350 • **ADMISSION:** 909-558-1100
FAX: 909-824-4146 • **E-MAIL:** ADMISSIONS.SM.APP@LLU.EDU • **WEBSITE:** WWW.LLU.EDU/LLU/MEDICINE

STUDENT BODY	
Type	Private
Enrollment	661
% male/female	59/41
% underrepresented minorities	6
# applied (total/out)	3,990/2,083

ADMISSIONS

Application Information

Regular application	11/1
Regular notification	12/15
Early application	6/1–8/1
Early notification	10/1
Are transfers accepted?	no
Admissions may be deferred?	yes
Interview required?	no
Application fee	$55

Academics

Joint-degree programs are offered to qualified students. Along with the MD, students may earn an MS or PhD degree in fields such as anatomy, biochemistry, genetics, immunology, microbiology, neuroscience, molecular biology, pharmacology, and physiology. Examinations and other methods of evaluation are given percentile scores, but the courses are graded as pass or fail. Passing the USMLE Step 1 is a requirement for promotion to the third year.

BASIC SCIENCES: Although Loma Linda's curriculum covers the basic science topics typical of most medical schools, its religious affiliation adds another dimension. In addition to learning about human biology, the nature of disease, and the appropriate treatment for disease, first- and second-year students participate in a course called whole person formation, which emphasizes biblical, ethical, and relational aspects of the practice of medicine. Patient contact occurs during the first year in physical diagnosis and interviewing. Other first-year courses are biochemistry/molecular biology, cell structure and function, gross anatomy and embryology, human behavior, information sciences and population-based medicine, medical applications of the basic sciences, and neuroscience. Second-year courses are human behavior, microbiology, pathology, physiology, pathophysiology and applied physical diagnosis, and pharmacology. First- and second-year instruction takes place in facilities located on the Loma Linda campus and close to the medical center, giving students access to university resources and clinical activities. Computers are available in a comprehensive computer lab and are used for instruction and research.

CLINICAL TRAINING

Third-year required rotations are orientation to clinical medicine/preventive medicine (4 weeks), family medicine (4 weeks), ob/gyn (6 weeks), internal medicine (12 weeks), pediatrics (8 weeks), psychiatry (6 weeks), and surgery (12 weeks). Half of the fourth year is reserved entirely for basic science and clinical electives, and half of the year is split between required clerkships and selectives. Required clerkships are sub internship selectives (8 weeks, selected from family medicine, internal medicine, ob/gyn, pediatrics, and surgery), intensive care unit (4 weeks), neurology (4 weeks), ambulatory care (4 weeks), and electives (16–22 weeks). Training takes place primarily at Loma Linda University Medical Center (500 beds), the Jerry L. Pettis Memorial Veterans Hospital, Riverside General Hospital, and the White Memorial Medical Center in Los Angeles. Other affiliated sites are San Bernardino County General Hospital, Kaiser Foundation Hospital, and Glendale Adventist Medical Center.

Students

Most students are members of the Seventh-Day Adventist Church. About 6 percent of students are underrepresented minorities, most of whom are African American. Generally, there is a wide age range among incoming students, with the average at about 24. Class size is 189.

STUDENT LIFE

For the most part, student life revolves around the medical school and the immediate community. When in need of a change of scenery, Los Angeles and beautiful southern California beaches are a short drive. Perhaps as a result of a shared religious background, students are cohesive. Alcohol is not a part of the social life, as it is prohibited in the Seventh-Day Adventist Church. Beyond extracurricular activities sponsored by the medical school, students are welcome to participate in university-wide events and organizations. Medical students have access to the university's athletic facilities, and are active in intramural sports. Students live both on and off campus, and virtually all students own cars.

GRADUATES

Graduates are successful in securing residencies in all specialty fields. Loma Linda Medical Center is a popular destination for postgraduate training, offering about 25 residency programs.

Admissions

REQUIREMENTS

Prerequisite course work is 8 semester hours each of biology, general chemistry, organic chemistry, and physics. Applicants should have met the English and religion requirements of their respective undergraduate institution. The MCAT is required, and scores should be no more than three years old. For applicants who have taken the test more than once, all sets of scores are considered.

SUGGESTIONS

Courses in the humanities and social sciences are recommended, and applicants are urged to take the April, rather than August, MCAT. For applicants who have taken time off after college, recent course work is important. Some involvement in health care delivery is valued by the Admissions Committee. Preference is given to qualified applicants who are members of the Seventh-Day Adventist Church. However, others who demonstrate a commitment to Christian principles are also considered favorably.

PROCESS

All AMCAS applicants are sent secondary applications. Of those returning secondaries, about 10 percent are invited to interview between November and March. Interviews consist of 1 or 2 hour-long sessions with faculty, students, and/or administrators. On interview day, lunch, a campus tour, and the opportunity to meet with current students are all provided. About 40 percent of interviewed candidates are accepted on a rolling basis, while others are rejected or wait listed. Wait-listed candidates may send updated transcripts.

Admissions Requirements (Required)

MCAT scores, science GPA, non-science GPA, letters of recommendation, state residency, extracurricular activities, exposure to medical profession.

Admissions Requirements (Optional)

Interview, essays/personal statement.

COSTS AND AID

Tuition & Fees

Tuition $24,949

LOUISIANA STATE UNIVERSITY
SCHOOL OF MEDICINE IN NEW ORLEANS

OFFICE OF ADMISSIONS, 1901 PERDIDO STREET, PO BOX P3-4, NEW ORLEANS, LA 70112 • ADMISSION: 504-568-6262
FAX: 504-568-7701 • E-MAIL: MS-ADMISSIONS@LSUHSC.EDU • WEBSITE: WWW.MEDSCHOOL.LSUHSC.EDU/ADMISSIONS

STUDENT BODY

Type	Public
Enrollment	712
% male/female	50/50
% underrepresented minorities	15
# applied	1,179

ADMISSIONS

Average GPA and MCAT Scores

Overall GPA	3.7
MCAT Bio	9.5
MCAT Phys	9.0
MCAT Verbal	9.0
MCAT Essay	P

Application Information

Regular application	11/15
Regular notification	rolling
Early application	9/1
Early notification	10/1
Are transfers accepted?	yes
Admissions may be deferred?	yes
Interview required?	yes
Application fee	$50

Academics

The course of instruction leading to the MD extends over a 4 year period. A revised first- and second-year curriculum was introduced and changes in the third- and fourth-year clinical curriculum were implemented. An honors program, which involves independent research and challenges the exceptional student, is open to those who excel during their first semester of medical school. For highly qualified students interested in careers in research, a combined MD/PhD program is available. Medical students are graded with honors, high pass, pass, and fail. All students are required to pass Step 1 of the USMLE following completion of year 2, and fourth-year students must pass Step 2 of the exam.

BASIC SCIENCES: Although most instruction uses a lecture format, small-group discussions and tutorials are also part of the curriculum. First-year courses are anatomy, biochemistry, cell biology and micro-anatomy, clinical correlation, human prenatal development, introduction to clinical medicine, neuroscience, medicine, medical ethics, physiology, psychiatry, and social issues in medicine. Electives are offered in community service, geriatrics, health promotion and wellness, and problem-based learning. Second-year courses are clinical pathology, immunology and parasitology, introduction to clinical medicine, microbiology, pathology, and pharmacology. Basic sciences are taught in a modern building that is part of the medical center complex. Important educational resources are maintained by the LSU Division of Learning Resources, which provides audiovisual and classroom services to the downtown campus of the LSU Health Sciences Center. The medical library in New Orleans has a total of about 188,000 volumes, nearly 4,000 audiovisual titles, and approximately 2,000 periodicals. The library is fully computerized and houses individual computers that are equipped with educational software programs.

CLINICAL TRAINING

The third and fourth years are devoted primarily to clinical rotations. Lectures, conferences, and small-group discussions supplement the hands-on clinical training. Year 3 consists of 8.5 days of ophthalmology course work in addition to rotations in medicine (12 weeks), general surgery (8 weeks), pediatrics (8 weeks), ob/gyn (6 weeks), psychiatry (6 weeks), family medicine (4 weeks), otolaryngology (2 weeks), and urology (2 weeks). The final year consists of 36 weeks divided into nine 4-week blocks, which include an acting internship, ambulatory care, general medicine, neural sciences, and special topics. The special-topics block includes drug and alcohol abuse, financial planning, geriatrics, human sexuality, nutrition, and office management. The remainder of the year may include electives either in basic or clinical sciences with 4 weeks allowed for vacation. Most training takes place at LSU-affiliated hospitals including Charity Hospital, which has a total of 2,200 beds. Elective requirements may be fulfilled at any accredited medical school or teaching hospital in the United States or Canada. With approval, electives may also be taken at foreign institutions.

Students

All students are Louisiana residents. Approximately 15 percent of students are under-represented minorities, most of whom are African American. The average age of entering students is about 23, and there are usually a number of students in their late 20s and 30s. Class size is 165.

STUDENT LIFE

Some medical students are active in the student government, which works closely with the faculty and the administration on a range of important issues. Others are involved in the student publication or in any number of professional clubs, honor societies, recreational groups, and community service projects. Extracurricular opportunities in New Orleans abound. The restaurants, music scene, historic and cultural sights, and annual festivals and events are world-renowned. Some students opt to live in the school's residence hall, which has its own student center. Others live off campus where housing is generally reasonably priced.

GRADUATES

The school assists and advises graduating students in obtaining suitable appointments in hospitals. LSU—New Orleans offers a comprehensive graduate medical education program in more than 20 specialty fields.

Admissions

REQUIREMENTS

Louisiana residency is a requirement. Prerequisite courses are 8 semester hours each of biology, chemistry, organic chemistry, and physics, all with associated labs. Strength in both written and spoken English is required. The MCAT is required, and scores should be from within the past three years. For applicants who have taken the exam more than once, the most recent set of scores is weighed most heavily.

SUGGESTIONS

A well-rounded undergraduate experience with course work in English, humanities, math, and social sciences is advised. Community service or medically related work or volunteer activities are valued.

PROCESS

All AMCAS applicants who are Louisiana residents are sent secondary applications. Of those returning secondaries, about 50 percent are invited to interview between October and April. The interview consists of two or three one-on-one sessions, each with a faculty member, student, or administrator. On interview day, candidates also have the opportunity to meet with students, tour the campus, and have lunch. About 60 percent of interviewed candidates are accepted on a rolling basis. Wait-listed candidates may send additional information to update their files.

Admissions Requirements (Required)

MCAT scores, science GPA, non-science GPA, letters of recommendation, interview, state residency, extracurricular activities, exposure to medical profession.

Admissions Requirements (Optional)

Essays/personal statement.

LOUISIANA STATE UNIVERSITY

SCHOOL OF MEDICINE IN SHREVEPORT

ADMISSIONS OFFICE, 1501 KINGS HIGHWAY, PO BOX 33932, SHREVEPORT, LA 71130-3932 • ADMISSION: 318-675-5190
FAX: 318-675-5244 • E-MAIL: SHVADM@LSUHSC.EDU • WEBSITE: WWW.LSUHSC.EDU

STUDENT BODY

Type	Public
Enrollment	391
% male/female	67/33
% underrepresented minorities	5
# applied (total/out)	1,046/272
# accepted (total/out)	27/0

ADMISSIONS

Application Information

Regular application	11/15
Regular notification	10/15
	until filled
Early application	6/1–8/1
Early notification	10/1
Are transfers accepted?	yes
Admissions may be deferred?	yes
Interview required?	no
Application fee	$50

Academics

The first two years are devoted to basic medical sciences with orientation to clinical applications. The second two years are devoted to clinical training and are spent primarily in hospitals and clinics. In addition to the MD degree, advanced studies leading to the MD/PhD are possible. The doctorate may be earned in anatomy, biochemistry, microbiology, pharmacology, and physiology. All medical students are encouraged to take advantage of the many research opportunities available during summers and year-round. Special funds are provided for this purpose, and medical students who complete prescribed research activities are awarded diplomas with the special designation Honors Research Participant. During summer terms, the school offers opportunities for rural, clinical electives. Medical students are evaluated with an A–F scale, with the exception of elective courses, which are pass/fail. Passing both steps of the USMLE is a graduation requirement.

BASIC SCIENCES: During the first year, students are in lectures, small-group seminars, labs, or other scheduled sessions for about 25 hours per week. Courses are biochemistry and molecular biology, biometry, CPR, ethics, family medicine and comprehensive care, histology, human anatomy, human embryology, introduction to computer-aided learning, library science, medical genetics, medical neuroscience, physiology and biophysics, psychiatry, and radiology. The second year is increasingly clinically oriented. Students are in class or other scheduled sessions for about 35 hours per week. Courses are clinical diagnosis, clinical neurology, clinical pathology, clinical-pathological conference, family medicine and comprehensive care, microbiology, pathology, perspectives in medicine, pharmacology, psychiatry, and radiology. A note-taking service, organized by and for students, assists with learning and retaining material. Computer-assisted instruction is a critical component of the basic science education, and all entering students are required to own a computer.

CLINICAL TRAINING

An unusual longitudinal clerkship called comprehensive care spans both the third and fourth years. In it, students work together and serve as the primary caregivers in a functioning clinic. Other third-year required rotations are family medicine (8 weeks), medicine (8 weeks), ob/gyn (8 weeks), surgery (4 weeks), pediatrics (4 weeks), psychiatry (4 weeks), and surgery subspecialties (3 weeks). A minimum of 16 weeks during the fourth year are reserved for electives. Required clerkships are medicine (6 weeks), surgery (3 weeks), pediatrics (3 weeks), and neuroscience (3 weeks). Most training takes place at the LSU Hospital (650 beds), the Shreveport Veterans' Administration Hospital, and the Comprehensive Care Clinic.

Students

All students are Louisiana residents. About 5 percent of students are underrepresented minorities. There is a wide age range among entering students, including those in their late 20s or 30s. Class size is 100.

STUDENT LIFE

Outside of class, LSU offers medical students a rich campus life. The university offers more than 60 student organizations in addition to intramural sports, performing arts events, visiting speakers, and social activities. The university center has dining facilities, a lounge, student activity rooms, and a bookstore, among other student services. Generally, it serves as a meeting place for students. The Health and Physical Education Building houses an indoor swimming pool; handball and racquetball courts; basketball; tennis, volleyball, and badminton courts; a dance studio; and fitness and weight training rooms. Shreveport is a historic southern city with a population of more than 370,000. Museums, art galleries, parks, gardens, restaurants, bars, and shopping areas are some of its many attractions. The cities of Baton Rouge and New Orleans are easily accessible. Houston, Memphis, Little Rock, and Jackson are also within driving distance. Most medical students live off campus.

GRADUATES

An increasing proportion of graduates are entering primary care fields. The majority of graduates return to Louisiana to practice.

Admissions

REQUIREMENTS

Admission to the School of Medicine is limited to Louisiana residents. Requirements are 1 year each of biology, chemistry, English, organic chemistry, and physics. All science courses must include laboratory work. The MCAT is required, and scores should be from within three years of application. For applicants who have taken the exam more than once, the most recent set of scores is generally weighed most heavily.

SUGGESTIONS

Once prerequisites are fulfilled, prospective applicants are encouraged to pursue their own interests and to develop their own special talents in gaining a broad educational background. In making admissions decisions, a candidate's motivation as well as his or her intellectual ability and preparation are assessed. Applicants must show potential of developing into mature, sensitive physicians who will inspire and deserve trust and confidence.

PROCESS

All AMCAS applicants who are Louisiana residents are sent secondary applications. Of those returning secondaries, about 30 percent are invited to interview between September and March. Interviews are given by members of the Admissions Committee, which is composed of Medical School faculty from the basic and clinical sciences as well as physicians from the community at large. The interview is used to assess personal traits and also allows candidates to see the facilities and to meet current students. Approximately 90 percent of interviewed candidates are accepted on a rolling basis. Others are rejected or wait listed.

Admissions Requirements (Required)

MCAT scores, science GPA, non-science GPA, letters of recommendation, state residency, extracurricular activities, exposure to medical profession.

Admissions Requirements (Optional)

Interview, essays/personal statement.

COSTS AND AID

Tuition & Fees

Out-of-state tuition	$7,900
Fees	$6,826

Financial Aid

% students receiving aid	81

LOYOLA UNIVERSITY CHICAGO
STRITCH SCHOOL OF MEDICINE

2160 SOUTH FIRST AVENUE, MAYWOOD, IL 60153 • ADMISSION: 708-216-3229
WEBSITE: WWW.MEDDEAN.LUMC.EDU

STUDENT BODY

Type	Private
Enrollment	544
% male/female	51/49
% underrepresented minorities	18
# applied (total/out)	4,413/3,574
# accepted (total/out)	290/188
# enrolled (total/out)	140/75
Average age	23

FACULTY

Total faculty (number)	1,323
% female	29
% minority	24
% part-time	52
Student-faculty ratio	2:1

ADMISSIONS

Average GPA and MCAT Scores

Overall GPA	3.62
MCAT Bio	10.2
MCAT Phys	9.9
MCAT Verbal	9.5
MCAT Essay	P

Application Information

Regular application	11/15
Regular notification	10/15
Are transfers accepted?	yes
Admissions may be deferred?	yes
Interview required?	yes
Application fee	$70

Academics

Students follow a 4 year curriculum leading to the MD degree. A dual degree MD/PhD program accepts up to three students each year. In this program, a doctorate degree may be earned in anatomy, biochemistry, cell biology, immunology, microbiology, molecular biology, neuroscience, pathology, pharmacology, or physiology. Evaluation of student performance uses honors/high pass/pass/fail. Students must pass USMLE Step 1 and USMLE Step 2 to graduate.

Stritch's curriculum relies on small-group sessions and problem-based learning as much as it does on traditional lectures and labs. Students are in class or other scheduled sessions for approximately 25 hours per week, discussing behavioral science and humanistic perspectives along with basic science concepts. First-year courses are host defense; molecular cell biology and genetics; structure of the human body; function of the human body; and patient-centered medicine I, a 3-year continuum that begins with the medical interview and later covers the physical diagnosis, health promotion, medical ethics, health care finance, and legal issues in medicine. As part of the course, each student participates in special mentoring programs, participating on hospital rounds with a primary care physician and chaplain. Second-year courses are neuroscience, mechanisms of human disease, pharmacology and therapeutics, behavioral development, and patient-centered medicine II. During years 2, 3, and 4, bioethics, professionalism, and ethics grand rounds take place. The Stritch facility includes classrooms of many different sizes to accommodate different instructional modalities, labs, video equipment, computer laboratories, lounges, study areas, and other spaces. The Health Sciences Library houses about 170,000 volumes and periodicals.

CLINICAL TRAINING

Required third-year rotations are surgery (12 weeks), internal medicine (12 weeks), family medicine (6 weeks), ob/gyn (6 weeks), pediatrics (6 weeks), and psychiatry (6 weeks). During the fourth year, requirements are sub internships (8 weeks), neurology (4 weeks), medical humanities (1 week), and 26 weeks of electives. Clinical facilities include Loyola University Hospital, Loyola Outpatient Center, Hines Veterans Affairs Hospital, Cardinal Bernardin Cancer Center, and a variety of community hospitals. Elective credits can be earned at other academic or clinical institutions.

Students
STUDENT LIFE

At Loyola, there is a very strong identity among each class. Class officers, including social chairs, promote numerous group activities, from small study groups to class-specific events to all-school social events. To help promote the interaction among classes, students from all classes are assigned to one of three communities. Each student has a wardrobe locker and mailbox within the community and shared study space along with a lounge area and kitchenette. Students also get to know one another through an active student government and almost 30 registered student organizations, which include professional, academic, social, and religious-based groups. Each organization has a faculty advisor, who in turn helps the student leaders and student members to direct their own organization. During the first two years, most pre-clinical courses end early enough to allow time for self-directed learning and extracurricular pursuits. Many students use this time to volunteer for public clinics, homeless shelters, senior centers, hospital-based pediatrics, school and reading programs, and to present educational health-related topics at various local schools. On- and off-campus events and programs also are sponsored by University Ministry, including international service experiences. In addition to student health and counseling services, there is a 62,000-square-foot health and fitness center adjacent to the medical school to help round out the physical well-being of the students. The center features various cardio equipment, a state-of-the-art aerobic/exercise studio, free weights and variable resistance equipment, basketball and volleyball court, aquatics area, elevated running track, racquetball courts, and spa and massage services. Off-campus activities are plentiful, as Chicago is easily accessible from the medical center. All students live off-campus and most within the western suburbs of Chicago.

GRADUATES

Graduates are successful in securing residency positions nationwide in primary care and specialized fields. In 2006, 72 percent of graduates remained in the Midwest, 12 percent went to the western United States, 10 percent to the East, and 6 percent to the South.

Admissions

REQUIREMENTS

Applicants must be U.S. citizens or hold a permanent resident visa. Prerequisites are one year each of biology, chemistry, organic chemistry, and physics, all with associated labs. One semester of biochemistry may be substituted for a semester of organic chemistry. The MCAT is required and scores should be from within four years of anticipated entrance to medical school.

SUGGESTIONS

Although state residents are given some preference, there are no positions reserved for them. Some recent course work is important for nontraditional applicants who have been out of school for a period of time. All students are advised to take the April MCAT so that the exam may be repeated in August if scores are not at the national average. Qualities that are sought in applicants are maturity, integrity, the ability to work with diverse populations, dedication to community service, and an awareness of the environment surrounding health care provision.

PROCESS

All applicants who meet minimum qualifications receive secondary applications. Of those returning secondaries, about 15 percent are interviewed between September and April. Interviews consist of two one-hour sessions, each with a faculty member, administrator, or student Committee on Admissions member. On interview day, candidates also have lunch with current medical students and tour the campus. Among interviewed candidates, about 50 percent are accepted on a rolling basis, with notification beginning in October. Wait-listed candidates, or those in a hold category, may send additional information to update their files and indicate interest in Loyola.

Admissions Requirements (Required)

MCAT scores, science GPA, non-science GPA, letters of recommendation, interview, essays/personal statement, extracurricular activities, exposure to medical profession, baccalaureate degree.

Admissions Requirements (Optional)

State residency.

COSTS AND AID

Tuition & Fees

Tuition	$34,500
Room and board (off campus)	$13,576
Cost of books	$3,810
Fees	$984

Financial Aid

% students receiving aid	94
Average grant	$10,886
Average loan	$41,128
Average debt	$136,791

MARSHALL UNIVERSITY
JOAN C. EDWARDS SCHOOL OF MEDICINE

OFFICE OF ADMISSIONS, 1600 MEDICAL CENTER DRIVE, HUNTINGTON, WV 25701 • ADMISSION: 800-544-8514
FAX: 304-691-1744 • E-MAIL: WARREN@MARSHALL.EDU • WEBSITE: WWW.MUSOM.MARSHALL.EDU

STUDENT BODY

Type	Public
Enrollment	211
% male/female	60/40
% underrepresented minorities	18
# applied (total/out)	785/618
# accepted (total/out)	102/19
# enrolled (total/out)	60/10
Average age	24

FACULTY

Total faculty (number)	239
% female	29
% minority	16
% part-time	17
Student-faculty ratio	1:1

ADMISSIONS

Average GPA and MCAT Scores

Overall GPA	3.5
MCAT Bio	8.9
MCAT Phys	8.2
MCAT Verbal	9.1
MCAT Essay	0

Application Information

Regular application	12/1
Regular notification	10/15
Are transfers accepted?	yes
Admissions may be deferred?	yes
Interview required?	yes
Application fee	$50

Academics

The academic curriculum is influenced by the needs of rural providers and the community's and the state's priorities. It is geared toward achieving greater retention of West Virginia trained physicians in underserved communities. Although most students complete a 4 year course of study leading to the MD degree, qualified students interested in research may concurrently pursue an MS or PhD in biomedical sciences. Evaluation of student performance uses an A–F scale. Passing Step 1 of the USMLE is required for promotion to year 3 and passing Step 2 is a graduation requirement.

BASIC SCIENCES: Basic science is taught primarily by using a lecture/lab format, although some time is spent in small-group discussions and clinical settings. Students are in scheduled sessions for about 30 hours per week. First-year courses are gross anatomy and embryology, behavioral medicine, biochemistry, human sexuality, introduction to patient care, medical cell and molecular biology, medical ethics, microanatomy and ultrastructure, neuroscience, and physiology. Second-year courses are community medicine, genetics, introduction to clinical medicine, immunology, introduction to patient care, microbiology, pathology, pharmacology, physical diagnosis, psychopathology, and medical ethics. The medical education building where basic sciences are taught is self-contained, with a library and other educational resources.

CLINICAL TRAINING

Third-year students participate in required third-year clerkships. These are medicine (8 weeks), ob/gyn (8 weeks), psychiatry (8 weeks), surgery (8 weeks), pediatrics (8 weeks), family practice (8 weeks), and clinical orientation (1 week). During the fourth year, required rotations are medicine (4 weeks), surgery (4 weeks), emergency medicine (4 weeks), and senior symposium (1 week). A full 23 weeks are reserved for elective study. During the third and fourth years, a total of 3 months must be taken in a rural area. Affiliated clinical teaching sites are numerous and include Cabell Huntington Hospital (300 beds), St. Mary's Hospital (440 beds), and the Veterans Affairs Medical Center (80 beds).

Students

Among entering students in a recent class, 37 percent graduated from Marshall's undergraduate college. A total of 28 other undergraduate institutions were represented in the class. Fifty-five percent majored in biology, 7 percent in chemistry, and the remainder in other disciplines. The average age of incoming students is about 25, with an age range of 20–45. About 17 percent are minorities, mostly Asians. Class size is 60.

STUDENT LIFE

The small class size at Marshall contributes to a supportive and friendly environment. Students are active in chapters of national organizations, and in groups like the Christian Medical Association, American Medical Women's Association, and the American Medical Student Association. Huntington is a small city, offering the amenities and resources that students need while providing easy access to rural areas. For more recreational and cultural opportunities, the larger cities of Pittsburgh and Cincinnati are each about a 4-hour drive away. Medical students have access to the athletic and recreational facilities of the main university and take part in university-wide events. University-administered housing options include university dormitories and units suitable for families. Off-campus housing is also affordable and readily available.

GRADUATES

Two-thirds of graduates enter primary care fields, which include family medicine, internal medicine, pediatrics, and ob/gyn. Graduates are successful in securing residencies inside and outside of West Virginia.

Admissions

REQUIREMENTS

Prerequisites are 8 semester hours each of biology, chemistry, organic chemistry, and physics. Six semester hours each of social or behavioral science and English are also required. An applicant's GPA is evaluated with consideration given to the academic institution and the rigor of courses taken. The MCAT is required and scores must be from within three years of matriculation. For applicants who have retaken the exam, the latest set of scores is weighed most heavily.

SUGGESTIONS

As a state school, Marshall gives preference to West Virginia residents. A maximum of 10 positions in each year's class are reserved for residents of states that border West Virginia, and for candidates with strong ties to the state. The April, rather than August, MCAT is recommended. In addition to the academic record, Marshall considers personal qualities such as judgment, responsibility, altruism, integrity, and sensitivity important. Strong communication skills are valued.

PROCESS

All West Virginia and bordering state AMCAS applicants receive secondary applications. Almost all West Virginia residents are interviewed, while only about 7 percent of out-of-state applicants are interviewed. Interviews take place between September and February and consist of two 30-minute sessions with members of the Admissions Committee. Acceptances are issued on a rolling basis. Wait-listed candidates may send information to update their files as the year progresses.

Admissions Requirements (Required)

MCAT scores, science GPA, non-science GPA, letters of recommendation, interview, extracurricular activities.

Admissions Requirements (Optional)

State residency, essays/personal statement, exposure to medical profession.

Overlap Schools

West Virginia University.

COSTS AND AID

Tuition & Fees

In-state Tuition	$14,200
Out-of-state Tuition	$36,400
Room and board (off campus)	$15,120
Cost of books	$2,000
In-state Fees	$888
Out-of-state Fees	$2,078

Financial Aid

% students receiving aid	94
Average grant	$6,093
Average loan	$33,396
Average debt	$132,857

MAYO CLINIC COLLEGE OF MEDICINE
MAYO MEDICAL SCHOOL

MAYO MEDICAL SCHOOL, 200 FIRST STREET, SW, ROCHESTER, MN 55905 • **ADMISSION:** 507-284-3671
FAX: 507-284-2634 • **E-MAIL:** MEDSCHOOLADMISSIONS@MAYO.EDU • **WEBSITE:** WWW.MAYO.EDU/MMS

STUDENT BODY

Type	Private
Enrollment	166
% male/female	51/49
% underrepresented minorities	13
# applied (total/out)	2,464/266
# accepted (total/out)	59/46
# enrolled (total/out)	42/25
Average age	26

FACULTY

Total faculty (number)	460
Student-faculty ratio	1:1

ADMISSIONS

Average GPA and MCAT Scores

Overall GPA	3.84
MCAT Bio	11.4
MCAT Phys	10.8
MCAT Verbal	10.6
MCAT Essay	Q

Application Information

Regular application	11/1
Regular notification	rolling
Early application	8/1
Early notification	10/1
Are transfers accepted?	no
Admissions may be deferred?	yes
Interview required?	yes
Application fee	$75

Academics

Each year, 34 students begin a 4 year curriculum, leading to the MD degree, and six students pursue a joint MD/PhD program in connection with the Mayo Graduate School. Through this program, a PhD may be obtained in biochemistry, biomedical engineering, cell biology and genetics, immunology, molecular neuroscience, molecular pharmacology and experimental therapeutics, tumor biology, and virology and gene therapy. Two students with DDS degrees are admitted each year for training toward careers in oral and maxillofacial surgery. Courses are grouped into units, which are the clinical experience, the organ, the patient, physician and society, the research quarter, and the scientific foundation of medical practice. All students are required to write a research paper while at Mayo, and 80 percent of these works are published. Evaluation of student performance uses honors, high pass, pass, marginal pass, and fail. The USMLE Steps 1 and 2 is a requirement for graduation.

Three weeks (held just prior to the third year) are devoted to preparation for the clinical clerkships in the third and fourth years. This includes the following: A radiology course, ECG course, survival skills workshop, and Breaking Bad News lecture.

BASIC SCIENCES: During the first 5 months of school, students take anatomy, immunology, molecular biology and genetics, and pathology and cell biology. The remainder of year 1 is organized around the following organ and physiological systems: Allergy, cardiovascular system, cutaneous system, digestive system, endocrine system, growth and development, hematopoietic system, musculoskeletal system, neuroscience, renal system, respiratory system. Patient contact begins in year 1, in Introduction to the Patient and Continuity of Care. Small groups and problem-based learning enhance the lecture/lab format and account for about one-third of the 28 hours per week of scheduled class time. The second year is split between clinical and basic science education. The first block of year 2 includes bioethics, ENT, microbiology and infectious disease, psychopathology, and sar/sexual medicine. In the next block, second-year students attend lectures and seminars and rotate through several clinical departments, evaluating patients under the guidance of a preceptor. Clinical rotations are medicine (9 weeks), pediatrics (6 weeks), dermatology (3 weeks), musculoskeletal medicine and rehabilitation (3 weeks), surgery (3 weeks), clinical skills aquisition (3 weeks), and family medicine (2 weeks). Tutoring and a wide variety of advising services are available to students, and a formal system is in place to identify and assist students who may be experiencing academic difficulties. Scheduled classes and labs take place on the Mayo campus, while independent and computer-aided instruction is offered in the Learning Resource Center located in the Mitchell Student Center. The Mayo Medical Library houses 353,000 volumes and subscribes to 4,300 journals.

CLINICAL TRAINING

The third year is divided into 4 quarters. The Research Quarter is a 13-week experience in which students participate in a biomedical research project and produce a related scientific paper. Three quarters are spent in clinical rotations: Medicine (6 weeks), surgery (6 weeks), pediatrics (6 weeks), ob/gyn (6 weeks), internal neurology (3 weeks), psychiatry (4 weeks), an elective at Mayo (3 weeks), and family medicine (2 weeks). Training takes place at the Mayo Clinic, Rochester Methodist, and Saint Mary's Hospitals, which together have 2,000 beds.

Students

The student body consists of about 170 students from more than 40 states. About 15 percent of a typical class are underrepresented minorities. Class size is 42.

STUDENT LIFE

The small class size facilitates cohesion among students. Mitchell Student Center, in addition to housing the Learning Resource Center, provides an area for relaxation and communal study. Students are involved in medically related organizations and societies, community service projects, and groups organized around athletic and cultural interests. Students also play an important role in the school's administration, participating in governing committees. Rochester's population is 80,000, offering concerts, theater, museums, golf courses, and parks, among other recreational opportunities. All students live off campus.

GRADUATES

In a class of recent graduates, 36 percent entered residencies in primary care. Specialties selected by more than one student were pediatrics (18 percent), diagnostic radiology (13 percent), anesthesiology (8 percent), internal medicine (8 percent), family medicine (5 percent), ob/gyn (5 percent), dermatology (5 percent), and radiation oncology (5 percent).

Admissions

REQUIREMENTS

Prerequisites are: Biochemistry (1 course), biology with lab (1 year), chemistry with lab (1 year), organic chemistry with lab (1 year), and physics with lab (1 year). The MCAT is required and must be no more than three years old.

SUGGESTIONS

Mayo is interested in undergraduate course work that demonstrates both aptitude in science and breadth of knowledge in social science and humanities. Substantial experience in community service and leadership are also very important considerations. Additionally, Mayo is committed to matriculating a diverse student body that includes students from racial and ethnic backgrounds, which are underrepresented in medicine.

PROCESS

No supplementary application is required. About 20 percent of AMCAS applicants are asked to submit letters of recommendation and participate in a telephone interview. About 50 percent of those screened applicants are invited to an on-campus interview. The interviews are scheduled between September and March. Applicants have two interviews about 30–45 minutes with faculty, students, community members, or administrators. Of interviewed applicants, about 20 percent are accepted on a rolling basis. Others are rejected or wait listed. Additional material from wait-listed candidates is not encouraged.

Admissions Requirements (Required)

MCAT scores, science GPA, non-science GPA, letters of recommendation, interview, essays/personal statement, extracurricular activities, telephone interview.

Admissions Requirements (Optional)

State residency, exposure to medical profession.

Overlap Schools

The University of Iowa; University of California—Irvine; University of California—Los Angeles; University of California—San Diego; University of Florida; University of Minnesota; University of Wisconsin—Madison.

COSTS AND AID

Tuition & Fees

Tuition	$24,500
Room and board (off campus)	$11,602
Cost of books	$1,846
Fees	$2,000

Financial Aid

% students receiving aid	100
Average grant	$18,375
Average loan	$22,150
Average debt	$84,604

McGill University
Faculty of Medicine

3655 Sir William Osler Promenade, Suite 602, Montreal, QC H3G 1Y6 • **Admission:** +1 514-398-3517
Fax: +1 514-398-4631 • **E-mail:** ADMISSIONS.MED@MCGILL.CA • **Website:** WWW.MEDICINE.MCGILL.CA/ADMISSIONS/

STUDENT BODY	
Type	Public
Enrollment	731
% male/female	45/55
# applied 1,044	
# accepted 253	
# enrolled (total/out)	173/32
Average age	21

FACULTY	
Total faculty (number)	824
% female	40

ADMISSIONS

Average GPA and MCAT Scores

Overall GPA	3.74
MCAT Bio	11.0
MCAT Phys	11.0
MCAT Verbal	10.0
MCAT Essay	P

Application Information

Regular application	11/15
Regular notification	3/31
Early notification	1/15
Are transfers accepted?	no
Admissions may be deferred?	yes
Interview required?	yes
Application fee	$80

Academics

CURRICULUM STRUCTURE: There are two central themes to the curriculum—physician as professional and physician as healer—which is grouped in four components brieflyoutlined below. The program utilizes a variety of teaching and evaluation methods, emphasizing small-group teaching.

The Basis of Medicine (16 months) covers the basic sciences, such as anatomy and physiology. The students have extensive opportunities for "hands-on" laboratory sessions, including cadaver dissection. The Introduction to Clinical Medicine component provides a clinical experience of 5 months duration in most of the core disciplines. Students are assigned to small groups in affiliated hospitals, community clinics, and in the offices of family physicians and are provided many opportunities to refine their clinical skills.

The Practice of Medicine (20 months) component begins with the core clerkships (internal medicine, pediatrics, general surgery, obstetrics and gynecology, psychiatry, and family medicine) followed by the senior clerkships including rotations in surgical subspecialties, geriatric medicine and emergency medicine. The clerkships all provide extensive clinical contact, under supervision by faculty members. The final component, physicianship & physician apprenticeship, is a unique component which spans all four years focusing on the cognitive aspects of the professional and healer roles of a physician. This component teaches the main elements of the clinical method including observation, skilful listening, medical history taking, physical examination, reasoning and hypothesis generation while the apprenticeship provides for mentoring and works for the gradual transition from layman to physician.

BASIC SCIENCES: The first academic period begins in September and continues through December of the second year. The theme of the first academic period is basis of medicine, and courses are organized into blocks. These are gas, fluids, and electrolytes (9 weeks); nervous system and special senses (8 weeks); host defense and host parasite (8 weeks); endocrinology, metabolism, and nutrition (7 weeks); molecules, cells, and tissues (4 weeks); musculoskeletal and blood (4 weeks); life cycle (3 weeks); and pathobiology, treatment, and prevention of disease.

CLINICAL TRAINING
The second academic period, introduction to clinical medicine (ICM), begins in January of the second year and goes through September of the third year. ICM takes place in hospitals and outpatient clinical settings. Topics covered are anesthesia, emergency medicine, family medicine, geriatric medicine, health law, introduction to clinical sciences, introduction to hospital practice, medical ethics, medicine, neurology, radiology, surgery, ob/gyn, pediatrics, psychiatry, and an elective. During the third academic period, practice of medicine, students rotate through required clerkships. These are medicine (8 weeks), surgery (8 weeks), psychiatry (8 weeks), ob/gyn (8 weeks), pediatrics (8 weeks), family medicine (4 weeks), and electives/selectives (16 weeks). The final academic period is called Back to Basics. During this 16-week session, students take medicine and society, topics in medical science, and ambulatory care. Teaching hospitals include Montreal General Hospital, Montreal Children's Hospital, Montreal Neurological Hospital, Sir Mortimer B. Davis-Jewish General Hospital, Douglas Hospital, and Royal Victoria Hospital. Training also takes place at a number of affiliated hospitals and other clinical care centers.

Students

Each entering class has about 172 students, with reservations for 12 students from the United States or other international applicants. The student body is among the most culturally diverse, and is approximately 55 percent women.

STUDENT LIFE

McGill is a large and active campus that offers social and recreational activities to a diverse student body. In addition, the city of Montreal itself is an interesting and exciting place for students to live. McGill offers three residence styles suited to your needs (including one women's residence), which are located on the main campus and are open to medical students. Information concerning apartments or flats located in the vicinity of the campus can be obtained from the Off-Campus Housing Office.

Admissions

REQUIREMENTS

The Faculty of Medicine offers a 4 year undergraduate medical curriculum. A premed (MED-P) program is available to Québec residents following an approved curriculum in the Québec Collegial system. The faculty does not accept transfers, part-time medical studies, or award advanced standing. Deferrals and leaves of absence may be granted on academic grounds. An MD/PhD program is offered for students interested in a research career in academic medicine. For students interested in both medicine and management, the faculties of medicine and management offer a five-year program leading to an MD/MBA degree. The language of instruction is English with option to submit papers and exams in French. Requirements include the following: Applicants must have received an undergraduate degree or be in the final year of a course of study at a recognized college or university leading to an undergraduate degree with at least 120 academic credits. Prerequisites include 1 year with laboratory work in each of general biology, general chemistry, and physics; and 1 semester with laboratory work in organic chemistry. The MCAT is required and applicants must have taken the exam no later than August 2004.

SUGGESTIONS

In addition to prerequisite science courses, some course work in biochemistry or molecular biology is strongly recommended. Applicants to the 4 year program should have undergraduate GPA of 3.5 or better and a total of 30 or more in the MCAT scores. In a recent entering class, the average GPA was a 3.75 and the average overall MCAT score was 31.10.

PROCESS

The deadline for receipt of applications to the regular MD/CM program is January 15 for Quebec residents and November 15 for all others. Applicants with strong academic qualifications submit an application that includes an autobiographical letter used to assess personal qualities and achievements. Selection for interview is based on grades, MCAT scores, letters of reference, and autobiographical letter. Once interviews have been completed, all the components of the application are considered in making admissions decisions. Residents of Quebec will be notified after May 1. Nonresidents will be notified as soon as possible after March 31.

Admissions Requirements (Required)

MCAT scores, science GPA, non-science GPA, letters of recommendation, interview, essays/personal statement, extracurricular activities, exposure to medical profession.

Admissions Requirements (Optional)

State residency.

Overlap Schools

Universite Laval, University of British Columbia, University of Montreal, University of Sherbrooke, University of Toronto.

COSTS AND AID

Tuition & Fees

In-state Tuition	$6,033
Out-of-state Tuition	$25,613
Cost of books	$850

McMaster University
Undergraduate Medical Programme

1200 Main Street, Room: 1M7 Hamilton, ON L8N 3Z5 • Admission: 905-525-9140
Fax: 905-546-0349 • E-mail: MDADMIT@MCMASTER.CA • Website: WWW.FHS.MCMASTER.CA/MDPROG

STUDENT BODY

Type	Public
# applied	3,732
# accepted	193
# enrolled	138
Average age	26

ADMISSIONS

Average GPA and MCAT Scores

Overall GPA	3.8

Application Information

Regular application	10/1
Regular notification	5/31
Are transfers accepted?	no
Admissions may be deferred?	yes
Interview required?	yes

Academics

The 3-year program in medicine uses a problem-based approach to learning that emphasizes skills, knowledge, critical thinking, independent study, professional behavior, and lifelong learning. The components have been organized in sequential units with early exposure to patients and case management. Flexibility is ensured to allow for the variety of student backgrounds and career goals. In addition to required units, electives form an integral part of the curriculum. Full-time elective blocks, ongoing horizontal electives, and special enrichment electives are all important components of the medical education. The 3-year program (130 weeks of instruction) uses an approach to learning that will apply throughout the physician's career. Flexibility is ensured to allow for the variety of student backgrounds and career goals. The graduates of McMaster's Undergraduate Medical Programme will have developed the knowledge, ability, and attitudes necessary to qualify for further education in any medical career. The general goals for students in the program include the following: the development of competency in problem-based learning and in problem solving; the development of the personal characteristics and attitudes compatible with effective health care; the development of clinical and communication skills; and the development of the skills to be a lifelong, self-directed learner. To achieve the objectives of the Undergraduate Medical Programme, students are presented with a series of health care problems and questions requiring the understanding of principles and data collection. Much of the students' learning occurs within the setting of the small-group tutorial. Faculty members serve as tutors/facilitators or as sources of expert knowledge. The Undergraduate Medical Programme is arranged as a four-unit pre-clerkship sequence followed by a clerkship; there are additional elective opportunities, both in block periods (totaling 27 weeks) and horizontal electives taken concurrently with ongoing units. Unit 1 is a 12-week introduction to concepts and information from three of the following knowledge perspectives: Behavior, biology, and population. In addition, a major theme of the entire curriculum, the life cycle, is developed as a perspective and anchors the three sub units of Unit 1 including early development, maturation, and aging units 2 + 3 are 14 weeks. Unit 4 is 13-week units organized on the basis of organ systems, in which biomedical and health care problems are analyzed in depth. The clerkship emphasizes the clinical application of concepts learned in the earlier units and consists of experience in inpatient and ambulatory settings. These concepts include family medicine, internal medicine, obstetrics-gynecology, pediatrics, psychiatry, and surgery. Unit 6, which follows the clerkship, is an interactive unit in which students will tackle issues derived from societal expectations of a practicing physician.

Students

Each entering class has 138 students. In a recent entering class, 130 were from Ontario, and 8 were from the rest of Canada. About one-third of the class is over 25, with an age range of 19–49. In this class, the male/female ratio was 32/106. Beginning in the Fall of 2000, McMaster has admited up to 10 students from a new International Applicant Pool.

STUDENT LIFE

The teaching methodology and general approach at McMaster fosters student interaction, which carries over outside of the classroom. Medical students take part in extracurricular activities including clubs, athletics, and community service. Off-campus housing is available.

GRADUATES

Postgraduate programs are offered at McMaster in anesthesia, community medicine, critical care, emergency medicine, family medicine, internal medicine, laboratory medicine, ob/gyn, pediatrics, psychiatry, radiology, and surgery.

Admissions

REQUIREMENTS

At the time of entrance, students must have completed a minimum of three years (30 full credits) of undergraduate work. Two years (20 full credits) must be above the year 1 level of courses. Only degree credit courses taken at an accredited university are considered. Applicants must have achieved an overall simple average of at least a 3.0 on a 4.0 scale in their academic work at the time of application. There are no specific prerequisite courses and the MCAT is not required. Students granted admission must be proficient in spoken and written English. All students are required to have obtained a current certificate in Basic Cardiac Life Support prior to registration in the medical program.

SUGGESTIONS

Priority is given to residents of Ontario and then to applicants from the rest of Canada. International students may choose to apply through this applicant pool.

PROCESS

The application and transcript deadline for submission to OMSAS is October 15. Approximately 400 applicants are invited for interviews at McMaster in March or April. All applicants are notified in writing on the last day of May as to the results of their application.

Admissions Requirements (Required)

Science GPA, nonscience GPA, letters of recommendation, interview, extracurricular activities.

Admissions Requirements (Optional)

MCAT scores, state residency, essays/personal statement, exposure to medical profession.

Overlap Schools

University of Ottawa.

COSTS AND AID

Tuition & Fees

In-state Tuition	$4,422

MEDICAL COLLEGE OF GEORGIA
SCHOOL OF MEDICINE

OFFICE OF ADMISSIONS, AA-2040, AUGUSTA, GA 30912 • ADMISSION: 706-721-3186
FAX: 706-721-0959 • E-MAIL: SCLMED.STDADMIN@MAIL.MCG.EDU • WEBSITE: WWW.MCG.EDU

STUDENT BODY

Type	Public
Enrollment	720
# applied (total/out)	1,742/769
# accepted (total/out)	258/3
# enrolled (total/out)	180/2

FACULTY

Total faculty (number)	595
% female	23
% minority	19
% part-time	13
Student-faculty ratio	1:1

ADMISSIONS

Average GPA and MCAT Scores

Overall GPA	3.66
MCAT Bio	10.37
MCAT Phys	9.88
MCAT Verbal	9.94

Application Information

Regular application	11/1
Regular notification	5/1
Early application	6/1–8/1
Early notification	10/1
Are transfers accepted?	yes
Admissions may be deferred?	yes
Interview required?	yes

Academics

The school emphasizes early patient contact, uses problem-based learning, and strives to educate physicians who will help meet the health care needs of Georgians. Students and applicants interested in earning both an MD and a PhD may apply to combined degree programs arranged with the School of Graduate Studies or with departments of the University of Georgia, Georgia Institute of Technology, or Georgia State University. Areas of doctorate study include, but are not limited to, anatomy, biochemistry, biomedical engineering, biophysics, cell biology, genetics, immunology, microbiology, molecular biology, neuroscience, pharmacology, and physiology.

BASIC SCIENCES: During the two pre-clinical years, students acquire the building blocks of basic science that underlie medical practice and the skills required for clinical decision-making and patient interaction. The modular content of the curriculum is taught in lectures, labs with integrated clinical conferences, and small-group activities. In the first semester of year 1, the introductory molecular cell biology module provides a foundation for the basic sciences and is followed by the cellular and systems structures module to introduce students to gross anatomy, histology, and development. In the second semester, biochemistry and physiology are taught in the cellular and systems processes module while the brain and behavior module gives students an understanding of the interplay between psychiatry and neuroscience. Offered concurrently with the basic science modules, the yearlong essentials of clinical medicine emphasizes family, cultural, and population aspects of health care, communication skills, and information retrieval and analysis, health promotion/disease prevention, ethics, history taking with children and adults, and a community project. The essentials of clinical medicine is a 2-year sequence that emphasizes skills needed for success in the third year. In year 2, essentials of clinical medicine addresses interviewing and physical examination, common medical problems, and interdisciplinary topics such as ethics, nutrition, and the impact of behavior on health while highlighting principles of patient care for each stage of life. Cellular and systems disease states is a yearlong module running in parallel so the students are exposed to the topics of medical microbiology, pathology, and pharmacology as the issues related to patient care throughout the stages of life. Teaching strategies, including interactive small groups, preceptor relationships, and lectures are linked to course objectives. On average, students are in scheduled activities for 26 hours per week during the first two years. Classes are held in the modern research and education building and the medical student resource area, which includes small group rooms with computers and Internet access. Each student is advised to purchase a computer capable of using relevant educational software. The Greenblatt Library maintains more than 1,800 current journal subscriptions and provides access to many external databases. Audiovisual learning aids are used in class and are available to the library. Grading is A–F with a C constituting a passing grade. Passing the USMLE Step 1 is a requirement for promotion to the third year.

CLINICAL TRAINING

Patient contact begins during year 1 in the essentials clinical medicine course, which extends through year 2. Year 3 consists of required core clerkships: internal medicine (12 weeks), surgery (8 weeks), pediatrics (6 weeks), family medicine (6 weeks), ob/gyn (6 weeks), psychiatry (6 weeks), and neurology (4 weeks). Core clerkships take place at the Medical College of Georgia Hospitals and Clinics, the Children's Medical Center, various affiliated hospitals, and community-based teaching sites throughout the state. Students may rotate to affiliated community hospitals for part of the core curriculum. During year 4, students must complete 4-week rotations in critical care, emergency medicine, and an acting internship in family medicine, gynecology, medicine, pediatrics, and surgery or obstetrics. The remainder of the fourth year is for elective study, which can include both clinical and research courses. Evaluation during the clinical years is based on assessment of knowledge, clinical skills, and professional behavior, and uses an A–F scale. Passing the USMLE Step 2 is a requirement for graduation.

Students

At least 95 percent of students are Georgia residents. Underrepresented minorities account for about 6 percent of the student body. About one-fourth of each class took time off after college, and there is a wide range of prior experiences within the student body. Class size is 180.

STUDENT LIFE

The campus is close to downtown Augusta, the second-largest metropolitan area in Georgia. Augusta offers a wide range of activities including museums, theater, restaurants, music, shopping, water skiing, sailing, tennis, and golf. Students are cohesive, brought together by popular on-campus housing and student groups. Students are involved in organizations focused on professional, social, athletic, and community service activities. Many on-campus housing options are available, including residency halls, 1- or 2-bedroom apartments, and family housing.

GRADUATES

In the past, the majority of graduates have selected specialized fields. As part of their generalist initiative, the Medical College encourages students to explore primary care. The goal of the initiative is for at least half of the graduates to enter residencies in family practice, internal medicine, or pediatrics. Students may remain at the Medical College of Georgia for their postgraduate study while others enter programs elsewhere in the state and the nation.

Admissions

REQUIREMENTS

Undergraduate preparation must include: Biology with lab (1 year), English (1 year), inorganic chemistry with lab (1 year), organic chemistry with lab (1 semester), physics with lab (1 year), additional upper-level chemistry (1 semester). Transcripts should have grades; pass/fail courses are not advised. The MCAT is required and must be no more than three years old.

SUGGESTIONS

The April, rather than August, MCAT is strongly advised. For students who have taken time off after college, recent course work is recommended. Experiences that involve patient contact is valuable. In addition to academic strength and general personal qualities, the Admissions Committee looks for an individual's potential for meeting the health care needs of Georgia.

PROCESS

All Georgia residents who submit AMCAS application are sent secondary applications, while only selected out-of-state residents receive secondaries. About half of in-state residents and less than 5 percent of out of state residents are interviewed. Interviews consist of two sessions that are a half hour each with faculty, administrators, or students. One interview is done by a member of the Admissions Committee and the other interview is done by a faculty member who is not a member of the Admissions Commitee. Interviews take place from October through March. Notification is rolling for regular admissions. After enough offers have been made to fill the class, an alternate list is established from which about 40–50 candidates are usually admitted.

Admissions Requirements (Required)

MCAT scores, science GPA, non-science GPA, letters of recommendation, interview, state residency, essays/personal statement, extracurricular activities, exposure to medical profession, completion of secondary application.

COSTS AND AID

Tuition & Fees

In-state Tuition	$11,850
Out-of-state Tuition	$30,976
Fees	$826

Financial Aid

% students receiving aid	90
Average grant	$2,663
Average loan	$22,674
Average debt	$90,696

MEDICAL UNIVERSITY OF OHIO
COLLEGE OF MEDICINE

3045 ARLINGTON AVENUE, TOLEDO, OH 43614 • ADMISSION: 419-381-4229
FAX: 419-381-4005 • E-MAIL: ADMISSIONS@MEDUOHIO.EDU • WEBSITE: WWW.MEDUOHIO.EDU

STUDENT BODY

Type	Public
Enrollment	565
% male/female	70/30
% underrepresented minorities	10
# applied (total/out)	3,698/2,472
# accepted (total/out)	37/6
# enrolled (out-of-state)	9

FACULTY

Total faculty (number)	335
% female	23
% minority	15
% part-time	10
Student-faculty ratio	2:1

ADMISSIONS

Application Information

Regular application	11/1
Regular notification	10/15
	until filled
Early application	6/1–8/1
Early notification	10/1
Are transfers accepted?	yes
Admissions may be deferred?	yes
Interview required?	no
Application fee	$30

Academics

Although most students follow a 4 year program, some educationally disadvantaged students enter the Flexible Curriculum Program, which permits extension of the MD curriculum over a 5-year period. Joint-degree programs offered in conjunction with affiliated schools are available, including the MD/MS and MD/PhD through which a doctorate degree may be earned in the following areas: anatomy, biochemistry, microbiology, neuroscience, pathology, pharmacology, physiology, and numerous other fields. Medical students are evaluated with ratings of honors, high pass, pass, and fail. Passing Step 1 of the USMLE is a requirement for promotion to year 3. In order to graduate, a score on Step 2 must be recorded.

BASIC SCIENCES: The first two years are devoted to an integrated approach to the basic sciences, behavioral sciences, primary care preceptorships, introductory clinical experiences, and Problem-Based Learning (PBL) for all students. First-year courses are the following: Cellular and molecular biology; human structure and development; neuroscience and behavioral science; Integrated Pathophysiology I (PBL); and physician, patient, and society I. During the first year, students are in class for about 30 hours per week, most of which is either lecture or lab periods. Second-year courses are introduction to primary care; immunity and infection; organ systems; integrated pathophysiology II (PBL); and physician, patient, and society II. Physician, patient, and society includes introduction to primary care; introduction to clinical medicine (ICM); and a series of courses that address topics in medical ethics, managed care, medical decision-making, nutrition, geriatrics, and substance abuse disorders. The ICM course covers practical skills such as taking patient histories and conducting physical examinations. It also serves as a forum for correlating basic science principles with clinical case studies and for discussing ethical issues related to practicing medicine. Second-year students are in class for about 20 hours per week. Basic science instruction takes place in the Health Sciences Teaching and Laboratory Building and the Health Education Building. The Mulford Library holds 125,000 volumes and 1,800 journals and, along with the Computer Learning Resource Center, provides educational and informational resources to students.

CLINICAL TRAINING

Third-year required clerkships are the following: Medicine (12 weeks), surgery (12 weeks), pediatrics (6 weeks), psychiatry (6 weeks), family medicine (6 weeks), and ob/gyn (6 weeks). During the fourth year, one basic science selective (4 weeks) and one neurology clerkship (4 weeks) are required. The remaining 28 weeks are reserved for elective study. Three teaching hospitals operate on campus, the Medical College of Ohio Hospital (258 beds), Coghlin Rehabilitation Hospital (36 beds), and Lenore W. and Marvin S. Kobacker Center (25 beds, a children's psychiatric hospital). Other associated hospitals include St. Vincent Mercy Medical Center, The Toledo Hospital/Children's Medical Center of Northwest Ohio, Flower Hospital, and Northwestern Psychiatric Hospital. Through the Area Health Education Center clerkships, MCO students also have the opportunity to train in rural and inner-city communities.

Students

At least 80 percent of students are Ohio residents although many attended undergraduate institutions outside of the state. Underrepresented minorities, mostly African Americans, account for approximately 10 percent of the student body. Among entrants, there are significant numbers of older individuals, some of whom are in their late thirties and early forties. Typically, about 80 percent of medical students were science majors in college.

STUDENT LIFE

In addition to providing academic resources, the Office of Student Affairs supports students inside and outside of the classroom, organizing events such as an annual orientation for incoming students. There are many student associations, ranging from one that administers a community care clinic to a student-to-student support group to organizations focused on personal, recreational, religious, cultural, and professional interests. MCO is situated on 475 acres of land, with ponds, streams, trees, and open areas. The campus offers extensive athletic and recreational facilities. Major attractions in Toledo are easily reached on public transportation and include riverside restaurants and bars, museums, parks with golf courses and other facilities, a zoo, theaters, and shopping areas. Further distraction is found in Detroit, Cincinnati, Pittsburgh, Cleveland, and Chicago, all of which are in driving distance of MCO. Students live off campus, usually in the surrounding residential neighborhood.

GRADUATES

About 40 percent of graduates go on to practice in Ohio. In recent years, about 60 percent of graduates have entered primary care fields.

Admissions

REQUIREMENTS

Prerequisites are 1 year each of biology, English, general chemistry, math, organic chemistry, and physics. All science courses must include labs. The MCAT is required. For applicants who have retaken the exam, the best set of scores is weighted most heavily. Thus, withholding scores is not advantageous.

SUGGESTIONS

As a state-supported institution, MCO gives preference to Ohio residents. Additional preparation in biology is recommended as are courses in the humanities and social sciences. For students who have been out of school for a significant period of time, some recent course work is advised. Community service and medically related experience involving patient contact are both considered valuable.

PROCESS

About 75 percent of AMCAS applicants are sent secondary applications. Of those returning secondaries, about 25 percent of Ohio residents and 10 percent of nonresidents are invited to interview. Interviews take place between October and April and consist of two hour-long sessions each with a faculty member, medical student, or school administrator. Also on interview day, candidates tour the campus, hear group informational sessions, and have the opportunity to meet informally with current students. About one-third of interviewees are accepted, with notification occurring throughout the year. Wait-listed candidates may send additional information, such as transcripts and test scores, to update their files.

Admissions Requirements (Required)

MCAT scores, science GPA, non-science GPA, state residency, extracurricular activities, exposure to medical profession.

Admissions Requirements (Optional)

Letters of recommendation, interview, essays/personal statement.

COSTS AND AID

Tuition & Fees

In-state Tuition	$10,512
Out-of-state Tuition	$22,966
Cost of books	$2,054
Fees	$741

Financial Aid

% students receiving aid	90
Average grant	$6,000
Average loan	$18,500

MEDICAL COLLEGE OF WISCONSIN

OFFICE OF ADMISSIONS, 8701 WATERTOWN PLANK ROAD, MILWAUKEE, WI 53226 • ADMISSION: 414-456-8246
FAX: 414-456-6505 • E-MAIL: WWW.MEDSCHOOL@MCW.EDU • WEBSITE: WWW.MCW.EDU

STUDENT BODY

Type	Private
Enrollment	811
% male/female	56/44
% underrepresented minorities	10
# applied (total/out)	5,645/5,093
# accepted (total/out)	475/315
# enrolled (total/out)	204/108
Average age	23

FACULTY

Total faculty (number)	1,100
Student-faculty ratio	0:1

ADMISSIONS

Average GPA and MCAT Scores

Overall GPA	3.72
MCAT Bio	10.0
MCAT Phys	10.0
MCAT Verbal	9.7
MCAT Essay	P

Application Information

Regular application	11/1
Regular notification	10/15
Early application	6/1-8/1
Early notification	10/1
Are transfers accepted?	yes
Admissions may be deferred?	yes
Interview required?	yes
Application fee	$60

Academics

The curriculum at the Medical College of Wisconsin leading to a doctor of medicine degree consists of a 4 year traditional program with two years of pre-clinical course work followed by two years of clinical rotations. The pre-clinical course work represents a combination of basic science courses plus a substantial amount of work in the clinical continuum, which represents interactive, experiential, and clinically-relevant opportunities to develop the skills and identity of a physician. The clinical continuum course work is taken in both the first and second years of the curriculum. An extended curriculum allows students to complete their first year course work over a 2-year period leading to graduation in five years. This program enables students to pursue research, employment, or other activities that may match their interests. Medical students are encouraged to participate in summer research programs following the completion of their first-year course work and many choose to complete a rigorous research program that leads to an additional honors designation. Qualified students may enter a combined MD/PhD degree program through the Medical Scientists Training Program (MSTP). The Graduate School of Biomedical Sciences offers additional degrees that include PhD, MS, MA, MPH, and joint-degree programs. The Graduate School offers programs in bioethics, biochemistry, biophysics, biostatistics, cell and developmental biology, epidemiology, functional imaging, microbiology and molecular genetics, pharmacology and toxicology, physiology, and public health. To earn the MD degree, students must successfully complete all of their course work, which is evaluated on a five-interval grading system. In addition, the students must successfully pass the Step 1 exam of the USMLE to be promoted to the fourth year of the curriculum and pass the USMLE Step 2 CS to graduate. They must take the Step 2 CS exam. They must pass an end-of-third-year OSCE exam in order to meet graduation requirements, as well.

BASIC SCIENCES: Basic sciences are taught during the first two years of the curriculum. The learning activities consist of a mix of traditional curriculum formats (lectures, labs, dissection, and discussion groups) and newer educational methods including Computer-Aided Instruction (CAI), Problem-Based Learning (PBL), and independent study options. First-year courses include biochemistry, clinical human anatomy, human development, cell and tissue biology, integrated medical neurosciences, and physiology. Second-year courses include a year-long pathology course, foundations in clinical psychiatry, microbiology, and pharmacology. Support services for medical students include individual and group advising and tutorials. Educational facilities include the Medical Education Building that provides a variety of learning settings and contains two large modern auditoriums, the Computer-Aided Instruction Laboratory, multi-use teaching spaces, and the recently completed state-of-the-art Standardized Teaching and Resource Center containing a center for assessment of history-taking and physical examination skills using standardized patients and simulation centers housing advanced human simulators. The Health Research Center contains an auditorium with state-of-the-art communication technology, small group teaching spaces, teleconferencing room with satellite capabilities and research laboratories. The MCW Libraries houses a collection of 250,000 volumes and subscribes to print and electronic medical journals, offering a comprehensive network of electronic databases and resources.

CLINICAL TRAINING

Exposure to the clinical environment begins shortly after entering medical school during the clinical continuum. This 2-year long course consists of introduction to patient care, medical interviewing, foundation of human behavior, medical information management, and the mentor course, which are all taken in the first year. In the second year, medical ethics and palliative care, clinical examination and reasoning, and health policy are taken. Third-year rotations include internal medicine (2 months), surgery (2 months), pediatrics (2 months), obstetrics and gynecology (1 and a half months), psychiatry (1 month), neurology (one-half month), clinical procedures rotation (1 month), family medicine (1 month), and 1 month of vacation, but most students choose to take an elective instead of the vacation. The fourth year consists of 4 months of required rotations that include internal medicine, medically-oriented sub internship, surgery-oriented sub internship, and an integrated selective. Five elective rotations may be chosen by the student, some of which may be taken as away rotations or international rotations. The Medical College of Wisconsin is the academic center of the Milwaukee Regional Medical Center campus, which includes Froedtert Hospital, Children's Hospital of Wisconsin, Curative Rehabilitation Center, Milwaukee County Mental Health Complex, the Blood Center of Southeastern Wisconsin Research Institute, and the Eye Institute. MCW is affiliated with numerous hospitals and clinics in and around Milwaukee and with rural care centers in other parts of the state.

Students

MCW is the eighth largest medical school and the second largest free-standing medical school in the country. As a free-standing institution, MCW attracts and enrolls students from across the country each year in its class of 2004 students. Located at the Milwaukee Regional Medical Center campus, the Medical College is able to provide all clinical clerkships and rotations at this location or in the metropolitan area.

STUDENT LIFE

Student organizations focus on professional and leadership development, community service, and recreational pursuits. The college is involved in more than 30 community service activities, including a student-run clinic for the uninsured, an AIDS interventions center, and health education programs in local schools. Organized social events include parties, dinners, and ongoing activities such as intramural sports. Along with the college's fitness center, these activities allow students to relax, socialize, or exercise between or after class. Located in a suburb 7 miles west of downtown Milwaukee, students live and go to school in a safe, comfortable environment. At the same time, they are also within easy access of the cultural, social, and sporting events offered in the metropolitan area.

GRADUATES

MCW students consistently perform at or better then the national average on the USLME. This coupled with the school's reputation for providing excellent clinical training results in an excellent placement record for graduates.

Admissions

REQUIREMENTS

Eligibility requirements to apply include the following: Candidates must have completed or are in the process of completing 90 or more undergraduate graded credits, including the prerequisites, at an accredited college/university in the United States or Canada. The MCAT is required and must have been taken no more then three years prior to matriculation. Prerequisites include 8 semester hours, two of which must be labs, in biology, inorganic chemistry, and organic chemistry, 8 semester hours of physics, four of college algebra and 6 of English. With the exception of organic chemistry, AP credit is accepted for prerequisites.

SUGGESTIONS

Beyond required courses, applicants are encouraged to present a well-rounded academic background with course work in public speaking, social studies, and the humanities. In addition to academic credentials, a mature sense of values, motivation, dedication, and a clear understanding of clinical medicine are important factors in the selection process.

PROCESS

Applications are reviewed on rolling, first come, first-serve basis by the completion date. Applicants are encouraged to apply early. Interviews are an integral part of the selection process and offers are made on a rolling basis until the class is filled.

Admissions Requirements (Required)

MCAT scores, science GPA, non-science GPA, letters of recommendation, interview, essays/personal statement, extracurricular activities, exposure to medical profession.

Admissions Requirements (Optional)

State residency.

COSTS AND AID

Tuition & Fees

Tuition	$33,370
Room and board (off campus)	$7,500
Cost of books	$1,522
Fees	$45

Financial Aid

% students receiving aid	95
Average grant	$10,234
Average loan	$38,210
Average debt	$131,700

MEDICAL UNIVERSITY OF SOUTH CAROLINA
COLLEGE OF MEDICINE

96 JONATHAN LUCAS STREET, SUITE 601, PO BOX 250617, CHARLESTON, SC 29425 • ADMISSION: 843-792-2055
FAX: 843-792-4262 • E-MAIL: TAYLORWL@MUSC.EDU • WEBSITE: WWW2.MUSC.EDU./COM/COM.HTML

STUDENT BODY	
Type	Public
Enrollment	584
% male/female	55/45
% underrepresented minorities	14
# applied (total/out)	1,746/1,324
# accepted (total/out)	179/5
# enrolled (total/out)	135/2
Average age	26

FACULTY	
Total faculty (number)	612
% female	32
% minority	13
Student-faculty ratio	2:1

ADMISSIONS

Average GPA and MCAT Scores

Overall GPA	3.6
MCAT Bio	9.4
MCAT Phys	9.8
MCAT Verbal	9.8
MCAT Essay	Q

Application Information

Regular application	12/1
Regular notification	rolling
Early application	6/1–8/1
Early notification	10/1
Are transfers accepted?	yes
Admissions may be deferred?	yes
Interview required?	yes
Application fee	$55

Academics

The goal of the College of Medicine is to produce caring and competent physicians capable of succeeding in their postgraduate career. The 4 year program, which leads to an MD degree, is divided into two years of pre-clinical instruction and consists of education in the basic sciences and an introduction into clinical medicine, followed by two years of clinical science education. The curriculum during the first two years addresses the following four major objectives: Provision of basic science concepts; acquisition of problem-solving strategies; development of skills, which permit the performance of an adequate history and physical examination; and an introduction to the role of the physician in society. Throughout the curriculum, emphasis is placed on small-group instruction. The curriculum was changed to expand and improve opportunities for independent, self-directed learning. As a result, students are being exposed earlier to clinical skills.

CLINICAL TRAINING

The junior year consists of eight clinical core clerkships. The clinical core consists of eight weeks each of internal medicine, obstetrics/gynecology, pediatrics, and surgery, as well as 4 weeks each of Dean's Rural Primary Care, family medicine, psychiatry, and neurology. During the clerkships, emphasis is placed on the development of clinical, interpersonal, and professional competence. In addition, students participate in the foundations in clinical medicine course. This course is designed to integrate basic and clinical sciences utilizing small group discussions and patient case scenarios. During the senior year, students take a minimum of eight 4-week rotations. The student is required to take one clinical externship and one month each of surgery, psychiatry, and internal medicine. The remaining four blocks are elective and, depending upon previous academic performance, can be taken at approved sites throughout the state or country. A complete listing of elective courses may be found in the Catalog of Electives at www.musc.edu/comelectives/index.html. In addition, students are required to complete and satisfactorily pass the Clinical Practice Exam (CPX).

Students

Over 95 percent of students are South Carolina residents. About 15 percent are underrepresented minorities, most of whom are African American. The average age of incoming students is typically around 25, and usually at least 10 percent of entering classes are over 30 years old. Class size is 135.

STUDENT LIFE

During orientation, incoming students are assigned to groups composed of first- and second-year students and a faculty member. The groups serve as informational resources for both academic and nonacademic matters. Also during the first week of school, the Activities Fair is held and introduces various student activities, groups, and events. Organizations that are popular with medical students include chapters of national medical fraternities, professionally oriented interest groups, and groups focused on health care related community service. Intramural sports are also popular. The Harper Student Center (HSC) houses student service offices, a student lounge, and a comprehensive fitness center with indoor and outdoor tracks, rooftop tennis courts, and a swimming pool, among other features. HSC is also a gathering site for students, offering happy hours and other social events. Beyond the campus, Charleston is a city known for its beauty and charm. Students enjoy the nearby beaches and other outdoor attractions. All students live off campus.

GRADUATES

Graduates are successful in securing residencies in all medical fields, with a significant number entering family medicine. MUSC itself offers more than 20 postgraduate training programs. More than 95 percent pass USMLE Step 2.

Admissions

REQUIREMENTS

No prerequisites are specified. An applicant's GPA is evaluated with consideration given to the undergraduate institution attended and the difficulty of the course load pursued. The MCAT is required, and scores must be from the past five years. For applicants who have taken the exam on multiple occasions, the best set of scores is used.

SUGGESTIONS

South Carolina residents are given strong preference. The MCAT requirement suggests that applicants should have a basic science background. However, breadth of course work, including courses in the humanities and social sciences, is also valued. Since the best set of MCAT scores is used, withholding scores has no advantage. Extracurricular activities, specifically those that are medically or research related are important. Community service is also considered important. During the interview, non-cognitive traits such as emotional stability, integrity, honesty, and enthusiasm are evaluated.

PROCESS

All applicants are asked to submit secondary applications. Of those returning secondaries, about 65 percent of state residents, and 3 percent of out-of-state residents are interviewed, if they are academically qualified. Interviews are conducted from September through March, and consist of three sessions, each with a faculty member or MUSC alumni. About one-third of interviewees are accepted on a rolling basis. Others are rejected or wait listed.

Admissions Requirements (Required)

MCAT scores, science GPA, non-science GPA, letters of recommendation, interview, essays/personal statement, extracurricular activities, exposure to medical profession. Preference is given to SC residents.

Admissions Requirements (Optional)

State residency.

Overlap Schools

Duke University, Emory University, University of South Carolina.

COSTS AND AID

Tuition & Fees

In-state Tuition	$13,302
Out-of-state Tuition	$37,622
Room and board (off campus)	$9,830
Cost of books	$3,890

Financial Aid

% students receiving aid	81
Average grant	$2,000
Average loan	$25,865
Average debt	$92,883

MEHARRY MEDICAL COLLEGE
SCHOOL OF MEDICINE

1005 Dr. D.B. Todd Jr. Boulevard, Nashville, TN 37208-3599 • **Admission:** 615-327-6223
Fax: 615-327-6228 • **E-mail:** ADMISSIONS@MMC.EDU • **Website:** WWW.MMC.EDU

STUDENT BODY	
Type	Private
Enrollment	343
% male/female	48/52
% underrepresented minorities	48
# applied (total/out)	3,542/3,323
# accepted (total/out)	145/120
# enrolled (total/out)	80/60
Average age	26

FACULTY	
Total faculty (number)	184
Student-faculty ratio	2:1

ADMISSIONS

Application Information

Regular application	12/1
Regular notification	10/15
Early application	6/1–8/1
Early notification	10/1
Are transfers accepted?	no
Admissions may be deferred?	no
Interview required?	yes
Application fee	$60

Academics

Meharry benefits from its proximity to Fisk University and Tennessee State University. The three schools share certain facilities and together provide an active academic community. Most medical students at Meharry complete their studies in four years, although some extend their first year over a longer period of time and complete medical training in five years. A combined MD/PhD program is offered in biochemistry, biomedical science, microbiology, pharmacology, and physiology. Grades are A, B, C, and F. All medical students must pass Step 1 of the USMLE to be promoted to year 3 and Step 2 to graduate.

BASIC SCIENCES: First-year courses are anatomy, biochemistry, introduction to clinical medicine I, and physiology. Students are in class or other scheduled sessions for 20–25 hours per week. Most instruction uses a lecture format, supplemented by labs and small-group discussions. Second-year courses are behavioral sciences, general and clinical pathology, genetics, microbiology, introduction to clinical medicine II, and pharmacology. During the second year, students are in class for about 30 hours per week, a significant proportion of which is devoted to small-group discussions. The Teaching and Learning Resource Center, located in the student center, serves as a comprehensive academic support unit and provides tutoring and board review, among other services. The library, holding more than 50,000 volumes and 1,000 journals, is located in the same complex.

CLINICAL TRAINING

Third-year required rotations are medicine (12 weeks), surgery (12 weeks), pediatrics (8 weeks), ob/gyn (8 weeks), family and preventive medicine (8 weeks), and psychiatry (4 weeks). Fourth-year sub internships are medicine (4 weeks), surgery (4 weeks), family and preventive medicine (4 weeks), radiology (4 weeks), and psychiatry (4 weeks). 12 weeks are reserved for electives. Major teaching hospitals are Metropolitan Nashville General Hospital, Alvin C. York Veterans Administration Medical Center, and Blanchefield Army Community Hospital. Other affiliated health care institutions are Centennial Medical Center, Vanderbilt Medical Center, Middle Tennessee Mental Health Hospital, and numerous clinics and health centers throughout the state. All students complete an ambulatory rotation in an underserved area.

Students

About 70 percent of students are African American. Students come from around the country, with about 20 percent of students from Tennessee. Class size is 80.

STUDENT LIFE

Students are supportive and cooperative, usually opting to study together in groups. There are a large number of student organizations, including honor societies, medical fraternities, support groups such as the Meharry Wives Club, groups focused on professional interests, such as the Family Practice Club, and societies focused on a common religion or ethnicity. The Daniel T. Rolfe Student Center accommodates student activities and organizations and provides a focal point for extracurricular life. Many students are involved in community activities, such as serving as mentors for high school students. Medical students interact with other Meharry students and also with peers at nearby universities. Nashville offers restaurants, nightlife, outdoor activities, and a generally student-friendly atmosphere. On-campus housing options are residence halls and apartment complexes with both 1- and 2-bedroom units.

GRADUATES

The College of Medicine has graduated more than 5,000 African American physicians, almost half of the total number of African American physicians who studied and who practice in the United States. About three-quarters of graduates go on to work in medically underserved rural and inner-city areas. Some graduates enter residency programs at Meharry, which has a total of 30 postgraduate positions in family practice, internal medicine, occupational medicine, preventive medicine, and psychiatry.

Admissions

REQUIREMENTS

Required course work is 8 semesters hours each of biology, general chemistry, organic chemistry, and physics, all with associated labs. Six semester hours of English are also required. The MCAT is required, and scores should be from within the past three years. The April, rather than August, MCAT is strongly advised. For applicants who have taken the exam on multiple occasions, all sets of scores are considered.

SUGGESTIONS

Special consideration is given to underrepresented minority students and students from disadvantaged backgrounds. Meharry is interested in applicants who are dedicated to improving health care for the underserved. In addition to academic credentials, medically related or community service activities are viewed as important.

PROCESS

All qualified AMCAS applicants are sent secondary applications. Of those returning secondaries, about 10 percent are interviewed between September and May. Interviews consist of two sessions, each with a faculty member, administrator, or current medical student. On interview day, applicants also have the opportunity to meet informally with students. About one-third of interviewed candidates are accepted on a rolling basis. Others are rejected or placed on a wait list. Wait-listed candidates may send additional information if it serves to update their files.

Admissions Requirements (Required)

MCAT scores, science GPA, non-science GPA, letters of recommendation, interview, extracurricular activities, exposure to medical profession.

Admissions Requirements (Optional)

State residency, essays/personal statement.

COSTS AND AID

Tuition & Fees

Tuition	$23,208
Cost of books	$1,528
Fees	$3,916

Financial Aid

% students receiving aid	79
Average grant	$1,000
Average loan	$28,893
Average debt	$125,339

MEMORIAL UNIVERSITY NEWFOUNDLAND
FACULTY OF MEDICINE

ROOM 1751, HEALTH SCIENCES CENTER, ST. JOHN'S, NF A1B 3V6 • **ADMISSION:** 709-777-6615
FAX: 709-777-8422 • **E-MAIL:** MUNMED@MUN.CA • **WEBSITE:** WWW.MED.MUN.CA/ADMISSIONS/

STUDENT BODY

Type	Public
Enrollment	244
% male/female	48/52
# applied	648
# accepted	77
# enrolled	60

FACULTY

Total faculty (number)	186
% female	31
% part-time	60

ADMISSIONS

Average GPA and MCAT Scores

Overall GPA	3.7
MCAT Bio	9.0
MCAT Phys	9.0
MCAT Verbal	9.0
MCAT Essay	0

Application Information

Regular application	11/15
Regular notification	3/1
Are transfers accepted?	no
Admissions may be deferred?	yes
Interview required?	yes
Application fee	$75

Academics

Each of the first two years is organized into three terms. Although the emphasis of the course work is on basic science, clinical medicine is also introduced. During the second two years, students perform clerkships in affiliated hospitals that provide both undergraduate and graduate medical education. In addition to the 4 year MD, MS, and PhD degree programs are also open to qualified students. Areas of academic strength include cardiovascular sciences including epidemiology; community medicine; endocrinology and metabolism; gastroenterology; human genetics; immunology; molecular biology; neurosciences.

BASIC SCIENCES: An important component of the first year is basic science of medicine. This course introduces students to the biology of the normal human and integrates anatomy, biochemistry, physiology, immunology, cell biology, genetics, microbiology, nutrition, pharmacology, pathology. Teaching methods include lectures, small group sessions, laboratories, seminars, and open discussions. Students have the opportunity to initiate basic science research, which can be pursued throughout medical school. First-year students also take integrated study of disease, which teaches pathology and pharmacology through the study of diseases of the major organ systems. In clinical skills, students are first introduced to the medical interview and techniques of counseling. The physical exam and important ethical issues are also part of the course. Community medicine is a unique course, which focuses on the contextual aspects of disease and introduces behavioral sciences, biostatistics, community nutrition, environmental and occupational health, epidemiology, preventive medicine, and social and organizational factors in health. The course includes visits to community-based hospitals and clinics. All courses continue in the second year, building on principles learned during the first year. On average, pre-clinical students are in class or other scheduled sessions for 23 hours per week.

CLINICAL TRAINING

Year 3 is a 12-month duration beginning in September and continuing to the following Fall. It is composed of the core clerkships and some electives. Core clerkships, typically 8 weeks in length, are internal medicine, ob/gyn, psychiatry, pediatrics, and surgery. A 4-week rural family medicine rotation is also required. The fourth year consists of electives and selectives, some of which may be completed at institutions other than those affiliated with the university. Teaching hospitals include General Hospital (531 beds), Grace General Hospital, Dr. Charles A Janeway Child Health Centre, St. Clare's Mercy Hospital, Waterford Hospital, and a number of institutions that are not under the Health Care Corporation of St. Johns.

Students

The school's class size is relatively small at 60 students. The male/female ratio within the student body is about 50/50.

STUDENT LIFE

On-campus housing is available for both single and married students. In addition, the university provides assistance in locating off-campus housing. Medical students benefit from an active counseling center, childcare services, learning enhancement programs, a career planning office, and a student health service. The student's union promotes artistic, educational, charitable, and social activities, and the graduate student union provides common areas for social and other activities. Medical students have access to the services and resources of the greater university.

GRADUATES

A significant proportion of graduates enter residencies at affiliated hospitals in areas such as anesthesia, internal medicine, neurology, ob/gyn, orthopedics, anatomic pathology, general pathology, pediatrics, psychiatry, radiology, and surgery. Most graduates enter clinical medicine, often in primary care fields.

Admissions

REQUIREMENTS

To be eligible for admission, a bachelor's degree is required in almost all circumstances. Requirements include two courses in English. The MCAT is also required, and must be taken prior to the application deadline, which is normally November 15. Transcripts and letters of reference must be submitted by November 29. Interviews are required of some candidates. The majority of places in each class are reserved for applicants who are residents of Newfoundland and Labrador. There are a limited number of places available for applicants from New Brunswick, from other Canadian provinces, and non-Canadians. Non-Canadians pay higher fees.

SUGGESTIONS

There are approximately 650 applications received for 60 places each year. Therefore, competition is high. Material submitted after the stated deadlines will not be considered. Academic achievement, MCAT scores, work or other experiences, and personal traits are all reviewed in admissions decisions. Though age itself is not used as a basis for selection, time away from academic studies may be taken into consideration.

PROCESS

Requests for applications should be directed to the address above. Applications are accepted until November 15 in the year preceding anticipated matriculation. Decisions are made in the spring. Notification of the committee's decision will be made to candidates by letter from the Admissions Committee. Applicants have 14 days in which to confirm acceptance.

Admissions Requirements (Required)

MCAT scores, letters of recommendation, interview, essays/personal statement, extracurricular activities.

Admissions Requirements (Optional)

Science GPA, nonscience GPA, state residency, exposure to medical profession.

COSTS AND AID

Tuition & Fees

In-state Tuition	$6,250
Out-of-state Tuition	$30,000
Room and board (off campus)	$9,000
Cost of books	$1,593
In-state Fees	$457
Out-of-state Fees	$645

Financial Aid

% students receiving aid	90
Average grant	$800
Average debt	$150,000

MERCER UNIVERSITY
SCHOOL OF MEDICINE

1550 COLLEGE STREET, MACON, GA 31207 • ADMISSION: 478-301-2542
FAX: 478-301-2547 • E-MAIL: FAUST_EK@MERCER.EDU • WEBSITE: HTTP://MEDICINE.MERCER.EDU

STUDENT BODY	
Type	Private
Enrollment	221
% male/female	58/42
# applied (total/out)	738/180
# accepted 60	
# enrolled (total/out)	60/0
Average age	25

ADMISSIONS

Average GPA and MCAT Scores

Overall GPA	3.4
MCAT Bio	8.65
MCAT Phys	7.8
MCAT Verbal	8.88
MCAT Essay	N

Application Information

Regular application	11/1
Regular notification	rolling
Early application	6/1–8/1
Early notification	10/1
Are transfers accepted?	yes
Admissions may be deferred?	yes
Interview required?	yes
Application fee	$50

Academics

Each entering student is assigned to a faculty advisor who assists with the transition to medical school, with strategies for pre-clinical studies, and later with decisions involved in elective and specialty selection. Almost all students complete the MD curriculum in four years. Evaluation uses satisfactory/unsatisfactory during the first two years, and honors/satisfactory/unsatisfactory during the third and fourth years. Self and peer evaluations are also used in some situations. Passing both steps of the USMLE is a requirement for graduation.

BASIC SCIENCES: Basic sciences are presented during the first two years as part of the Biomedical Problems Program, which uses case-based instructional techniques and computer-assisted, self-directed study. The curriculum is organized around physiological systems or "phases," which are biology of reproduction, brain and behavior, cardiology, cells and metabolism, gastrointestinal, genetics and development, hematology, host defense, infectious disease, musculoskeletal, neurology, pulmonology, and renal endocrinology. Issues related to medical ethics are also discussed in the context of case studies. Community science is another important part of the first two years. Courses included in this category are clinical biostatistics, community epidemiology, managed care and physician workforce, rural preceptorship, and research design and the medical literature. Clinical training begins during the first year, when students learn interviewing and examination skills by working with simulated patients. Actual patient contact occurs through the Community Office Practice Program (COPP) in which students work directly with community physicians. Most basic science instruction takes place in the Medical Education Building, which, in addition to classrooms, houses the Medical Library; Mercer Health Systems, which provides clinical services; the Health Education Center; and the school's administrative offices. This physical arrangement, with basic science and clinical facilities in the same building, guarantees first- and second-year students an integrated educational experience. The library has over 90,000 volumes, 2,500 audiovisuals, and 850 current subscriptions. The Learning Resource Center offers computers and labs.

CLINICAL TRAINING

Third-year required rotations are internal medicine (12 weeks), surgery (8 weeks), pediatrics (8 weeks), ob/gyn (6 weeks), family medicine (8 weeks), and psychiatry (6 weeks). During the fourth year, students choose among fields within surgical subspecialities (4 weeks). They also complete clerkships in community science (4 weeks), substance abuse (2 weeks), and critical care (2 weeks). The remainder of the year is reserved for elective study. The primary teaching hospitals are the Medical Center of Central Georgia in Macon (518 beds) and the Memorial Health University Medical Center in Savannah (530 beds). Other major affiliates are Floyd Medical Center in Rome, Phoebe Putney Memorial Hospital in Albany, and the Medical Center in Columbus. Training also takes place outside of major hospitals, at sites such as community hospitals, clinics, and physicians' offices throughout the state.

Students

All students are Georgia residents. About 4 percent are underrepresented minorities. The average age of incoming students is around 24, and at least 20 percent of a typical entering class took significant time off between college and medical school.

STUDENT LIFE

Medical students have access to the facilities of the greater university. These include cafeterias, athletic facilities, and recreational centers. Medical students also have their own student center, which has a snack bar and functions as a meeting place. Students may join chapters of national medical student organizations, including those that focus on the needs of women and minority medical students. Mercer offers conveniently located, campus-owned apartments to medical students on a limited basis. Affordable accommodations are also available in and around Macon. The Office of Admissions and Student Affairs helps students find suitable housing.

GRADUATES

Most graduates enter residency programs in Georgia and go on to practice in primary care fields within the state.

Admissions

REQUIREMENTS

Generally, only residents of Georgia are accepted. Required course work is 1 year each of biology, physics, chemistry, and organic chemistry. The MCAT is required and scores must be no more than two years old.

SUGGESTIONS

In addition to required preparatory courses, biochemistry is recommended. The April MCAT is strongly advised, as files are not reviewed until MCAT scores are available. The Admissions Committee is interested in students who are strongly motivated to work with underserved populations and in rural areas. For applicants who have taken time off after college, some recent course work is important.

PROCESS

Secondary applications are sent to AMCAS applicants who meet minimum requirements. Typically, about 70 percent of Georgia residents who apply receive secondary applications. Of those returning secondaries, about 20 percent are invited to interview. Interviews take place between October and March, and consist of two sessions with faculty. About one-third of interviewees are accepted. All decisions are made before March 15, at which point a wait list is formed.

Admissions Requirements (Required)

MCAT scores, science GPA, non-science GPA, letters of recommendation, interview, state residency, essays/personal statement, extracurricular activities, exposure to medical profession, practice vision statement.

COSTS AND AID

Tuition & Fees

Tuition	$26,372
Room and board (off campus)	$12,970
Cost of books	$1,700

Financial Aid

% students receiving aid	95
Average grant	$5,452
Average loan	$27,149
Average debt	$135,438

MICHIGAN STATE UNIVERSITY
COLLEGE OF HUMAN MEDICINE

A-239 LIFE SCIENCES EAST, LANSING, MI 48824 • ADMISSION: 517-353-9620
FAX: 517-432-0021 • E-MAIL: MDADMISSIONS@MSU.EDU • WEBSITE: MDADMISSIONS.MSU.EDU

STUDENT BODY

Type	Public
Enrollment	454
% male/female	43/57
% underrepresented minorities	36
# applied (total/out)	3,165/2,123
# accepted (total/out)	180/49
# enrolled (total/out)	106/23
Average age	24

FACULTY

Total faculty (number)	308
% part-time	11

ADMISSIONS

Average GPA and MCAT Scores

Overall GPA	3.52
MCAT Bio	9.9
MCAT Phys	9.1
MCAT Verbal	9.2
MCAT Essay	P

Application Information

Regular application	11/15
Regular notification	rolling
Early application	8/1
Early notification	10/1
Are transfers accepted?	yes
Admissions may be deferred?	yes
Interview required?	yes
Application fee	$60

Academics

The 4 year curriculum is modern and highly innovative. While the first two years are spent at MSU's main campus in East Lansing, students are assigned to 1 of 6 community-based programs for clinical training during the third and fourth years. These communities are the following: Kalamazoo, Upper Peninsula, Grand Rapids, Flint, Lansing, and Saginaw. Special clinical programs include the Rural Physician Program and Leadership in Medicine for the Underserved. Along its focus on primary care, the College of Human Medicine welcomes students seeking a dual degree. Fields in which graduate degrees may be earned include the following: Biochemistry/molecular biology, bioethics/humanities/society, epidemiology, health communication, microbiology/molecular genetics, pharmacology/toxiocology, and physiology. Medical students are evaluated with a modified pass/no pass system.

BASIC SCIENCES: In addition to mastering basic science concepts, first-year students address the doctor/patient relationship in clinical skills. A unique mentor program assigns small groups of students to a preceptor, allowing the groups to explore patient care and the complex roles of the physician. Students accompany their mentor for hospital rounds and patient visits. The course integrative clinical correlations, taught by basic science faculty members and clinicians, develops problem-solving skills and allows students to apply basic science concepts to clinical case studies. Other first-year courses are the following: Biochemistry, biostatistics and epidemiology, cell biology and physiology, clinical skills, gross anatomy, human development and behavior in society, neuroscience, molecular biology and genetics, microbiology and immunology, pathology, pharmacology, and radiology. The second year is organized around body systems and general disease categories. These are the following: cardiovascular, digestive, disorders of development and behavior, hematopoietic/neoplasia, infectious diseases, major mental disorders, metabolic endocrine reproductive, neurological/musculoskeletal, pulmonary, urinary tract. In the social context of clinical decisions, students take part in a series of small-group seminars dealing with the concepts of medical ethics; epidemiology; biostatistics; critical reasoning; humanities; and social, economic, and organizational issues in medicine. The primary mode of instruction during the second year is small-group discussions/tutorials. Students are in scheduled sessions for fewer than 20 hours per week, allowing ample time for individual and group study. Academic facilities include the Echt Computer Lab, which offers computer-based instructional programs and audio/visual aids, a 24 hour exclusive and comprehensive Student Learning Center, and MSU's main library.

CLINICAL TRAINING

Most clerkship requirements are fulfilled during the third year and the early part of year 4. Students move to one of six communities during the summer of their third year. They then rotate through 8 weeks of each of the following: family practice, internal medicine, ob/gyn, pediatrics, psychiatry, and surgery. Four weeks of advanced medicine and advanced surgery are also required. Throughout the period in which students complete required clerkships, students also participate in a core competency seminar, which requires 2 hours per week and provides a forum for discussion of interdisciplinary topics important to the care and health management of patients. A total of 20 weeks are reserved for elective experiences. Students may rotate to other communities in the state, to hospitals and academic centers in other states, and to clinical sites overseas.

Students

At least 80 percent of students are Michigan residents. Class size is 106. In a recent class, the average age of incoming students was 25.

STUDENT LIFE

First- and second-year students enjoy the activities, facilities, resources, and social life of a Big Ten university. Medical students are also involved in the greater community, volunteering at clinics and as health educators in schools. Professionally focused and special-interest organizations are numerous, as are athletic opportunities such as intramural sports. A variety of campus-owned housing options are available. Some single students live in a graduate/professional student residence hall. Apartments of all sizes are also available, accommodating single and married students, and students with larger families. Where students spend their third and fourth years is largely determined by a lottery, with consideration given to special circumstances and preferences.

GRADUATES

Students typically score above the national average on the USMLE, contributing to their success in securing top-choice residency positions. A recent 3 year average of residency choices are in the following: Family practice (27 percent), internal medicine (15 percent), surgery (13 percent), pediatrics (15 percent), ob/gyn (10 percent), psychiatry (3 percent), and other programs (17 percent). About 50 percent of graduates remained in Michigan for residency programs.

Admissions

REQUIREMENTS

Prerequisites are eight semester credits of biology, chemistry, organic chemistry, and physics, all with associated labs. Eight semester credits in English and social science, one upper-level biology course, and college algebra or statistics and probability are also required. The MCAT is required, and scores must be no more than four years old. For applicants who have retaken the exam, the most recent set of scores is used. Applicants should be United States or Canadian citizens, hold a permanent resident visa, or have asylum in the United States.

SUGGESTIONS

Though Michigan residents are given preference, about 20 percent of the positions in an entering class are available to highly qualified nonresident applicants. MSU is focused on training generalist physicians and seeks applicants with an interest in primary care and community-based medicine. Applicants should have medical/clinical experience. Important personal traits are excellent interpersonal communication skills, leadership, social responsibility, and compassion.

PROCESS

About one-fourth of AMCAS applicants are sent secondary applications. Of those returning secondaries, about one-third are interviewed. Interviews are conducted on Thursdays and Fridays, from September through March. Interviews consist of two sessions, one with a faculty member and one with a current medical student. On interview day, candidates attend informational sessions and have a social hour with medical students. About one-third of interviewees are accepted on a rolling basis.

Admissions Requirements (Required)

MCAT scores, science GPA, non-science GPA, letters of recommendation, interview, essays/personal statement, extracurricular activities, exposure to medical profession, U.S. resident, U.S. Perm. Res., Visa, or Canadian.

Admissions Requirements (Optional)

State residency.

Overlap Schools

University of Michigan—Ann Arbor; Wayne State University.

COSTS AND AID

Tuition & Fees

In-state Tuition	$22,377
Out-of-state Tuition	$50,277
Room and board (on campus)	$12,024
Cost of books	$3,200
Fees	$1,323

Financial Aid

% students receiving aid	93
Average grant	$3,500
Average loan	$26,000
Average debt	$140,000

MOREHOUSE COLLEGE
SCHOOL OF MEDICINE

ADMISSIONS AND STUDENT AFFAIRS, 720 WESTVIEW DRIVE, SW, ATLANTA, GA 30310 • ADMISSION: 404-752-1650
FAX: 404-752-1512 • E-MAIL: SROAF@MSM.EDU • WEBSITE: WWW.MSM.EDU

STUDENT BODY

Type	Private
Enrollment	182
% male/female	37/63
% underrepresented minorities	87
# applied (total/out)	2,047/1,736
# accepted (total/out)	116/43
# enrolled (total/out)	52/25
Average age	23

FACULTY

Total faculty (number)	260
% female	43
% minority	85
% part-time	14
Student-faculty ratio	1:1

ADMISSIONS

Application Information

Regular application	12/1
Regular notification	11/1
Early application	6/1–8/1
Early notification	10/1
Are transfers accepted?	yes
Admissions may be deferred?	yes
Interview required?	yes
Application fee	$50

Academics

Most students follow a 4 year curriculum leading to a MD, although some pursue joint-degree programs of MD/MPH or MD/PhD. To be considered for these programs, applications must be submitted to the appropriate graduate department at the time of application to medical school. Medical students are evaluated on an A–F scale. Passing the USMLE Step 1 is a requirement for promotion to year 3, and passing Step 2 is a requirement for graduation.

BASIC SCIENCES: Instruction uses a lecture/lab format, and students are in class or laboratories for about 30 hours per week. First-year courses are fundamentals of medicine I, human morphology, medical biochemistry, community health, medical physiology, neurobiology, and a weekly preceptorship with a community physician. Second-year courses are fundamentals of medicine II, pathology, pathophysiology, microbiology and immunology, nutrition, and pharmacology. During the second year, students learn patient interview and examination techniques. Instruction takes place in the Basic Medical Sciences Building, which contains classrooms, laboratories, and administrative offices in the adjacent Medical Education Building.

CLINICAL TRAINING

Third- and fourth-year required clerkships are psychiatry (7 weeks), internal medicine (2 months), pediatrics (2 months), ob/gyn (2 months), surgery (2 months), family medicine (1 month), ambulatory medicine (1 month and a year long fundamentals of medicine III Series), maternal child health (1 month), and rural primary care (1 month). Five months are reserved for electives. Third-year rotations take place primarily at Grady Memorial Hospital (1,000 beds), a full-service facility for indigent patients that, for training purposes, is shared with Emory University. A portion of elective credit may be earned at accredited medical schools other than Morehouse and at a wide range of clinical institutions.

Students

Approximately 67 percent of students are African American. About 51 percent of students are from Georgia, while others are from a wide geographic area. Class size is 52.

STUDENT LIFE

Community service is an important part of student life, and virtually all students are involved in some sort of volunteer activity while in medical school. Students are cohesive both in and out of the classroom. A demonstration of cooperation between students is the large percentage of students who are in study groups. Students participate in local chapters of national medical school organizations and in student groups focused on professional interests. Atlanta is the cultural, financial, and industrial hub of the Southeastern United States and offers a wide range of activities and attractions including arts, sports, recreation, dining, and entertainment. The city is accessible by public transportation. Although there is no school-owned housing, students are able to locate affordable housing off campus.

GRADUATES

Graduates are successful in securing residencies in prestigious programs nationwide. Approximately 75 percent of graduates enter primary care fields, one of the highest percentages among medical schools. Most go on to work with underserved populations, either in inner cities or in rural areas.

Admissions

REQUIREMENTS

Required courses are biology (1 year), general chemistry (1 year), organic chemistry (1 year), physics (1 year), college-level math (1 year), and English (1 year). All science courses must include associated labs. Grades are assessed with consideration given to academic improvement, balance and depth of academic program, difficulty of courses taken, and overall achievement. The MCAT is required, and scores must be from within the past two years. Applicants who have taken the exam on multiple occasions are not penalized, but the most recent set of scores is weighed most heavily.

SUGGESTIONS

Of the 52 spots in a class, at least 20 are reserved for Georgia residents. Thus, competition for out-of-state residents can be intense. For all applicants, the April, rather than August, MCAT is advised. Beyond academic achievement, the committee is interested in extracurricular activities, research projects and experiences, and evidence of pursuing interests and talents in depth. Compassion, honesty, motivation, and perseverance are qualities that are considered important to the practice of medicine.

PROCESS

About 80 percent of AMCAS applicants are sent secondary applications. Of those returning secondaries, about 8 percent are invited to interview between October and March. Of Georgia residents, about 25 percent are invited to interview. Interviews generally consist of one 30-minute session with a faculty member. On interview day, candidates receive a campus tour, group orientation sessions, lunch, and the opportunity to meet with current medical students. About 10–20 percent of interviewees are accepted, with notification beginning in December. Wait-listed candidates may send supplementary material to update or strengthen their files.

Admissions Requirements (Required)

MCAT scores, science GPA, non-science GPA, letters of recommendation, interview, essays/personal statement, extracurricular activities, exposure to medical profession.

Admissions Requirements (Optional)

State residency.

COSTS AND AID

Tuition & Fees

Tuition	$20,966
Room and board (on campus)	$10,970
Cost of books	$8,779
Fees	$4,405

Financial Aid

% students receiving aid	96
Average grant	$18,477
Average loan	$30,384
Average debt	$118,091

New York Medical College
School of Medicine

Office of Admissions, Administration Building, Valhalla, NY 10595 • Admission: 914-594-4507
Fax: 914-594-4976 • E-mail: MDADMIT@NYMC.EDU • Website: WWW.NYMC.EDU

STUDENT BODY

Type	Private
Enrollment	765
% male/female	50/50
% underrepresented minorities	10
# applied (total/out)	7,073/565
# accepted (total/out)	743/598
# enrolled (total/out)	186/129
Average age	26

FACULTY

Total faculty (number)	2,933
% female	28
% minority	32
% part-time	4

ADMISSIONS

Average GPA and MCAT Scores

Overall GPA	3.5
MCAT Bio	10.5
MCAT Phys	10.2
MCAT Verbal	9.5
MCAT Essay	Q

Application Information

Regular application	12/15
Regular notification	rolling
Early application	8/1
Early notification	10/1
Are transfers accepted?	yes
Admissions may be deferred?	yes
Interview required?	yes
Application fee	$100

Academics

Students have an opportunity to earn joint degrees, combining the MD with an MPH, which is of great value considering the increased awareness of public health issues, or a PhD in the basic medical sciences. Grading is honors/high pass/pass/fail. Passing Step 1 and 2 of the USMLE is a graduation requirement. In recent years, the pass rate has been at or near 100 percent .

BASIC SCIENCES: The curriculum of the first two years, although focused on the basic sciences, maintains a consistent clinical orientation. The program has been revised to bring clinical relevance and small-group teaching into all courses. The first two years focus on developing a thorough understanding of the sciences basic to clinical medicine. The core of the first-year curriculum—anatomy, behavioral science histology, biochemistry, neural science, and physiology—is supplemented by clinical case correlations and courses in epidemiology and biostatistics. The second-year curriculum, with its strong focus on pathology/pathophysiology, emphasizes small-group discussion, problem-based learning, and self-study, with only 25 percent of class time spent in large lectures. Clinical skills training, pharmacology, and medical microbiology prepare students for the clerkship experience of the next two years.

CLINICAL TRAINING

While immersed in the basic science curriculum, all first-year students have ongoing, direct patient contact, working in the office of a primary care physician. This one-on-one placement gives students clinical exposure and a personal mentor relationship. This preceptorship experience continues throughout the second year. Third-year clinical clerkships are the following: Medicine (12 weeks), surgery (8 weeks), pediatrics (8 weeks), ob/gyn (6 weeks), psychiatry (6 weeks), neurology (4 weeks), family medicine clerkship (4 weeks). The school's location in the suburban New York area and large hospital network afford clinical-training opportunities in demographically and clinically diverse settings. About half of the third-year class moves into New York City for their clinical years. Fourth-year requirements are the following: Medicine or pediatrics sub internship (4 weeks), ambulatory surgical subspecialties (4 weeks), geriatrics or chronic care pediatrics (4 weeks), and anesthesiology/rehabilitation medicine (2 weeks). The 18 weeks of electives can be taken anywhere. About 15–20 students take international electives each year.

Students

The school's student body is generally representative of the demographic diversity of the country. The first-year class size is 190 students; in recent years, it has been fairly equally divided by gender, with the proportion of females increasing incrementally. About half come from public colleges and universities.

STUDENT LIFE

Most first- and second-year students live on campus in attractive, unfurnished garden apartments, or furnished suite-style apartment shares in a suburban setting that encourages a sense of community. Students gather for pick-up football, soccer, and basketball games outdoors when the weather permits. Students can participate in more than 40 clubs and organizations groups focused on professional, cultural, social, educational, and athletic interests. These include The Arrhythmias, an a cappella singing group, a chamber music club, and other cultural groups. Project Sunshine works to better the lives of children in hospitals, and AMSA, AMA, AMWA, and SMNA—student chapters of major professional organizations—offer students an opportunity to represent the school at regional and national student conferences.

GRADUATES

The School of Medicine encourages students to aim high in applying for residency matches. While a large number of students choose to match in primary care disciplines, there are equally impressive matches in highly competitive specialty programs. Matches for the current year can be viewed on the school's website. Some 10,000 alumni are supported by alumni association chapters in major cities. Alumni can track university announcements of upcoming events on the website, and a special alumni section allows them to post news and read about other alumni. Alumni can also keep current on their classmates' activities via the university magazine, *Chironian*, which is mailed to all alumni and is also available for viewing on the Web.

Admissions

REQUIREMENTS

All applicants must have taken the MCAT within the last three years and must have completed or have in progress the following prerequisites: 2 semesters of biology, chemistry, organic chemistry, and physics. Each of these must have been completed with lab work. Two semesters of English are also required. The most recent MCAT scores are given greatest weight. While most students have majored in the sciences, the school encourages those with strong humanities backgrounds and the necessary science requirements to apply.

SUGGESTIONS

In addition to purely academic factors, we look for students who show clear evidence through their activities of strong motivation toward medicine and a sense of dedication to the service of others. Personal qualities of character and personality are evaluated from letters of recommendation, from the personal statement, and from the interview. New York Medical College does not deny admission to any applicant on the basis of race, color, creed, religion, national or ethnic origin, age, sex, sexual orientation, or disability.

PROCESS

All AMCAS applicants are requested to complete an online secondary application. After the completed secondary application and all letters of recommendation have been processed, the applicant's file is reviewed for consideration. Interviews are by invitation and are conducted on campus. We generally interview from October through April and decisions are made on a rolling basis.

Admissions Requirements (Required)

MCAT scores, science GPA, non-science GPA, letters of recommendation, interview, essays/personal statement, extracurricular activities, exposure to medical profession.

COSTS AND AID

Tuition & Fees

Tuition	$37,200
Room and board (on campus)	$17,326
Room and board (off campus)	$17,326
Cost of books	$1,650
Fees	$3,076

Financial Aid

% students receiving aid	90
Average grant	$20,000
Average loan	$45,000
Average debt	$163,000

NEW YORK UNIVERSITY
MOUNT SINAI SCHOOL OF MEDICINE

ANNENBERG 5-04A, PO BOX 1002, 1 GUSTAVE L. LEVY PLACE, NEW YORK, NY 10029-6574
ADMISSION: 212-241-6696 • FAX: 212-828-4135 • E-MAIL: ADMISSIONS@MSSM.EDU • WEBSITE: WWW.MSSM.EDU/BULLETIN

STUDENT BODY	
Type	Private
Enrollment	473
% male/female	48/52
% underrepresented minorities	35
# applied (total/out)	4,272/3,198
# accepted (total/out)	329/191
# enrolled (total/out)	120/73
Average age	23

FACULTY	
Total faculty (number)	1,922
% female	36
% minority	25
% part-time	13
Student-faculty ratio	4:1

ADMISSIONS

Average GPA and MCAT Scores

Overall GPA	3.67
MCAT Bio	11.4
MCAT Phys	11.0
MCAT Verbal	10.6
MCAT Essay	Q

Application Information

Regular application	11/1
Regular notification	rolling
Early application	8/1
Early notification	10/1
Are transfers accepted?	yes
Admissions may be deferred?	yes
Interview required?	yes
Application fee	$10

Academics

Mount Sinai's approach to medical education emphasizes cooperative, rather than competitive learning to prepare students for the lifelong learning that is essential for the modern medical career. Group study, small classes and, for the past 30 years, a pass/fail grading system for the first- and second-year students contribute to this emphasis. The majority of the students' time in the first 2 (pre-clinical) years is focused on the core biomedical knowledge and the basic skills of the doctor-patient relationship. Through direct patient contact during the third and fourth (clinical) years in inpatient and ambulatory settings, students develop the skills necessary for the practice of medicine. We offer the following joint-degree programs: MS/MD, MD/MPH, MD/MBA. In addition, 8–10 students each year pursue an MSTP-sponsored PhD degree along with the MD in conjunction with the Mount Sinai Graduate School of Biological Sciences. The PhD may be earned in biochemistry, biomathematical sciences, cell biology and anatomy, genetics, immunobiology, microbiology, molecular biology, neuroscience, pharmacology, or physiology/biophysics. Evaluation of student performance uses pass/fail for the pre-clinical courses and honor/high pass/pass/fail for clinical training. Students must pass Step 1 of the USMLE for promotion to year 3, and Step 2 to graduate.

BASIC SCIENCES: Basic sciences are taught through a combination of lectures, small-group discussions, labs, and clinical correlates. Lecture time is kept to 2 hours per day and students typically have 3 mornings or afternoons per week study time. Beginning on day one, the art and science of medicine, taught in both the first and second years, introduces students to the skills needed to care for patients. Throughout both years, the emphasis is on case-based learning. Integrated with every course are numerous means for providing clinical relevance for the basic science being studied. Topics—such as ethics, radiology, and palliative care—that overlap many areas are incorporated into the curriculum of all four years through courses without walls. First-year courses are embryology, first aid, genetics, histology and physiology, host defense mechanisms, molecules and cells, and pathogenesis. The year ends with an integrative core that focuses on translational topics, allowing students to work with faculty from the bench to the bedside on a selected and structured topic. Extensive study of mechanisms of disease and therapy is the major focus of the second year. This sequence of courses addresses each of the major pathophysiology topics essential to the practice of medicine. Organs and systems covered include breast, cardiovascular, endocrine, gynecologic, hematologic, musculoskelatal, renal/genitourinary, skin, and respiratory. A section on brain and behavior encompasses both psychopathology and neurology, and at the end of the year, the focus shifts to epidemiology and biostatistics.

CLINICAL TRAINING

The curriculum in the third year is composed of four 12 week modules of clinical clerkships. The modules are pediatrics, obstetrics, nursery, and gynecology; medicine and geriatrics; surgery and psychiatry; and neurology, anesthesia and family practice. Four weeks of electives are also offered in the third year. As in the first two years, an integrated case-based curriculum enriches the learning opportunities throughout the year. The fourth year begins with a four week preparation period for Step 2 of the USMLE followed by an emergency rotation and a sub internship in medicine. A clinical translational fellowship combines the clinical practice of medicine with the relevant basic science. A 4 week required post-match integrated selective addresses issues essential for students to explore before going on to residency. A significant portion of clinical training takes place at The Mount Sinai Hospital, which includes the 625-bed Guggenheim Pavilion and a Primary Care Building with an expansive ambulatory care program. Affiliated teaching facilities include, but are not limited to, Bronx Veterans Affairs Medical Center (561 beds); Elmhurst Hospital Center, Queens, (526 beds); Englewood Hospital and Medical Center, New Jersey, (520 beds); North General Hospital, Central and East Harlem; and Maimonedes Medical Center.

Students

The class entering in 2005 came from 46 different undergraduate institutions and pursued 54 undergraduate majors. Underrepresented minorities accounted for 21 percent of the students. The average age of incoming students was 23.

STUDENT LIFE

Mount Sinai provides a healthy environment and encourages the development of life-long, healthy habits. Cultural diversity is respected and supported, both in and out of the classroom. Students are active in a wide range of school-related organizations, particularly those focused on community service activities, and New York City is a rich source of extracurricular life. The Recreation Office provides discounted tickets to theater, movies, sporting events, and concerts. The Aron Residence Hall offers more than 600 furnished suites for single students. It is conveniently located and features a fitness center, among other amenities. School-owned housing for couples is also available.

GRADUATES

Among those who graduated in 2005, 21 percent entered internal medicine, 19 percent entered surgical specialties, 8 percent entered pediatrics, and 5 percent entered ob/gyn. The remainder entered a broad range of other postgraduate programs.

Admissions

REQUIREMENTS

Prerequisites are 1 year each of biology, general chemistry, organic chemistry and college-level math, English, and physics. The MCAT is required, and scores from 2000 onward are acceptable.

SUGGESTIONS

Students who have taken significant time off after college should have some recent course work. No particular extracurricular activities are specified, although successful applicants usually have some community service, research, or medically-related experience.

PROCESS

All AMCAS applicants receive secondary applications. Of those returning secondaries, about 17 percent are interviewed. Interviews are conducted from September through March, and consist of two 30-minute sessions, either with two faculty members or one faculty member and one medical student. Candidates are notified of the committee's decision with 2–6 weeks after the interview. Wait-listed candidates may send supplementary material to update their files. An early assurance program admits a limited number of sophomores with admission contingent upon completing undergraduate requirements.

Admissions Requirements (Required)

MCAT scores, science GPA, non-science GPA, letters of recommendation, interview, essays/personal statement, extracurricular activities, exposure to medical profession.

Admissions Requirements (Optional)

State residency.

COSTS AND AID

Tuition & Fees

Tuition	$33,250
Room and board (on campus)	$13,800
Cost of books	$1,220
Fees	$3,800

Financial Aid

% students receiving aid	87
Average grant	$19,429
Average loan	$35,825
Average debt	$104,730

NEW YORK UNIVERSITY
SCHOOL OF MEDICINE

550 FIRST AVENUE, NEW YORK, NY 10016 • **ADMISSION:** 212-263-5290
FAX: 212-263-0720 • **E-MAIL:** ADMISSIONS@MED.NYU.EDU • **WEBSITE:** WWW.MED.NYU.EDU

STUDENT BODY

Type	Private
Enrollment	702
% male/female	51/49
% underrepresented minorities	9
# applied (total/out)	8,028/6,561
# accepted (total/out)	468/330
# enrolled (total/out)	160/93
Average age	21

FACULTY

Total faculty (number)	1,344
% female	33
% minority	18
% part-time	22

ADMISSIONS

Average GPA and MCAT Scores

Overall GPA	3.73
MCAT Bio	11.3
MCAT Phys	11.1
MCAT Verbal	10.4
MCAT Essay	Q

Application Information

Regular application	10/15
Regular notification	2/15
Are transfers accepted?	no
Admissions may be deferred?	yes
Interview required?	yes
Application fee	$100

Academics

The goal of the curriculum is to train physician-scholars who will approach the profession of medicine with intellectual rigor and who also understand the humanistic and ethical aspects of the field. Selected students may pursue a curriculum leading to both MD and PhD degrees. The PhD degree is earned in a basic medical science field. The honors program permits students who are following the standard 4 year MD curriculum to supplement formal class work with summer research or ongoing projects and to receive credit. Grading during the pre-clinical years is pass/fail. Letter grades are given during the clinical clerkship.

BASIC SCIENCES: The School of Medicine's basic science curriculum is organized into interdisciplinary modules. Year 1 has three modules. The first module is comprised of anatomy, embryology, and molecular biology/genetics and biochemistry. Module 2 includes cellular biology, histology, immunology, and physiology. Module 3 is histology of tissues/organs, immunology and parasitology, microbiology, and organ physiology. Throughout the first year, students take behavioral science/introduction to clinical medicine, which addresses the interrelationship among patients, their families, environments, their particular illness, and their care. The first year also includes the skills and science of doctoring. This includes a preceptorship in the office of a practicing physician and serves to integrate basic science concepts with clinical applications. First-semester, second-year courses are the following: General pathology, neuroscience, and psychopathology. In the second semester, pathophysiology, pharmacology and biostatistics/epidemiology, and systemic pathology are integrated in a human organ system module. During the first two years, class time is divided between lectures and small-group discussions. Laboratory work and computer-assisted instruction enhance learning. In total, first- and second-year students are in class or other scheduled sessions for about 20 hours per week. Our division of academic computing has resulted in increased integration of bioinformatics into the curriculum. Each of the courses has a Web page, and students can access all course materials, including lecture slides, through the Web. Instruction takes place in the Medical Science Building and adjacent facilities, which provide laboratory space, lecture halls, rooms for small-group discussions, and conference rooms. The Frederick L. Ehrman Medical Library occupies three stories in the Medical Science Building and has areas that are open to students 24 hours a day. Its collection includes over 160,000 volumes and 2,000 current serial titles.

CLINICAL TRAINING

Required clerkships must be completed during year 3 and the first part of year 4. These are the following: medicine (10 weeks), surgery (10 weeks), pediatrics (8 weeks), ob/gyn (6 weeks), psychiatry (6 weeks), neurology (4 weeks), and ambulatory care medicine (4 weeks). During the fourth year, all students take 6 weeks of advanced medicine. The remainder of the year is reserved for elective study, which typically involves a research project. Clinical training takes place at Bellevue Hospital Center and New York University Medical Center Complex and at affiliated institutions. A portion of electives may be taken at other hospitals in the United States or abroad.

Students

Approximately 50 percent of students are New York residents. Others come from all regions of the country. Though the majority of students are in their early twenties, each class has several nontraditional students who pursued careers or other activities between college and medical school. Class size is 160.

STUDENT LIFE

NYU School of Medicine (SoM) is located in one of the most vibrant and centrally located neighborhoods in New York City. The area's many resources are easily accessible to NYU's campus, so that our students are presented with a vast array of cultural, social, and recreational opportunities. By way of the NYU SoM student ticket office, students are able to take advantage of the city's many cultural events and performances at discounted prices. The NYU SoM is easily accessible to other parts of the city. Midtown and Union Square are within walking distance, and other popular neighborhoods are only a short subway ride away. The SoM operates housing facilities for students, assuring that all NYU medical students can afford convenient and comfortable housing. Both residence halls and apartments are available.

GRADUATES

Of the 2005 graduates, the most prevalent fields for postgraduate training were the following: Internal medicine (18 percent), pediatrics (10 percent), diagnostic radiology (10 percent), and emergency medicine (7 percent). Most graduates enter residency programs at top institutions nationwide.

Admissions

REQUIREMENTS

Prerequisites are 6 semester hours each. They include the following: Biology, English, general chemistry, organic chemistry, and physics. All science courses must include laboratory work. The MCAT is required and must be taken no more than three years prior to application. For applicants who have taken the exam more than once, the best set of scores is considered.

SUGGESTIONS

Biochemistry is strongly recommended. Other recommended courses are calculus, embryology, genetics, Spanish, and quantitative and physical chemistry particularly if the applicant intends to practice in New York City. Experience in health care, research, and community service are considered valuable.

PROCESS

NYU Medical School participates in the AMCAS program. About 15 percent of applicants are invited to interview between September and December. Interviews consist of one session with a faculty member. On interview day applicants tour the campus and have lunch with current students. About 35 percent of interviewed candidates are accepted, with notification occurring by late January. Others are either wait listed or rejected. Wait-listed candidates can be selected for admission up until the first day of class in August.

Admissions Requirements (Required)
MCAT scores, science GPA, non-science GPA, letters of recommendation, interview, essays/personal statement, extracurricular activities, exposure to medical profession.

Admissions Requirements (Optional)
State residency.

Overlap Schools
Columbia University, Cornell University, Harvard University, Johns Hopkins University, Stony Brook University, UMDNJ, University of Pennsylvania.

COSTS AND AID

Tuition & Fees

Tuition	$30,625
Room and board (on campus)	$13,750
Cost of books	$1,200
Fees	$7,550

Financial Aid

% students receiving aid	75
Average grant	$9,250
Average loan	$34,500
Average debt	$128,000

NORTHEASTERN OHIO UNIVERSITIES COLLEGE OF MEDICINE

PO Box 95, ROOTSTOWN, OH 44272-0095 • ADMISSION: 330-325-6270
FAX: 330-325-8372 • E-MAIL: ADMISSION@NEOUCOM.EDU • WEBSITE: WWW.NEOUCOM.EDU

STUDENT BODY

Type	Public
Enrollment	430
% male/female	46/54
% underrepresented minorities	6
# applied (total/out)	1,402/524
# accepted (total/out)	254/20
# enrolled (total/out)	102/7
Average age	22

FACULTY

Total faculty (number)	1,905
% female	19
% minority	15
% part-time	86

ADMISSIONS

Average GPA and MCAT Scores

Overall GPA	3.66
MCAT Bio	9.0
MCAT Phys	9.1
MCAT Verbal	9.3
MCAT Essay	P

Application Information

Regular application	11/1
Regular notification	3/21
Early application	6/1–8/1
Early notification	10/1
Are transfers accepted?	yes
Admissions may be deferred?	no
Interview required?	yes
Application fee	$30

Academics

While most students participate in the 6 or 7 year BS/MD program, about 15–25 students each year enter the 4 year MD program. A combined MD/PhD program is offered in collaboration with either Kent State or the University of Akron, leading to the doctorate degree in biomedical engineering or a number of medically related science fields. A summer fellowship program provides a stipend to selected medical students who undertake research or clinical education projects related to community health. Medical students are evaluated with marks of honors, satisfactory, conditional-unsatisfactory, or unsatisfactory for most courses. Passing the USMLE Step 1 is a requirement for promotion to year 3, and passing Step 2 is a requirement for graduation.

BASIC SCIENCES: Basic sciences are taught primarily in a lecture/lab format, although some courses also utilize small-group discussions and tutorials. On average, students are in class or other scheduled sessions for 32 hours per week. First-year courses are behavioral science, biochemistry and molecular pathology, developmental medicine, human anatomy/embryology, infectious diseases, introduction to physical exam and ambulatory care experience, immunobiology, microscopic anatomy, medical neuroscience, physiology, and problem-based learning. Second-year courses are infectious disease 2, Introduction to Clinical Medicine (ICM), M2 ambulatory care experience, pharmacology, principles of medical sciences, radiology, and systemic pathology. The ICM course focuses on clinical problems, fundamental doctor-patient communication skills, the physical examination, and clinical evaluation. NEOUCOM's approach to instruction in this transitional year allows for extensive clinical exposure and patient contact. As part of ICM, students spend time each week in family practice centers. Students benefit from academic support and counseling services offered by the Office of Academic Affairs. The Oliver Ocasek Regional Medical Information Center, on the Rootstown campus, houses more than 91,000 books and journals in addition to computerized information systems. The center is electronically linked to libraries in the teaching hospitals and consortium universities.

CLINICAL TRAINING

Third-year required rotations are internal medicine (10 weeks), surgery (10 weeks), general pediatrics (8 weeks), ob/gyn (8 weeks), psychiatry (6 weeks), and family medicine (6 weeks). During the fourth year, additional requirements are primary care preceptorship (4 weeks), medical humanities (4 weeks), community medicine clerkship (4 weeks), and 20 weeks of electives. Training takes place at the following affiliated hospitals: Lodi Community Hospital, Wadsworth-Rittman Hospital, Akron General Medical Center, Barberton Citizens Hospital, Children's Hospital Medical Center, Edwin Shaw Hospital, Summa Health System, Robinson Memorial Hospital, Hillside Rehabilitation Hospital, Trumbull Memorial Hospital, St. Elizabeth Health Center, Western Reserve Care System, Salem Community Hospital, Aultman Hospital, Massillon Psychiatric Center, and Columbia Mercy Medical Center. In addition, students train at community-based centers that are part of the Area Health Education Center Program.

Students

Approximately 95 percent of students are Ohio residents. About 105 students in each class are admitted through the BS/MD program, and up to 25 are admitted through the traditional route. Although most entering students are in their early twenties, there are a few older or nontraditional students in each class. Underrepresented minorities account for about 4 percent of the student body.

STUDENT LIFE

Rootstown is a small town located about 15 miles east of Akron. On the medical school campus are recreation and exercise centers, student lounges, a picnic area, and tennis, basketball, and volleyball courts. Student groups include chapters of national medical student organizations, groups focused on professional interests, student-to-student support groups, and a recreation club. On-campus housing, including residence halls and apartments, is available on all three campuses.

GRADUATES

NEOUCOM graduates usually score well above the national average on the USMLE. Of the 1,350 graduates currently in residency or practice, 55 percent have remained in Ohio. About half of graduates enter primary care fields.

Admissions

REQUIREMENTS

Prerequisites are 1 year each of organic chemistry and physics, although success on the MCAT probably requires preparation in biology and general chemistry as well. The MCAT is required, and scores must be no more than two years old. For applicants who have retaken the exam, the most recent set of scores is considered. Thus, there is no advantage to withholding scores.

SUGGESTIONS

Ohio residents are given strong preference in the admissions process, and slight preference is given to graduates of consortium schools. Highly qualified applicants are encouraged to apply to the early decision program. Beyond requirements, recommended course work includes biochemistry, calculus, community health, embryology, general biology, general chemistry, humanities, microbiology, molecular biology, physiology, psychology, sociology, and statistics. For applicants who have taken time off after college, some recent course work is advised.

PROCESS

High school students interested in the combined BS/MD program apply to NEOUCOM in the Fall of senior year and complete a condensed undergraduate experience at Kent State, University of Akron, or Youngstown State before arriving at the Rootstown campus. As a result of attrition from this program, a limited number of seats are available for college graduates interested in the 4 year MD program. These applicants must apply through AMCAS. About 30 percent of AMCAS applicants are sent secondary applications. Of those returning secondaries, about 40 percent are interviewed between November and March. On interview day, candidates receive one interview with a panel of members of the Admissions Committee, a tour of the campus, lunch with current students, and a group informational session. Of interviewed candidates, about 10 percent are accepted on a rolling basis. Wait-listed candidates may update their files with transcripts.

NORTHWESTERN UNIVERSITY
FEINBERG SCHOOL OF MEDICINE

ADMISSIONS OFFICE, 1ST FLOOR, ROOM 606, 303 EAST CHICAGO AVENUE, CHICAGO, IL 60611-3008 ADMISSION: 312-503-8206
FAX: 312-503-0550 • E-MAIL: MED-ADMISSIONS@NORTHWESTERN.EDU • WEBSITE: MED-ADMISSIONS.NORTHWESTERN.EDU

STUDENT BODY

Type	Private
Enrollment	678
% male/female	51/49
% underrepresented minorities	12
# applied	6,817
# accepted (total/out)	399/356
# enrolled (total/out)	171/124
Average age	23

FACULTY

Total faculty (number)	3,929
% female	37
% minority	4
% part-time	51
Student-faculty ratio	6:1

ADMISSIONS

Average GPA and MCAT Scores

Overall GPA	3.72
MCAT Bio	11.5
MCAT Phys	11.6
MCAT Verbal	10.7
MCAT Essay	Q

Application Information

Regular application	10/15
Regular notification	12/15
Are transfers accepted?	yes
Admissions may be deferred?	yes
Interview required?	yes
Application fee	$75

Academics

The Feinberg medical curriculum retains the best aspects of traditional medical education and incorporates innovative, interactive methods designed for the independent adult learner. The curriculum is designed to cultivate leaders who will effect change in their communities and in the profession. Approximately 20 percent enter joint degree programs. The MD/MPH (masters in public health), MD/MA (masters in medical humanities and bioethics) and MD/MS (masters in health care quality and patient safety) can be completed in four years. The MD/MBA, offered in conjunction with the Kellogg School of Management, requires five years. The Medical Scientist Training Program leading to both MD and PhD degrees requires a minimum of seven years. Many other students conduct research during the summer after the first year; this can lead to ongoing research involvement in the Research Thesis Program. A number of students also undertake extended research opportunities during an additional year at Feinberg or in extramural programs. International academic and clinical opportunities are provided through a network of over a dozen partner institutions around the world.

BASIC SCIENCES: The first- and second-year curriculum is composed of 4 major courses, each presented in a series of discreet, topically focused units. Each course and nearly every unit is interdisciplinary and draws faculty from a number of departments. There is one integrated course in the basic medical sciences in each of the first two years, involving approximately 10 hours of lecture per week, complemented by problem-based learning sessions, laboratories, and small-group discussions and tutorials. Structure-function, the first-year course, begins with a review of cell and molecular biology, genetics, and signal transduction, then addresses gross and microscopic anatomy, biochemistry, and physiology in a consecutive sequence of organ systems. The second year basic science course, scientific basis of medicine, begins with an overview of immunology, microbiology, and infectious diseases and then details the pathology, pathophysiology, and pharmacology specific to each organ system. The medical decision-making course occupies 3 short blocks of time: The initial week of the first year, 1 week later in the first year, and the final portion of the second year. This innovative course allows students to develop the knowledge and skills in information management, epidemiology and biostatistics, and clinical problem solving essential to the contemporary practice of medicine. The fourth major course, patient, physician and society, is devoted to the development of clinical skills and professional perspectives and provides each student the opportunity to develop mentoring relationships with a variety of faculty preceptors. The class is divided into four colleges, each led by an experienced clinician. Colleges meet two afternoons per week throughout the first two years, and continue to meet on a regular basis through the third and fourth years (see below). One afternoon offers learning experiences centered around clinical skills development and the provision of an integrated biopsychosocial perspective on illness and patient care. The second afternoon's course sequence addresses medical ethics and humanities, public health, and health policy. Activities in both afternoon tracks incorporate health promotion and disease prevention as a guiding principle of the practice of medicine.

CLINICAL TRAINING

The third year consists of 49 weeks of required clerkships. Students gain experience in: medicine (12 weeks), surgery (12 weeks), pediatrics (6 weeks), ob/gyn (6 weeks), psychiatry (4 weeks), neurology (4 weeks), and primary care (4 weeks). A 1 week introduction to clinical clerkships provides orientation to the clerkship environment. During the fourth year, students complete a 6 week acting internship in medicine or pediatrics, 4 weeks in emergency medicine, 4 weeks in intensive care, and 2 weeks in physical medicine and rehabilitation.

Most clinical rotations are conducted within a consortium of major clinical affiliates, known as the McGaw Medical Center, that also sponsors one of the largest graduate medical education (residency) programs in the country. These clinical affiliates include Northwestern Memorial Hospital, Children's Memorial Hospital, the Rehabilitation Institute of Chicago, Evanston Northwestern Healthcare, and VA Chicago Health care System. The remainder of the fourth year is elective, and many students use this opportunity to explore extramural and international experiences.

Students

The 175 students in Feinberg's entering class typically represent 60 or more undergraduate institutions, more than 30 states, and several foreign countries. Approximately half the students are female. Over the last few years, about a fourth of each class has been made up of students with at least one year of experience in another field between undergraduate school and medical school matriculation. Admission deferments of one year are routinely available, and a special arrangement with Teach for America allows students accepted into that program to defer admission for two years. Within each class of about 175 students, 10 to 12 are admitted through the Medical Scientist Training Program (MD/PhD), and 35 to 40 are from the Honors Program in Medical Education (HPME), a combined BA/MD program through Northwestern University.

STUDENT LIFE

Northwestern students spend less time in class than students at many other schools, and more time in outside preparation and independent learning. Students are encouraged to pursue supplemental academic interests, community service endeavors, and other activities. The school's location is an important asset. Chicago is one of the most vibrant and diverse cities in the world, offering students a variety of community service learning activities as well as access to world-class museums, theaters, restaurants and other attractions. About half the medical students live within walking distance of the school and Northwestern Memorial Hospital. Others live in a variety of neighborhoods throughout the city, and take advantage of Chicago's excellent public transportation system.

GRADUATES

Northwestern graduates are accepted to competitive residencies throughout the nation. Today there are more than 12,000 medical school alumni living in the United States and around the world. Northwestern alumni are particularly well represented in academic medicine.

Admissions

REQUIREMENTS

There are no specific course requirements, but a full year each of modern biology, organic chemistry, inorganic chemistry, general physics, and English are recommended. The MCAT is required, with scores no more than three years old at the time of application. A minimum of three years of college (135 quarter hours/90 semester hours) is required for admission; a bachelor's degree is preferred.

SUGGESTIONS

The Feinberg School seeks applicants who have demonstrated academic excellence, leadership qualities, intellectual curiosity, and personal maturity. Applicants should be liberally educated men and women who have studied a discipline in some depth beyond the conventional premedical courses. The school has a particular interest in students with promise as physician-scholars. Experience in research and evidence of commitment to medicine as a service profession are positive factors in selection.

PROCESS

All qualified AMCAS registrants applying to Feinberg are sent a supplemental application. Of those returning the supplemental, about 10 percent are interviewed between October and February. The medical school uses a combined interview approach, with both individual and panel interview. The individual interview is conducted by a member of the dean's administration or Committee on Admissions, and a panel of three to four candidates is interviewed by three members of the Interview Committee (usually two faculty and one medical student).

Admissions Requirements (Required)

MCAT scores, science GPA, non-science GPA, letters of recommendation, interview, essays/personal statement.

Overlap Schools

Case Western Reserve University, New York University—Mount Sinai School of Medicine, New York University—School of Medicine, The University of Chicago, University of Michigan—Ann Arbor, University of Pittsburgh, Vanderbilt University, Washington University.

COSTS AND AID

Tuition & Fees

Tuition	$37,308
Room and board (on campus)	$14,625
Cost of books	$2,577
Fees	$2,693

Financial Aid

% students receiving aid	76
Average grant	$9,933
Average loan	$45,573
Average debt	$103,253

THE OHIO STATE UNIVERSITY
COLLEGE OF MEDICINE

155 D MEILING HALL, 370 WEST 9TH AVENUE, COLUMBUS, OH 43210 • ADMISSION: 614-292-7137
FAX: 614-247-7959 • E-MAIL: MEDICINE@OSU.EDU • WEBSITE: WWW.MEDICINE.OSU.EDU

STUDENT BODY

Type	Public
Enrollment	839
% male/female	63/37
% underrepresented minorities	32
# applied (total/out)	4,180/3,159
# accepted (total/out)	400/217
# enrolled (total/out)	210/91
Average age	22

FACULTY

Total faculty (number)	2,731
% part-time	49
Student-faculty ratio	0:1

ADMISSIONS

Average GPA and MCAT Scores

Overall GPA	3.72
MCAT Bio	11.22
MCAT Phys	10.92
MCAT Verbal	10.34
MCAT Essay	P

Application Information

Regular application	12/1
Regular notification	10/15
Early application	8/1
Early notification	10/1
Are transfers accepted?	yes
Admissions may be deferred?	yes
Interview required?	yes
Application fee	$60

Academics

All students begin with a 14-week course in human anatomy. This includes cadaver dissection, cross-sectional anatomy, multimedia for self-directed learning, imaging technology, and clinical correlations, as well as histology and embryology. Students also initiate their study of the medical humanities and behavioral sciences during this period in courses called patient-centered medicine and physician development. After the conclusion of the first 14-week academic experience, students enter one of two pre-clinical pathways: integrated pathway or independent study. A program emphasizing a family medicine enrichment experience is also available. Passage of Step 1 of the USMLE is required for progression to year three. A hallmark of Ohio State's MD curriculum is the opportunity for students to select experiences that fit with their individual learning styles and long-term career goals. The curriculum provides a variety of analytical and managerial skills specifically designed to be applicable in the health services setting.

BASIC SCIENCES: Joint-degree programs include four options. The Medical Scientist Program (MSP), a 7 year combined MD/PhD degree for highly-qualified and motivated students who have excellent academic backgrounds, motivation for a career in academic medicine, and a commitment to or demonstrated aptitude for a research career. The Master of Public Health (MPH), a combined five-year program allows students to simultaneously earn the MD and MPH degrees, with instruction in epidemiology/biometrics, environmental health sciences, health promotion, and health services management/policy. The Master of Health Administration (MHA) is a joint five-year program that allows students to simultaneously earn the MD and MHA degrees. The Master of Business Administration (MBA) is a five-year degree program designed to prepare future physicians to meet the challenges of business administration and financial issues in the practice of medicine in physician offices, hospitals, and health care systems. The Doctor of Medicine/Juris Doctor (MD/JD) combined 7 year degree program has been designed to prepare future physicians to meet the challenges of legal issues in physician offices, hospitals, comprehensive medical centers, and health care-related industries.

CLINICAL TRAINING

Clinical rotations begin with the introduction to clinical medicine (ICM). The goal of this clerkship is to enable students to better use their major and elective experiences to become excellent physicians. The third-year required clerkships consist of: Ambulatory medicine, family medicine, general internal medicine, internal medicine, pediatrics, surgery, ob/gyn, psychiatry, neurology, and one elective. Curriculum in the fourth year includes four selective experiences called the differentiation of care selectives (DOCS). DOC 1 is the undifferentiated patient; DOC 2 is the differentiated ambulatory patient; DOC 3 is the chronic care patient; DOC 4 is the sub-internship in a chosen specialty. Other fourth-year requirements include the Dean's Colloquium, other elective opportunities, and vacation allowances. Training occurs in 24 affiliated hospitals, including the University Hospital, University Hospital-East, The Arthur G. James/Richard J. Solove Cancer Hospital and Research Institute, and Children's Hospital. Passage of Step 2 of the USMLE is required for graduation.

Students

The class profile for 2005 reflects a class size of 210 entering students, with 57 percent from Ohio, 33 percent women, and 9 percent underrepresented minority students. The average GPA was 3.72 with an MCAT average of 11 in the subscores.

STUDENT LIFE

There are more than 40 medical student organizations. Medical students have access to all of the resources and facilities of the university. Campus and city bus transportation is free with the presentation of student ID. Computerized housing opportunities are available free of charge through the Off-Campus Student Services. University graduate residence halls and family housing are also available.

GRADUATES

PGY-1 Match Results for 2005 reflect 44 percent of the graduating class plan to enter primary care residencies, and 41 percent matched with Ohio residency programs.

Admissions

REQUIREMENTS

One year of biology with labs, chemistry, organic chemistry with labs, and physics are required. Also recommended are courses in biochemistry and molecular genetics. Application through AMCAS and MCAT test with scores that are no more than three years old are required.

SUGGESTIONS

The Admissions Committee evaluates candidates according to competitive standards. Applicants are judged on the basis of academic performance as well as personal qualities such as integrity, leadership, and interpersonal skills. Clinically related experiences, as well as research positions, are encouraged.

PROCESS

Applications are reviewed upon receipt from AMCAS. Competitive applicants are sent secondary applications. Approximately 680 applicants are interviewed between September and March. On interview day, applicants tour the medical center and have lunch with current medical students.

Admissions Requirements (Required)

MCAT scores, science GPA, non-science GPA, letters of recommendation, interview, essays/personal statement, extracurricular activities, exposure to medical profession.

COSTS AND AID

Tuition & Fees

In-state Tuition	$22,833
Out-of-state Tuition	$35,644
Room and board (on campus)	$13,560
Cost of books	$4,134
Fees	$573

Financial Aid

% students receiving aid	89
Average grant	$6,014
Average loan	$28,524
Average debt	$123,015

OREGON HEALTH AND SCIENCE UNIVERSITY

SCHOOL OF MEDICINE

OFFICE OF EDUCATION & STUDENT AFFAIRS, L102, 3181 SOUTHWEST, PORTLAND, OR 97201 **ADMISSION:** 503-494-2998
FAX: 503-494-3400 • **E-MAIL:** MDADMISS@OHSU.EDU • **WEBSITE:** WWW.OHSU.EDU/EDU/SOM-DEAN/ADMIT.HTML

STUDENT BODY

Type	Public
Enrollment	452
% male/female	52/48
% underrepresented minorities	14
# applied (total/out)	3,601/3,292
# accepted (total/out)	184/110
# enrolled (total/out)	112/44
Average age	25

FACULTY

Total faculty (number)	1,066
% female	40
% minority	3
% part-time	4
Student-faculty ratio	4:1

ADMISSIONS

Average GPA and MCAT Scores

Overall GPA	3.6
MCAT Bio	10.16
MCAT Phys	10.2
MCAT Verbal	10.15
MCAT Essay	P

Application Information

Regular application	10/15
Regular notification	rolling
Are transfers accepted?	yes
Admissions may be deferred?	no
Interview required?	yes
Application fee	$75

Academics

Although most students complete a 4 year MD curriculum, others follow alternative courses of study, including joint-degree programs. The 5 year MD/MPH degree program is offered by the School of Medicine's Department of Public Health and Preventive Medicine in conjunction with appropriate departments at Oregon State University and Portland State University. Generally, students indicate their interest in this program when they apply to the School of Medicine. First-year medical students may pursue an epidemiological and biostatistical track, which also serves as preparation for careers in public health. The joint-degree program is the MD/PhD in the following fields: Biochemistry and molecular biology, cell biology and anatomy, molecular and medical genetics, medical psychology, molecular microbiology and immunology, neuroscience, and pharmacology and physiology. Grades are honors, near honors, satisfactory, marginal, and fail. Step 1 and Step 2 of the USMLE is a requirement for graduation.

BASIC SCIENCES: Students spend 2 hours per day in lecture. An additional 2 hours each day are used for small-group sessions and/or laboratory activities. One afternoon each week is devoted to principles of clinical medicine in which students work one-on-one with physicians and an additional afternoon studying issues related to public health, behavioral sciences, history taking and learning physical diagnosis skills. First-year courses are anatomy, embryology, and imaging; biological basis of disease; cell structure and function; systems process and homeostasis; and principles of clinical medicine, which continues into the second year. The second year is organized around organ systems and physiological concepts, which include blood, circulation, neuroscience and behavior, metabolism, and human development and life cycle. The first two years are spent largely in the Basic Sciences and Education Buildings, which have facilities for lectures, discussions, computer learning, and laboratories. The library contains more than 150,000 volumes and 2,500 periodicals.

CLINICAL TRAINING

Required third-year rotations are medicine (12 weeks), primary care (6 weeks), ob/gyn (6 weeks), child health (6 weeks), psychiatry (6 weeks), family medicine (6 weeks), surgery (6 weeks), and transition to clerkship (1 week). During the fourth year, students fulfill advanced clerkship requirements in medicine, surgery, child health, and neurology (4 weeks each) in addition to selectives and electives. The fourth year culminates in transition to physician, a week-long experience. Clinical training takes place at the University Hospital and Clinics and at affiliated institutions, which include Doernbecher Children's Hospital and Portland's Veterans Affairs Medical Center. The School of Medicine's research touches all realms of modern medical sciences. Some investigate the causes and treatments of learning disorders, addiction, heart disease, stroke, cancer, infertility, movement disorders, and emotional disorders. Others work at the molecular and cellular levels to unravel the most basic aspects of human health.

Students

About 6 percent of students at OHSU are from underrepresented minority backgrounds. The average age of incoming students is around 25. Class size is 96.

STUDENT LIFE

Portland is an ideal location for students, offering the comforts of a medium-sized city and proximity to spectacular outdoor destinations. Close to campus are parks and other places to run, walk, or bike ride. A bit further are mountains for hiking and skiing. For an urban area, Portland is relatively affordable and safe. On-campus activities are also popular with medical students. The newly renovated fitness and sports center includes a full weight room, racquetball and squash courts, aerobics classes, swimming pools, and a spa. The Office of Multicultural Affairs supports students of ethnic and international backgrounds with supplemental counseling services, recreational activities, workshops, and classes. Numerous clubs and organizations bring students together around professional or extracurricular interests. Although student housing is available on a limited basis in the residence hall, most opt to live off campus.

GRADUATES

Graduates are successful in securing residency positions at prestigious institutions all over the country. However, most enter programs in the Western United States. More than half enter primary care residencies.

Admissions

REQUIREMENTS

Required courses are chemistry/organic chemistry (two years), biology (1 year), physics (1 year), English (1 year), humanities (1 year), social science (1 year), and college-level math (1 semester). GPAs from all 4 year undergraduate institutions are evaluated equally, although factors such as the breadth of education, rigor of major, GPA trends, course load, and extracurricular activities are considered. The MCAT is required and scores must be from within three years of the year of matriculation.

SUGGESTIONS

Preference is given to Oregon, WICHE-certified residents of Montana and Wyoming, MD/PhD and MD/MPH candidates, and nonresident applicants with superior achievements in academics and other related experiences. The School of Medicine Admissions Committee fully recognizes the importance of diversity in its student body and in the physician workforce in providing for effective delivery of health care. Accordingly, the OHSU School of Medicine strongly encourages applications from persons from all socioeconomic, racial, ethnic, religious, and educational backgrounds and persons from groups underrepresented in medicine. The committee adheres to a policy of equal opportunity and non-discrimination on the basis of sex, age, race, ethnic origin, religion, or sexual orientation.

PROCESS

About half of AMCAS applicants receive secondaries, and about 40 percent of candidates in this group are interviewed. Interviews consist of two 30 minute sessions with members of the faculty or Admissions Committee. Interviewees are invited to lunch with medical students and are given a tour of the campus. Approximately 20 percent of interviewees are accepted on a rolling basis. Wait-listed candidates are ranked and have a fairly good chance of being accepted later in the spring.

Admissions Requirements (Required)

MCAT scores, science GPA, non-science GPA, letters of recommendation, interview, essays/personal statement, extracurricular activities, exposure to medical profession.

Admissions Requirements (Optional)

State residency. Preference is given to Oregon residents.

Overlap Schools

Stanford University.

COSTS AND AID

Tuition & Fees

In-state Tuition	$21,000
Out-of-state Tuition	$31,500
Cost of books	$2,800
Fees	$3,517

Financial Aid

% students receiving aid	90
Average grant	$2,000
Average loan	$30,000
Average debt	$112,000

PENNSYLVANIA STATE UNIVERSITY
COLLEGE OF MEDICINE

OFFICE OF STUDENT AFFAIRS, PO BOX 850, HERSHEY, PA 17033 • ADMISSION: 717-531-8755
FAX: 717-531-6225 • E-MAIL: HMCSAFF@PSU.EDU • WEBSITE: WWW.HMC.PSU.EDU/COLLEGE

STUDENT BODY	
Type	Private
Enrollment	423
% male/female	50/50
% underrepresented minorities	13
# applied (total/out)	6,615/5,509
# enrolled (out-of-state)	135
Average age	23

FACULTY	
Total faculty (number)	155
% female	18
% minority	23

ADMISSIONS

Average GPA and MCAT

GPA	3.65
MCAT Bio	10.05
MCAT Phys	9.51
MCAT Verbal	9.06
MCAT Writing	P

Application Information

Regular application	11/15
Regular notification	until filled
Early application	6/1–8/1
Early notification	10/1
Are transfers accepted?	yes
Admissions may be deferred?	yes
Interview required?	no
Application fee	$40

Academics

Penn State was one of the first medical schools in the country to institute departments of humanities and behavioral science and to incorporate these perspectives into the basic science and clinical education programs. The College of Medicine was also among the first to develop a separate family and community medicine department. A combined MD/PhD program is offered, allowing students to earn the doctorate degree in biochemistry, biomedical engineering, cell biology, genetics, immunology, microbiology, molecular biology, pharmacology, and physiology. There are also numerous opportunities to pursue discrete research projects as electives or during summers. Grading designations are honors, high pass, pass, and fail. Students must pass USMLE Step 1 after the pre-clinical years, and Step 2 to graduate.

BASIC SCIENCES: During the first and second years, students are in class or other scheduled sessions for approximately 23 hours per week. This schedule gives students the opportunity for independent and collaborative study. Clinical problems are used as a means of applying and correlating the basic science information that is presented in lectures or discussions. Labs and computer-assisted learning are also important parts of the curriculum. First-year courses are biological basis of disease; cellular and molecular basis of medical practice; humanistic aspects of medicine; physicians, patients and society, which touches on the psychological, social, ethical, and legal; and structural basis of medical practice. Second-year courses are immunology, issues in medical practice, introduction to medicine III and IV, microbiology, pathology, pharmacology, physical diagnosis, and psychiatry. Instruction takes place in the Medical Sciences Building, which houses classrooms and laboratories. The Harrell Library is open 24 hours a day and holds approximately 125,000 volumes, 2,000 periodicals, and modern computer and audiovisual resources.

CLINICAL TRAINING

Third-year required clerkships are internal medicine (8 weeks), selectives (8 weeks), surgery (8 weeks), pediatrics (6 weeks), ob/gyn (6 weeks), psychiatry (4 weeks), family and community medicine (4 weeks), and primary care (4 weeks). The fourth year is devoted to electives and selectives, which are chosen from clinical or research departments. An overseas elective program allows a number of fourth-year students to fulfill elective requirements at clinical sites in Asia, Africa, and Latin America. Generally, clinical training takes place at the University Hospital (463 beds), Children's Hospital, the Rehabilitation Center, and at other hospitals and clinics affiliated through an organized health network called Alliance Health. Additional facilities on campus are a sports medicine center, the General Clinical Research Center, an animal research center, and a trauma center.

Students

About 40 percent of students are Pennsylvania residents. More than 25 percent of students are underrepresented minorities, a tribute to the school's commitment to recruiting a diverse student body. The average age of incoming students is 23, with a wide age range. Class size is 110.

STUDENT LIFE

Educational facilities, clinical teaching sites, campus housing, and recreational centers are within walking distance of one another. The College of Medicine is an attractive campus, occupying 550 acres. Hershey provides a comfortable, student-friendly community that is relatively safe. As a tourist destination, Hershey offers a variety of dining and entertainment possibilities. Medical students are involved in organizations such as honor societies, professional interest groups, local chapters of national organizations, and groups focused on community service or recreational pursuits. When in need of urban distractions, the state capital, Harrisburg, is 12 miles away, and both Philadelphia and Pittsburgh are easily accessible. On-campus housing options include 1-, 2-, and 3-bedroom apartments.

GRADUATES

Graduates are successful at securing residencies nationwide. Penn State emphasizes primary care and encourages students to consider postgraduate training programs in primary care fields.

Admissions

REQUIREMENTS

Prerequisites are 1 year each of biology, chemistry, college-level math, organic chemistry, physics. All science courses should have associated labs. One semester each of social sciences and humanities is also required. The MCAT is required, and scores must be no more than two years old. For applicants who have taken the exam on multiple occasions, all sets of scores are considered.

SUGGESTIONS

Beyond requirements, course work in anthropology, calculus, genetics, psychology, sociology, and statistics are recommended. The April, rather than August, MCAT is strongly advised. Health care related experience is valued, as are interpersonal and communication skills. State residency is not a consideration in the application process.

PROCESS

All AMCAS applicants are sent secondary applications. About 10 percent of those returning secondaries are interviewed between September and March. Interviews consist of two or three sessions each with a faculty member. On interview day, candidates also tour the campus and have lunch with current medical students. About one-third of interviewees are accepted on a rolling basis. Another group is wait listed. Wait-listed candidates are not encouraged to send supplementary material.

Admissions Requirements (Required)

MCAT scores, essays/personal statement, extracurricular activities, exposure to medical profession.

Admissions Requirements (Optional)

Science GPA, nonscience GPA, letters of recommendation, interview, state residency.

COSTS AND AID

Tuition & Fees

Room and board (on campus)	$6,144
Cost of books	$1,205

Financial Aid

% students receiving aid	91
Average grant	$10,248
Average loan	$23,500
Average debt	$98,061

PONCE SCHOOL OF MEDICINE

PO BOX 7004, PONCE, PR 00732 • **ADMISSION:** 787-840-2575
FAX: 787-842-0461 • **E-MAIL:** ADMISSIONS@PSM.EDU • **WEBSITE:** WWW.PSM.EDU

STUDENT BODY	
Type	Private
# applied (total/out)	968/690
# accepted (total/out)	148/47
# enrolled (total/out)	66/17

ADMISSIONS

Average GPA and MCAT Scores

Overall GPA	3.25
MCAT Bio	7.8
MCAT Phys	7.0
MCAT Verbal	7.2
MCAT Essay	M

Application Information

Regular application	12/15
Regular notification	rolling
Early application	8/1
Early notification	10/5
Are transfers accepted?	yes
Admissions may be deferred?	no
Interview required?	yes
Application fee	$100

Academics

The primary goal of the Ponce School of Medicine is to provide quality medical education to bilingual students, with an emphasis on primary care and family medicine. The curriculum includes a strong emphasis on basic sciences, enabling students to get the most out of their clinical training. Longitudinal programs in preventive medicine and medical ethics are integrated into the 4 year curriculum.

BASIC SCIENCES: Basic sciences are taught during the first two years. Year 1 courses include the following: Behavioral science, biochemistry, bioethics, cellular biology and histology, general pathology, gross anatomy imaging and embryology, human genetics, microbiology and immunology, neuroscience, physiology, and a year-long session devoted to clinical correlation. Second-year courses are bioethics, family and community medicine, infectious diseases, introduction to clinical medicine, pathophysiology, pathology, pharmacology, and psychiatry. Instructional methods include computer-assisted learning, lectures, labs, and problem-based learning. Standardized patients are used for teaching and evaluation of basic clinical skills. During the first two years, students are in class or other scheduled sessions for about 30 hours per week. Students must pass Step I of the USMLE for promotion to year 3.

CLINICAL TRAINING

The third year begins in July with 2 weeks of a course called introduction to hospital life. Following this orientation, students begin required clerkships. These are: Internal medicine (10 weeks), surgery (10 weeks), pediatrics (10 weeks), ob/gyn (5 weeks), psychiatry (5 weeks), and family medicine (5 weeks). The third year also includes a dean's hour, which emphasizes bioethics, health economics, law, literature, and medical humanities. In the fourth year, students participate in a required clerkship in medicine (4 weeks); a sub internship (medicine, ob/gyn, pediatrics, or family medicine); a clerkship in emergency medicine (4 weeks); and a primary care selective (4 weeks). Students are also required to complete 16 weeks of elective rotations, of which 5 weeks may be completed at sites other than Ponce. USMLE Step II must be passed prior to graduation.

Students

STUDENT LIFE

The relatively small class size of 60 students encourages communication among students and faculty. The school's location is an asset, offering a pleasant environment for living and studying.

Admissions

REQUIREMENTS

Required undergraduate course work includes 8 semester credits in biology, general chemistry, organized chemistry, and physics in addition to 6 credits in advanced math and Spanish. Twelve credits in both behavioral sciences and English are also required. Behavioral science includes anthropology, economics, political sciences, psychology, and sociology. Applicants must have a minimum overall grade point average of 2.7 and an average of 2.5 in science courses. The MCAT is required, and scores should be from within one year of application. Applicants should have at least the mean on all sections of the MCAT.

SUGGESTIONS

In evaluating applicants, the Admissions Committee considers academic achievements, MCAT scores, interview reports, letters of recommendation, and other supplementary information. Preference is given to residents of Puerto Rico.

PROCESS

Ponce takes part in the AMCAS application process. The deadline for submission to AMCAS is December 15. Secondary applications are sent to all qualified applicants, and interviews are conducted throughout the spring.

Admissions Requirements (Required)

MCAT scores, science GPA, non-science GPA, letters of recommendation, interview, essays/personal statement.

Admissions Requirements (Optional)

State residency, extracurricular activities, exposure to medical profession.

COSTS AND AID

Tuition & Fees

Tuition	$25,304
Fees	$1,761

Financial Aid

Average grant	$8,000
Average loan	$35,954
Average debt	$96,931

QUEEN'S UNIVERSITY
SCHOOL OF MEDICINE

68 BARRIE STREET, KINGSTON, ON K7L 3N6 • ADMISSION: 613-533-2542
FAX: 613-533-6190 • E-MAIL: JEB8@POST.QUEENSU.CA • WEBSITE: HTTP://MEDS.QUEENSU.CA

STUDENT BODY

Type	Public
Enrollment	100
% male/female	52/48
% underrepresented minorities	2
# applied	1,388
# accepted	175
# enrolled	100

ADMISSIONS

Average GPA and MCAT Scores

Overall GPA	3.6
MCAT Bio	11
MCAT Phys	11.11
MCAT Verbal	10.84
MCAT Essay	P

Application Information

Regular application	10/1
Regular notification	5/31
Are transfers accepted?	no
Admissions may be deferred?	yes
Interview required?	yes
Application fee	$250

Academics

Most students follow a 4 year curriculum leading to an MD degree. Masters and Doctoral degree programs are also offered in biochemistry, biostatistics, environmental and occupational health, epidemiology, general community health, health-care systems, pathology, and preventive medicine. Although there are no formally structured combined programs, superior students may be permitted the flexibility to work toward an MSc or a PhD concurrently with the MD. Grading uses a honors/pass/fail system.

BASIC SCIENCES: Most basic science instruction takes place during the first three years. First-year course starts with phase I, introduction to the sciences relevant to medicine, an introduction to the fundamental language and concepts of medical science, and communication/clinical skills. Phase IIA includes allergy and immunology, clinical skills, dermatology/musculoskeletal systems, haematology and oncology, and microbiology and infectious diseases. Second-year courses are clinical skills, genitourinary/cardiovascular/ respirology, and psychiatry/neuroscience/ophthalmology/ENT. In addition, 8 weeks are left open for an elective. Third year courses are clinical skills, endocrine/metabolism/ reproduction, and gastrointestinal. In addition to problem-based learning, teaching methods include lectures, seminars, small group discussions, laboratory experience, and computer-based instruction. Basic science instruction takes place primarily at Botterell Hall, which also houses administrative offices and Bracken Library. The Clinical Learning center is an important educational facility within the Faculty of Health Sciences specifically designed for the teaching, learning, and evaluation of important clinical skills, and is used during both pre-clinical and clinical years. The Health Sciences Library subscribes to approximately 844 serials, and its total collection consists of 156,000 volumes. In the library is the Multimedia Learning Centre, which offers both video- and computer-assisted instruction.

CLINICAL TRAINING

Clerkships begin in January of the third year. They are: Medicine (12 weeks), surgery (8 weeks), psychiatry (6 weeks), ob/gyn (6 weeks), pediatrics (6 weeks), family medicine (4 weeks), geriatrics (2 weeks), and emergency medicine (2 weeks). Four weeks of selectives and 12 weeks of electives are also required. Clerkships takes place at a number of affiliated hospitals, including Kingston General Hospital, Hotel Dieu Hospital, St. Mary's of the Lake Hospital, Kingston Psychiatric Hospital, and Ongwanada Hospital. The provision of health care services in Kingston is presently being restructured and will change over the next few years.

Students

Each class has 90 students, about 50 of whom are typically from the province of Ontario. The student body is approximately 50 percent women.

STUDENT LIFE

Medical students enjoy the recreational, cultural, social activities of the greater university, and the city of Kingston. On-campus attractions include museums, concert halls, cinema, and an observatory. Student services include a child care resource center, a foundation supporting women, comprehensive health services, an international center, a physical education center, and a student center. The university provides accommodations in single and double occupancy rooms for approximately 300 graduate students. In addition, the Apartment and Housing Office manages university-owned rentals in the area.

Admissions

REQUIREMENTS

In order to apply, students must have completed three years of full-time study at a university. In addition, 1 year each of biological sciences, physical sciences, and humanities/social sciences are required. The MCAT is required. To be eligible for admission, applicants must be Canadian citizens, Canadian permanent residents, or children of Queen's University alumni.

SUGGESTIONS

The Admissions Committee looks for both academic abilities, such as commitment, achievement, critical thinking, and self-directed learning, and personal characteristics such as communication skills, creativity, and sensitivity. No preference is given to a particular undergraduate program of studies, and college students seeking admission are encouraged to pursue studies in their area of interest.

PROCESS

Applicants seeking further information about admission should contact the School of Medicine. Applications are made through the following: Ontario Medical Schools' Application Service, 70 Research Lane, Guelph, Ontario N1G 5E2. The deadline is October 15. The first admissions cutoff is based on the cumulative converted grade point average, and the second is made on the basis of MCAT scores. Those applicants who qualify are interviewed. Applicants are then ranked according to evaluation of letters of reference, autobiographic sketch, and interview results.

Admissions Requirements (Required)

MCAT scores, science GPA, non-science GPA, letters of recommendation, interview, essays/personal statement, extracurricular activities.

Overlap Schools

McMaster University, University of Ottawa, University of Toronto, University of Western Ontario.

COSTS AND AID

Tuition & Fees

Tuition $13,500

ROSALIND FRANKLIN UNIVERSITY OF MEDICINE AND SCIENCE

OFFICE OF ADMISSIONS, 3333 GREEN BAY ROAD NORTH, CHICAGO, IL 60064 • ADMISSION: 847-578-3204
FAX: 847-578-3284 • E-MAIL: CMS.ADMISSIONS@ROSALINDFRANKLIN.EDU • WEBSITE: WWW.ROSALINDFRANKLIN.EDU

STUDENT BODY

Type	Private
Enrollment	757
% male/female	55/45
% underrepresented minorities	6
# applied (total/out)	6,447/5,449
# accepted	442
# enrolled (total/out)	185/148
Average age	24

FACULTY

Total faculty (number)	674
% female	27
% part-time	44
Student-faculty ratio	1:1

ADMISSIONS

Average GPA and MCAT Scores

Overall GPA	3.59
MCAT Bio	10.36
MCAT Phys	10.13
MCAT Verbal	9.08
MCAT Essay	P

Application Information

Regular application	11/15
Regular notification	10/15
Early application	6/1–8/1
Early notification	10/1
Are transfers accepted?	yes
Admissions may be deferred?	yes
Interview required?	yes
Application fee	$95

Academics

Founded in 1912, Rosalind Franklin University of Medicine and Science has been dedicated to excellence in medical education for nearly a century. The school has educated thousands of professionals with recognized innovation in health education, excellence in the creation of knowledge, and scientific discovery focused on prediction and prevention of disease, outstanding clinical programs, and compassionate community service. Major hospital affiliates include Advocate Lutheran General Hospital, John H. Stroger, Jr., Hospital of Cook County, Mount Sinai Hospital and Medical Center, and the North Chicago Veterans Affairs Medical Center (NCVAMC). The university's clinical campus consists of the NCVAMC and The Clinics at Rosalind Franklin University.

BASIC SCIENCES: The Rosalind Franklin University of Medicine and Science curriculum offers a strong grounding in the sciences basic to medicine along with assuring competency in skills necessary for the practice of medicine. The curriculum features a unique interprofessional approach with interaction among a broad range of health professional students and practitioners. The curriculum is a mix of lectures, labs, small group discussions, team based learning, and opportunities for peer to peer learning. Our educational information system, Desire to Learn (D2L), provides 24 hour a day access to learning materials. Topic integration across courses and a unique interprofessional teams course are the hallmark of the M1 curriculum.

CLINICAL TRAINING

Students have early clinical experiences in our state of the art evaluation and education center, as well as opportunities to connect with physician preceptors. The required junior clinical clerkships include ambulatory care, family medicine, medcore, medicine, neurology and emergency medicine, obstetrics/gynecology, psychiatry, pediatrics, and surgery. The senior requirements include 4 weeks in a medicine or pediatrics sub internship, plus 32 weeks of approved electives (14 of which must be intramural). The elective period gives students an opportunity, through both intramural and extramural experiences, to explore and strengthen their personal career interests.

Students

Rosalind Franklin University of Medicine and Science is situated in the northern suburbs of Chicago, with easy access to downtown Chicago and the surrounding areas by car or public transportation. The university's main campus comprises a four-story Basic Sciences Building and a newly constructed Health Sciences Building. State-of-the-art facilities include a recently completed $10 million research wing expansion, multimedia classrooms and gross anatomy laboratory, and an Education and Evaluation Center for physical examination skills training. Recreation facilities include an exercise room, game room, and the Student Union (home to the University Bookstore, Union Café, and dedicated e-mail stations). Underrepresented minorities, mostly African American students, account for about 8 percent of the student body. Of the class entering in 2005, 20.5 percent were in-state residents. The entering class size in 2005 was 185.

STUDENT LIFE

Most first- and second-year students live in the vicinity of campus and drive to school. On-campus housing is available at Rosalind Franklin University. Each of the university's three apartment buildings has five floors and consists of 60 1- and 2-bedroom apartments. Individual apartments feature a variety of amenities, such as kitchen appliances, fully networked Internet connectivity, and washer/dryer hookups. Each apartment building also includes study and lounge areas, shared laundry facilities on every floor, and individual storage units. Often, third- and fourth-year students elect to live in Chicago, where they are closer to clinical training sites. Public transportation from downtown Chicago to campus facilitates such living arrangements. Chicago is one of the largest and most culturally rich cities in the country, providing a wealth of entertainment, museums, theater, restaurants, nightlife, indoor and outdoor athletic activities, and spectator sporting events. The city provides distraction for medical students when they need it. Students have a voice in school administrative affairs through the university student council and through participation on various boards and committees. The Rosalind Franklin University has chapters of most national medical student associations and has special interest clubs and organizations based on recreational activities, professional interests, and ethnic/social background.

GRADUATES

Of the 2005 graduating class, the most popular specialty choices were internal medicine (22.7 percent), pediatrics (10.2 percent), emergency medicine (9.7 percent), family practice (9.1 percent), anesthesia (6.8 percent), general surgery (5.7 percent), ob/gyn (5.1 percent), and orthopedics (5.1 percent).

Admissions

REQUIREMENTS

One year of biology, chemistry, organic chemistry, and physics, all with labs, are required. The MCAT is required and must be no more than three years old at time of matriculation. For multiple exams, the most recent set of scores are used.

SUGGESTIONS

In addition to requirements, courses in math, social sciences, English, and the arts are recommended. A solid preparation in science, accompanied by a broad background in the liberal arts, is recommended. The Admissions Committee also puts strong emphasis on other non-academic factors, such as an applicant's motivation, character, personality, experience, and achievements.

PROCESS

In addition to the AMCAS, a secondary application is required. Interviews take place from October through May and consist of two sessions with faculty, administrators, and/or medical students. Notification of acceptance begins in November and is an ongoing process until the class is filled. Candidates awaiting a decision may submit supplemental information about course work, activities, or new MCAT scores.

RUSH UNIVERSITY
RUSH MEDICAL COLLEGE

OFFICE OF ADMISSIONS, 524 AAC, 600 SOUTH PAULINA, CHICAGO, IL 60612 • ADMISSION: 312-942-6913
FAX: 312-942-2333 • E-MAIL: RMC_ADMISSIONS@RUSH.EDU • WEBSITE: WWW.RUSHU.RUSH.EDU/MEDCOL

STUDENT BODY

Type	Private
# applied	2,023
# accepted	290
# enrolled (total/out)	120/25
Average age	23

ADMISSIONS

Average GPA and MCAT Scores

Overall GPA	3.5
MCAT Bio	10.0
MCAT Phys	10.0
MCAT Verbal	9.5
MCAT Essay	P

Application Information

Regular application	11/1
Regular notification	rolling
Early application	6/1–8/1
Early notification	10/1
Are transfers accepted?	no
Admissions may be deferred?	yes
Interview required?	yes
Application fee	$65

Academics

Students follow a 4 year curriculum, except those pursuing a PhD along with the MD degree. Joint MD/PhD programs are offered in many disciplines, including anatomy, biochemistry, immunology, microbiology, neuroscience, pharmacology, and physiology. Medical students are evaluated with honors/pass/fail, and passing the USMLE Step 1 is a requirement for promotion to year 3. Entering students are assigned a faculty member as an academic advisor to assist with education and career development.

BASIC SCIENCES: Students learn basic sciences through the traditional curriculum, which relies on lectures and labs for instruction, or the alternate curriculum, which is entirely case-based and emphasizes self-directed learning and problem-solving skills. About 24 students enter the alternate curriculum each year. all students participate in the generalist curriculum, which involves one-on-one mentorships with physician preceptors. Topics covered in the first year are anatomy, behavioral science, biochemistry, ethics and law in medicine, general pathology, health and the public, histology, interviewing and communication, neurobiology, physiology, primary care preceptorship, and physical diagnosis. Second-year subjects are clinical pathophysiology, immunology, interviewing and communication, microbiology, pathology, pharmacology, physical diagnosis, preventive medicine, primary care preceptorship, and psychopathlgy. To enhance classroom instruction, the McCormick Learning Resource Center offers audiovisual and computer-based learning aids. Academic Computer Resources operates a personal computer laboratory and a computer-assisted instruction laboratory that is available 24 hours a day. The tutoring program provides additional instruction and study tips from faculty, classmates, or upperclass students.

CLINICAL TRAINING

All students fulfill the same clerkship requirements during the third and fourth years. Third-year rotations are internal medicine (12 weeks), surgery (12 weeks), ob/gyn (8 weeks), pediatrics (8 weeks), psychiatry (6 weeks), family practice (6 weeks), and neurology (4 weeks). Fourth-year students participate in an advanced, primary care sub internship, choosing from family medicine, internal medicine, or pediatrics (4 weeks). At least 18 weeks are reserved for electives. Most clinical training takes place at Rush-Presbyterian-St. Luke's Hospital (903 beds), a nonprofit hospital with more than 30 specialty areas. Other affiliated institutions, in urban, suburban, and rural locations, are Illinois Masonic Medical Center, Rush North Shore Medical Center, Rush-Prudential Health Plans, Cook County Hospital, Hinsdale Hospital, LaGrange Memorial Hospital, MacNeal Memorial Hospital, and Westlake Hospital.

Students

Approximately 85 percent of students are Illinois residents. About 10 percent of students are underrepresented minorities, and about 30 percent are older or nontraditional, having taken time off between college and medical school. Class size is 120.

STUDENT LIFE

Student life, both on and off campus, is varied and exciting. Campus facilities are designed to encourage student interaction. For example, student lounges provide space for socializing, relaxing between classes, or special events. The Academic Facility is open to Rush students 24 hours a day and is a good spot for group or individual study. Student organizations are numerous, ranging from the Rush Golf Club to the Multicultural Affairs Coalition to chapters of national medically oriented organizations. The Rush Community Service Initiative Program (RCSIP) is a student-run umbrella organization for many projects and activities, all of which allow students to contribute to the community. RCSIP activities include free clinics, health education programs, and big sibling relationships with children who have HIV. Students have access to athletic and recreational facilities at Rush and at the University of Illinois, including indoor tennis courts, swimming pools, a bowling alley, and pool tables. Chicago is an ideal city for students, as it is relatively affordable and can be accessed with public transportation. Convenient and comfortable housing options are available both on and off campus.

GRADUATES

Rush has met its stated goal that at least 50 percent of graduates will enter primary care fields. Graduates are successful in securing residencies all over the country. Rush graduates practice in 50 states and in a number of foreign countries.

Admissions

REQUIREMENTS

Prerequisites are 8 semester hours each of biology, general chemistry, organic chemistry, and physics. The MCAT is required and scores must be from within the past four years. For applicants who have retaken the exam, recent scores are most heavily weighed.

SUGGESTIONS

Preference is given to residents of Illinois, although up to 20–30 out-of-state applicants are accepted each year. Beyond requirements, Rush suggests undergraduate courses in English, math, and social sciences. The Admissions Committee looks for social and intellectual maturity, personal integrity, motivation, and concern in applicants. Applicants are encouraged to take the MCAT in April of the year of application.

PROCESS

All AMCAS applicants receive secondary applications. About 500 applicants, or 10 percent of the applicant pool, are interviewed between September and March. Interviews consist of two sessions with faculty members, in addition to a tour of the campus and the opportunity to meet with current students. Of interviewed candidates, about half are accepted on a rolling basis. Wait-listed candidates may submit supplementary material to update their files.

Admissions Requirements (Required)

MCAT scores, science GPA, non-science GPA, letters of recommendation, interview, state residency, essays/personal statement, extracurricular activities, exposure to medical profession.

COSTS AND AID

Tuition & Fees

Tuition	$32,268
Cost of books	$1,050
Fees	$1,530

Financial Aid

% students receiving aid	80

SAINT LOUIS UNIVERSITY
SCHOOL OF MEDICINE

COMMITTEE ON ADMISSIONS, 1402 SOUTH GRAND BLVD., M226, ST. LOUIS, MO 63104 • ADMISSION: 314-977-9870
FAX: 314-977-9825 • E-MAIL: SLUMD@SLU.EDU • WEBSITE: HTTP://WWW.MEDSCHOOL.SLU.EDU/ADMISSIONS

STUDENT BODY

Type	Private
Enrollment	616
% male/female	53/47
% underrepresented minorities	11
# applied (total/out)	4,193/3,888
# accepted (total/out)	493/407
# enrolled (total/out)	153/104

FACULTY

Total faculty (number)	1,723
% female	30
% minority	20
% part-time	68

ADMISSIONS

Average GPA and MCAT Scores

Overall GPA	3.7
MCAT Bio	10.84
MCAT Phys	10.38
MCAT Verbal	10.13
MCAT Essay	P

Application Information

Regular application	12/15
Regular notification	10/15
Early application	6/1–8/1
Early notification	10/1
Are transfers accepted?	yes
Admissions may be deferred?	yes
Interview required?	yes
Application fee	$100

Academics

The medical curriculum is continually evolving to respond to the rapid changes in the health care field and to reflect national trends in medical education. Current students enjoy a program of study that uses a block schedule, system based learning and emphasizes small-group and independent study. SLU offers several options for students interested in research. The doctorate is offered in anatomy, biochemistry, cell biology, genetics, immunology, microbiology, molecular biology, neuroscience, pathology, pharmacology, health care ethics, and physiology.

BASIC SCIENCES: The first and second years each consist of 36 weeks of instruction, which includes laboratories, demonstrations, discussion groups, didactic lecture sessions, and preceptorships at clinical sites. Students are in class or other scheduled sessions for about 20 hours per week, providing ample time for self-directed learning. First-year courses are introduction to human anatomy; cell biology; metabolism; microbes and host responses; molecular biology and genetics; principles of pharmacology; health information resources; and patient, physician, and society, which covers topics such as bioethics, community medicine, medical communication, and the physical diagnosis. Second-year courses are introduction to clinical psychiatry; introduction to medicine; microbiology; neuroscience; pathology; pharmacology; preventive and social medicine; and patient, physician, and society, which includes both clinical and sociological/psychological topics. An important resource for students is the Learning Resources Center, which houses both the Health Sciences Center Library and the Clinical Skills Center, where both diagnostic and treatment skills are taught.

CLINICAL TRAINING

The third year consists of core clerkships in most basic medical fields. These are internal medicine (12 weeks), surgery (8 weeks), ob/gyn (6 weeks), pediatrics (8 weeks), family medicine (4 weeks), psychiatry (6 weeks), and neurology (4 weeks). The fourth year is flexible, allowing students to pursue elective opportunities in both clinical and research areas. A minimum of 36 weeks of instruction must be completed. Required rotations are in intramural floor service (4 weeks) and surgery subspecialty selective (4 weeks). Most training is conducted at the St. Louis University Hospital, a 365-bed tertiary care facility. It is also a Level I trauma center. Other affiliated institutions include the Cardinal Glennon Children's Hospital, the Anheuser-Busch Eye Institute, David P. Wohl Mental Health Institute, St. Elizabeth's Hospital, St. John's Mercy Medical Center, St. Mary's Hospital, Bethesda Cancer Research Ceneter, and the St. Louis Veterans Affairs Medical Center. A portion of electives may be taken at other academic and clinical institutions.

Students

Although students come from all regions of the country, a large number are from the Saint Louis area. About 10 percent of students are underrepresented minorities and about 30 percent are nontraditional, having pursued other careers or interests between college and medical school.

STUDENT LIFE

SLU students can pursue their health-related interests by taking part in research forums or by participating in the school's many organizations. The campus ministry is particularly strong. Those who need a break from academic and career pursuits can take advantage of the resources of the main campus, including the award-winning Simon Recreational Center or the well-subscribed intramural sports program. St. Louis also offers a wide variety of extracurricular activities. Tower Grove Park and the Missouri Botanical Gardens are a few blocks from the Medical School. Nearby Forest Park, one of the nation's largest metropolitan parks, is the home of the St. Louis Zoo, the Art Museum, and the Science Center. St. Louis also has its own opera, theater, and ballet, in addition to professional baseball and hockey teams. Although the school has some housing facilities, most medical students choose to live off campus, where housing is affordable and comfortable.

GRADUATES

About 50 percent of graduates enter primary care residencies. Students are competitive applicants for specialty and surgical fields as well.

Admissions

REQUIREMENTS

Requirements are 1 year with lab of biology, chemistry, organic chemistry, and physics. In addition, 6 semester hours of English and 12 hours of humanities or behavioral science are expected. The MCAT is required, and scores must be from the new version of the test. For applicants who have taken the exam more than once, the best set of scores is considered.

SUGGESTIONS

Students should apply early in the application cycle as interviews and acceptances are given on a rolling basis. Both hospital and research experience are valuable. Activities that demonstrate a commitment to serving others is also useful.

PROCESS

All AMCAS applicants receive secondary applications. Of the approximately 4,200 students who return secondaries, about 23 percent are interviewed on a rolling basis. Interviews are 1 hour in length and are conducted by a faculty member. The remainder of the interview day includes a tour of the campus, group informational sessions, and lunch with current students. Applicants are notified of committee decisions within 6–8 weeks of the interview and are either accepted, rejected, or put into a hold category. Approximately 45 percent of the interviewed group is accepted. For wait-listed applicants, additional grades, awards, and honors are useful supplementary information.

Admissions Requirements (Required)

MCAT scores, science GPA, non-science GPA, letters of recommendation, interview, essays/personal statement.

Admissions Requirements (Optional)

State residency, extracurricular activities, exposure to medical profession, exposure to research, volunteer experience.

Overlap Schools

Creighton University; Georgetown University; Loyola University Chicago; Rush Medical College of Rush University; The University of Iowa; University of Illinois at Chicago; University of Missouri—Columbia.

COSTS AND AID

Tuition & Fees

Tuition	$38,960
Room and board (off campus)	$8,400
Cost of books	$1,368
Fees	$2,132

Financial Aid

% students receiving aid	63
Average grant	$9,511
Average loan	$40,000
Average debt	$148,000

SOUTHERN ILLINOIS UNIVERSITY
SCHOOL OF MEDICINE

PO Box 19624, Springfield, IL 62794-9624 • Admission: 217-545-6013
Fax: 217-545-5538 • E-mail: ADMISSIONS@SIUMED.EDU • Website: WWW.SIUMED.EDU

STUDENT BODY

Type	Public
Enrollment	291
% male/female	48/52
% underrepresented minorities	15
# applied (total/out)	1,013/40
# accepted (total/out)	192/2
# enrolled (total/out)	72/0
Average age	24

FACULTY

Total faculty (number)	336
% female	37
% minority	19
% part-time	6
Student-faculty ratio	1:1

ADMISSIONS

Average GPA and MCAT Scores

Overall GPA	3.5
MCAT Bio	8.97
MCAT Phys	8.47
MCAT Verbal	8.9
MCAT Essay	0

Application Information

Regular application	11/15
Regular notification	10/15
Are transfers accepted?	yes
Admissions may be deferred?	yes
Interview required?	yes
Application fee	$50

Academics

SIU offers a case-based, small group-oriented curriculum with an abundance of patient contact and early clinical exposure. In cooperation with the SIU School of Law, a joint MD/JD degree program is also offered. Medical students are evaluated on pass/fail and with honors system. The USMLE Step 1 must be passed as a graduation requirement.

BASIC SCIENCES: The instructional format not only emphasizes small-group instruction, self-directed study, and a case-based approach but also incorporates lectures and an organ system organizational scheme. Topics covered in the first year are cardiovascular, respiratory, renal, endocrine, reproductive, gastrointestinal, and sensorimotor systems and behavior. In Carbondale, basic science instruction takes place in Lindegren Hall. Early clinical experiences are offered at Memorial Hospital in Carbondale (151 beds), the Carbondale Clinic, offices of local physicians, and at the VA Hospital (171 beds). In Springfield, the Medical Instructional Facility contains lecture halls, classrooms, labs, and a teaching museum. A 4 year doctoring curriculum (physicians conduct and attitude, clinical skills development, and medical humanities issues) begins immediately. Both simulated and real patients are used. Topics covered in the second year include circulation, infection, and host diseases, medicine and behavior, neoplasia, neuromuscular, population health, and preventive medicine. Computer assisted instruction is used as a learning aid, and computers are available in the student computer lab and at other sites. The Morris Library at Carbondale houses more than 100,000 volumes, while the Medical Instruction Facility in Springfield contains 113,000.

CLINICAL TRAINING

Third-year required multidisciplinary rotations are family and community medicine, gynecology obstetrics, internal medicine, pediatrics, psychiatry, and surgery. Four weeks of electives, which may include anesthesiology, emergency medicine, and radiology, are allowed in the third year. The doctoring curriculum continues during this year. At the conclusion of the third year, students must pass an examination that evaluates their skills in assessing and managing patient problems. During the fourth year, students complete one additional required clerkship in neurology (4 weeks). Thirty-one weeks are reserved for elective studies. Clinical training sites include Memorial Medical Center (580 beds), St. John's Hospital and Pavilion (715 beds), and the clinics and offices of faculty and community physicians. Electives may be taken off compus, and SIU has an institutional agreement with overseas universities—including locations in Germany and the Netherlands—that facilitate training overseas.

Students

At least 95 percent of students are Illinois residents. The average age of incoming students is 24. Underrepresented minorities account for 10 percent of the student body. Class size is 72.

STUDENT LIFE

On-campus recreational facilities at Carbondale include a complete fitness room, swimming pools, racquetball courts, and a student center. Taking part in intramural sports and attending intercollegiate sporting events are popular extracurricular activities for medical students. St. Louis, with the amenities of a large city, is a 2 hour drive. The surrounding area features a state park and the Shawnee National Forest, where the students can hike, bike, camp, canoe, or enjoy the beach. In Springfield, medical students enjoy discounts to health clubs such as the YMCA. Lake Springfield offers fishing, swimming, boating, and sailing. Parks, golf courses, and cultural and historical sites are other local attractions. All students live off campus in both Carbondale and Springfield.

GRADUATES

Among the 2004 graduating class, the most prevalent fields for postgraduate training were internal medicine (19 percent); pediatrics (19 percent); and emergency medicine, family medicine, and ob/gyn (all 9 percent). Students generally score around the national mean on the USMLE Part 1, and above the mean on Part 2, making them well-positioned for securing residency positions.

Admissions

REQUIREMENTS

To do well on the MCAT, students should have taken at least 1 year each of biology, chemistry, English, math, organic chemistry, and physics—the last of which should have included some statistics. The MCAT is required and scores must be no more than two years old. For applicants who have taken the exam on multiple occasions, the most recent set of scores is considered.

SUGGESTIONS

As a state school, preference is given to applicants from Central and Southern Illinois who are interested in practicing in the region. Applicants are expected to have a good foundation in the humanities, natural sciences, and social sciences in addition to sound English skills. The Admissions Committee looks beyond scholastic achievement for evidence of responsibility, integrity, compassion, motivation, interest in medicine, community service, and sound interpersonal skills. The Medical Education Preparatory Program (MEDPREP) is a nondegree post-baccalaureate program that assists disadvantaged students with meeting the requirements for the SIU School of Medicine.

PROCESS

About one-fourth of AMCAS applicants are interviewed, the vast majority of them Illinois state residents. Interviews are conducted between August and April, and consist of two sessions with individual faculty and/or administrators. About 30 percent of interviewed candidates are accepted on a batch basis. Others are rejected or wait listed. Wait-listed candidates may send supplemental material to update their files.

Admissions Requirements (Required)

MCAT scores, science GPA, non-science GPA, letters of recommendation, interview, state residency, essays/personal statement, extracurricular activities, volunteer/employment experience.

Admissions Requirements (Optional)

Exposure to medical profession.

Overlap Schools

University of Illinois at Chicago.

COSTS AND AID

Tuition & Fees

In-state Tuition	$18,312
Out-of-state Tuition	$54,936
Room and board	
(off campus)	$6,956
Cost of books	$5,021
Fees	$1,673

Financial Aid

% students receiving aid	94
Average grant	$12,938
Average loan	$29,338
Average debt	$121,274

SPARTAN HEALTH SCIENCES UNIVERSITY
SCHOOL OF MEDICINE

PO BOX 324 VIEUX FORT, ST. LUCIA, WEST INDIES • ADMISSION: 758-454-6128 • FAX: 758-454-6811
E-MAIL: SPARTANMED@AOL.COM • WEBSITE: WWW.SPARTANMED.ORG

STUDENT BODY

Type	Private
Enrollment	250
% male/female	65/35
% underrepresented minorities	90
# applied (total/out)	170/240
# accepted (total/out)	50/32
# enrolled (total/out)	30/27
Average age	28

FACULTY

Total faculty (number)	14
% female	18
% minority	100
% part-time	2
Student-faculty ratio	7:1

ADMISSIONS

Average GPA and MCAT Scores

Overall GPA	3.0

Application Information

Regular application	7/15
Regular notification	3/15
Are transfers accepted?	yes
Admissions may be deferred?	yes
Interview required?	yes
Application fee	$60

Academics

Spartan Health Sciences University, School of Medicine, offers a four academic year (36 calendar month) program leading to the Doctor of Medicine degree (MD), and is taught on a trimester (four months) schedule. The curriculum of the university's Doctor of Medicine degree program encompasses a comprehensive course of Basic Sciences (BS), Pre-clinical, and Clinical Sciences (CS) that lasts for four (4) academic years. The trimester periods start in January, May, and September of each year. A student may elect to enter in any one of the three trimesters. To provide the best possible medical education to the students, the curriculum is under continuous review by the Deans of Basic and Clinical Sciences in conjunction with the faculty. All students are required to demonstrate competency in the basic medical sciences before being permitted to begin clinical rotations. Competency is assessed from the university administered and required Comprehensive Exit Examination at the end of the Basic Sciences program. No student will be eligible for graduation until all academic requirements and financial obligations to the university have been fulfilled.

BASIC SCIENCES: The initial four trimesters of the program represent an integrated course presentation of the Basic Sciences (BS) which include anatomy, physiology, pharmacology, biochemistry, immunology, pathology, microbiology, behavioral sciences, neuroanatomy, and general introduction to medicine, including physical diagnosis. Didactic lectures in internal medicine, pediatrics, psychiatry, obstetrics/gynecology, and surgery are offered. Clinical correlated conferences are conducted for related basic sciences to clinical medicine.

CLINICAL TRAINING

The final five trimesters are committed to broad clinical exposure in the major clinical disciplines of internal medicine (12 weeks), surgery and its sub-specialties (20 weeks), pediatrics (6 weeks), obstetrics and gynecology (8 weeks), psychiatry (6 weeks), family medicine (6 weeks), radiology (4 weeks), pathology (4 weeks), and clinical electives (14 weeks).

Students

The university's student body is made up of multiracial backgrounds. Some of the students were professionals in their fields before they were admitted; some were pharmacists, biochemists, and researchers with postgraduate degrees. The university is a microcosm of the United Nations in the pursuit of eradication of diseases that plague the human race. Students come from different continents around the world (90 countries): North and South America, Africa, Europe, Asia, and Australia.

STUDENT LIFE

Spartan Health Sciences University, School of Medicine, is located in the former British Colony of Saint Lucia. The people of Saint Lucia are English speaking, friendly, and very accommodating. The population of St. Lucia at the end of 2000 was 163,819. The local language is Creole (or Patois, an adulterated French), and emerged as a result of British and French influences with English as the official language. Outside of the classroom, students are involved in various community health care events. Medical students take advantage of the fitness center, tennis courts on school premises, and a cricket and soccer field behind the school. All students live off campus, within walking or biking distance of campus.

Admissions

REQUIREMENTS

The minimum requirement for admission is 90 semester credit hours of college level work. Prerequisites are 1 year each of general chemistry, organic chemistry, biology, physics, English, and mathematics. The MCAT is recommended. Applicants from the United Kingdom, British Commonwealth of Nations, and other countries with similar educational standards must possess a baccalaureate degree and have completed courses in biology, chemistry, mathematics, and physics. However, applicants with high grades in the General Certificate of Education (G.C.E.) advanced level with courses in the sciences may be considered. Prospective students from other countries with educational systems different from the British or U.S. will be evaluated on their own merits.

SUGGESTIONS

The Mission of Spartan Health Sciences University, School of Medicine, is to train doctors of all races and nations for the world rather than indulgence in parochialism of medical education. The primary objective of the university is to provide qualified students an opportunity to fulfill their lifelong ambition of serving humanity with medical education and prolongation of human life through medical care and research. The university strives to attain a high standard of education with affordable tuition fees ever since its inception, without compromising the standard of medical education offered. The university is dedicated to training its graduates with excellent medical knowledge and competent skills in order to assure that the medical profession meets the health care demands of the societies to which it belongs.

PROCESS

In evaluating individual applicant's credentials, Admissions Committee looks for the applicant's capacity to do academic work for absorption of the material needed for sound foundation in the basic medical sciences. Evaluation is also carried out on Grade Point Average (GPA) from individual colleges and universities, and letters of recommendation. However, academic background is not the main criterion for selection; the individual's character and motivation to become a physician are essential determinants for admission.

Admissions Requirements (Required)

Science GPA, nonscience GPA, letters of recommendation, interview, essays/personal statement, official transcripts.

Admissions Requirements (Optional)

MCAT scores, state residency, extracurricular activities, exposure to medical profession.

COSTS AND AID

Tuition & Fees

Tuition	$8,500
Room and board (off campus)	$4,000
Cost of books	$1,000

Financial Aid

% students receiving aid	60
Average loan	$20,000

STANFORD UNIVERSITY
SCHOOL OF MEDICINE

OFFICE OF MD ADMISSIONS, 251 CAMPUS DR, MSOB XC301 STANFORD, CA 94305-5404 **ADMISSION:** 650-723-6861
FAX: 650-725-7855 • **E-MAIL:** MDADMISSIONS@STANFORD.EDU • **WEBSITE:** WWW.MED.STANFORD.EDU

STUDENT BODY

Type	Private
Enrollment	462
% male/female	53/47
% underrepresented minorities	22
# applied (total/out)	5,445/3,421
# accepted (total/out)	186/115
# enrolled (total/out)	87/53
Average age	24

FACULTY

Total faculty (number)	710
% female	33
% minority	5

ADMISSIONS

Average GPA and MCAT Scores

Overall GPA	3.8
MCAT Bio	11.83
MCAT Phys	11.56
MCAT Verbal	10.18
MCAT Essay	R

Application Information

Regular application	10/15
Regular notification	rolling
Early application	6/1–8/1
Early notification	10/15
Are transfers accepted?	yes
Admissions may be deferred?	yes
Interview required?	yes
Application fee	$75

Academics

Generally, about 60 percent of Stanford students receive their MD in five rather than four years, which allows for individual research and elective study. In addition to the MD, departmental joint-degrees include an MD/PhD in biochemistry, developmental biology, genetics, microbiology and immunology, molecular and cellular physiology, molecular pharmacology, and structural biology. Interdepartmental joint-degrees are also possible and include an MS in biomechanical engineering and health services research, an MS and PhD in epidemiology and medical information sciences, and a PhD in biophysics, cancer biology, immunology, and neuroscience. There are about 6–8 MSTP slots available. In addition to formal degree programs, students may take electives in nonmedical departments. Through the Medical Student Scholars Program and other programs, students enjoy a range of research opportunities, most of which are remunerated.

BASIC SCIENCES: Stanford operates on a quarter system, and pre-clinical studies are organized into 6 quarters. During this period of rigorous science course work, students are gradually introduced to clinical care and have clinical training opportunities throughout. Classes demand 20–35 hours per week, with considerable variation from quarter to quarter. During the fall, first quarter of the first year, students typically take human anatomy and development, which includes an introduction to the physical examination; introduction to psychiatry, which involves patient interviews; and structure of cells and tissues. Winter, second quarter, offers biochemistry; biostatistics and epidemiology; clinical psychiatry; health systems/policy; neurobiology; and physicians and patients, a course exploring interdisciplinary topics and continuing medical interviews. During the spring, third quarter, students take cardiovascular physiology, genetics, host parasites and defense, molecular biology, and pathology. The second-year fall, fourth quarter, introduces students to infectious basis of disease, more pathology, pharmacology, and physiology. In addition, preparation for clinical medicine begins. The fifth quarter includes endocrine physiology, pathophysiology, and more pharmacology and pathology. Students make the transition into their clinical studies during this quarter and the second year, sixth quarter, with clinical problem solving, presented in a case-based, small-group format and a preceptor program including general and psychiatric patient care. The Lane Medical Library, which is soon to benefit from substantial remodeling and enlargment, currently houses 3,000 journal titles, 350,000 volumes, and online data management services. Computer, audiovisual, and other learning aids are accessible to students at the Fleischmann Learning and Resource Center. Videotapes of most pre-clinical courses are available and appear to substitute for student-organized note services. Grading is strictly pass/fail, and mid-quarter exams are optional. A week-long reading period prior to final exams allows students uninterrupted study time. Step 1 of the USMLE must be passed no later than 1 year prior to graduation, and Step 2 must be passed to graduate.

CLINICAL TRAINING
Patient contact begins in the Fall quarter of the first year, and there are opportunities for clinical experiences during the first two years. Third- and fourth-year clerkships take place at the major affiliated teaching hospitals, which include Stanford Hospital (479 beds), the Lucile Salter Packard Children's Hospital (162 beds), Santa Clara Valley Medical Center (644 beds), three VA Hospitals, Kaiser Permanente (336 beds), and

Columbia San Jose Medical Center (529 beds). These facilities serve both rural and urban populations with diverse needs. Students complete 15 months of clinical clerkships, including 9 months of required core clerkships in family medicine, medicine, ob/gyn, pediatrics, psychiatry, and surgery. Three months are spent training in areas related to required clerkships through selectives, in which students choose from ambulatory care, basics in clinical care, and sub internship. The final 3 months are designated as elective clerkships.

Students

Stanford students are often characterized as being less cutthroat than those attending other top-ranked schools, perhaps because the flexible curriculum encourages students to focus beyond the classroom. Special effort is made to recruit students from underrepresented minority backgrounds, and student organizations support these and other student groups. With 86 students per class, Stanford is relatively small.

STUDENT LIFE

The campus and the surrounding area offer excellent sports and other outdoor activities. San Francisco is one hour away and is accessible by train. Numerous on-campus housing options exist, including family housing, apartments, dormitories, and co-ops. However, high rent in the vicinity of Stanford makes student housing competitive.

GRADUATES

Stanford itself offers excellent residency programs, and many graduates opt for postgraduate training at Stanford. Perhaps as a result of the teaching and research experience students gain while in school, many go on into academic medicine. Increasingly, graduates are entering primary care fields.

Admissions

REQUIREMENTS

Biology with lab (1 year), chemistry/organic chemistry with labs (two years), and physics with lab (1 year). The MCAT must be no more than three years old. The most recent set of scores is used.

SUGGESTIONS

Biochemistry, behavioral sciences, and calculus are recommended, as is knowledge of a second language. No preference is given to California residents or to Stanford undergraduates. Successful applicants generally have significant medical, health-related, research, or community service experience.

PROCESS

Secondary applications are sent out on a rolling basis, with information due in 2 weeks. Interviews involve two semi-structured, 60-minute sessions, one with a faculty member and one with a medical student. Of interviewed candidates, about one-third are accepted, one-third rejected, and one-third put on a wait list, with responses given within 4–6 weeks of the interview. During the past few years, from 0–15 applicants were eventually accepted off of the wait list.

Admissions Requirements (Required)

MCAT scores, science GPA, non-science GPA, letters of recommendation, interview, essays/personal statement, extracurricular activities, exposure to medical profession.

Admissions Requirements (Optional)

State residency.

Overlap Schools

Harvard University, University of California—San Francisco.

COSTS AND AID

Tuition & Fees

Tuition	$34,716
Room and board (on campus)	$14,500
Room and board (off campus)	$19,333
Cost of books	$1,500
Fees	

Financial Aid

% students receiving aid	66
Average grant	$28,705
Average loan	$14,849
Average debt	$63,695

STATE UNIVERSITY OF NEW YORK—DOWNSTATE MEDICAL CENTER

OFFICE OF ADMISSIONS, 450 CLARKSON AVENUE, PO BOX 60M, BROOKLYN, NY 11203 • ADMISSION: 718-270-2446
FAX: 718-270-7592 • E-MAIL: ADMISSIONS@DOWNSTATE.EDU • WEBSITE: WWW.HSCBKLYN.EDU

STUDENT BODY

Type	Public
Enrollment	757
% male/female	50/50
% underrepresented minorities	15
# applied (total/out)	3,505/1,159
# enrolled	185
Average age	24

ADMISSIONS

Application Information

Regular application	12/15
Regular notification	10/15
	until filled
Early application	6/1–8/1
Early notification	10/1
Are transfers accepted?	no
Admissions may be deferred?	yes
Interview required?	no
Application fee	$65

Academics

The curriculum emphasizes the development of clinical reasoning and problem-solving skills. It integrates basic and clinical sciences and exposes students from the first year to patient care. Each student spends one afternoon biweekly in a physician's private office or clinic; the practicing physician serves as the student's clinical mentor for the entire year. Students are also encouraged to participate in research. Opportunities are available throughout the four years of medical school. Those who make a significant research contribution are eligible to graduate with distinction in research. A MD/PhD program is open in one of two modern biomedical science areas, neuroscience, or molecular and cell biology. Medical students are evaluated with an honors/high pass/pass/fail system. Students must pass Step 1 of the USMLE to be promoted to year 3. Students are encouraged to take Step 2 prior to graduation, but it is not a requirement.

BASIC SCIENCES: Basic science courses have been integrated into topics or blocks. Each block is taught using a combination of traditional lectures, case-based, small-group sessions, laboratories, conferences, and a weekly clinical experience. First year topics are blood/hematopoiesis/lymphoid, cardiovascular system, endocrine and reproduction systems, gastrointestinal system/intermediary metabolism, genes to cells, head and neck, musculoskeletal system, neuroscience, renal/urinary system, respiratory system, and skin and connective tissue. The current second-year curriculum includes courses in microbiology and immunology, nutrition, pathology, pathophysiology, pharmacology, preparation for clinical medicine, preventive medicine, and psychopathology. With the exception of the last two, each course runs throughout the full academic year, with each discipline presenting material related to specific organ systems. The Office of Academic Development promotes students' academic success through seminars, workshops, and individual tutoring. The Health Science Education Building holds two floors of study carrels, which serve as home base to students during the first two years. In the same building is the Medical Research Library, one of the largest medical school libraries in the country, and a 500-seat auditorium. A Learning Resource Center has 90 computer work stations loaded with an array of medical applications.

CLINICAL TRAINING

The current clerkships are medicine (10 weeks), surgery (8 weeks), pediatrics (6 weeks), ob/gyn (6 weeks), psychiatry (6 weeks), neurology (4 weeks), and anesthesia (2 weeks). Also included are primary care, a sub internship (4 weeks), and at least 20 weeks of electives. Training takes place at a number of major affiliates, University Hospital, and Kings County Hospital. Electives can be completed at those institutions or at extramural hospitals or medical centers.

Students

This year's first-year class is 185 students from more than 60 individual colleges. About 93 percent are New York State residents. Approximately 13 percent of students are underrepresented minorities. The age range of the 2001 entering class is 20–35, with a median of 22.

STUDENT LIFE

All entering students are assigned a clinical faculty mentor who provides guidance and support throughout the first year. The focal point for recreational, social, and cultural activities on campus is the Student Center, which has lounges, a piano room, an athletic center, a swimming pool, squash courts, and a spa. Student organizations focus on professional, ethnic, service related, social, and recreational interests, and also provide support for groups of students. For example, the Daniel Hale Williams Society, named for a prominent black physician, is a voice for minority students on campus and also brings students together to participate in educational, social, and service-related goals. Brooklyn is a culturally rich, active community that provides an exciting extracurricular life for medical students. Manhattan is easily accessible on the subway. On-campus housing options are single or shared studios or dormitory rooms. Students who live off campus often reside in the nearby neighborhood of Park Slope.

GRADUATES

SUNY Downstate graduates perform above the national average in terms of securing residency positions at top institutions nationwide. Alumni hold faculty positions at universities such as Harvard, Case Western, Stanford, Yale, Hopkins, Columbia, Cornell, and the University of Pennsylvania, among other prestigious institutions. Forty percent of 2002 graduating students entered residency programs in primary care. More than 69 percent of graduates chose to stay within New York State.

Admissions

REQUIREMENTS

Fifteen positions in each class are reserved for students in a BA/MD program organized with Brooklyn College. Five positions are reserved for early assurance applicants from Queens College and the College of Staten Island. New York residents are given strong preference for the remaining spots. Prerequisites are 8 semester credits each of biology, chemistry, organic chemistry, and physics, all with associated labs. Six semester hours of English are also required. The MCAT is required and scores must be from within three years of the date of anticipated enrollment. Component scores for each MCAT series are looked at individually.

SUGGESTIONS

In addition to required courses, 1 year each of biochemistry, college-level math, and another advanced science are recommended. Medically related experience and demonstrated commitment to social service and community outreach activities are important factors in admission.

PROCESS

All AMCAS applicants are sent secondary applications. About 20 percent of those returning secondaries are interviewed between September and April. Interviews consist of one session for one hour with a faculty member. On interview day, candidates also have a group orientation session, lunch with current students, and a campus tour. Of interviewed candidates, about 40 percent are accepted on a rolling basis. Wait-listed candidates are not encouraged to send supplementary information.

Admissions Requirements (Required)

MCAT scores, science GPA, non-science GPA, letters of recommendation, state residency, extracurricular activities, exposure to medical profession.

Admissions Requirements (Optional)

Interview, essays/personal statement.

COSTS AND AID

Tuition & Fees

In-state Tuition	$10,840
Out-of-state Tuition	$21,940
Fees	$220

Financial Aid

Average debt	$59,906

STATE UNIVERSITY OF NEW YORK—STONY BROOK UNIVERSITY
SCHOOL OF MEDICINE

COMMITTEE ON ADMISSIONS, LEVEL 4, RM 147, HEALTH SCIENCES, STONY BROOK, NY 11794 • ADMISSION: 631-444-2113
FAX: 631-444-6032 • E-MAIL: SOMADMISSIONS@STONYBROOK.EDU • WEBSITE: WWW.HSC.SUNYSB.EDU/SOM/

STUDENT BODY

Type	Public
Enrollment	447
% male/female	53/47
% underrepresented minorities	14
# applied (total/out)	1,934/876
# accepted (total/out)	263/125
# enrolled (total/out)	101/2
Average age	24

FACULTY

Total faculty (number)	574
% female	35
% part-time	13

ADMISSIONS

Average GPA and MCAT Scores

Overall GPA	3.6
MCAT Bio	11.0
MCAT Phys	12.0
MCAT Verbal	10.0
MCAT Essay	Q

Application Information

Regular application	12/15
Regular notification	10/15
Early application	6/1–8/1
Early notification	10/1
Are transfers accepted?	yes
Admissions may be deferred?	yes
Interview required?	yes
Application fee	$75

Academics

Most students earn the MD degree in four years. Students who engage in relevant projects or course work may be eligible for the MD with recognition in research, the MD with recognition in primary care, or the MD with recognition in humanities. A combined MD/PhD program is offered as part of the MSTP. The doctorate degree may be earned in anatomy, biochemistry, biomedical engineering, cell biology, genetics, immunology, microbiology, molecular biology, neuroscience, pathology, pharmacology, and physiology. Medical students are evaluated with honors/pass/fail and must take Step 1 and 2 of the USMLE to graduate.

The curriculum of the School of Medicine provides the opportunity for extensive training in the basic medical sciences and teaching in the clinical disciplines of medicine. The curriculum requires the acquisition and utilization of a variety of skills in basic and clinical sciences. The official grading system is honors/pass/fail. The first two years are devoted to basic sciences and the integrated Foundations of Medicine course. This latter course teaches medical ethics, patient assessment skills, preventative medicine, human behaviour, and nutrition. The second year focuses on an organ system-based pathophysiology and therapeutics course. Third-year students complete core clerkships in medicine pediatrics, family medicine, obstetrics-gynecology, psychiatry, and surgery. One month of elective time is available. Fourth-year students are offered selectives and electives. Core clerkships are completed at University Hospital or one of three teaching affiliates. Electives can be completed at other sites.

USMLE, Step 1: Required. Students must record a passing score for promotion.

USMLE, Step 2: Required. Students must record a passing total score to graduate.

Students

Typically, 90–95 percent of students are New York residents. About 15 percent are underrepresented minorities. There is a wide age range among students, and at least 5–10 students in each class are in their thirties. Class size is 100.

STUDENT LIFE

Stony Brook is located on the North Shore of Long Island, just more than a one hour train ride from Manhattan. Students enjoy both the comfort of their school's suburban location and its proximity to the city. The campus offers a vast sports complex, and the immediate area offers bike trails, beaches, and parks. The Stony Brook Union is the campus center for hundreds of activities, including eating, socializing, watching TV, taking art and other noncredit classes, playing billiards and table tennis, and shopping. It is also the home of student organizations, student government, and informational services. On-campus child care is available to students. University-owned housing includes residence halls and several apartment complexes with units of all sizes. Most students own cars, which are particularly important during the clinical years.

GRADUATES

Among 2006 graduates, the most prevalent fields for residencies were medicine (30 percent), anesthesiology (14 percent), pediatrics (12 percent), emergency medicine (10 percent), and surgery (2 percent). About 15 percent entered programs at university-affiliated hospitals.

Admissions

REQUIREMENTS

Academic prerequisites are 1 year each of biology, chemistry, English, organic chemistry, and physics. Science courses must include associated labs. The MCAT is required, and scores must be no more than five years old. For applicants who have taken the exam more than once, the best scores are considered. Thus, there is no advantage in withholding scores.

SUGGESTIONS

Applicants who have taken significant time off after college should have some recent course work. For all applicants, some medically related experience is important, and patient contact is particularly valued.

PROCESS

All AMCAS applicants receive secondary applications. About 25 percent of those returning secondaries are interviewed between September and March. Interviews consist of one session with a member of the Admissions Committee in addition to a group orientation session, tour, and the opportunity to meet with current medical students. About 40 percent of interviewed candidates are accepted, with notification occurring on a rolling basis. An alternate admissions path is through the BA/MD scholars for the medicine program, which admits a limited number of high school students via the Honors College into an 8 year combined program. In addition, seven post-baccalaureate programs, including Bryn Mawr, Goucher, Stony Brook, NYU, Queens, Hunter, and Columbia have admission arrangements with Stony Brook through a linkage program.

STATE UNIVERSITY OF NEW YORK—UNIVERSITY AT BUFFALO
SCHOOL OF MEDICINE AND BIOMEDICAL SCIENCES

131 BEB, BUFFALO, NY 14214-3013 • ADMISSION: 716-829-3466
FAX: 716-829-3849 • E-MAIL: JJROSSO@BUFFALO.EDU • WEBSITE: WWW.SMBS.BUFFALO.EDU

STUDENT BODY

Type	Public
Enrollment	575
% male/female	50/50
% underrepresented minorities	7
# applied (total/out)	2,772/1,134
# accepted (total/out)	358/63
# enrolled (total/out)	136/22
Average age	23
Student-faculty ratio	1:1

ADMISSIONS

Average GPA and MCAT Scores

Overall GPA	3.57
MCAT Bio	10.1
MCAT Phys	9.83
MCAT Verbal	9.2
MCAT Essay	P

Application Information

Regular application	11/15
Regular notification	10/15
Early application	8/1 or 8/31
Early notification	10/1
Are transfers accepted?	no
Admissions may be deferred?	yes
Interview required?	yes
Application fee	$65

Academics

In addition to the MD, the School of Medicine and Biomedical Sciences awards the PhD, MA, MS, and the combined MD/PhD. There are four MSTP-sponsored MD/PhD positions available each year. Departments awarding graduate degrees include anatomy, biochemistry, biophysics, cell biology, genetics, immunology, microbiology, molecular biology, neuroscience, pathology, pharmacology, and physiology. A new joint-degree program, leading to the MD/MBA began in 1997. Evaluation of medical students uses honors/pass/fail. Passing the USMLE Step 1 is required before matriculants can enter third year.

BASIC SCIENCES: Basic sciences are taught through a combination of lectures, labs, small group sessions, problem-based learning and clinical experiences. On average, students are in class or scheduled sessions for about 20 hours per week. First-year courses are biochemistry; embryology; gross anatomy; histology; human behavior; medical genetics; neuroscience, physiology; scientific basis of medicine; social and preventive medicine; and clinical practice of medicine, which provides early patient-contact experiences. Second-year courses are genetics, hematology, human behavior, microbiology, pathology, pharmacology, scientific basis of medicine, social and preventive medicine, and the continuation of clinical practice of medicine. Summer externships, which allow up to 60 first- and second-year medical students to shadow primary care physicians are available with stipends. Stipends are also available on a limited basis for summer research projects. The Health Sciences Library features a Media Resources Center with approximately 2,000 multimedia items, a History of Medicine Collection with 12,000 volumes, and a comprehensive general medicine/scientific book and journal collection.

CLINICAL TRAINING

Third-year required rotations are internal medicine (8 weeks), surgery (8 weeks), ob/gyn (7 weeks), pediatrics (7 weeks), psychiatry (7 weeks), and family medicine (7 weeks). The Family Medicine Clerkship includes six sessions in a community-based family physician's office, two sessions in a problem-based learning format, one session focusing on a community project, and one session devoted to independent learning. During the third year, students also choose a week-long seminar from diverse selective offerings. Fourth-year requirements are 4 weeks each of neurology, medicine, and surgery, and 4 weeks of an ambulatory experience. Four year electives are also available. Training takes place at The Buffalo General Hospital, Children's Hospital of Buffalo, Erie County Medical Center, Mercy Hospital, Millard Fillmore Health System, Sisters of Charity Hospital, Roswell Park Cancer Institute, and the Buffalo VA Medical Center. The Community Academic Practice Program identifies community-based sites for clinical training. With faculty approval, up to 16 weeks of electives may be taken at other academic institutions.

Students

All but five or six students in each class are New York residents. About 20 percent of entering students are over 25 years old. Approximately 5 percent of students are underrepresented minorities. Class size is 135.

STUDENT LIFE

The first year begins with a relaxed orientation week that allows students to get acquainted with one other and their new surroundings. Several student centers serve as focal points for student life on campus. The Student Union houses more than 75 clubs and organizations in addition to recreational facilities, dining areas, and a theater. The Oasis Recreation Center features pool tables, music, and a TV room. The Harriman Student Activities Center is an alternate student union, and the Creative Craft Center provides ongoing craft programs and courses. The Living Well Center (LWC) is dedicated to improving students' overall health and wellness. It offers a range of services to students, including counseling, health education, fitness assessments, seminars on personal health issues, relaxation services such as massage, and special events with outside speakers. For medical students, the LWC also provides opportunities for volunteer work in areas related to preventive medicine. Buffalo is an affordable and student-friendly community. Residence Halls and graduate student apartments are available close to campus.

GRADUATES

Among graduates in a recent class, the most prevalent specialty fields were internal medicine (28 percent), pediatrics (25 percent), family practice (15 percent), ob/gyn (10 percent), surgery (11 percent), and emergency medicine (5 percent). Approximately half of graduates entered residency programs in New York State.

Admissions

REQUIREMENTS

Prerequisites are chemistry (4 semesters, including 2 of organic chemistry); biology (2 semesters); physics (2 semesters); and English (2 semesters). The MCAT is required, and must be from after 2003. For applicants who have taken the exam on multiple occasions, the best set of scores is generally considered. Thus, there is no advantage in withholding scores.

SUGGESTIONS

In addition to science requirements, two years of course work in social sciences and 1 year in the humanities are advised. For applicants who have taken time off after college, some recent course work is recommended. Medically related experience is important.

PROCESS

All applicants are sent secondary applications. Between 500 and 600 applicants are interviewed from September through February. These candidates are selected from a pool of about 3,000, meaning that about 20 percent of applicants make it to the interview stage. Interviews consist of 2 sessions each with a faculty member or medical student. On interview day, there are also group informational sessions, a campus tour, and the opportunity to have lunch with current medical students. The first acceptance letters are mailed in October, with subsequent batches of letters sent at 4–6 week intervals throughout the year. Approximately 30 percent of interviewees are accepted initially. Others are rejected or placed on a wait list. Supplementary material from wait-listed candidates is not encouraged. Usually 60 percent of interviewees are eventually offered an acceptance before orientation begins.

Admissions Requirements (Required)

MCAT scores, science GPA, letters of recommendation, interview, essays/personal statement.

Admissions Requirements (Optional)

Nonscience GPA, state residency, extracurricular activities, exposure to medical profession.

Overlap Schools

SUNY Upstate Medical University, University of Rochester.

COSTS AND AID

Tuition & Fees

In-state Tuition	$18,800
Out-of-state Tuition	$33,000
Room and board (off campus)	$8,000
Cost of books	$3,500
Fees	$1,115

Financial Aid

% students receiving aid	85
Average grant	$2,000
Average loan	$30,000

STATE UNIVERSITY OF NEW YORK—UPSTATE MEDICAL UNIVERSITY
COLLEGE OF MEDICINE

OFFICE OF STUDENT ADMISSIONS, 766 IRVING AVENUE, SYRACUSE, NY 13210 • ADMISSION: 315-464-4570
FAX: 315-464-8867 • E-MAIL: ADMISS@UPSTATE.EDU • WEBSITE: WWW.UPSTATE.EDU

STUDENT BODY

Type	Public
Enrollment	652
% male/female	54/46
% underrepresented minorities	8
# applied (total/out)	3,227/1,352
# accepted (total/out)	396/92
# enrolled (total/out)	153/31
Average age	23

FACULTY

Total faculty (number)	366
% part-time	49
Student-faculty ratio	1:1

ADMISSIONS

Average GPA and MCAT Scores

Overall GPA	3.54
MCAT Bio	10.1
MCAT Phys	9.91
MCAT Verbal	9.58
MCAT Essay	Q

Application Information

Regular application	12/1
Regular notification	5/1
Early application	8/1
Early notification	10/1
Are transfers accepted?	yes
Admissions may be deferred?	yes
Interview required?	yes
Application fee	$100

Academics

The College of Medicine curriculum integrates the basic and clinical sciences with basic science courses teaching the clinical implications of the material and provides clinical experience starting in the first semester.

All courses are aligned by organ systems. For example, in the first year, students learn the structure and function of the brain in February, the heart in March and the lungs in April. Similarly, the second year aligns the pharmacology, microbiology, and pathology of each organ system.

The curriculum also addresses the humanistic aspects of medicine, including its ethical, legal, and social implications. Throughout their four years at Upstate, students acquire the knowledge, skills, and attitudes necessary to become competent, caring physicians.

All College of Medicine students spend their first two years on the Upstate campus in Syracuse. At the start of the third year, one-fourth of the class moves to the Binghamton Clinical campus. The rest of the class remains in Syracuse and completes clinical education at University Hospital and its clinical affiliates. Students learn the same skills at both campuses, but the ambiance is different.

Much of the clinical training in Syracuse takes place in a tertiary care setting, the special focus of a university hospital. In Binghamton, most of the training occurs in a community-based setting that is more akin to the environment in which most physicians will practice later on. Applicants indicate their campus preference within 2 weeks of the admissions interview and are assigned to a clinical campus upon acceptance to the College of Medicine.

Students

Eighty percent of students are New York residents; however, admissions decisions are merit based and state of residency is not a factor considered when making a decision on an application. Applications from non-New York state residents are welcome. About 12 percent of students are underrepresented minorities, and about 15 percent took some significant time off between college and medical school. Class size is 152.

STUDENT LIFE

A large part of college life takes place outside the classroom, and Upstate is no exception. We offer 45 student clubs and organizations, including ballroom dancing, student government, special events, and athletic programs.

The Campus Activities Governing Board schedules social, cultural, and recreational programs for students including first-run movies on weekends, a guest lecture series, comedy hours, weekend getaways, and discount tickets to local sports and cultural events. The Campus Activities Building (CAB), located next door to our residence hall, has a computer lounge, snack bar, bookstore, TV lounge, pool, sauna, gym, squash and racquetball courts, treadmills, step machines, Nautilus, tennis courts, billiards, ping pong, and more. Our intramural sports program runs men's, women's, and/or coed leagues in basketball, volleyball, softball, football, racquetball, and soccer.

Syracuse is a medium-sized city surrounded by countryside. It is a one hour drive to Lake Ontario's beaches and four hours to New York City. The Binghamton campus is conveniently situated about three hours from New York City, Philadelphia, and Buffalo. Modern residence halls at the Syracuse campus provide dormitory rooms, studios, and 1-bedroom apartments for single and married students. Off-campus housing is readily available for students choosing to attend the Binghampton campus during their last two years of study.

GRADUATES

Graduates are successful in securing residencies in all fields.

Admissions

REQUIREMENTS

Prerequisites are general chemistry (6–8 hours); organic chemistry (6–8 hours); general biology (6–8 hours); general physics (6–8 hours); and English (6 hours, at least 3 of which must be composition).

SUGGESTIONS

Academic work in the humanities and social sciences is considered equally as important as science course work.

PROCESS

All applicants are sent secondary applications. Of those returning secondaries, about 20 percent are invited to interview between September and March. Interviews consist of two sessions each with faculty members, administrators, students, or alumni. About 20 percent of interviewed candidates are accepted on a rolling basis, while others may be admitted later in the year.

Admissions Requirements (Required)

MCAT scores, science GPA, non-science GPA, letters of recommendation, interview, essays/personal statement, extracurricular activities, exposure to medical profession.

Admissions Requirements (Optional)

State residency.

Overlap Schools

Stony Brook University, University at Buffalo, State University of New York.

COSTS AND AID

Tuition & Fees

In-state Tuition	$18,800
Out-of-state Tuition	$33,500
Cost of books	$2,000
Fees	$1,090

Financial Aid

% students receiving aid	87
Average grant	$6,205
Average loan	$31,736
Average debt	$113,231

TEMPLE UNIVERSITY
SCHOOL OF MEDICINE

3340 NORTH BROAD STREET, SFC SUITE, 305 PHILADELPHIA, PA 19140 • ADMISSION: 215-707-3656
FAX: 215-707-6932 • E-MAIL: MEDADMISSIONS@TEMPLE.EDU • WEBSITE: WWW.TEMPLE.EDU/MEDICINE

STUDENT BODY

Type	Private
# applied (total/out)	7,504/6,556
# accepted (total/out)	889/366
# enrolled (total/out)	176/83
Average age	24

FACULTY

Total faculty (number)	527
% female	27
% minority	5
% part-time	13
Student-faculty ratio	2:1

ADMISSIONS

Average GPA and MCAT Scores

Overall GPA	3.59
MCAT Bio	10.4
MCAT Phys	10.1
MCAT Verbal	9.5
MCAT Essay	P

Application Information

Regular application	12/15
Regular notification	10/15
Early application	8/1
Early notification	10/1
Are transfers accepted?	yes
Admissions may be deferred?	yes
Interview required?	yes
Application fee	$70

Academics

The primary educational goals of Temple University School of Medicine are to teach students to provide outstanding medical care to a culturally diverse population and to be exceptionally well-prepared for further training and life-long career development. This education is based upon a solid foundation in the basic sciences, extensive hands-on clinical training, the principles of evidence-based medicine, and integration of basic science and clinical medicine throughout the curriculum. Students will develop the skills necessary to continually update their knowledge base and healthcare delivery after graduation, and will be prepared for careers in clinical medicine, medical education and medical research. Qualified students may pursue an MPH, MBA, or PhD concurrently with an MD. PhD degrees may be obtained in anatomy and cell biology, biochemistry, microbiology and immunology, molecular biology and genetics, neuroscience, pathology and laboratory medicine, pharmacology, or physiology. Temple's system of student evaluation uses honors/high pass/pass/condition/fail. A grade of pass or higher is required for promotion, and passing the USMLE Step 1 and 2CK are required for graduation. Students must also take Step 2CS.

BASIC SCIENCES: The first two years are taught in an integrated approach, closely tying basic science concepts to clinical medicine, professionalism, and medical ethics. The clinical years are marked by extensive hands-on experience in caring for patients. The new Clinical Simulation and Skills Center allows students to learn basic clinical skills in a safe learning environment throughout the curriculum. Thus, graduates are exceptionally well prepared to pursue residency training. The major goal of year 1 is normal structure, function, and development. Year 2 focuses on the causes, mechanisms, identification, and treatment of major human diseases. A doctoring course, to run throughout the curriculum, will enable students to learn the basics of history-taking, physical exam skills, and professionalism. The course uses clinical cases to integrate the teaching and evaluation of clinical skills with the basic science concepts in each of the blocks, and utilizes the Clinical Simulation and Skills Center to aid learning through interactive clinical scenarios. Faculty preceptors will provide individualized mentoring and career advising. In year 2, the doctoring course will enable students to practice and improve their clinical skills through closely supervised rotations in both ambulatory and hospital settings.

CLINICAL TRAINING

During year 3, beginning in late May of the second year, students rotate through core clerkships in ambulatory medicine (4 weeks), family medicine (6 weeks), internal medicine (8 weeks), neurology (4 weeks), ob/gyn (6 weeks), pediatrics (6 weeks), psychiatry (6 weeks), and surgery (8 weeks). The third year doctoring course emphasizes career advising, evidence-based medicine, and clinical decision-making. Beginning in May in year 4, students can focus on areas of interest through a large variety of electives, and enhance their clinical skills through two sub internships: Surgical Subspecialties and Intensive Care and Radiology. The School of Medicine maintains affiliations with several major urban and suburban Pennsylvania hospitals, each with a long history of academic and clinical excellence. This provides medical students with an opportunity to see a wide range of medical disorders in people who have varied social, economic and cultural backgrounds, and to learn the management of those disorders in diverse ambulatory and inpatient settings. Four of these institutions—Crozer-Chester Medical Center in Upland, Geisinger Medical Center in Danville, St. Luke's Hospital in Bethlehem, and the Western

Pennsylvania Hospital in Pittsburgh—are comprehensive clinical campuses to which students may commit for all of their third and fourth year clinical rotations. Several other sites—Abington Memorial Hospital in Abington Township, Conemaugh Memorial Medical Center in Johnstown, Lehigh Valley Hospital in Allentown, Mercy Hospital in Scranton, and Reading Hospital and Medical Center in Reading—offer required and elective clerkships and sub internships.

Students

Approximately 50 percent of students are Pennsylvania residents. About 15 percent of students in a typical class are underrepresented minorities. In particular, Temple has a strong contingent of African American and Latino students. Class size is 180.

STUDENT LIFE

Temple students benefit from rich, extracurricular offerings both on and off campus. Both Temple's Health Science campus and the main campus have comprehensive athletic and recreational facilities. Medical students are active in school governance and are members of the curriculum, financial affairs, and Admissions Committees. There are numerous student organizations that range from support groups for minority medical students to community outreach organizations to a rugby club. Philadelphia is a historically and culturally rich city. It is also a very student-friendly city in which medical students in particular abound. Most students live off campus.

GRADUATES

For the 2006 graduating class, 53 percent will be staying in Pennsylvania for residency training. The most prevalent specialty choices were internal medicine (28 percent), surgery (13 percent), pediatrics (12 percent), emergency medicine (10 percent), family medicine (10 percent), psychiatry (5 percent), and orthopedics (3 percent).

Admissions

REQUIREMENTS

One year each of biology, chemistry, organic chemistry, and physics are required as well as 6 semester hours of humanities. The MCAT is required, and scores must be no more than three years old.

SUGGESTIONS

As a state-related school, Temple gives slight preference to Pennsylvania residents, but significant numbers of out-of-state applicants are admitted. For applicants who have been out of college for a period of time, some recent course work is important. The April, rather than August, MCAT is advised. Medically-related and community-service activities are valued, and the Admissions Committee is serious about selecting students who will make supportive class members and caring physicians.

PROCESS

There is no GPA or MCAT cut off, and all applications are reviewed by a member of the Admissions Committee. All AMCAS applicants receive requests for secondary application materials, and about 20 percent of those returning secondaries are invited to interview. Interviews take place between September and April and consist of a half-hour session with a faculty member or administrator. On interview day, applicants meet with the Admissions Director, receive a campus tour, and have lunch with second-year medical students. About one-third of interviewees are accepted, with notification occurring on a rolling basis. Admission may also be gained through programs with post-baccalaureate, premedical programs at Temple, Goucher, Duquesne, Bryn Mawr, Columbia, Scripps, Brandeis, West Chester, Scranton, and the University of Pennsylvania. Early assurance programs exist with premedical programs at Duquesne and Washington-Jefferson. Uniquely qualified high school students may apply for BA/MD programs with Temple, Washington Jefferson, Duquesne, Scranton, and Widener.

Admissions Requirements (Required)

MCAT scores, science GPA, non-science GPA, letters of recommendation, interview, essays/personal statement, extracurricular activities, exposure to medical profession, 6 semester hours of humanities.

COSTS AND AID

Tuition & Fees

Tuition	
(in-state)	$33,730
(out-of-state)	$41,310
Room and board	
(off campus)	$13,580
Cost of books	$1,598
Fees	$575

Financial Aid

% students receiving aid	89
Average grant	$7,039
Average loan	$38,500
Average debt	$150,946

TEXAS A&M UNIVERSITY SYSTEM HEALTH SCIENCE CENTER
COLLEGE OF MEDICINE

159 JOE H. REYNOLDS MB, COLLEGE STATION, TX 77843 • ADMISSION: 979-845-7743
FAX: 979-845-5533 • E-MAIL: ADMISSIONS@MEDICINE.TAMHSC.EDU • WEBSITE: WWW.MEDICINE.TAMHSC.EDU

STUDENT BODY

Type	Public
Enrollment	300
% male/female	52/48
% underrepresented minorities	14
# applied (total/out)	2,746/225
# accepted (total/out)	245/16
# enrolled (total/out)	81/8
Average age	24

FACULTY

Total faculty (number)	844
% female	20
% minority	16
% part-time	10
Student-faculty ratio	1:1

ADMISSIONS

Average GPA and MCAT Scores

Overall GPA	3.73
MCAT Bio	9.7
MCAT Phys	9.3
MCAT Verbal	8.7
MCAT Essay	Q

Application Information

Regular application	10/15
Regular notification	11/15
Are transfers accepted?	yes
Admissions may be deferred?	yes
Interview required?	yes
Application fee	$45

Academics

As one of the most ambitious and comprehensive medical colleges in the nation, the College of Medicine offers the Doctor of Medicine, Doctor of Philosophy, and combined MD/PhD, MD/MBA, and MD/MPH degrees. Active research programs are currently underway in the departments of molecular and cellular medicine, microbial and molecular pathogenesis, neuroscience and experimental therapeutics, and systems biology and translational medicine. The college is committed to providing an environment which promotes integrity, compassion, and excellence in its future physicians and scientists.

BASIC SCIENCE: The first year is organized into blocks that span 36 weeks beginning in late July. Year one consists of the following blocks with some overlapping each other and others spanning entirely over the 36 weeks: 14 weeks of gross anatomy and embryology; 18 weeks of molecular and cellular foundations of medicine; 14 weeks of human organ systems (cardiovascular, gastrointestinal, respiratory, renal, endocrine, and reproduction); 10 weeks of neuroscience; and, 36 weeks of becoming a clinician I (which includes the following courses: working with patients, medical humanities, gross anatomy, clinical correlations, leadership in medicine, introduction to physical diagnosis, evidence-based medicine, and introduction to behavioral medicine). Year two is also organized into blocks that span 36 weeks. Year two consists of the following distinct blocks with no overlap except for becoming a clinician II: 12 weeks of basic which encompasses medical microbiology/immunology, pathology/laboratory medicine, and medical pharmacology/toxicology; 2 weeks of hematology; 1 week of respiratory; 2 weeks of cardiovascular; 1 week of renal, 2 weeks of emergency preparedness; 2 weeks of gastrointestinal/nutrition; 3 weeks of endocrine/reproduction; 1 week of integument/musculoskeletal; 2 weeks of neurology/psychiatry; and 36 weeks of becoming a clinician II (which includes the following courses: emergency preparedness, evidence-based medicine, humanities in medicine, introduction to clinical psychiatry, introduction to clinical medicine, introduction to reproductive medicine and human sexuality, introduction to pediatrics, and preceptorship). An emphasis in organ systems-based instruction in the medical sciences produces individuals with the knowledge, expertise, and vision to meet the challenge facing modern medicine in the twenty-first century.

CLINICAL TRAINING

The College of Medicine is the result of a unique affiliation between the Texas A&M Health Science Center and several well established clinical affiliates. Scott and White Memorial Hospital and Clinic in Temple, Texas; the Central Texas Veterans Health Care System-Olin E. Teague Veterans Center in Temple, Texas; Darnall Army Community Hospital in Fort Hood, Texas; Driscoll Children's Hospital in Corpus Christi, Texas, Christus-Spohn Health Care System in Corpus Christi, and John Peter Smith Health Care System in Fort Worth, Texas. These affiliations of a highly ranked research-oriented state university, a comprehensive private sector health care provider, two of the largest federal health service agencies in the world, and regional comprehensive multi-specialty centers in Corpus Christi and Fort Worth, Texas integrate the strengths and resources of each institution. Combined, these clinical facilities treat approximately 3 million outpatients and another 50,000 inpatients each year, giving our medical students excellent learning opportunities. The goal of the curriculum is to produce undifferentiated physicians of the highest caliber. Years 1 and 2 are taught on the campus in College Station and includes organ systems curriculum, which integrates the traditional basic sciences along with instruction in behavioral science, working with patients, physical diagnosis, humanities in medicine, community medicine, leadership in medicine, evidence-based medicine, and epidemiology. Correlation of the basic sciences with clinical medicine is achieved from the start, with clinical instruction in both year 1 and 2. Years 3 and 4 are taught on the clinical campus in Temple and consist of traditional clerkships and a mixed rotation of ambulatory care experiences.

Students

The vast majority of students are from Texas. About 10 percent of students are underrepresented minorities, most of whom are of Mexican American descent. About 90 percent of the student body were science majors of some type as undergraduates.

STUDENT LIFE

Each medical school class selects and sponsors human service organizations, at which students volunteer. This, along with social activities sponsored by the school and the university, unifies the class and gives students extracurricular activities to pursue together. The university's recreational facilities are outstanding, offering every possible athletic activity. Students live off campus, generally in apartments.

GRADUATES

Our medical students continue to enter a broad spectrum of good residency programs across the state and nation. Between the years of 2002 and 2006, 43 percent entered primary care residency training programs (family medicine, pediatrics, internal medicine, and medicine-pediatrics) throughout the state and country. Of those who graduated between 2002 and 2006, the following residencies were the most popular: Internal medicine, pediatrics, anesthesiology, obstetrics/gynecology, family medicine, surgery, emergency medicine, and psychiatry. Forty-seven percent of the graduates matched into residencies in Texas and 15 percent into Scott and White residency programs.

Admissions

REQUIREMENTS

The College of Medicine considers for enrollment individuals who have completed at least 90-credit hours of undergraduate course work. By state mandate, enrollment of out-of-state residents may not exceed 10 percent. Each year 100 entering students are enrolled. The following courses are required with at least a grade of C: General biology with lab (8 hours), additional biological sciences (3 hours), general chemistry with lab (8 hours), organic chemistry with lab (8 hours), general physics with lab (8 hours), English (6 hours), and calculus (3 hours). The MCAT is required and must have been taken no earlier than five years before the expected date of enrollment. The best set of test scores is considered in the evaluation process. Applicants should not withhold previous test scores.

SUGGESTIONS

Although the MCAT is offered twice each year, in April and August, we strongly encourage applicants to take the MCAT in April. Official scores must be released directly to the Texas Medical and Dental Schools Application Service in Austin, Texas. Involvement in community service and health-related work that involves patient and physician contact are helpful. For applicants who have been out of school for several years, some recent course work is recommended.

PROCESS

Approximately 30 percent of Texas applicants are interviewed, and 20 percent of those interviewed are offered a place in the class. About 5 percent of out-of-state residents are interviewed, and only a few are accepted each year. Interview sessions typically are scheduled from August to December. Each applicant is given two 30-minute interviews. The earliest date of acceptance is November 15. The College of Medicine participates in the Texas Medical Schools Matching Program employed by the Texas Medical and Dental Schools Application Service. A ranked wait list is established in February. The Texas Medical and Dental Schools Application Service (TMDSAS) processes all applications. Application materials may be obtained after May 1 online at http://dpweb1.dp.utexas.edu/mdac.

Admissions Requirements (Required)

MCAT scores, science GPA, non-science GPA, letters of recommendation, interview, state residency, essays/personal statement.

Admissions Requirements (Optional)

Extracurricular activities, exposure to medical profession.

Overlap Schools

Rush Medical College of Rush University, Texas Tech University, University of Texas.

COSTS AND AID

Tuition & Fees

In-state Tuition	$7,750
Out-of-state Tuition	$19,650
Room and board (off campus)	$11,874
Cost of books	$2,428
Fees	$1,262

Financial Aid

% students receiving aid	96
Average grant	$4,000
Average loan	$23,000
Average debt	$90,000

TEXAS TECH UNIVERSITY
TTU HEALTH SCIENCES CENTER SCHOOL OF MEDICINE

3601 4TH STREET, 2B116 LUBBOCK, TX 79430 • ADMISSION: 806-743-2297
FAX: 806-743-2725 • E-MAIL: TREVOR.YATES@TTUHSC.EDU • WEBSITE: WWW.TTUHSC.EDU

STUDENT BODY

Type	Public
Enrollment	490
% male/female	44/56
% underrepresented minorities	22
# applied	2,850
# accepted	300
# enrolled	140
Average age	24

FACULTY

Total faculty (number)	527
% female	29
% minority	31
% part-time	9
Student-faculty ratio	1:1

ADMISSIONS

Average GPA and MCAT Scores

Overall GPA	3.5
MCAT Bio	9.7
MCAT Phys	9.5
MCAT Verbal	9.5
MCAT Essay	O

Application Information

Regular application	12/1
Regular notification	rolling
Early application	8/1
Early notification	10/1
Are transfers accepted?	yes
Admissions may be deferred?	yes
Interview required?	yes
Application fee	$40

Academics

Most students complete a 4 year curriculum designed to prepare physicians with a broad base of medical knowledge and sound analytic and problem-solving skills. It is organized in two stages: basic science and clinical training. Some students devote an additional year to research and earn an MD degree in five years. Others are involved in summer research projects. Qualified students interested in biomedical research or academic medicine can earn a PhD along with the MD degree. To address the needs of a rapidly changing health care system, students can participate in an MD/MBA joint-degree program in which both degrees are earned in four years. Medical students are graded on a numerical system and must maintain a weighted average of 75 for promotion and graduation.

BASIC SCIENCES: First year courses are biochemistry; gross anatomy; histology; neuroscience; physician in society; physiology; and concepts in community and ambulatory care, which serves as an introduction to clinical medicine and uses physician community mentors. First-year students also have the opportunity to take an elective. Second-year courses are integrated approach to patient care, introduction to medicine, introduction to psychiatry, microbiology, pathology, and pharmacology. During the first and second years, instruction primarily uses a lecture/lab format. However, some concepts are addressed in small-group sessions. Students are in classes or other scheduled sessions for about 27 hours per week. All instruction takes place in medical education buildings on the Lubbock campus.

CLINICAL TRAINING

Third-year required rotations are internal medicine (12 weeks), surgery (12 weeks), pediatrics (6 weeks), family medicine (6 weeks), ob/gyn (6 weeks), and psychiatry (6 weeks). Fourth-year requirements are neurology (4 weeks), selectives (8 weeks), a sub internship (4 weeks), and 16 weeks of electives. After successful completion of years 1 and 2, approximately 35 students go on to Amarillo for clinical training, 35 stay in Lubbock, and 50 go to El Paso. Amarillo, El Paso, and Lubbock all serve both urban and rural populations. Multiple clinical affiliations of each site provide a wealth of training opportunities for students. El Paso serves an urban border population of more than 700,000 and provides a unique multicultural educational opportunity. Training sites include Thomason Hospital and other community and military facilities. In Lubbock, students benefit from recreational and cultural opportunities available on the Texas Tech University campus of the main university. The primary teaching hospital is University Covenant Health-Lakeside. Other affiliated hospitals include Mary of the Plains Hospital, Charter Plains Hospital, and the Veterans Administration Outpatient Clinics. Amarillo provides exposure to medicine primarily from a private hospital perspective. Teaching hospitals include Northwest Texas Health Care System, Baptist St. Anthony Health Care System, and Veterans Administration Hospital. In total, Texas Tech affiliates provide almost 3,000 teaching beds.

Students

The entering class had the following characteristics: 100 percent Texas residents, 23 percent underrepresented minorities, and 75 percent science majors. Typically, about 20 percent of students in an entering class are a bit older, having taken time off after college. Class size is 120.

STUDENT LIFE

During their first two years, students benefit from the resources of the Health Science Center and from being adjacent to Texas Tech University, a major undergraduate institution. Medical students are supportive of one another, as demonstrated by a student-initiated, peer-tutoring program. First and second-year students are often involved in community-service projects, which provide early clinical exposure. Student life during the third and fourth years varies according to location.

GRADUATES

Approximately 21 percent of graduates enter Texas Tech residency programs, which operate on all four campuses. Others are successful in obtaining positions throughout Texas and at institutions in other regions of the country. Eighty-one percent of graduates matched with one of their top three residency choices.

Admissions

REQUIREMENTS

Requirements are biology (12 semester hours), biology lab (2 semester hours), general chemistry with lab (8 semester hours), organic chemistry with lab (8 semester hours), physics with lab (8 semester hours), English (6 semester hours), and calculus (3 semester hours). All prerequisite courses require a grade of C or better. The MCAT is required and should be taken within the past five years. For applicants who have taken the exam more than once, the most recent set of scores is weighed most heavily, but all scores must be reported. Texas residents and residents of neighboring counties in New Mexico and Oklahoma, which comprise the service areas of the school, are given preference in admission. Only nonresident applicants with GPAs of 3.6 or higher, and MCAT scores of 29 or higher will be considered for admission.

SUGGESTIONS

The April, rather than August, MCAT is advised. In addition to high intellectual ability and a record of strong academic achievement, the Admissions Committee looks for qualities and traits such as compassion, motivation, communication skills, maturity, and personal integrity.

PROCESS

Texas Tech does not participate in AMCAS. Texas Tech participates with five other state-supported medical schools in the Texas Medical and Dental Application Service (TMDAS). A single application is sent to the TMDAS for processing and then is forwarded to any or all of the participating schools as requested by the applicant. A secondary application is also required by Texas Tech. Both applications will be available via the Internet. In addition, application forms may be requested from Texas Medical and Dental Application Service, 702 Colorado Street, Suite 6400, Austin, TX 78701. About 38 percent of applicants are interviewed between September and January. Interviews consist of two sessions, each with an Admissions Committee/faculty member. On interview day, applicants tour the campus, attend group information sessions, meet current students, and have the opportunity to attend classes. Notification begins on October 15 and continues until the class is filled.

Admissions Requirements (Required)

MCAT scores, science GPA, non-science GPA, letters of recommendation, interview, essays/personal statement, extracurricular activities, exposure to medical profession.

Admissions Requirements (Optional)

State residency.

COSTS AND AID

Tuition & Fees

In-state Tuition	$7,654
Out-of-state Tuition	$20,754
Room and board (off campus)	$11,000
Cost of books	$1,271
Fees	$1,226

Financial Aid

% students receiving aid	85
Average grant	$1,600
Average loan	$20,084
Average debt	$100,000

THOMAS JEFFERSON UNIVERSITY

JEFFERSON MEDICAL COLLEGE

1015 WALNUT STREET, ROOM 110, PHILADELPHIA, PA 19107 • ADMISSION: 215-955-6983
FAX: 215-955-5151 • E-MAIL: JMC.ADMISSIONS@JEFFERSON.EDU • WEBSITE: WWW.JEFFERSON.EDU/JMC/

STUDENT BODY

Type	Private
Enrollment	935
% male/female	51/49
% underrepresented minorities	26
# applied (total/out)	7,702/6,739
# accepted (total/out)	517/334
# enrolled (total/out)	254/147
Average age	24

FACULTY

Total faculty (number)	2,408
% female	27
% minority	3
% part-time	24
Student-faculty ratio	3:1

ADMISSIONS

Average GPA and MCAT Scores

Overall GPA	3.6
MCAT Bio	10.4
MCAT Phys	10.0
MCAT Verbal	10.2
MCAT Essay	Q

Application Information

Regular application	11/15
Regular notification	rolling
Early application	6/1–8/1
Early notification	10/1
Are transfers accepted?	yes
Admissions may be deferred?	yes
Interview required?	yes
Application fee	$80

Academics

Along with basic science and clinical training, Jefferson's curriculum emphasizes the social and public health issues related to medicine. Students with solid science backgrounds may pursue an MD and a PhD in one of the departments of the College of Graduate Studies. These include biochemistry and molecular biology, genetics, immunology and microbial pathologies, joint-PhD programs, molecular cell biology, molecular pharmacology and structural biology, neuroscience, physiology, and tissue engineering and regenerative medicine. A joint-MD/MBA degree is offered in conjunction with Widener University in Chester, Pennsylvania, as is a combined MD/Masters in Hospital Administration. A 5 year program is available in which Jefferson students have the opportunity to earn an MPF at Johns Hopkins School of Hygiene and Public Health while earning their MD degree at Jefferson Medical College. This program is offered to students with special interests such as community health and in recognition of the increasing importance of population medicine. Pennsylvania State University and Jefferson Medical College allow students to pursue a combined BS/MD program, which grants both degrees in a 6 or 7 year period. Jefferson has special arrangements with the University of Pennsylvania's, Bryn Mawr's, and Columbia University's post-baccalaureate programs through which highly-qualified students may be admitted to Jefferson prior to completion of their premedical requirements.

BASIC SCIENCES: We believe that the first year of medical school sets the stage for at least the first four years of medical education, if not for one's entire professional career. During this year, Jefferson students focus on the structure and function of the human organisim in its physical and psychosocial context. Course work in the basic sciences of human gross anatomy, biochemistry, cell biology, genetics, microscopic anatomy, neuroscience, and physiology provides first-year students with a strong basic science grounding. Practice-related topics such as medical informatcs, evidence-based medicine, health policy, and ethics are also introduced during the first year. Clinical course work focuses on the patient-doctor relationship, medical interviewing, and history-taking, the human developmental trajectory, and behavioral science principles. This curricula provides students with both a behavioral science foundation and a clinical framework; it establishes an educational bridge between lay perspectives and the realities of medical practice. In addition to increasing emphasis on the study of bedside skills, the curriculum shifts in the second year to the study of pathophysiology and disease. After an introductory block of clinical medicine, general pathology and general pharmacology, the subjects of immunology, microbiology, pathology, physical diagnosis, and systems-based pharmacology are presented as an interdisciplinary curriculum. The curriculum includes small group sessions focusing on the problem-solving evidence-based medicine and service-based learning. Grades are honors/pass/fail. Pre-clinical studies take place in the central Medical College Building Complex, which includes administrative offices, labs, lecture halls, common areas, and recreational facilities. The Scott Library includes 200,000 print volumes, a Learning Resources Center and computer labs in addition to videos, slides, and supplemental learning materials. MEDLINE and other electronic data systems are available, as well as more than 500 electronic journals and books. The Rector Clinical Skill Center occupies more than 900 square feet and houses a 14-room standardized patient suite and classrooms for high-tech simulators.

CLINICAL TRAINING

Patient contact officially begins in the first year, with medical practice in the twenty-first century. There are also ongoing opportunities for medical students interested in volunteer clinical experience or clinical research through summer programs and part-time jobs. Formally, the clinical portion of the curriculum begins in year 3 with required rotations. These are family medicine (6 weeks), general surgery (6 weeks), internal medicine (12 weeks), pediatrics (6 weeks), psychiatry and human behavior (6 weeks), and ob/gyn (6 weeks). Phase II of clinical rotations are selectives in which students choose specialties within broadly defined categories. 12 weeks are also designated as purely elective. Training sites include Albert Einstein Medical Center; Bryn Mawr Hospital (383 beds); Bryn Mawr Rehabilitation Hospital; Christiana Care Medical Center; DuPont Hospital for Children; Geisinger Medical Center (in Danville, Pennsylvania, providing rural exposure); Lankenau Hospital (475 beds); Latrobe Hospital (280 beds, family medicine); Magee Rehabilitation Hospital; Mercy Hospital, Pittsburgh; Wills Eye Hospital; and West Jersey Health System. The patients come from several states and represent extremely diverse populations.

Students

About 30 states are represented by the students within a class, mostly those of the eastern part of the country. About 40 percent of the students are Pennsylvania state residents. Applicants underrepresented in medicine make up about 9 percent of each class. Class size is 255. Approximately 20 percent of each class is over 25 years of age upon matriculation. In recent years, about 5 percent of matriculates have held advanced degrees.

STUDENT LIFE

Numerous professional, athletic, and cultural student organizations exist on campus. Beyond campus, the city of Philadelphia provides ample recreational and cultural possibilities and New York is just about one hour away. On-campus housing options include residence halls and apartments of all sizes; housing is guaranteed to first-year students. With Jefferson's central and urban location, a car is unnecessary in the first two years.

GRADUATES

More than 70 percent of Jefferson graduates enter residency programs at university-affiliated hospitals around the nation. Jefferson graduates do very well in the residency-matching program, both in primary care and in more specialized fields.

Admissions

REQUIREMENTS

Required course work is 1 year of biology with lab, chemistry with lab, organic chemistry with lab, and physics with lab.

SUGGESTIONS

Applicants should demonstrate problem-solving capability, success in a range of subjects, and some in-depth knowledge of one or a few subjects. Strong writing skills are also valued. Experience in a medical or research environment is important. Delaware residents are given preference, as are applicants from programs that have special arrangements with Jefferson. Applicants are advised to submit all materials in a timely fashion.

PROCESS

On receipt of the verified AMCAS application, Jefferson will send, via e-mail, notification of receipt. The Committee of Admissions will begin reviewing the application when all supplementary materials have been received, including the following: The Jefferson Medical College Secondary Application Form, the nonrefundable $80 application fee, MCAT scores, and the required letters of recommendation. Interviews are conducted from September through March, and about 10 percent of the applicant pool is eventually interviewed. Interviews are approximately 30–45 minutes in length and are conducted by a member of the faculty or administration. Admissions are rolling. About 50 percent of those who interview are accepted. Others are either rejected or wait listed. When places become available later in the cycle, wait-listed applicants will be notified and offered positions. Indicating interest in Jefferson may help the prospects of wait-listed candidates.

Admissions Requirements (Required)

MCAT scores, science GPA, letters of recommendation, interview, essays/personal statement, extracurricular activities, exposure to medical profession, secondary application.

Admissions Requirements (Optional)

Nonscience GPA, state residency.

COSTS AND AID

Tuition & Fees

Tuition	$38,316
Room and board (on campus)	$15,609
Cost of books	$5,880

Financial Aid

% students receiving aid	99
Average grant	$4,500
Average loan	$37,030
Average debt	$145,472

TUFTS UNIVERSITY
SCHOOL OF MEDICINE

OFFICE OF ADMISSIONS, 136 HARRISON AVENUE, STEARNS 1, BOSTON, MA 02111 • ADMISSION: 617-636-6571
E-MAIL: SGP@COR.CDM.NEMC. • WEBSITE: WWW.TUFTS.EDU/MED

STUDENT BODY	
Type	Private
Enrollment	695
% male/female	54/46
% underrepresented minorities	11
# applied (total/out)	8,277/8,336
# accepted	473
# enrolled (total/out)	168/113

ADMISSIONS

Average GPA and MCAT Scores

Overall GPA	3.5
MCAT Bio	10.5
MCAT Phys	10.3
MCAT Verbal	9.9

Application Information

Regular application	11/1
Regular notification	rolling
Early application	8/1
Early notification	10/1
Are transfers accepted?	yes
Interview required?	yes
Application fee	$95

Academics

The majority of students follow a 4 year curriculum leading to the MD degree. Students with an interest in public health have the opportunity to earn an MPH along with their MD. This combined MD/MPH program may be completed in four years. Other combined-degree programs include the 4 year MD/MBA in health management in partnership with Brandeis University and Northeastern University; the MD/PhD in conjunction with the Sackler School of Graduate Biomedical Sciences; and the BS in engineering and combined MS/MD in an engineering degree program, a collaborative effort of the Tufts College of engineering and the Tufts University School of Medicine. The doctorate may be earned in the following fields: Anatomy, biochemistry, biophysics, cell biology, genetics, immunology, microbiology, molecular biology, neuroscience, pathology, pharmacology, and physiology. Each year, four funded MD/PhD positions are available. A primary care preceptorship program allows students with a particular interest in primary care to experience early patient contact.

BASIC SCIENCES: In addition to required courses, first- and second-year students choose among pre-clinical selectives. These are graded as pass/fail and allow students to explore their interests early on in the program. A new Principles and Practice of Medicine Program (PPM) was developed to enhance the first- and second-year curriculum. PPM integrates basic science topics with interdisciplinary subjects such as computer literacy, ethics, health care economics, information management, and negotiation/team building skills. PPM also introduces important clinical techniques such as the patient interview, examination, and physical diagnosis. First-year courses are the following: Biochemistry, cell biology, epidemiology biostatistics, genetics, gross anatomy, hematology, histology, immunology, molecular biology, physiology, pre-clinical selectives, problem-based learning, and PPM. Second-year courses are the following: Addiction medicine, microbiology, neuroscience, pathology, pathophysiology/infectious disease, pharmacology, pre-clinical selectives, problem-based learning, psychopathology, and PPM, which focuses on clinical skills and serves as an important transition to third-year clerkships. During the first and second years, instruction involves lectures, labs, and small-group sessions. As an important learning aid, Tufts Health Sciences Library developed the Health Sciences Database. It contains the full text of many syllabi, lecture slides, reserve slide collections, lecture recordings, and other multimedia and resource materials.

CLINICAL TRAINING

Third-year required clerkships are the following: medicine (12 weeks), surgery (12 weeks), ob/gyn (6 weeks), pediatrics (6 weeks), and psychiatry (6 weeks). About 4 weeks are available for elective study during the third year. Fourth-year requirements are a 4 week primary care clerkship and a 4 week neurology elective. At least 32 weeks of electives are also required, 20 of which must be completed at Tufts facilities. Twelve weeks of electives may be taken at other academic and clinical institutions. Some students fulfill a portion of elective requirements overseas.

Students

In last year's entering class, about 28 percent of students were Massachusetts residents, and about 14 percent of students went to Tufts as undergraduates. Another 28 percent of students were California residents, and 10 percent were New York residents. Approximately 30 percent of students were at least 23 years old, and 15 percent were 25 or older. Women accounted for 41 percent of the class, and underrepresented minorities accounted for about 11 percent.

STUDENT LIFE

Medical students at Tufts are generally cohesive and supportive of one another. Some students are involved in clubs or in local chapters of national medical student organizations. Off campus, students enjoy the offerings of Boston, a city filled with students, bookstores, coffee shops, restaurants, parks, and cultural activities. Residence facilities are available on a limited basis in Posner Hall, located close to the medical school campus. Students who live off campus generally share apartments in neighborhoods that are convenient to the school.

GRADUATES

Graduates are successful in securing residency positions at institutions in all regions of the country. Tufts prepares graduates for careers in both primary care and specialty areas.

Admissions

REQUIREMENTS

Requirements are 8 semester credits of biology, chemistry, organic chemistry, and physics all with associated labs. Applicants must possess the ability to speak and write English correctly. The MCAT is required, and scores should be from within the past three years. For applicants who have taken the exam on multiple occasions, the best scores are used.

SUGGESTIONS

In addition to prerequisite courses, recommended course work includes biochemistry, calculus, computer science, English, and statistics. The selection of candidates for admissions is based not only on performance in the required premedical courses but also on the applicant's entire academic record and extracurricular experiences.

PROCESS

All AMCAS applicants are sent secondary applications. Of those returning completed applications, about 12 percent are invited to interview between November and March. Interviews consist of two sessions, each with a faculty member, school administrator, or senior medical student. On interview day, applicants also attend informational sessions and a reception with current medical students. Approximately half of interviewed candidates are accepted. Notification occurs on a rolling basis and is completed by May. Wait-listed candidates are generally not encouraged to send additional information.

Admissions Requirements (Required)

MCAT scores, science GPA, non-science GPA, letters of recommendation, interview, state residency, extracurricular activities, exposure to medical profession.

Admissions Requirements (Optional)

Essays/personal statement.

COSTS AND AID

Tuition & Fees

Tuition	$39,579
Room and board (on campus)	$9,864
Cost of books	$1,500
Fees	$2,679

Financial Aid

% students receiving aid	75
Average grant	$6,867
Average loan	$24,383

TULANE UNIVERSITY
SCHOOL OF MEDICINE

OFFICE OF ADMISSIONS, 1430 TULANE AVENUE, SL67 NEW ORLEANS, LA 70112 • ADMISSION: 504-588-5187
FAX: 504-599-6735 • E-MAIL: MEDSCH@TMCPOP.TMC.TULANE.EDU • WEBSITE: WWW.MCL.TULANE.EDU

STUDENT BODY

Type	Private
Enrollment	599
% male/female	58/42
% underrepresented minorities	12
# applied	6,503
# enrolled	155
Age	24

ADMISSIONS

Average GPA and MCAT Scores

GPA	3.5
MCAT Bio	10.5
MCAT Phys	10.5
MCAT Verbal	10.0
MCAT Writing	R

Application Information

Regular application	12/15
Regular notification	10/15
	until filled
Early application	6/1–8/1
Early notification	10/1
Are transfers accepted?	yes
Admissions may be deferred?	yes
Interview required?	no
Application fee	$95

Academics

The School of Medicine is one part of the Tulane University Health Sciences Center. In addition to the School of Medicine, the Health Sciences Center includes the School of Public Health and Tropical Medicine, the Tulane University Hospital and Clinic, the Tulane Hospital for Children, the University Health Service, the Primate Research Center and the U.S.-Japan Biomedical Research Laboratories. The following programs and centers of excellence are located within the Health Sciences Center: Center for Gene Therapy, the Center for Infectious Diseases, General Clinical Research Center, the Hayward Genetics Center, Hypertension and Renal Center, Tulane Center for Clinical Effectiveness and Prevention, the Center for Bioenvironmental Research at Tulane and Xavier University, DePaul-Tulane Behavioral Health Center, Tulane Cancer Center, the Tulane Center for Abdominal Transplant, the Tulane Institute of Sports Medicine, the Tulane-Xavier National Women's Center, and Tulane Cardiovascular Center of Excellence.

BASIC SCIENCES: First-year courses include anatomy, biochemistry, embryology, histology, neuroscience, and physiology. Multimedia lectures, problem-based learning sessions, small group discussions, laboratories, and clinical correlations are all employed by these first-year courses. An emphasis is placed upon the clinical application of the basic science material. The second year takes a systems-oriented approach that integrates immunology, microbiology, pathology, pathophysiology, pharmacology, and physical diagnosis. During the second semester of the first year and throughout the entire second year, students choose from an extensive offering of both basic and clinical science electives, including many research opportunities. Each year, many students will use some of their elective time to take courses in the School of Public Health and Tropical Medicine; approximately 30–35 students each year graduate with the MD and the MPH degrees. Basic science instruction takes place in the Medical School Building, which is central to both the research and clinical facilities. Computers are used as learning aids and research tools; a computing center serves the needs of the campus. The Rudolph Matas Library houses 130,000 volumes and receives 1,200 periodicals. The grading scale is honors/high pass/pass/conditional/fail. This grading scale, which is employed throughout all four years of medical school, is honors/high pass/pass/conditional/fail. Students are required to record a grade on USMLE Step 1 but are not required to pass for promotion. The USMLE Step 2 is not required for graduation.

CLINICAL TRAINING

During the first two years, clinical training is integrated with the basic science curriculum, with patient contact beginning immediately in year 1 through the foundations in medicine program. During these two years, students work with actual patients in hospitals near the school (the Tulane University Hospital, the Medical Center of Louisiana, University Hospital, and the Veterans Affairs Hospital) and with surrogate, or standardized, patients. Formal clinical training begins with the third year and consists of the following required 8 week rotations: Family/community medicine, internal medicine, obstetrics and gynecology, pediatrics, psychiatry and neurology, and surgery. During the fourth year, students do a 4 week clerkship focusing on the undifferentiated patient; this internship allows students to experience ambulatory care medicine in several settings. Also in the fourth year, students do a 4 week sub internship in ward management. Fourth-year students also have 6 selectives, which may include locations either domestically or internationally.

Students

Students of the class of 2005 entering class represented 31 states and 5 countries. Of a class of 155 students, 32 came from the State of Louisiana, 27 from California and 7 each from

Massachusetts and Utah. They received their undergraduate training at 88 different colleges and/or universities, with 15 earning the bachelor's degree from Tulane University. The average age of the class was 24, with a range of 21 to 34. About 14 percent of the class is from an underrepresented minority population.

STUDENT LIFE

Students are very much involved in life both on- and off-campus. Medical school extracurricular groups dedicated to student social life include medart, music and medicine, the Tulane chorale, and students against right brain atrophy. Organizations based upon academics, specialty interests, religion, hobbies, ethnicity, and athletics bring medical students together around shared interests. An expansive support program is available for students experiencing problems, be those of an academic or personal nature. The medical school is within walking distance of the world famous French Quarter and Superdome, and New Orleans has many parks and areas suitable for fishing, biking, running, tennis and other outdoor activities, which are possible year-round. A housing facility, located adjacent to the Tulane University Health Sciences Center, makes more than 250 apartments available to medical students, although most students choose to live off campus in which houses and apartments are affordable and attractive. At the uptown or university campus, a large athletic facility, which includes an indoor track, two swimming pools, basketball and handball courts, and a very large selection of exercise equipment, is available for medical student use.

GRADUATES

Of the 2002 graduating class, the most popular residencies were family practice and psychiatry, internal medicine, pediatrics, and surgery. Approximately 50 percent of the class entered specialties considered to be primary care. Graduates from the class of 2002 will be pursuing residency training in 29 different states, with 33 staying in the State of Louisiana. Other popular states for residency training were Texas, California, Washington, Pennsylvania, Massachusetts, and Maryland.

Admissions

REQUIREMENTS

All students must have completed the following prerequisites prior to matriculation: Biology (6 semester hours), English (6 semester hours), general chemistry (6 semester hours), organic chemistry (6 semester hours), and physics (6 semester hours). All required sciences courses must include a laboratory. The MCAT is required and should be no more than three years old; if the MCAT is taken more than once, the best set of scores is considered.

SUGGESTIONS

It is strongly advised that applicants take the MCAT in April of the year in which they intend to apply to medical school and not wait until the August administration. Tulane's admission policy has no preference for any particular major; about one-third of the student body majored in a discipline other than science. While volunteer work in a hospital is useful, Tulane is more interested in seeing that applicants have an established history of providing service to a community, be it the college campus, church, or hometown, rather than a one-time exposure to a clinical environment. Activities that demonstrates strong interpersonal skills and/or evidence of self-discipline are valued, as are leadership positions.

PROCESS

Tulane University is an AMCAS school and, therefore, the process begins with the student submitting an AMCAS application. All who submit an AMCAS application receive a Tulane secondary application and, of those who return the secondary, about 20 percent are interviewed. Interviews take place from September through February and consist of three one-on-one interviews; two with faculty and one with a Tulane medical student. After the interview, the applicant's file is submitted to the Admissions Committee, which is an action committee. Notification of the Admission Committee's action occurs on a rolling basis with every effort made to inform the applicant of the committee's decision within 2 weeks of the interview. Of those interviewed, about 30 percent are offered a place in the class; candidates who are wait listed are invited to send additional information if they feel it will strengthen their files.

Admissions Requirements (Required)

MCAT scores, science GPA, non-science GPA, letters of recommendation, state residency, extracurricular activities, exposure to medical profession.

Admissions Requirements (Optional)

Interview, essays/personal statement.

COSTS AND AID

Tuition & Fees

Cost of books	$1,000

Financial Aid

% students receiving aid	87
Average grant	$10,000
Average loan	$29,704
Average debt	$90,000

UNIFORMED SERVICES UNIVERSITY OF THE HEALTH SCIENCES
F. EDWARD HEBERT SCHOOL OF MEDICINE

4301 JONES BRIDGE ROAD, ROOM A1041, BETHESDA, MD 20814 • **ADMISSION:** 301-295-3101 OR 800-772-1743
FAX: 301-295-3545 • **E-MAIL:** ADMISSIONS@USUHS.MIL • **WEBSITE:** WWW.USUHS.MIL

STUDENT BODY

Type	Public
Enrollment	665
% male/female	69/31
% underrepresented minorities	20
# applied	1,725
# accepted	263
# enrolled	169
Average age	25

FACULTY

Total faculty (number)	2,713
% female	22
% minority	9
% part-time	88
Student-faculty ratio	4:1

ADMISSIONS

Average GPA and MCAT Scores

Overall GPA	3.5
MCAT Bio	10.0
MCAT Phys	9.5
MCAT Verbal	9.7
MCAT Essay	0

Application Information

Regular application	11/1
Regular notification	rolling
Are transfers accepted?	no
Admissions may be deferred?	yes
Interview required?	yes

Academics

Incoming students without prior uniformed service experience attend a professional orientation course during the summer before entering the School of Medicine. Most classes and rotations are evaluated with an A–F scale. Passing Step 1 and 2 of the USMLE is a requirement for graduation.

BASIC SCIENCES: Lectures and labs are the primary means of instruction during the first two years, and students are in scheduled sessions for about 25 hours per week. In addition to a solid grounding in the basic sciences, students receive interdisciplinary instruction that includes sociological, historical, ethical, and legal perspectives on medicine. First-year courses are biochemistry; clinical head, neck, and functional neuroscience; diagnostic parasitology and medical zoology; fundamentals of epidemology and biometrics; human context in health care; introduction to clinical medicine I; introduction to structure and function; medical psychology; medical history; military studies; military medical field studies—summer; physiology II; and structure and function of organ systems. During the summer following the first academic year, students take part in a hands-on field experience that serves as an introduction to military operations. Students who have a background in this area use the summer for research or other activities. Second-year courses are ethical, legal, and social aspects of medical care; human behavior; introduction to clinical medicine II and III; introduction to clinical reasoning; microbiology and infectious diseases; military studies II; pathology; pharmacology; preventive medicine; and radiographic interpretation. Instruction takes place on the grounds of the National Naval Medical Center, in Bethesda, Maryland. Educational resources include the Multidisciplinary Laboratories and the Anatomical Teaching Laboratories, both of which are open 24 hours a day. The Learning Resource Center serves as the library, and has 120,000 volumes, journals, slides, videotapes, CDs, microcomputer programs, and online informational programs.

CLINICAL TRAINING
Third-year required clerkships are medicine (12 weeks), surgery (12 weeks), ob/gyn (6 weeks), pediatrics (6 weeks), psychiatry (6 weeks), and family practice (6 weeks). During the fourth year, 20 weeks are reserved for clinical electives or research. Required fourth-year clerkships are military contingency medicine, military emergency medicine, military preventive medicine, neurology, and a sub internship. The main teaching hospitals are Walter Reed Army Medical Center; National Naval Medical Center; and Malcolm Grow USAF Medical Center, which are all in the Washington, DC area; and the Wilford Hall USAF Medical Center in San Antonio, Texas. In total, these hospitals provide more than 3,000 beds. Electives may be fulfilled at clinical sites nationwide and overseas.

Students

In a recent class, 42 percent had no prior military experience. Others have backgrounds in service academies, ROTC activities, as active and prior duty officers and enlisted service members, and as reservists. Students are from all over the country and represent a large number of undergraduate institutions. The most prevalent undergraduate majors were biology (41 percent), chemistry (12 percent), engineering (7 percent), and biochemistry (5 percent). About 10 percent of students are underrepresented minorities. The average age of entering students is about 25. Class size is 169.

STUDENT LIFE

USUHS student groups include chapters of national organizations in addition to organizations focused on professional or service-oriented goals. These organizations are devoted to activities such as journalism, providing support to women medical students or spouses of medical students, and recreational pursuits. The school sponsors intramural athletic programs for men and women and offers comprehensive athletic facilities. Nearby military posts and bases provide recreational and social activities for students and their families. Washington, DC, with its museums, sites, parks, events, and diverse population, is an important resource and enriches the lives of medical students. All students live off campus, most in the immediate vicinity of the school or in metro-accessible areas.

GRADUATES

Graduates must select residency programs at military hospitals and often enter programs at the hospitals where they performed clerkships. Residencies vary in length, depending on the medical specialty. The residency period does not fulfill the 7 year commitment involved in attending USUHS. The military branch in which a graduate will serve is determined when he or she enters the School of Medicine and reflects both the student's preference and the needs of the organization.

Admissions

REQUIREMENTS

Applicants must be citizens of the United States, be at least 18 years old at the time of matriculation (but no older than 30 as of June 30) in the year of admission, meet military regulations related to physical health, possess a baccalaureate degree by 6/15 in the year of admissions, and fulfill academic prerequisites. These are one year each with lab of biology, general chemistry, organic chemistry, and physics. One year of English composition and/or literature and one semester of calculus are required. The MCAT is required, and scores must be from within three years of desired matriculation. For applicants who have retaken the exam, the best set of scores is used.

SUGGESTIONS

Although a broad undergraduate background, with courses in economics, foreign languages, history, literature, philosophy, political science, psychology, and sociology is considered valuable, it is essential that an applicant have a strong background in the sciences. Applicants must be dedicated both to the medical profession and to the idea of serving the country.

PROCESS

About 80 percent of AMCAS applicants are sent secondary applications. Of those returning secondaries, about 25 percent are invited to interview. Interviews take place between September and February and consist of two 30-minute sessions with practicing physicians. About one-third of interviewees are accepted, with notification occurring on a rolling basis. Wait-listed candidates may send supplementary material to enhance their files.

Admissions Requirements (Required)

MCAT scores, science GPA, non-science GPA, letters of recommendation, interview, essays/personal statement, exposure to medical profession, military motivation.

Admissions Requirements (Optional)

Extracurricular activities.

COSTS AND AID

Financial Aid

% students receiving aid   100

UNIVERSIDAD CENTRAL DE CARIBE

UNIVERSIDAD CENTRAL DEL CARIBE, CALL BOX 60-327, BAYAMON, PR 00960-6032 • ADMISSION: 787-798-3001 EXT. 2403
FAX: 787-269-7550 • E-MAIL: ICORDERO@UCCARIBE.EDU • WEBSITE: WWW.UCCARIBE.EDU

STUDENT BODY

Type	Private
Enrollment	240
% male/female	49/51
% underrepresented minorities	5
# applied (total/out)	806/592
# accepted (total/out)	126/24
# enrolled (total/out)	64/14
Average age	22

FACULTY

Total faculty (number)	332
% female	52
% minority	12
% part-time	31
Student-faculty ratio	1:1

ADMISSIONS

Average GPA and MCAT Scores

Overall GPA	3.31
MCAT Bio	7.75
MCAT Phys	6.84
MCAT Verbal	6.47
MCAT Essay	M

Application Information

Regular application	12/15
Regular notification	2/15
Are transfers accepted?	yes
Admissions may be deferred?	no
Interview required?	yes
Application fee	$50

Academics

The mission of the School of Medicine is to develop competent physicians with an outstanding preparation within a humanistic and holistic framework. A guiding principle of our mission is to ensure that our graduates possess a strong sense of professionalism and commitment to social duties and service to Puerto Rico and Hispanic communities throughout the United States mainland. The curriculum emphasizes techniques and values related to the provision of primary medical care. The first two years primarily teach basic medical sciences with a strong introduction to the clinical sciences through a longitudinal primary care preceptorship, human behavior, and clinical skills. The second two years are devoted to clinical rotations and to continuing interdisciplinary instruction.

BASIC SCIENCES: Basic sciences are taught primarily through lectures. Labs and small-group sessions are also utilized. First-year courses consist of behavioral sciences, bioethics and humanities in medicine I, histology, human gross anatomy, introduction to clinical skills, LPCP I, neurosciences, physiology, and problem-based learning I. Second-year courses are bioethics and humanities in medicine II, clinical skills, LPCP II, microbiology and immunology, pathology, pathophysiology, physiopathology, pharmacology, problem-based learning II, and psychopathology. Most instruction during the first two years takes place in the new Biomedical Sciences Building, which also houses laboratories and research facilities.

CLINICAL TRAINING

Clinical clerkships begin in the third year. These are comprised of internal medicine (10 weeks), family medicine (6 weeks), surgery (10 weeks), pediatrics (6 weeks), psychiatry (6 weeks), ob/gyn (6 weeks), and radiology/emergency medicine (2 weeks). Major teaching hospitals are the Dr. Ramon Ruiz Arnau University Hospital, San Pablo Hospital, First Hospital Panamericano, San Jorge Children's Hospital, San Juan Veterans Administration Hospital, and the San Juan City Hospital.

Students

Around 51 percent of students are women. Virtually all students are from underrepresented minority groups.

STUDENT LIFE

To help students acclimate to medical school, an orientation is given to the entering first-year class. This also serves as an opportunity for students to interact with one other and with faculty members and administrators. Students are encouraged to develop an interest in culture and the arts. With this in mind, the Dean of Student Affairs sponsors an extracurricular activities program for medical students. Counseling services are aimed at helping students take advantage of the extensive educational opportunities at the medical school. A comprehensive health plan is offered to all medical students. Housing facilities are available through individual arrangements in areas adjacent to the medical school and the University Hospital.

GRADUATES

The Medical School has graduated about 1,832 physicians who serve the Commonwealth of Puerto Rico and Hispanic communities in the United States.

Admissions

REQUIREMENTS

Applicants must demonstrate proficiency in both Spanish and English. This is essential, as lectures are conducted in the language preferred by the respective professor, most often Spanish. In addition, Spanish is necessary for all clinical work. Applicants must complete a minimum of 90 credits at an institution of higher education. A baccalaureate degree is highly recommended. Required premedical courses are English (12 credit hours), behavioral sciences and social sciences (12 credit hours), general biology (8 credit hours), general chemistry (8 credit hours), organic chemistry (8 credit hours), physics (8 credit hours), college-level math (6 credit hours), and Spanish (6 credit hours). The MCAT is required. Official exam results from within the past two years must be submitted to the School of Medicine.

PROCESS

The Universidad Central del Caribe School of Medicine participates in the American Medical College Application Service (AMCAS). All applicants must file an AMCAS application. In addition, applicants should contact the School of Medicine for additional application materials and a processing fee, photograph (optional), an essay, and a Certificate of Police Record. After applications, MCAT scores and transcripts are given an initial review. Applicants who are under consideration will be invited for personal interviews with members of the faculty.

Admissions Requirements (Required)
MCAT scores, science GPA, non-science GPA, letters of recommendation, interview, essays/personal statement.

Admissions Requirements (Optional)
State residency, extracurricular activities, exposure to medical profession.

Overlap Schools
University of Puerto Rico.

COSTS AND AID

Tuition & Fees

Tuition	$20,000
Room and board (on campus)	$6,000
Cost of books	$1,800
Fees	$4,490

Financial Aid

% students receiving aid	94
Average grant	$38,500
Average loan	$38,500
Average debt	$132,000

UNIVERSITE LAVAL
FACULTÉ DE MÉDECINE

PAVILLON VANDRY, U. LAVAL STE FOY, QC G1K 7P4 • ADMISSION: 418-656-2131
FAX: 418-656-2733 • E-MAIL: GUY.LABRECQUE@FMED.ULAVAL.CA • WEBSITE: WWW.FMED.ULAVAL.CA

STUDENT BODY	
Type	Public
# applied (total/out)	1,508/123
# accepted	208
Average age	20

FACULTY	
Total faculty (number)	208
% female	74

ADMISSIONS

Application Information

Regular application	3/1
Regular notification	5/15
Are transfers accepted?	no
Admissions may be deferred?	no
Interview required?	yes
Application fee	$30

Academics

Laval offers a 4 year curriculum leading to the MD degree. In addition, academic programs are available in a number of health and medical science fields including community health, epidemiology, molecular biology, occupational health and safety, and physiology. Research is an important part of the academic experience at Laval, and students are encouraged to pursue research during summers and throughout the academic year.

BASIC SCIENCES: The first two years involve basic science instruction and opportunities for addressing clinical problems. The first year includes courses in biochemistry, histology-pathology, introduction to problems, microbiology-immunology, physiology, and pharmacology. During the second part of the first year, instruction is organized around anatomical systems and medical concepts. These are cardiovascular system, microbiology/infectious disease, physiological/sociological, respiratory system, and uronephrology. Introduction to problems continues during the second semester. Students also study endocrinology, growth/development, and ob/gyn during their first year. Year 2 subjects are ENT, gastroenterology, hematology, locomotor system, medical ethics, nervous system, ophthalmology, preventive medicine, problem discussion, psychopathology, skin, and the art of interviewing. Laval's library system is an important academic resource for students, holding millions of volumes and periodicals.

CLINICAL TRAINING

Years 3 and 4 are devoted to clinical rotations. Required clerkships are medicine (8 weeks), surgery (8 weeks), pediatrics (8 weeks), psychiatry (8 weeks), ob/gyn (8 weeks), introduction to clinical medicine (5 weeks), preventive medicine (4 weeks), geriatrics/rehabilitation medicine (4 weeks), family practice (4 weeks), and emergency medicine (4 weeks). In addition, up to 20 weeks are open for various clinical and basic science electives. Training takes place at a number of affiliated hospitals including Centre Hospitalier de l'Universite Laval, Hopital Laval, Hopital de l'Enfant-Jesus, Hotel-Dieu de Levis, Hotel-Dieu de Quebec, Hopital du Saint-Sacrement and Hopital Saint-Francois d'Assie.

Students

Each entering class at the Faculty of Medicine is comprised of about 112 students. Typically, all but a few are from within the province of Quebec. Students from other provinces must be French speakers. Within the student body are a limited number of international, French-speaking students. Women make up about 60 percent of the students.

STUDENT LIFE

Laval supports medical students both inside and outside the classroom. Programs offered include orientation and counseling services, religious organizations, career place-ment services, social and athletic organizations, childcare, and attractive, low-cost student housing. The Laval campus is situated in an urban environment.

GRADUATES

Graduates of Laval Faculty of Medicine enter both clinical and academic medicine. The teaching hospitals affiliated with Laval offer many programs for graduate medical training.

Admissions

REQUIREMENTS

Generally, all applicants must have completed at least two years of college to be considered for admission. Required undergraduate courses are biology (8 semester hours), general chemistry (8 semester hours), organic chemistry (8 semester hours), general physics (2 hours), and mathematics including calculus (2 hours). In addition, some course work in French, humanities, and social sciences is required. Fluency in French is a requirement for admission.

SUGGESTIONS

Priority is given to residents of the province of Quebec. Candidates are evaluated on the basis of academic achievement, interpersonal skills, experience, and personal characteristics. Although two years of college is the minimum requirement, additional schooling serves to strengthen applications.

PROCESS

Applications are coordinated in part by the organization of Quebec Colleges and Universities. For entrance in the fall, the application deadline is March 1. In addition to a written application, interviews are an important part of the selection process. Generally, about 10–15 percent of applicants are accepted in a given year.

Admissions Requirements (Required)

Science GPA, nonscience GPA, interview, state residency, essays/personal statement, extracurricular activities.

COSTS AND AID

Tuition & Fees

In-state Tuition	$1,964
Out-of-state Tuition	$7,927
Fees	$200

University of Alabama at Birmingham
School of Medicine

Medical Student Services, VH 100, 1530 Third Avenue South, Birmingham, AL 35294-0019 • Admission: 205-934-2433 Fax: 205-934-8740 • E-mail: MEDSCHOOL@UAB.EDU • Website: WWW.UAB.EDU/UASOM/

STUDENT BODY

Type	Public
Enrollment	685
% male/female	59/41
% underrepresented minorities	22
# applied (total/out)	1,734/1,298
# accepted (total/out)	213/33
# enrolled (total/out)	160/16
Average age	23

FACULTY

Total faculty (number)	1,113
% female	29
% minority	21
% part-time	4
Student-faculty ratio	2:1

ADMISSIONS

Average GPA and MCAT Scores

Overall GPA	3.72
MCAT Bio	10.4
MCAT Phys	10.1
MCAT Verbal	9.8
MCAT Essay	P

Application Information

Regular application	11/1
Regular notification	11/15
Early application	8/1
Early notification	10/1
Are transfers accepted?	yes
Admissions may be deferred?	yes
Interview required?	yes
Application fee	$70

Academics

Basic sciences are taught during the first two years, primarily through lectures and small group case studies. Clinical techniques are introduced early and are often taught in small groups. The curriculum is particularly rich in relevant humanities and social sciences courses such as ethics and behavioral sciences. Joint graduate/MD degrees are offered in many fields, notably the MPH/MD combination. About eight students a year are accepted into joint MD/PhD programs as MSTP candidates. A combined undergraduate/medical school program is offered at the University of Alabama at Birmingham to which high school seniors who are Alabama residents may apply.

BASIC SCIENCES: First-year students take the following courses: Behavioral sciences, biochemistry, gross anatomy, human sexuality, medical ethics, medical cell and tissue biology, physiology, pharmacology, neurosciences, and nutrition. Throughout the first year, students participate in a course called introduction to clinical medicine, which addresses doctor/patient interaction including professionalism, history-taking, and physical examinations. During the Fall of year 2, pharmacology continues and microbiology/immunology is introduced. Pathology is a year-long course, taken throughout year 2. Introduction to clinical medicine continues in year 2, focusing on physical diagnosis. The Lister Hill Library at the Birmingham campus houses 240,000 volumes and uses computer online search services. Pre-clinical performance is evaluated on a pass/fail by quartile scale. The USMLE Step 1 is required following completion of the pre-clinical studies and before promotion to the third year.

CLINICAL TRAINING

Clinical training begins well before the required clerkships of the third year. In addition to the introductory clinical course work of the first two years, some students are involved in community programs, which provide patient exposure to public health programs, such as the AIDS Care Team and other projects aimed at young or homeless populations. The final two years are essentially combined, with required clerkships and acting internships filling all of the third year and part of the fourth year. Students choose a primary campus for clerkships prior to acceptance. Each campus has unique strengths. Required clerkships are family medicine, medicine, neurology, ob/gyn, pediatrics, psychiatry, rural medicine, and surgery. Each campus is affiliated with several teaching hospitals, and rotations take students to a variety of learning environments ranging from large Veterans Affairs Hospitals to small, rural clinics. For required rotations, grading is pass/fail by quartile and for electives. The School of Medicine established a Medical Student Enrichment Program, which encourages and facilitates overseas clinical experience. In addition to providing elective opportunities to medical school seniors, medical students may apply to the program or placements during the summer between their first and second years. The USMLE Step 2 is required for graduation.

Students

About 75 percent of the matriculates majored in a scientific field during their undergraduate studies. The school seeks a diverse student body to reflect the diverse health care needs of the state of Alabama. The school has special programs to promote both clinical and basic science research as well as address unmet health care needs of the State of Alabama.

STUDENT LIFE

Outside of class, students are often involved in recreational and volunteer activities. Some are active in student organizations such as national medical groups. The Student Government Association consists of elected members of each class. The Birmingham campus, with its many departments, provides a community beyond that of medical students alone. Most students choose to live off campus where housing is ample and relatively affordable. Most students have cars.

GRADUATES

Primary care residencies are popular among graduates. Although graduates are competitive for residencies nationwide, a significant number enter residency programs in Alabama, at university-affiliated hospitals, or other locations in the state.

Admissions

REQUIREMENTS

Undergraduate requirements are biology or zoology (8 semester hours), chemistry with lab (8 semester hours), organic chemistry with lab (8 semester hours), physics with lab (8 semester hours), math (6 semester hours), and English (6 semester hours). Academic work accomplished overseas may be acceptable, depending on the institution and the course. A minimum total MCAT score, not more than two years old at the time of application, is required. The spring MCAT is strongly recommended. The AMCAS application is required.

SUGGESTIONS

The Admissions Committee values experience with patient care and exposure to health care environments. The University of Alabama School of Medicine welcomes nontraditional applicants. Alabama residents are given significant preference in the admissions process.

PROCESS

All qualified Alabama AMCAS applicants, and approximately one-third of out-of-state applicants, receive a secondary application. Generally, about 70 percent of in-state applicants are interviewed. About 2–10 percent of out-of-state applicants are interviewed. In 2005, about 66 percent of the in-state applicants interviewed were accepted, while about 44 percent of the out-of-state applicants interviewed were accepted. Notification begins in October, and the class is generally filled by April. Interviews consist of three 30-minute sessions with faculty members.

Admissions Requirements (Required)

MCAT scores, science GPA, non-science GPA, letters of recommendation, interview, essays/personal statement, extracurricular activities, exposure to medical profession.

Admissions Requirements (Optional)

State residency.

Overlap Schools

Emory University, University of South Alabama, Vanderbilt University.

COSTS AND AID

Tuition & Fees

In-state Tuition	$12,161
Out-of-state Tuition	$36,483
Room and board (off campus)	$11,868
Cost of books	$2,200
Fees	$6,182

Financial Aid

% students receiving aid	80
Average grant	$6,528
Average loan	$12,593
Average debt	$90,742

UNIVERSITY OF ALBERTA
FACULTY OF MEDICINE AND DENTISTRY

2-45 MEDICAL SCIENCES BUILDING, EDMONTON, AB T6G 2H7 • ADMISSION: 780-492-6350
FAX: 780-492-7303 • E-MAIL: DEAN@MED.UALBERTA.CA • WEBSITE: WWW.MED.UALBERTA.CA

STUDENT BODY

Type	Public
# applied	1,095

ADMISSIONS

Average GPA and MCAT Scores

MCAT Bio	10.8
MCAT Phys	11.3
MCAT Verbal	9.7

Application Information

Regular application	1/31
Admissions may be deferred?	yes
Interview required?	yes
Application fee	$60

Academics

Alberta's curriculum reflects the school's emphasis on clinical care and research. The pre-clinical curriculum has been revised and is largely centered on organ systems. It is multidisciplinary, including both biological and social science perspectives. Although basic sciences are the focus of study during the first two years, courses are taught with clinical applications in mind. The second two years integrate classroom and hospital-based instruction. While most medical students earn an MD degree in four years, qualified students may pursue joint degrees such as the MD/PhD or MD/MPH in a longer period of study.

BASIC SCIENCES: Basic sciences are taught in a variety of forums, including lectures, small-group discussions, laboratories, problem-based learning, independent study, and computer-based instruction. The academic period begins in August, covers 35 weeks, and includes courses in cardiology, renal, and pulmonary; endocrine and metabolism; immunity, infection, and inflammation; introduction to medicine; and practice of medicine (part I). On average, students are in class or other scheduled sessions for about 25 hours per week. The second academic period also begins in August and includes gastroenterology, musculoskeletal, neurosciences, oncology, practice of medicine (part II), and reproduction and urology, in addition to a systems-based curriculum. Systems studied are cardiovascular, endocrinology, gastrointestinal, hematology, medical ethics, nephrology, ophthalmology, pediatrics, pulmonary, surgery, and urology. Basic science instruction takes place mainly at the medical sciences building and uses the resources of the John W. Scott Health Sciences Library. Medical students may use all university libraries and computer facilities. All enrolled students have access to free online service.

CLINICAL TRAINING

The third and fourth academic periods primarily teach clinical skills and consist of classroom instruction, required rotations, electives, and selectives. Required clerkships are surgery (10 weeks), medicine (10 weeks), obstetrics/gynecology (8 weeks), pediatrics (8 weeks), psychiatry (8 weeks), rural family medicine (4 weeks), radiology (2 weeks), anesthesia (2 weeks), and geriatrics (2 weeks). Selectives include 2 weeks in internal medicine and 2 weeks in surgery. Training takes place at the University of Alberta hospitals, the Royal Alexandra Hospital, Edmonton General Hospital, Misericordia Hospital, Alberta Hospital, Glenrose Hospital, Cross Cancer Institute, and Grey Nuns Hospital. A certain number of electives may be taken at nonaffiliated institutions.

Students

STUDENT LIFE

Campus housing is available, although most students opt to live off campus in the surrounding area. The students' union provides a registry informing students of available housing. Medical students participate in clubs, events, and recreational activities geared toward medical students and the student body in general. Counseling and other support services are available to students, as are groups focused on special interests and minority groups. Edmonton is a mid-size city, offering plenty of restaurants, shops, parks, theaters, sporting events, and outdoor activities. Although public transportation is available, most medical students own cars.

GRADUATES

Graduates enter both clinical medicine and research-oriented careers.

Admissions

REQUIREMENTS

Only Canadian applications are accepted. All applicants should have completed at least 60 units of university course work (approximately two years of full-time studies). Requirements are six units each of biology, English, general chemistry, organic chemistry, and physics along with three units each of statistics and biochemistry. The MCAT is required and scores are valid for three years after the exam is taken. In addition to an application form, an autobiographical essay, and two letters of reference are required.

SUGGESTIONS

Residency is an important consideration in admissions decisions. For admissions purposes, a resident of Alberta is defined as a Canadian Citizen or permanent resident who has lived in the Province of Alberta or Yukon or Northwest Territories for at least one continuous year immediately prior to the date of intended matriculation. At least 85 percent of available positions in an entering class are reserved for Alberta residents. The remaining 15 percent are available to other Canadians. Typically, successful applicants have completed four years of university with a grade point average of 7.0 on the University of Alberta's nine point grading system. An MCAT score of less than seven in any category is not accepted.

PROCESS

Requests for applications should be directed to the address above. Applications are accepted between July 1 and November 1 in the year preceding anticipated matriculation. The essay and reference letters must be received by January 15, and transcripts must be submitted by January 15. Interviews are conducted between February and March, and admissions decisions are made between May and July. Applicants who feel that they may merit special consideration (because of studies in a nontraditional area or unusual pattern) should write to the Admissions Officer outlining their situation and goals. All native (Aboriginal) students who are interested in medical studies are encouraged to contact the coordinator at the Native Health Care Careers Program in care of the address above.

Admissions Requirements (Required)

Interview.

COSTS AND AID

Tuition & Fees

In-state Tuition	$6,066
Cost of books	$900
Fees	$6,000

University of Arizona
College of Medicine

Admissions Office, Room 2106, PO Box 245075, Tucson, AZ 85724 • Admission: 520-626-6214
Fax: 520-626-4884 • E-mail: ADMISSIONS@MEDICINE.ARIZONA.EDU • Website: WWW.MEDICINE.ARIZONA.EDU

STUDENT BODY

Type	Public
Enrollment	406
% male/female	52/48
% underrepresented minorities	15
# applied (total/out)	608/71
# accepted	51

ADMISSIONS

Application Information

Regular application	11/1
Regular notification	1/30
	until filled
Are transfers accepted?	no
Admissions may be deferred?	yes
Interview required?	yes
Application fee	$75

Academics

Students may apply to joint PhD/MD programs in the following: Anatomy, biochemistry, cell biology, genetics, immunology, microbiology, molecular biology, neuroscience, pharmacology, and physiology. Combined studies in other fields are possible as well, including a collaborative program with Arizona State University, Northern Arizona University, and the College of Medicine at the University of Arizona. This program focuses on the health needs of underserved communities and leads to a MPH along with the MD. Through this and other venues, medical students at the University of Arizona take advantage of the resources of the academic and medical institutions throughout the state.

BASIC SCIENCES: The basic sciences are taught in the Basic Science Building of the Tucson campus. Traditional lectures with labs are the primary mode of instruction, occupying about 24 hours per week. Alternative teaching methods, including small-group and case-based learning, account for the remaining 6 hours per week of structured classroom time. First-year courses are anatomy, biochemistry, histology and cell biology, medical and molecular genetics, neuroscience, physiology, preparation for clinical medicine, and social and behavioral science. During year 2, students take microbiology, pathology, pharmacology, preparation for clinical medicine, and social and behavioral science. In the course preparation for clinical medicine, students focus on clinical problem-solving and learn patient evaluation skills. This course links basic science principles with clinical applications. Computers, located in the Learning Resource Center, supplement lectures and are an important component of the basic science education. The Arizona Health Science Library houses nearly 200,000 volumes, operates extensive online database and informational services, and is connected electronically to the library system of the greater university. To accommodate the study schedules of all students, the library is open 24 hours a day. Students are evaluated with an honors/pass/fail scale. The USMLE Step 1 is required upon completion of basic science course work.

CLINICAL TRAINING

Patient contact begins during year 1 in preparation for clinical medicine. Throughout the four years, there are opportunities for clinical exposure through volunteer and outreach programs. In addition, clinical research is often community-based and gives medical students a chance to help others while they learn. The Commitment to Underserved People (CUP) is a program through which many medical students volunteer. In CUP, students are involved in health education for, and supervised treatment of, people in underserved communities. The formal clinical curriculum begins in year 3, when students rotate through the following clerkships: Medicine (12 weeks), pediatrics (6 weeks), family medicine (6 weeks), ob/gyn (6 weeks), psychiatry (6 weeks), surgery (6 weeks), specialty surgery (3 weeks), and neurology (3 weeks). Year 4 is composed of electives, many of which can be taken at alternate locations throughout the state. Clinical facilities in Tucson are the University Medical Center, the University Outpatient Clinic, the Children's Research Center, and the Arizona Cancer Center. The hospitals serve managed care participants, and the medical school seeks to respond to the ongoing changes in the economics of health care, as seen in the public health/health policy components of medical school training. Evaluation of clinical performance is honors/pass/fail. Passing the USMLE Step 2 is a requirement for graduation.

Students

Students are either Arizona residents, or are from western states that do not have their own medical schools. Generally, about 15 percent of the student body are underrepresented minorities, most of whom are of Mexican American descent. Older students comprise about one-third of each class. A wide range of undergraduate institutions and majors are represented in a typical class. Class size is 100.

STUDENT LIFE

With access to both the campus community of more than 36,000 students and a medium-sized urban community, students have active social lives. Recreational facilities are extensive at the university. The Medical School's emphasis on community involvement promotes extracurricular activities that are medically related. Student clubs also provide mechanisms for support and social interaction. The Chicano/Latino Club is linked to similar organizations at California universities, providing a larger network for those involved. On-campus housing options include apartments and dorms. Most students, however, opt to live off campus.

GRADUATES

At least 60 percent of graduates enter primary care fields, which include family medicine, internal medicine, ob/gyn, and pediatrics. About 50 percent of graduates enter residency programs within the state.

Admissions

REQUIREMENTS

Applicants should have completed 1 year of each of the following subjects: Biology, chemistry, English, organic chemistry, physics. In addition, at least 30 hours of upper-division course work as part of the undergraduate record is required. For older applicants, recent science course work is necessary. The MCAT is required, and only the best scores are considered, suggesting that applicants should not withhold scores. Together, the MCAT and college record are used for initial screening.

SUGGESTIONS

Hands-on clinical experience is important, as are other activities that demonstrate an applicant's commitment to community service. The Admissions Committee is interested in applicants whose undergraduate records include significant course work in the humanities and social sciences. Applicants are advised to take the April rather than August MCAT.

PROCESS

All AMCAS applicants receive secondary applications, and virtually all who meet residency requirements are interviewed. Interviews are conducted from September through March and consist of three short meetings with faculty members and one longer session with a practicing clinician from the area. About one-fourth of those who interview are accepted, with notifications occurring on a rolling basis. A ranked wait list is established, but those who find themselves on this list are not encouraged to send additional information.

Admissions Requirements (Required)

MCAT scores, science GPA, non-science GPA, letters of recommendation, interview, state residency, extracurricular activities, exposure to medical profession.

Admissions Requirements (Optional)

Essays/personal statement.

COSTS AND AID

Tuition & Fees

In-state Tuition	$7,860
Fees	$72

Financial Aid

% students receiving aid	87

UNIVERSITY OF ARKANSAS FOR MEDICAL SCIENCES
COLLEGE OF MEDICINE

4301 WEST MARKHAM STREET, SLOT 551, LITTLE ROCK, AR 72205-7199 • ADMISSION: 501-686-5354
FAX: 501-686-5873 • E-MAIL: SOUTHTOMG@UAMS.EDU • WEBSITE: WWW.UAMS.EDU/COM

STUDENT BODY

Type	Public
Enrollment	576
% male/female	56/44
% underrepresented minorities	10
# applied (total/out)	675/343
# accepted (total/out)	171/6
# enrolled (total/out)	140/2
Average age	24

ADMISSIONS

Average GPA and MCAT Scores

Overall GPA	3.6
MCAT Bio	9.0
MCAT Phys	9.0
MCAT Verbal	9.0
MCAT Essay	O

Application Information

Regular application	11/1
Regular notification	2/15
Are transfers accepted?	yes
Admissions may be deferred?	yes
Interview required?	yes
Application fee	$100

Academics

The College of Medicine, along with the schools of Nursing, Pharmacy, Public Health, Health Related Professions, and Graduate Studies, comprise the University of Arkansas for Medical Sciences, one of six campuses of the University of Arkansas system. Most students complete the MD curriculum in four years, but a few students each year take part in joint MD/PhD or MD/MPH, and MD/MBA programs. Joint-degrees can be pursued in the following fields: Anatomy, biochemistry, immunology, microbiology, neuroscience, pharmacology, and physiology.

BASIC SCIENCES: Throughout year 1, students learn skills related to patient care in introduction to clinical medicine. Fall semester courses are cell biology, genetics, gross anatomy, and microscopic anatomy. Spring semester courses are biochemistry, neuroscience, and physiology. In the fall semester of year 2, students take behavioral sciences, medical ethics, microbiology, and pathophysiology I. In the spring, classes are introduction to clinical medicine II, pathophysiology II, and pharmacology. Scheduled class time accounts for about 20 hours per week, most of which is devoted to lecture and lab. Alternately, for perhaps 2 hours per week, small groups are used as the instructional format. Grading uses an A–F scale. Passing the USMLE Step 1 is a requirement for promotion to year 3, and USMLE 2 for graduation. Basic-science teaching facilities, including libraries and labs, are part of the medical complex, which includes the main hospitals as well as residence halls.

CLINICAL TRAINING

Patient contact begins in year 1, in introduction to clinical medicine. The third year consists of required clerkships in the following: internal medicine (12 weeks), surgery (8 weeks), ob/gyn (6 weeks), psychiatry (6 weeks), pediatrics (8 weeks), specialties (4 weeks), family medicine (4 weeks), and geriatrics (unspecified). During year 4, students choose among primary care selectives (8 weeks) and specialties clerkships (4 weeks). The remainder of the year is designated as elective study, some of which may be taken off campus, out-of-state, or overseas. Training takes place primarily at the University Hospital (400 beds), located in the Medical Center complex. Other training sites are the Arkansas Children's Hospital (the sixth largest children's hospital in the country) and two VA hospitals (500 and 2,000 beds). In addition, outreach training sites in small communities around the state provide exposure to rural medicine. The primary care clerkships involve rotations to these sites, located in El Dorado, Fayetteville, Fort Smith, Jonesboro, Pine Bluff, and Texarkana. Specialized research institutes in Little Rock include The Child Study Center, The Ambulatory Care Center, The Arkansas Cancer Research Center, and the Jones Eye Institute. Evaluation of clinical progress in required clerkships uses an A–F scale, and electives are graded as pass/fail. Students must pass the USMLE Step 2 as a requirement for graduation.

Students

Virtually all students are Arkansas residents. About 70 percent of students earned undergraduate degrees in Arkansas. Approximately 79 percent of incoming students in a recent class had undergraduate majors in science disciplines. Classes include a significant number of older students, including some who were older than 50 years old at the time of admission. Class size is 150.

STUDENT LIFE

Little Rock is a small but lively city, with indoor and outdoor recreational activities. Students take part in volunteer and community activities. Many single first- and second-year students live on campus in residence halls. Most upperclass students and married students live off campus.

GRADUATES

Many graduates enter postgraduate programs in Arkansas. Programs in about 20 specialty areas are offered at university-affiliated hospitals in Little Rock. In addition, a number of family practice residencies are available at rural locations around the state. At least half of the graduates of the School of Medicine enter primary care fields.

Admissions
REQUIREMENTS

Within each class, 70 percent of students must be equally divided from among the four congressional districts in the state. The College of Medicine is allowed to admit a few out-of-state applicants each year but only if they do not displace Arkansas residents with equal qualifications. Out-of-state applicants should be highly qualified and have close ties to Arkansas. Students must have successfully completed the following courses prior to matriculation: Biology (1 year), chemistry (1 year), organic chemistry (1 year), physics (1 year), English (1 year), and math (1 year) or through calculus I. The MCAT is required, and scores must be no more than three years old. Scores from all sections of the MCAT, including the writing sample, are considered.

SUGGESTIONS

Other courses deemed helpful are anthropology, biochemistry, botany, calculus, composition, embryology, genetics, histology, history, human ecology, literature, logic, physical chemistry, psychology, sociology, speech, statistics, and zoology. For students who graduated from college several years ago, some recent course work is useful. All medically related extracurricular activities are valued.

PROCESS

All AMCAS applicants are asked to submit secondary applications. All Arkansas residents and highly qualified out-of-state residents are interviewed, with interviews taking place between October and January. Team interviews consist of a 1-hour session with faculty. All applicants are notified by February 15. A ranked wait list is established, and about 25 students from the list are usually admitted. Wait-listed candidates who commit to practicing in underserved areas of Arkansas may improve their chances of admission.

Admissions Requirements (Required)

MCAT scores, science GPA, non-science GPA, letters of recommendation, interview, state residency, essays/personal statement, extracurricular activities, exposure to medical profession.

COSTS AND AID

Tuition & Fees

In-state Tuition	$11,642
Out-of-state Tuition	$23,284
Cost of books	$1,600

Financial Aid

Average grant	$3,000
Average loan	$25,000
Average debt	$88,000

University of British Columbia

Faculty of Medicine

317-2194 Health Sciences Mall, British Columbia, BC V6T 1Z3 • Admission: 604-822-2421
Fax: 604-822-6061 • E-mail: Admissions.md@ubc.ca • Website: www.med.ubc.ca

STUDENT BODY

Type	Public
Enrollment	120
# applied (total/out)	621/145
Average age	23

ADMISSIONS

Average GPA and MCAT Scores

MCAT Bio	10.4
MCAT Phys	10.1
MCAT Verbal	9.5
MCAT Essay	Q

Application Information

Regular application	10/1
Regular notification	3/1
Are transfers accepted?	yes
Admissions may be deferred?	yes
Application fee	$105

Academics

The 4 year program leading to the MD degree is integrated and comprehensive, designed to take advantage of the vast resources of the faculty of medicine, and incorporates a case-based curriculum that emphasizes problem-solving and lifelong learning. In addition to the MD program, graduate programs leading to master's, doctorate, and combined degrees are available.

BASIC SCIENCES: Basic sciences are taught along with introductory clinical concepts during the first two years. First-year courses include cardiovascular systems; doctor/dentist; family practice continuum; fluids, electrolytes, and renal; host defenses and infection; introductory clinical skills and systems I; patient and society; principles of human biology; and pulmonary. Second-year courses include blood and lymphatic; brain and behavior and reproduction; clinical skills and systems II; doctor/dentist, patient, and society; family practice continuum; GI/nutrition; growth and development; integument; metabolism and endocrine; and musculoskeletal and locomotor. Basic sciences are taught primarily through small group forums, through lectures, computer-based instruction and labs also utilized.

CLINICAL TRAINING

The third academic period begins with courses in health care epidemiology, radiology, and therapeutics. Following these three courses, students enter a sequence of required clerkships. These are medicine (10 weeks), ob/gyn (8 weeks), pediatrics (8 weeks), psychiatry (8 weeks), surgery (8 weeks), emergency medicine (4 weeks), orientation (4 weeks), anesthesia (2 weeks), orthopedics (2 weeks), dermatology (1 week), and ophthalmology (1 week). Six weeks are left open for electives during the third academic period. Sixteen weeks are left open for electives during the fourth academic period. A portion of electives may be completed at sites outside of the network of affiliated institutions including the University Hospital, St. Paul's Hospital, British Columbia Children's Hospital, Vancouver General Hospital, British Columbia Women's Hospital and Health Center, British Columbia Cancer Center Agency, G. F. Strong Rehabilitation Center, and the Canadian Arthritis and Rheumatism Society Center.

Students

Each entering class has about 120 students. Approximately 50 percent of students are women. Typically, all but a handful of students in each class are from British Columbia.

STUDENT LIFE

Beyond a rich, academic life, medical students enjoy the resources, facilities, and surroundings of the Health Science Center, the University of British Columbia, and the city of Vancouver. The Faculty of Medicine and greater university offer a wide range of support services including counseling, special interest clubs and organizations, resources for minorities and international students, and day care. There are ample opportunities for athletic, social, and recreational activities on campus. Students also enjoy the cultural and recreational aspects of Vancouver.

GRADUATES

A significant number of graduates enter residency programs at hospitals affiliated with the University of British Columbia. Though most graduates enter clinical medicine, others successfully pursue research and academic medicine.

Admissions

REQUIREMENTS

Applicants should have successfully completed a minimum of 90 credits or the equivalent of three years of full-time course work in any degree program at an accredited university. A minimum of 70 percent academic average is required and all undergraduate courses are included in this average. Prerequisites are 1 year each of university-level biochemistry, biology, chemistry, English literature and composition, and organic chemistry. The MCAT is required. The exam should be taken no later than August of the year of application.

SUGGESTIONS

There is no preferred program of study for preparation for medical school. Often, due to the large number of applicants, the competitive average for successful applicants is much higher than 70 percent. MCAT scores of a recently admitted class averaged about 10. In addition to excellent academic qualifications, admission decisions are based on the applicant's personal characteristics, such as motivation and integrity. Last year, 695 applications were recieved for 120 positions.

COSTS AND AID	
Tuition & Fees	
In-state Tuition	$4,000
Cost of books	$1,200
Fees	$256

UNIVERSITY OF CALGARY
FACULTY OF MEDICINE

3330 HOSPITAL DRIVE NORTHWEST, ALBERTA, T2N 4N1 • ADMISSION: 403-220-4262

STUDENT BODY

Type	Public
Enrollment	234
% male/female	48/52
# applied (total/out)	1,314/784
Average age	25

ADMISSIONS

Average GPA and MCAT Scores

Overall GPA	3.5
MCAT Bio	10.67
MCAT Phys	10.48
MCAT Verbal	9.77
MCAT Essay	Q

Application Information

Regular application	11/15
Regular notification	5/14
Are transfers accepted?	yes
Admissions may be deferred?	yes
Interview required?	yes
Application fee	$65

Academics

Medical students follow an intensive, 11-month curriculum for a period of three years. Learning is based in part on clinical case presentations. In addition to the standard MD course of study, programs are offered in conjunction with the Faculty of Graduate Studies in Biomedical and Health Sciences with the objective of training clinician-scientists for academic medical research and those who will design, manage, and implement health care delivery programs. MD/PhD and MD/MSc are available in biochemistry and molecular biology, cardiovascular/respiratory sciences, community health sciences, gastrointestinal sciences, medical science, microbiology and infectious diseases, and neuroscience.

BASIC SCIENCES: First-year courses are based on organ systems and are taught primarily through lectures and small group discussions. Subjects are blood, cardiovascular, endocrine metabolic, integrative, medical skills program, musculoskeletal and skin, principles of medicine, renal-electrolyte, and respiratory. The second academic period begins in July. Subjects are gastrointestinal, human development, medical skills program, neuroscience, reproduction, and the mind. Throughout the first and second years, students also take part in independent research projects. Courses are taught in the Calgary Health Sciences Center, about 1.5 km from the main campus of the University of Calgary. The medical library is fully computerized, receives more than 1,000 serials, and houses approximately 130,000 books. It serves medical and nursing students as well as the greater university and the medical community. Other important facilities include the Medical Learning Resource Center, which houses instructional tools geared toward learning anatomical systems, and the Medical Skills Center for improving clinical skills and techniques.

CLINICAL TRAINING

Required clerkships are internal medicine (12 weeks), surgery (8 weeks), ob/gyn (6 weeks), pediatrics (6 weeks), psychiatry (6 weeks), family medicine (4 weeks), and anesthesia (2 weeks). Ten weeks are available for clinical electives. Training takes place primarily at the facilities of the Foothills Hospital, the Peter Lougheed Center, the Alberta Children's Hospital, and the Rockyview Hospital. In addition, the University of Calgary Medical Clinic allows medical students to learn about outpatient service delivery, preventative programs, and travel medicine.

Students

While medical students are primarily Canadian, the student body at the University of Calgary includes several hundred international students. Within the Faculty of Medicine, women compromise about 50 percent of students. The majority of medical students are from within the province of Alberta.

STUDENT LIFE

Student life is enhanced by campus activities, the resources of the community and city of Calgary, and the wide range of outdoor activities available. Nearby national parks, such as Banff and Jasper, offer skiing and hiking. The region also has vibrant wildlife and areas for fishing, swimming, and canoeing. In addition to its academic facilities, the Health Sciences Center includes a medical bookstore, exercise room, student lounge, cafeteria, and mall area. Medical students also have access to the resources of the greater university, including complete athletic and recreational facilities, intramural sports programs, outdoor programs, arts, and theater. The University Student Union organizes events and activities and operates a bookstore, cafe, and bar, along with other services. On-campus housing is available for single and married students. An off-campus registry is managed by the student union.

GRADUATES

Though most graduates enter postgraduate training that leads to careers in clinical medicine, some go on to pursue research and academic medicine. Increasingly, graduates are entering primary care fields.

Admissions

REQUIREMENTS

Students must have completed at least two full years of university education before being considered for admission. The minimum grade requirement for a Canadian citizen or landed immigrant resident of Alberta is an average of 3.0/4.0, which translates to a grade of B or at least 78 percent for each year of study. The minimum grade point average required of Canadians from other provinces is 3.5/4.0. The MCAT is required, and applicants should have at least an average score of 8. In addition to transcripts and a completed application form, three letters of reference are required.

SUGGESTIONS

Although the faculty has no prescribed prerequisites, 1 year of each of the following courses is strongly recommended: Biology, biochemistry, calculus, English, general chemistry, organic chemistry, physics, physiology, and pyschology/sociology. Presently, spaces for international students are limited to those students who come from institutions and/or countries with which the Faculty of Medicine at the University of Calgary has a formal, contractional agreement. All international students must sign an acknowledgment that the MD program would not lead to an opportunity for postgraduate training through the Canadian Resident Matching Service.

PROCESS

The application is available at www.med.ucalgary.ca/admissions. It requires information about all university courses taken, MCAT test dates/results, employment history, extracurricular activities, and an essay. The completed application is due November 15. The deadline for receipt of the three letters of reference, all official transcripts, and official MCAT scores is January 4. Applicants will be notified by March 15 whether or not they will be invited for an interview. In a recent year, there were 1,300 applicants for 100 positions.

Admissions Requirements (Required)

Interview.

COSTS AND AID

Tuition & Fees

In-state Tuition	$6,519
Out-of-state Tuition	$30,000
Cost of books	$1,200
Fees	$333

UNIVERSITY OF CALIFORNIA—DAVIS
SCHOOL OF MEDICINE

1 SHIELDS AVENUE, DAVIS, CA 95616-8661 • ADMISSION: 530-752-2717
FAX: 530-754-6252 • E-MAIL: MEDADMSINFO@UCDAVIS.EDU • WEBSITE: WWW.SOM.UCDAVIS.EDU

STUDENT BODY

Type	Public
Enrollment	403
% male/female	52/48
% underrepresented minorities	14
# applied (total/out)	4,109/775
# accepted (total/out)	204/11
# enrolled (total/out)	93/3
Average age	25

FACULTY

Total faculty (number)	690
% female	24
% part-time	15
Student-faculty ratio	1:1

ADMISSIONS

Average GPA and MCAT Scores

Overall GPA	3.61
MCAT Bio	11.0
MCAT Phys	10.0
MCAT Verbal	10.0
MCAT Essay	P

Application Information

Regular application	11/1
Regular notification	10/15
Are transfers accepted?	yes
Admissions may be deferred?	yes
Interview required?	yes

Academics

The School of Medicine is well-integrated into the UC Davis campus and benefits from the academic programs of the university. About 10 percent of each class extend their first two years in three, extend their fourth year, or take time off from the standard curriculum at some point. This "Enrichment Option" allows students to pursue research or attend to other academic and personal goals. Joint-degree programs organized in conjunction with graduate departments at UC Davis lead to an MBA, MA, or PhD along with the MD degree. In addition, the MPH degree may be earned through the School of Medicine's Department of Public Health Sciences or at UC Berkeley School of Public Health. Those interested in careers as physician-scientists may apply for programs leading to doctorates in the following fields: Biochemistry, biomedical engineering, cell biology, genetics, immunology, molecular biology, neuroscience, pathology, pharmacology, physiology and in the humanities or social sciences. Beginning in the fall of 2006, all four years of medical school will take place on the Sacramento Medical campus in a new Medical Education Center.

BASIC SCIENCES: The first basic science block (August through December) coordinates anatomy, physiology, cell biology, and biochemistry, and approaches the topic of cell biology systematically for the first time. Organ systems are studied together, including gross and microanatomy and function is integrated with structure. These courses will continue to be administered by basic science departments.

The second block features two new concurrent integrated basic and clinical science courses. In metabolism, endocrinology and reproduction, the various topics progress in a logical, integrated manner from normal function to disease models. In microbiology-immunology-pathology-host defense, the emphasis will be on how immunologic processes mediate response to infection and autoimmune disease and how the body responds to injury.

Year two starts with a summer block that combines neurobiology, clinical neurosciences, neuropathology, and neuropharmacology courses. The close temporal proximity of lectures in these areas will help students better appreciate how breakdowns in the normal structure and function of the nervous system cause disease and how these diseases can be treated. The remainder of year two places courses in better order to facilitate integration and learning. For example, cardiology/pulmonary/renal are concurrent and hematology and oncology are placed together.

An earlier start to the school year (August) allows an earlier start to the clinical clerkships (May of the second year). This will increase the number of eight-week blocks in the third year from six to seven (the six required third year clerkships will not change). The additional block will enable students to take sub-specialty clerkships (important for "early match" specialties) or other electives during their third year. The integrated 3 year doctoring curriculum will continue to run alongside the above courses and link to the concurrent basic science and pathophysiology content.

CLINICAL TRAINING

Third-year required clerkships are surgery (8 weeks), medicine (8 weeks), pediatrics (8 weeks), ob/gyn (8 weeks), psychiatry (8 weeks), and primary care plus (8 weeks), which includes 4 weeks in a family-practice setting and introduces primary care components of certain specialties. Required fourth-year clerkships are emergency medicine (4 weeks), physical medicine and rehabilitation (2 weeks), ophthalmology (2 weeks) neurology (2 weeks), and otolaryngology (2 weeks). A 2 week course that discusses the legal, ethical, and economic issues related to medicine is also required. Most of the fourth year is reserved for selectives, chosen by the student within the directives of an oversight committee and electives, which are unrestricted. Required clerkships take place at UC Davis Medical Center in Sacramento (528 beds), Kaiser Permanente Hospital, David Grant Hospital (Travis Air Force Base), Sutter Hospital, Highland General (Oakland), and at community physician sites. Other clinical facilities include a new Shriners Hospital opened on the Sacramento campus to provide care to children with orthopedic and other disorders, an expanded hospital, the Ellison Ambulatory Care Center, and the establishment of the Mather VA Hospital. Among these sites, students serve a diverse patient population. Selectives may be taken at any LCME-accredited medical school. Overseas clinical activities may be taken as elective programs organized by the Departments of Family Practice and Public Health Sciences, and through individual student efforts. Students must take and pass the USMLE Step 2 in order to graduate.

Students

All but a few students in each class are California residents. There is also significant diversity in the age of incoming students, the average being 25 or 26. Class size is 93.

STUDENT LIFE

As stated earlier, the School of Medicine in Davis will be moving to the new Medical Education Center located on the Sacramento Medical Center campus. The classrooms, lecture halls, library, and student resource facilities will be found in the new facility. All medical students will continue to have access to recreational facilities, housing, intramural sports program, and activities offering support and social opportunities to students in Davis. Students are encouraged to reside in Sacramento close to the medical center and nearby communities.

GRADUATES

Close to 50 percent of graduates enter primary care fields. The UC Davis Health System has at least 20 residency programs. Davis graduates are successful at obtaining residency position in prestigious programs all over the country.

Admissions

REQUIREMENTS

The following courses must be completed prior to matriculation: English (1 year), Biology with lab (1 year), upper-division biology (6 months, no lab required; can be satisfied with course work in genetics, biochemistry, molecular or cellular biology), General chemistry with lab (1 year), Organic chemistry with lab (1 year), Physics with lab (1 year) and college level math—calculus and/or statistics (1 year). The MCAT is required and should have been taken within the past three years. For those who have repeated the MCAT, the most recent scores are considered.

SUGGESTIONS

Additional helpful courses are biochemistry, genetics, and embryology. For students who have been out of school for a period of time, some recent course work is recommended. While no activities or qualities are specified, successful applicants demonstrate interpersonal skills, leadership potential, and the ability to work with diverse populations.

PROCESS

About 2,000 applicants, or roughly 50 percent of AMCAS applicants, receive secondaries. Secondary applications must be returned within a month; 400–500 applicants are interviewed, with interviews held from October through April. Interviews consist of two 1-hour sessions with faculty members and/or medical students. About one-third of those interviewed are accepted on a rolling basis. Others are rejected or put on a wait list that is split into thirds, depending on the candidate's prospect for admission. Wait-listed candidates are not advised to send supplementary material.

Admissions Requirements (Required)

MCAT scores, science GPA, non-science GPA, letters of recommendation, interview, essays/personal statement, extracurricular activities, exposure to medical profession, strong leadership background, community service.

Admissions Requirements (Optional)

State residency.

Overlap Schools

University of California—Irvine; University of California—San Francisco; University of California—Los Angeles; University of California—San Diego; University of Southern California.

COSTS AND AID

Tuition & Fees	
Room and board	
(off campus)	$9,728
Cost of books	$2,280
In-state fees	$21,176
Out-of-state fees	$33,421

Financial Aid

% students receiving aid	95
Average grant	$7,000
Average loan	$26,000
Average debt	$69,345

UNIVERSITY OF CALIFORNIA—IRVINE
COLLEGE OF MEDICINE

MEDICAL EDUCATION BUILDING 802, ROOM 100, IRVINE, CA 92697-4089 • ADMISSION: 949-824-5388
FAX: 949-824-2485 • E-MAIL: MEDADMIT@UCI.EDU • WEBSITE: WWW.UCIHS.UCI.EDU/ADMISSIONS

STUDENT BODY

Type	Public
Enrollment	372
% male/female	54/46
% underrepresented minorities	8
# applied (total/out)	3,400/369
# accepted (total/out)	244/0
# enrolled (total/out)	92/0
Average age	23

FACULTY

Total faculty (number)	788
% female	29
% minority	6
% part-time	18
Student-faculty ratio	2:1

ADMISSIONS

Average GPA and MCAT Scores

Overall GPA	3.7
MCAT Bio	11.0
MCAT Phys	11.0
MCAT Verbal	10.0
MCAT Essay	P

Application Information

Regular application	11/1
Regular notification	rolling
Are transfers accepted?	no
Admissions may be deferred?	yes
Interview required?	yes
Application fee	$60

Academics

For those that meet the requirements, six students each year are accepted into the Medical Scientist Training Program (MSTP), leading to a combined MD/PhD degree. The PhD can be earned in a number of fields, including all of the biological sciences, engineering sciences, information and computer sciences, and physical sciences. For those who meet requirements, a joint-MBA/MD program can be pursued in conjunction with UCI's Graduate School of Management. Most students follow a 4 year curriculum, throughout which a course called patient-doctor integrates clinical, social, and basic science concepts.

BASIC SCIENCES: For the duration of two years, the course patient-doctor gives students an opportunity for interaction with real patients in a clinical setting and with simulated patients in a closely monitored learning environment. During the first year, students also take anatomy and embryology, biochemistry, histology, immunology, medical genetics, medical neurosciences, molecular cell biology, and physiology/pathophysiology. All are taught primarily in a lecture/lab format. The patient-doctor course continues throughout year 2, by placing students in clinical service experiences within community physician offices. During the second-year students also take clinical pathology, general and systematic, medical microbiology, medical pharmacology, pathology, and topics in medicine, tutorial programs, academic monitoring, and study-skills workshops promote student success in the basic sciences. The Medical Center Library (MCL) is located at the UCI Medical Center and meets the research, education, and patient care needs of the Medical Center staff and the UCI College of Medicine. The College of Medicine is fully computerized with an internal electronic informational network. Students are evaluated with honors, pass, or fail.

CLINICAL TRAINING

Patient contact begins during the first year when students participate in the patient, doctor, and society course and the patient-doctor course. Standardized patients and surrogate patients are employed throughout the four years to enhance interactive experience. During the fourth year, the patient-doctor course continues, teaching students to apply basic science concepts to clinical situations. Required clerkships begin in year 3 and include the following: Inpatient and ambulatory medicine (12 weeks), ob/gyn (8 weeks), surgery (8 weeks), psychiatry (6 weeks), family medicine (4 weeks), and pediatrics (4 weeks). Year 4 rotations are intensive care unit (4 weeks), neuroscience (4 weeks), emergency medicine (2 weeks), radiology (2 weeks), a musculoskeletal elective (2 weeks), and substance abuse (2 weeks). The primary training sites are UCI Medical Center in the City of Orange, which includes several specialized clinical and research centers; the Veterans Administration Medical Center in Long Beach; and the College of Medicine's affiliated hospitals and clinics. Affiliates are located in Orange, Los Angeles, and San Bernardino counties, serving both rural and urban communities. During the clinical years, narrative evaluations supplement the honors/pass/fail grading system. Passing the USMLE Step 1 and Step 2 is a requirement for graduation.

Students

On and off campus, medical students can find a wide variety of recreational and extracurricular activities to help keep overall balance in their lives and discover new outlets for fitness and fun.

STUDENT LIFE

UCI has many student-interest groups, including those that provide support to minority students and to students with children. Other groups are geared toward volunteer and community activities. Medical students have access to a wide variety of resources at UCI, including cultural events, intramural athletics, and all facilities. On-campus, graduate-student housing is affordable, comfortable, and allows medical students to interact with students from other departments. Apartments, residence halls, and residential communities that feature living spaces of all sizes are available. The city of Irvine and surrounding communities, such as Newport Beach, provide recreational opportunities and attractive housing options.

GRADUATES

A large proportion of graduates enter postgraduate programs at UCI, which has one of the nation's largest residency programs in primary care disciplines and internal medicine. Most graduates enter programs in California, but seniors have been successful in obtaining residencies all over the country.

Admissions

REQUIREMENTS

The following must be completed prior to matriculation: General chemistry (2 semesters), organic chemistry (2 semesters), physics (2 semesters), biology (3 semesters, with a minimum of 1 upper-division biology class), biochemistry (1 semester), and calculus (1 semester). The MCAT is required, and scores should be no more than three years old. For those who have retaken the exam, the most recent set of scores is considered.

SUGGESTIONS

No specific major is required. In addition to the requirements for admission the following classes are also recommended: Molecular biology, cell biology, genetics, psychology, Spanish, and vertebrate embryology.

PROCESS

The UCI College of Medicine seeks to admit students who are highly qualified to be trained in the practice of medicine and whose backgrounds, talents, and experiences contribute to a diverse student body. The Admissions Committee carefully reviews all applicants whose undergraduate record and scores on the MCAT indicate that they will be able to handle the rigorous curriculum of medical school. Careful consideration is given to applicants from disadvantaged backgrounds (i.e., disadvantaged through social, cultural, and/or economic conditions). In addition to scholastic achievement, attributes deemed desirable in prospective students include leadership ability and participation in extracurricular activities, such as exposure to clinical medicine and/or medically related research, as well as community service. Preference is given to California residents and applicants who are either U.S. citizens or permanent residents. The College of Medicine does not accept transfer students.

Information provided by the AMCAS applicaion is used for the preliminary screening. Based on decisions reached by the Admissions Committee, applicants may be sent a secondary application. A limited number of applicants (approximately 500) are invited to be interviewed. The Admissions Committee reviews the academic records, letters of recommendation, and the results of personal interviews before making its final selections.

Admissions Requirements (Required)

MCAT scores, science GPA, non-science GPA, letters of recommendation, interview, essays/personal statement.

Admissions Requirements (Optional)

State residency, extracurricular activities, exposure to medical profession, community service, research.

COSTS AND AID

Tuition & Fees

Out-of-state tuition	$12,245
Room and board (on campus)	$10,913
Room and board (off campus)	$13,244
Cost of books	$1,799
Fees	$16,202

Financial Aid

% students receiving aid	92
Average grant	$4,200
Average loan	$27,122
Average debt	$79,186

UNIVERSITY OF CALIFORNIA—LOS ANGELES
DAVID GEFFEN SCHOOL OF MEDICINE AT UCLA

CENTER FOR HEALTH SCIENCES, LOS ANGELES, CA 90095-1720 • ADMISSION: 310-825-6081
FAX: 310-825-6081 • E-MAIL: SOMADMISS@MEDNET.UCLA.EDU • WEBSITE: WWW.MEDSTUDENT.UCLA.EDU

STUDENT BODY

Type	Public
Enrollment	674
% male/female	58/42
% underrepresented minorities	30
# applied	5,046
# enrolled	121

ADMISSIONS

Application Information

Regular application	11/1
Regular notification	1/15
Are transfers accepted?	yes
Interview required?	yes
Application fee	$40

Academics

Each year, 10 students are admitted to an extended curriculum program, which spreads the first two years of the standard curriculum over three years, creating opportunities for special projects or supplemental instruction. In each class, as many as 24 students who are interested in practicing in underserved communities spend their first two years at UCLA School of Medicine, and then complete clinical requirements at Drew University facilities. Drew University is a predominantly African American medical institution. Several joint-degree programs are offered to medical students, including an MD/MPH with the School of Public Health, an MD/MBA with the School of Management, and an MSTP-sponsored MD/PhD. All entering students are required to purchase a computer because both the basic science and clinical curriculum emphasize its applications.

BASIC SCIENCES: During the first two years, students are in scheduled sessions for about 26 hours per week. In addition to required courses, selectives give students an opportunity to explore topics of interest such as health care reform, addiction, and AIDS. First-year courses include the following: Anatomy, basic neurology, biological chemistry, biomathematics, clinical applications of basic sciences (CABS), doctoring I, micro-anatomy and cell biology, organ system physiology, topics in physiology. Doctoring I is the beginning of the doctoring curriculum, which uses a case-based approach and addresses the interdisciplinary issues that pertain to practicing medicine. In this course, the cultural, ethical, legal, economic, and social perspectives on medicine are considered. In CABS, students participate in community-based, health education, or health care projects and learn to apply basic science concepts to real-life clinical problems. Year 2 courses are the following: Doctoring II; genetics; microbiology; pathology; pathophysiology; psychopathology; pharmacology; and clinical fundamentals, which covers physical diagnosis and takes place largely at clinical sites. Both university-sponsored and student-initiated study and tutorial groups are available. Most classes are taught in the Health Sciences Building, a large structure on the UCLA campus in Westwood. The Biomedical Library is nearby and serves faculty, students, and the community with a collection of 500,000 volumes and 6,000 current journals. Grading is pass/fail, with written citations for outstanding achievement. Promotion to year 3 requires a passing score on the USMLE Step 1.

CLINICAL TRAINING
Outside of traditional clerkships, students gain experience with patients in doctoring and through the extensive volunteer opportunities. Some students identify volunteer opportunities with the assistance of the Community Service Compendium, a list of community outreach sites. Formal clinical training takes place during the third and fourth years, which are treated as a continuum. Fifty-seven weeks of the third and fourth years are reserved for the following required rotations: Medicine (12 weeks), surgery (12 weeks), pediatrics (6 weeks), ob/gyn (6 weeks), psychiatry (6 weeks), family medicine (6 weeks), radiology (4 weeks), neurology (2 weeks), and ophthalmology (2 weeks). Clerkships take place primarily at the University Hospital (517 beds). Other affiliated sites are Harbor General (800 beds), Cedars-Sinai, Kaiser Sunset, Kaiser West LA, Kern Medical Center (Bakersfield), King/Drew Medical Center, Olive View-UCLA Medical Center (Sylmar), Sepulveda Veterans Affairs, St. Mary Medical Center (Long Beach), and West LA Veterans Affairs Medical Center. Doctoring III is taken throughout the years, occupying students for one full day every other week. This segment of the course takes students to community-based medical sites and uses a small-group format to discuss various patient

problems. Twenty-seven weeks remain for electives. Some of the elective requirement may be fulfilled around the country or overseas. Grading is pass/fail supplemented with written evaluations. The USMLE Step 2 is required for graduation.

Students

The students reflect the multicultural population of Los Angeles, with underrepresented minorities accounting for one-third of the student body. In entering classes, the average age is 22, and there are usually no more than a few students over 28 years old. Eighty-five percent of the students are California residents. Class size is 145.

STUDENT LIFE

In addition to the beaches and beautiful weather of Southern California and Los Angeles, the UCLA campus itself offers excellent athletic facilities and plenty of entertainment. Student-led groups and activities within the medical school are numerous, ranging from the Iranian/American Medical Organization to the Salvation Army Outreach Clinic. The medical school also sponsors activities that encourage cohesion between faculty and students. Although residence halls and married-student housing are available, most medical students opt to live off campus.

GRADUATES

Graduates are well-prepared for careers in primary care, more specialized clinical fields, and research. About half of the graduates enter primary care fields, which is roughly the current national average. Many enter residencies at UCLA or affiliated hospitals.

Admissions

REQUIREMENTS

Admissions requirements are chemistry (two years, including inorganic and organic); English (1 year); college math (1 year, includes calculus and statistics); physics (1 year); and biology (1 year). Science courses must have associated labs, and AP credits are not counted. The MCAT is required, and scores must be no more than three years old. Generally, if a student has retaken the exam, the best set of scores is used.

SUGGESTIONS

Courses in humanities and social sciences, as well as Spanish and computer skills are highly recommended. Undergraduate courses that overlap with those in the medical school curriculum, such as anatomy, are not recommended. For applicants who graduated college several years ago, recent course work is expected. The April, rather than August, MCAT is advised. Extracurricular activities that are medically related, or that involve research or patient contact, are useful. UCLA is unusual among state-affiliated medical schools in California in that it welcomes applications from well-qualified, out-of-state residents.

PROCESS

Typically, 55 percent of AMCAS applicants are asked to submit supplementary information. Of those returning secondaries, about 20 percent are invited for interviews. Interviews take place from November through May and consist of 1 or 2 sessions with faculty members and/or medical students. Notification begins in January and continues until enough offers have been made to fill the class. About 25 percent of interviewees are accepted, and another group is wait listed. Wait-listed candidates may send additional information about academic or extracurricular achievements. The UCLA/UC Riverside Biomedical Sciences Program allows 24 admitted students to obtain both the BS and MD degrees in seven years. In this program, students enter UCLA School of Medicine after completing three years of undergraduate preparation at UC Riverside.

Admissions Requirements (Required)

MCAT scores, science GPA, non-science GPA, letters of recommendation, interview, state residency, extracurricular activities, exposure to medical profession.

Admissions Requirements (Optional)

Essays/personal statement.

COSTS AND AID

Tuition & Fees

In-state Tuition	$15,173
Out-of-state Tuition	$27,418
Room and board (on campus)	$14,000
Room and board (off campus)	$4,620
Cost of books	$4,360

University of California—San Diego

School of Medicine

9500 Gilman Drive, MC 0621, La Jolla, CA 92093-0621 • Admission: 858-534-3880
Fax: 858-534-5282 • E-mail: somadmissions@ucsd.edu • Website: www.meded.ucsd.edu/admissions/

STUDENT BODY

Type	Public
Enrollment	503
% male/female	51/49
% underrepresented minorities	18
# applied (total/out)	5,018/1,769
# accepted (total/out)	301/40
# enrolled (total/out)	121/9
Average age	24

ADMISSIONS

Average GPA and MCAT Scores

Overall GPA	3.73
MCAT Bio	11.5
MCAT Phys	11.3
MCAT Verbal	10.19
MCAT Essay	Q

Application Information

Regular application	11/1
Regular notification	10/15
Are transfers accepted?	no
Admissions may be deferred?	yes
Interview required?	yes
Application fee	$60

Academics

In addition to fulfilling course requirements, students must complete an Independent Study Project to graduate. These projects allow students to explore and define their own interests, and to collaborate with faculty members who share these interests. The medical school benefits from the resources of other parts of UCSD. Joint-MD/PhD programs are possible with UCSD Graduate Departments in biochemistry, biomedical engineering, biophysics, cell biology, genetics, immunology, microbiology, molecular biology, neuroscience, pathology, pharmacology, and physiology. Normally, these degrees are MSTP sponsored. Students can earn an MPH in conjunction with nearby San Diego State University Graduate School of Public Health.

BASIC SCIENCES: The first two years are organized into quarters. Electives are an important supplement to basic science requirements and account for about 20 percent of scheduled course time. During the fall quarter of year 1, cell biology and biochemistry is the principal endeavor. This lecture course is referred to as a block, which means that the material is covered intensely during 1 or 2 quarters. Students also begin a sequence in social and behavioral sciences, taught mostly through small-group sessions. Winter-quarter courses are introduction to clinical medicine, which continues throughout the basic science curriculum and prepares students for third-year rotations; pharmacology; and physiology. The spring quarter courses are endocrinology, metabolism, neurology, pharmacology, and reproductive biology, all of which are taught primarily through lectures. Year 2 begins with anatomy, biostatistics, histology, and a social/behavioral science course on health care systems. The winter quarter consists of hematology, human disease, and psychopathology. The second-year, spring quarter curriculum is human disease, lab medicine, and neurology. During the basic science years, there are, on average, 34 scheduled hours per week. Instruction takes place in the modern Basic Science Building, which is adjacent to the Biomedical Library (holds 100,000 volumes). Computers with access to online informational services and curricular programs are available for student use in the library and in the School's Learning Resource Center. Grading uses an honors/pass/fail system. The USMLE Step 1 is required for promotion to year 3.

CLINICAL TRAINING

Supervised patient contact begins in January of year 1, in introduction to clinical medicine. The physical examination is taught in conjunction with the study of individual organ systems in the first year, and together with the history, refined in the second basic science year. In addition, a simulated-patient program provides students the opportunity to improve their history-taking and physical-examination skills, as well as to obtain feedback from faculty mentors and view videotapes of their patient interaction. Required third-year rotations are medicine (12 weeks), surgery (12 weeks), neurology (4 weeks), ob/gyn (6 weeks), pediatrics (8 weeks), psychiatry (6 weeks), and primary care (1 afternoon per week all year). Students design their fourth-year curricula by selecting courses from within broad subject areas. Twelve weeks are selected from direct patient care clerkships, 4 weeks must be a primary care experience, 4 weeks inpatient training, and 4 weeks outpatient training. An additional twelve weeks of pure elective, clinical clerkships are also required. Clinical training takes place at large hospitals and small clinics including UCSD Medical Centers (577 beds total), VA Hospital (606 beds), Navy Hospital (750 beds), Children's Hospital (154 beds), Kaiser Foundation Hospital (1,285 beds),

Sharp Memorial Community Hospital (1,415 beds), Clinica De Salubridad de Campesinos, and the U.S. Public Health Service Outpatient Clinic. Electives may be taken from the various departments of UCSD or may be carried out in conjunction with community organizations. Most students take advantage of additional clinical training opportunities through volunteer work, some of which takes them across the border in Mexico. The USMLE Step 2 is required for graduation. UCSD students do exceptionally well on both parts of the USMLE.

Students

Students are predominantly Californians. There is a wide age range among students, and it is very common for them to have taken one or two years off after college for research or other activities. About 60 percent of incoming students in a recent class were science majors. Class size is 122.

STUDENT LIFE

On-campus housing is convenient, attractive, and popular with students. Modern apartments of all sizes are available for single and married students and for those who have children or pets. Some students rely on bicycles or shuttle buses, while others own cars. UCSD's location affords many recreational possibilities. Year-round outdoor activities include swimming, surfing, biking, sailing, rollerblading, running, and walking. Other activities are the San Diego Symphony, the zoo, and the Padres professional baseball team. Medical student organizations and events also contribute to students' extracurricular lives.

GRADUATES

Of the graduating class of 2005, the most popular fields for postgraduate training were internal medicine (25 graduates), pediatrics (17), family medicine (13), emergency medicine (13), psychiatry (8), radiology (7), anesthesiology (7), surgery (6), dermatology (4), ophthalmology (4), ob/gyn (4), pathology (4), orthopedic surgery (3), and neurology (3). Students also matched into neurosurgery, otolaryngology, plastic surgery, and urology. Many entered programs in San Diego, Oakland, San Jose, Los Angeles, and other California locations.

Admissions

REQUIREMENTS

One year of biology, chemistry, math, organic chemistry, and physics are all required. Strong written and spoken English is a requirement, and the ability to communicate in a second language is preferred. The rigor of an applicant's undergraduate institution is considered in assessing GPA. The MCAT is required, and the spring exam is advised.

SUGGESTIONS

Breadth of academic experience is important. Extracurricular activities are also important, particularly those that involve some sort of medical exposure, community involvement, or leadership.

PROCESS

About 40 percent of applicants receive a secondary application. Of those returning secondaries, about 550 are interviewed. Interviews take place from October through May and consist of two 1-hour sessions with faculty members. Following interviews, candidates are accepted, rejected, or put on hold for later notification. About half of those interviewed are eventually accepted. An extensive wait list is established.

Admissions Requirements (Required)

MCAT scores, science GPA, non-science GPA, letters of recommendation, interview, essays/personal statement.

Admissions Requirements (Optional)

State residency, extracurricular activities, exposure to medical profession.

Overlap Schools

Stanford University; University of California—Davis; University of California—Irvine; University of California—San Francisco; University of California—Los Angeles.

COSTS AND AID

Tuition & Fees

Out-of-state tuition	$12,245
Room and board (on campus)	$7,722
Room and board (off campus)	$11,043
Cost of books	$1,976
In-state fees	$22,008
Out-of-state fees	$12,245

Financial Aid

% students receiving aid	94
Average grant	$17,096
Average loan	$21,406
Average debt	$72,844

UNIVERSITY OF CALIFORNIA—SAN FRANCISCO

SCHOOL OF MEDICINE

SCHOOL OF MEDICINE ADMISSIONS, C-200, PO BOX 0408, SAN FRANCISCO, CA 94143-0408 • **ADMISSION:** 415-476-4044
FAX: 415-476-5490 • **E-MAIL:** ADMISSIONS@MEDSCH.UCSF.EDU • **WEBSITE:**WWW.MEDSCHOOL.UCSF.EDU/ADMISSIONS

STUDENT BODY	
Type	Public
Enrollment	600
% male/female	44/56
% underrepresented minorities	18
# applied (total/out)	5,298/2,520
# accepted (total/out)	257/73
# enrolled (total/out)	141/22
Average age	24

FACULTY	
Total faculty (number)	1,682
% female	36
% minority	19
% part-time	4
Student-faculty ratio	1:3

ADMISSIONS

Average GPA and MCAT Scores

Overall GPA	3.79
MCAT Bio	11.7
MCAT Phys	11.5
MCAT Verbal	10.6
MCAT Essay	P

Application Information

Regular application	11/1
Regular notification	rolling
Are transfers accepted?	no
Admissions may be deferred?	yes
Interview required?	yes
Application fee	$60

Academics

The standard curriculum for the MD degree may be completed in four years. However, approximately 40 percent of UCSF students remain in school for additional time to pursue advanced studies in research or a scholarly project, international health, or additional clinical rotations. Students may spend 1 year in the Certificate in Biomedical Research Program, giving them time to complete a substantial research project and to earn the MD with thesis degree. UCSF has a joint-MD/MPH degree program with UC Berkeley that allows up to 10 students per year to spend 2 semesters in Berkeley earning a master's degree from the School of Public Health. In addition, each year 12 students are admitted to the UCSF/UC Berkeley Joint Medical Program in which they complete the pre-clinical, problem-based curriculum and fulfill requirements for a master's of science degree in either public health or health and medical sciences. Upon completion, they transfer to UCSF to complete the third and fourth years. Up to 12 students enter the Medical Science Training Program (MSTP) joint-PhD/MD program yearly. Participants may earn a PhD from the following UCSF programs: Biochemistry, biophysics, cancer biology, cell biology, chemistry, developmental biology, endocrinology, genetics, immunology, neuroscience, stem cell biology, vascular and cardiac biology, virology and medical anthropology.

BASIC SCIENCES: The first two years form the essential core, and they are organized into 8 block courses, each about 8 weeks long. These courses deal with major themes and draw together a range of interdisciplinary topics. The first-year courses are brain, mind, and behavior; cancer; major organ systems; and prologue. In the second year, students take infection, inflammation, and immunity; life cycle; metabolism; and consolidation cases. Essential core lectures, labs, and small-group sessions account for about 20 hours a week, and they integrate subjects from the basic, social, and clinical sciences. All courses include supplementary resources on a Web-based system that forms the e-curriculum. The essential core comprises a course called foundations of patient care, which offers students exposure to the clinical setting. This course also allows students to explore issues of professional development, ethics, and doctor-patient interaction.

CLINICAL TRAINING

Patient contact begins during year 1 in foundations of patient care and in the week-long immersion in the hospital wards called the clinical interlude. Clinical elements are wholly integrated into the basic science curriculum, allowing for a smooth transition into the third year. Likewise, the clinical years include segments of classroom instruction that focus on basic and social science concepts. For example, the third year includes three intersessions, which occur between clerkship rotations and offer lectures and small-group discussions of basic science connections to the clinical experiences, ethics, evidence-based medicine, and health policy. Required third-year core clerkships are medicine (8 weeks), neurology and psychiatry (8 weeks), family and community medicine (6 weeks), ob/gyn (6 weeks), pediatrics (6 weeks), surgery (8 weeks), anesthesia (2 weeks), and surgical subspecialties (2 weeks). Teaching sites are primarily in San Francisco, Oakland, and Fresno and include the California Pacific Medical Center, Children's Hospital, Kaiser Foundation Hospitals, San Francisco City Clinics, San Francisco General Hospital, Veterans Affairs Medical Centers in San Francisco and Fresno, UCSF Medical Center including Mount Zion Hospital, University Medical Center-Fresno, and Langley Porter Neuropsychiatric Institute. Year 4 is primarily elective study, which may entail international work or research in addition to traditional advanced clinical rotations. Evaluation of students during years 3 and 4 includes an honors/pass/fail system enhanced with narrative comments. Outside of clerkships, students gain clinical experience through volunteer work and community service at any number of UCSF-affiliated projects.

Students

Twenty percent of the students are out-of-state residents. More than half are nonwhite, and approximately 17 percent are underrepresented minorities, mostly African and Hispanic Americans. Virtually all undergraduate majors are represented in the student body. Class size is 141.

STUDENT LIFE

University-owned housing appropriate for both married and single students is available. Many students take part in community programs, which provide not only an opportunity to contribute but also a chance for student-student and student-faculty interaction in an extracurricular setting. Students have access to school athletic facilities and to many local outdoor activities, including running in Golden Gate Park, surfing at Ocean Beach, mountain biking in Marin County, and skiing around Lake Tahoe, 3 hours away by car.

GRADUATES

Of the graduating class of 2005, the following specialties were selected by the indicated number of students: Family practice (8), internal medicine (23), internal medicine/primary care (10), pediatrics (19), emergency medicine (20), anesthesiology (12), psychiatry (10), ob/gyn (8), surgery (7), ophthalmology (5), pathology (4), radiation oncology (4), orthopedic surgery (3), neurology (3), otolaryngology (3), radiology (3), dermatology (2), neurosurgery (1), physical medicine (1), urology (2), and other (2). In total, 41 percent entered residencies in fields classified as primary care. See http://medschool.ucsf.edu/medstudents/resources/match/summary _table.html for details.

Admissions

REQUIREMENTS

To be considered for admission, applicants must complete the following courses by June of the year they expect to matriculate: General chemistry with lab (3 quarters, equal to 1 year); organic chemistry (2 quarters); physics and biology (equal to 1 year). Applications are welcome from candidates who have taken time off between college and applying to medical school. The MCAT is required, and the spring MCAT is strongly advised. For those who retake the test, the most recent scores are considered. MCAT scores must be no more than three years old. California residents are given preference.

SUGGESTIONS

Beyond requirements, applicants should have taken college-level math, English, and humanities courses. Upper-division biology is also recommended. All extracurricular activities that reveal an applicant's interests and demonstrate his or her commitment strengthen the application. Some exposure to medical issues or to patient care is also valuable.

PROCESS

GPA, MCATs, residency, and the AMCAS application are used to screen for secondary applications. The secondary application is straightforward and does not require additional essays for the MD program. Applicants have 3 weeks from the date of receipt of the secondary application to return the secondary and have their letters of recommendation sent. Letters of recommendation sent prior to receipt of the secondary will be destroyed. About 30 percent of applicants receive a secondary application and about one-third of those returning secondaries are invited to interview. There is also a hold category, which indicates that while the applicant is not in the top group, he or she may be interviewed as the year progresses. Interviews take place between September and March, and consist of two 1 hour blind sessions each with a faculty member or one faculty member and one student. After offers have been made to fill the class, some remaining candidates are placed on a ranked wait list and may be offered a spot as late as August, depending on accepted students' matriculation rate.

Admissions Requirements (Required)

MCAT scores, science GPA, letters of recommendation, interview, essays/personal statement.

Admissions Requirements (Optional)

nonscience GPA, state residency, extracurricular activities, exposure to medical profession.

Overlap Schools

Harvard University, Stanford University.

COSTS AND AID

Tuition & Fees

Out-of-state tuition	$12,245
Room and board	
(off campus)	$18,105
Cost of books	$1,800
Fees	$22,328

Financial Aid

% students receiving aid	89
Average grant	$8,358
Average loan	$18,592
Average debt	$76,573

UNIVERSITY OF CHICAGO
PRITZKER SCHOOL OF MEDICINE

OFFICE OF MEDICAL EDUCATION, BSLC 104W, 924 EAST FIFTY-SEVENTH ST., CHICAGO, IL 60637-5416 • ADMISSION: 773-702-1937
FAX: 773-834-5412 • E-MAIL: PRITZKERADMISSIONS@BSD.UCHICAGO.EDU • WEBSITE: WWW.PRITZKER.BSD.UCHICAGO.EDU

STUDENT BODY

Type	Private
Enrollment	432
% male/female	48/52
% underrepresented minorities	15
# applied (total/out)	3,830/2,914
# accepted (total/out)	277/216
# enrolled (total/out)	104/66
Average age	23

FACULTY

Total faculty (number)	982
% female	32
% minority	24
% part-time	6
Student-faculty ratio	2:1

ADMISSIONS

Average GPA and MCAT Scores

Overall GPA	3.74
MCAT Bio	11.3
MCAT Phys	11.0
MCAT Verbal	10.5
MCAT Essay	Q

Application Information

Regular application	10/15
Regular notification	rolling
Early application	8/1
Early notification	10/1
Are transfers accepted?	yes
Admissions may be deferred?	yes
Interview required?	yes
Application fee	$75

Academics

Pritzker offers a curriculum best characterized as modified traditional. Although most pre-clinical topics are presented in lecture, case-based methods and clinical exposure supplement lectures. For example, as students study particular parts in anatomy, they view afflictions of that body part in a clinical setting. About 24 percent of the students in each class earn a graduate degree in addition to the MD degree. Some of these students are MSTP participants; others are privately funded MD/PhD students and still others earn a JD or an MBA along with the MD. Pritzker students are well prepared by the curriculum as evidenced by their strong board exam performances.

BASIC SCIENCES: Chicago follows a quarter system. Fall quarter, first-year medical students study biochemistry and molecular biology; cell and organ physiology; and clinical skills 1A, which introduces students to the patient interview; and human morphology I. During the winter, first-year students study clinical skills, which covers social issues related to medicine; doctor/patient relationship; human morphology II; molecular and cell biology; and organ physiology and endocrinology. Spring curriculum includes development and psychopathology, medical genetics, neurobiology, nutrition and epidemiology and clinical investigation, and an opportunity for elective study. Second-year, fall quarter curriculum includes immunobiology, microbiology, pharmacology, and cell pathology. Winter quarter includes clinical pathophysiology and clinical skills 2A, which is called physical diagnosis. The final quarter of pre-clinical studies includes therapeutics, more clinical skills, review of basic sciences, and electives. Most students use a student-run, note-taking co-op in which each participating student is responsible for providing notes on a lecture assigned to him or her. First- and second-year students spend their time in the new Biological Sciences Learning Center, which is both a center for instruction and research. Classrooms are equipped with audio/video technology, and excellent computer-based learning tools are available. The Knapp Center is a new medical research facility with modern laboratory space. The Crerar Library has one of the largest science collections in the country and houses almost 1 million volumes. Grading is pass/fail, although students receive graded feedback on exams. Tutoring is available for students who are in danger of failure. Passage of the USMLE is not required for promotion or graduation although most students choose to take Step 1 after year 2.

CLINICAL TRAINING

Students are introduced to clinical techniques and experiences during their first quarter at Pritzker, with Clinical Skills 1A. Year 3 is composed of a series of clerkships with short breaks between rotations. Clerkships take place at the University of Chicago Hospitals and Health Systems and the new Comer Childrens Hospital. These hospitals serve a broad community, and students learn to treat a diverse patient population. Students rotate through the following departments: Internal medicine (3 months), surgery (3 months), pediatrics (2 months), ob/gyn (1.5 months), psychiatry (1.5 month), and family medicine (1 month). During the fourth year, students choose selectives from the following categories: Anesthesia, inpatient/sub internship, neurology, and scientific basis of medical practice. The fourth year is also an opportunity for students to pursue individual research projects or to study overseas. The University of Chicago Medical facilities have expanded significantly during the past decade, suggesting a strong patient base and economic situation. Evaluation of clinical performance uses marks of honors, high pass, pass, low pass, and fail. Though the USMLE II is not required for graduation, it may be substituted for a comprehensive exam, which is otherwise required.

Students

Typically, Pritzker attracts research-oriented students. Underrepresented minorities have accounted for about 14 percent of the student body and women about 50 percent. Class size is 104. The unique feature of the Pritzker School of Medicine is its integration into the rest of the University of Chicago. It is geographically, administratively, and programmatically integrated. As a consequence, it attracts students and faculty who have broader scholarly interests and who see the entire university as a resource for their academic goals. More than 24 percent of Pritzker's graduates leave with two degrees, and Pritzker is among the top schools in training faculty for academic medicine. Pritzker students obtain additional degrees in biological sciences, business, humanities and public health, law, physical sciences, and social sciences.

STUDENT LIFE

The University of Chicago is located in Chicago's Hyde Park neighborhood, a diverse and interesting community. Students are active in curriculum development and have representatives on important administrative councils. Student volunteer organizations are involved in projects such as organizing and implementing health education into public schools. Medical students take part in university-wide activities such as intramural sports. Many students also take national leadership in organizations such as SNMA and AMSA.

GRADUATES

During the past five years, the residency programs that attracted the most Pritzker graduates were the University of Chicago Hospitals; UCSF; University of Michigan; Mass General; University of Washington; University of Penn; Brigham and Women's Boston; McGaw Medical Center; Beth Israel, Boston; Barnes Hospital; Washington University; and UCLA. The following specialties were the most popular within the 2000 graduating class: Internal medicine (24), pediatrics (10), surgery (5), ob/gyn (5), dermatology (4), ophthalmology (4), anesthesiology (4), emergency medicine (4), orthopedic surgery (4), family practice (3), and internal medicine/pediatrics (2). About 20 percent of Pritzker graduates ultimately serve as faculty members at universities.

Admissions

REQUIREMENTS

One year of lecture plus lab is required in biology, general chemistry, organic chemistry, and physics. Biochemistry with lab may be substituted for one semester or quarter of organic chemistry. For applicants who graduated from college more than three years prior, recent science course work is important. The MCAT is required and should be no more than three years old.

SUGGESTIONS

Biochemistry is strongly recommended, as is significant course work in social sciences and humanities. The Admissions Committee is interested in what factors motivated applicants to pursue medicine and is also concerned with demonstrated problem-solving skills, leadership, experience with persons different from themselves, and experience in research.

PROCESS

Secondary applications are available to all AMCAS applicants and should be completed as soon as possible, no later than December 1. About 18 percent of applicants returning secondaries are interviewed, with interviews held between September and March. Interviewees participate in two one-on-one sessions with faculty members and medical students. Of those interviewed, about two-fifths or 40 percent are accepted on a rolling basis, and the rest are placed on a wait list. Wait-listed candidates are encouraged to submit information that will strengthen their application and will indicate their interest in the school.

Admissions Requirements (Required)

MCAT scores, science GPA, non-science GPA, letters of recommendation, interview, essays/personal statement, extracurricular activities, exposure to medical profession.

Admissions Requirements (Optional)

State residency.

Overlap Schools

Columbia University; Cornell University; Harvard University; Stanford University; University of Michigan—Ann Arbor; Washington University; Yale University.

COSTS AND AID

Tuition & Fees

Tuition	$32,022
Room and board (off campus)	$16,462
Cost of books	$1,600
Fees	$2,679

Financial Aid

% students receiving aid	87

UNIVERSITY OF CINCINNATI
COLLEGE OF MEDICINE

OFFICE OF ADMISSIONS, PO BOX 670552, CINCINNATI, OH 45267-0552 • ADMISSION: 513-558-7314
FAX: 513-558-1165 • E-MAIL: COMADMIS@UCMAIL.UC.EDU • WEBSITE: WWW.MED.UC.EDU

STUDENT BODY

Type	Public
Enrollment	629
% male/female	55/45
% underrepresented minorities	13
# applied (total/out)	2,971/2,017
# accepted (total/out)	343/109
# enrolled (total/out)	160/40
Average age	22

FACULTY

Total faculty (number)	1,372
% female	30
% minority	19
% part-time	8

ADMISSIONS

Average GPA and MCAT Scores

Overall GPA	3.59
MCAT Bio	10.5
MCAT Phys	10.1
MCAT Verbal	9.7

Application Information

Regular application	11/15
Regular notification	rolling
Early application	6/1–8/1
Early notification	10/1
Are transfers accepted?	yes
Admissions may be deferred?	yes
Interview required?	yes
Application fee	$25

Academics

Most students follow a 4 year curriculum leading to the MD degree. There is also a combined MD/MBA program with a five-year curriculum. Up to 6 positions a year are available in a combined MD/PhD program, an NIH funded Physician Scientist Training Program (PSTP), which has a 7- to 8-year curriculum. The PhD may be earned in one of the following disciplines: Cell and molecular biology; environmental health sciences (includes clinical/genetic epidemiology); molecular and developmental biology; molecular, cellular, and biochemical pharmacology; molecular and cellular physiology; molecular genetics, biochemistry, and microbiology; neuroscience; pathobiology and molecular medicine; biomedical engineering; and immunobiology. Medical students interested in shorter-term research projects may pursue them during the summer or as electives. Course grades are honors/high pass/pass/fail. Passing the USMLE Step 1 is a requirement for advancing to year 3 and passing Step 2 is a requirement for graduation.

BASIC SCIENCES: During the first and second years, courses are integrated around content blocks that foster critical thinking skills and problem solving. In both years, a major effort is made to limit lecture and laboratory time to use more small-group activities and ensure sufficient daily free time for active, independent learning. First-year classes are biochemistry, brain and behavior I, gross anatomy, microscopic anatomy, and physiology. Clinical foundations of medical practice, also in the first year, includes history-taking, interviewing, and basic physical examination skills, as well as biopsychosocial issues, death and loss, ethics, and human sexuality. It also provides each student with a one-on-one clinical experience in a physician's practice. Second-year courses are brain and behavior II; clinical foundations of medical practice II, which expands physical diagnosis and clinical skills training; microbiology; pathology; and pharmacology. An average of 20 contact hours per week and ample study time before each exam allows time for self-directed learning, group study, volunteering, and other activities in the basic science years. Computer-based tests have been developed and are used during the first and second year curriculum. There continues to be a concerted effort to vertically integrate content blocks between the basic science and clinical science years. The Office of Student Affairs Academic Support Programs provides tutoring services, academic counseling and training, and preparation seminars for the USMLE Step 1. Pre-clinical instruction takes place in the Medical Sciences Building, which is central to the medical center. Academic IT & Libraries (AIT&L), which is also in the building, has a wealth of health sciences information resources. The College of Medicine has renovated the pathology teaching laboratories into a digital learning environment. Each student has a computer for digital images.

CLINICAL TRAINING

Third-year required clerkships are internal medicine (8 weeks), surgery (8 weeks), pediatrics (8 weeks), obstetrics/gynecology (8 weeks), psychiatry (6 weeks), family medicine (4 weeks), radiology (2 weeks), and 2 specialty electives (2 weeks each). During the fourth year, students complete an 8-week internal medicine acting internship, a 4-week neuroscience selective, and 24 weeks of electives, some of which must be in primary care fields. Most clinical training takes place at University Hospital, Veterans Administration Medical Center, Children's Hospital Medical Center, the Christ Hospital, the Good Samaritan Hospital, and the Jewish Hospital. Half of the elective credits may be earned at other institutions in the area, around the country, or abroad. One organized overseas program is the international health elective, which involves hands-on clinical experience in Honduras.

Students

Among students in the 2005 entering class, 75 percent were Ohio residents, 13 percent were minorities, and 14 percent were 26 years of age or older at the time of application. Seven percent of the class had earned a master's degree. Seventy-nine percent of students were science majors, and a total of 63 undergraduate institutions were represented. The 2005 entering class size was 160.

STUDENT LIFE

Medical students enjoy a cooperative and supportive environment. There are more than 30 student organizations, clubs, and service groups available. Clubs include Family Practice, Cultural Diversity, Complementary Medicine, International Health and Medical Volunteers. Medical students have access to a UC Fitness Center and other campus athletic and recreational facilities. Cincinnati offers many attractions including theaters, restaurants and bars, museums, parks, bookstores, and professional sporting events. University-owned apartments for single and married students are available.

GRADUATES

Of those who graduated in 2005, 34 percent entered residency programs in Cincinnati, 15 percent entered programs elsewhere in Ohio, and the remainder were successful in securing positions nationwide. The most prevalent fields for postgraduate study were internal medicine (all types, 17.2 percent); pediatrics (11.3 percent); psychiatry (10 percent); surgery (7.3 percent); emergency medicine (6.6 percent); family medicine (6.6 percent); and radiology (6.6 percent).

Admissions

REQUIREMENTS

The MCAT is required, and scores should be from within the past three years. (For example, if you are applying for the 2007 entering class, you must submit scores from the 2006, 2005, or 2004 administration). Ohio residents are given preference. Although no courses are specified, applicants are expected to have the knowledge usually gained in a 1 year lecture and laboratory course in biology, general chemistry, organic chemistry, math, and physics. Applicants are expected to have an undergraduate preparation that provides insight into behavioral, social, and cultural issues. Academically, applicants are evaluated based on the following: GPA; MCAT scores; and undergrad, graduate, and post-baccalaureate achievement.

PROCESS

All applicants must submit an AMCAS application and complete the UC secondary online application available at www.med.uc.edu. Approximately 650 applicants are invited to interview. Interviewees attend an informational program, eat lunch, and tour the college. Notification of the Committee's decision occurs on a monthly basis, beginning on October 15 until May 15. After that time, students are accepted from the alternate list as openings occur until the class is filled. The College of Medicine also has a Dual Admissions Program for exceptional high school seniors who know they want to pursue a career in medicine. These 8 year programs are in conjunction with the University of Dayton (JAMS), Miami University, Xavier University, and the University of Cincinnati (Connections). There is also a 9 year Medicine and Engineering Dual Admissions Program (Connections E), which involves five years of undergraduate/ graduate engineering studies at the University of Cincinnati College of Engineering and four years of medical school. The University of Cincinnati College of Medicine and College of Business Administration have partnered to develop a joint-MD/MBA degree program. Students should apply for the program after their first year of medical school. The MD/MBA program is designed for highly qualified students who desire to complement standard medical training with a greater understanding of the economics, finance, marketing, and management of the health care system. Graduates of the combined degree program will have expanded career options, including management positions in major health care organizations. The College of Medicine has an NIH funded Medical Scientist Training Program (MD/PhD). The program is seven to eight years in length. Students applying to the program should have considerable research as an undergraduate and demonstrate excellence in their academic record.

Admissions Requirements (Required)

MCAT scores, science GPA, non-science GPA, letters of recommendation, interview.

Admissions Requirements (Optional)

State residency, essays/personal statement, extracurricular activities, exposure to medical profession, optional experiences are strongly encouraged.

COSTS AND AID

Tuition & Fees

In-state Tuition	$22,452
Out-of-state Tuition	$39,876
Room and board (on campus)	$15,191
Room and board (off campus)	$15,391
Cost of books	$3,016
Fees	$1,128

Financial Aid

% students receiving aid	89
Average grant	$11,000
Average loan	$13,000
Average debt	$119,355

UNIVERSITY OF COLORADO
SCHOOL OF MEDICINE

MEDICAL SCHOOL ADMISSIONS, 4200 EAST NINTH AVENUE, C-297, DENVER, CO 80262 • **ADMISSION:** 303-315-7361
FAX: 303-315-1614 • **E-MAIL:** SOMADMIN@UCHSC.EDU • **WEBSITE:** WWW.UCHSC.EDU/SOM/ADMISSIONS

STUDENT BODY

Type	Public
Enrollment	547
% male/female	54/46
% underrepresented minorities	15
# applied (total/out)	2,526/1,943
# accepted (total/out)	246/105
# enrolled (total/out)	156/35
Average age	24

FACULTY

Total faculty (number)	1,375

ADMISSIONS

Average GPA and MCAT Scores

Overall GPA	3.68
MCAT Bio	10.95
MCAT Phys	10.61
MCAT Verbal	10.3
MCAT Essay	P

Application Information

Regular application	11/1
Regular notification	rolling
Are transfers accepted?	no
Admissions may be deferred?	yes
Interview required?	yes
Application fee	$100

Academics

The School of Medicine is part of the University of Colorado at Denver and Health Sciences Center, which includes the schools of dentistry, nursing, pharmacy, and the graduate school. A combined MD/PhD program through the MSTP is available in the following fields: Biochemistry, cell biology, immunology, molecular biology, microbiology, pharmacology, and physiology. A Rural Track was instituted in 2005 with foundation funding. The academic training for the 12 students in the Rural Track in each class is the same as for the rest of the students, but those in the track commit to spending the summer after first year in a one-on-one rural preceptorship. The entire HSC campus—the health professional schools, the University of Colorado Hospital, the Children's Hospital of Denver, and the Denver Veterans' Administration hospital—will be moving to the new 210 acres Fitzsimons campus in Aurora, Colorado in 2007. The Fitzsimons campus is 11 miles from the Denver International Airport.

BASIC SCIENCES: The curriculum was revised beginning with the 2005 entering class. The first two years—now called Phases 1 and 2—are taught in systems blocks. The blocks in the first phase are human body (9 weeks), molecules to medicine (9 weeks), disease and defense and blood and lymph (taught simultaneously, 10 weeks), and cardiovascular, pulmonary, renal (11 weeks). Foundations of doctoring, which places each student in a one-on-one mentoring relationship with a community physician, begins at the start of the first year and continues for three years. The summer between Phases 1 and 2 is free though many students remain on campus to do research. The Phase 2 blocks are nervous system (9 weeks), metabolism (9 weeks), and life cycle and infectious disease (taught simultaneously, 10 weeks). Phase 2 ends in mid-March and the core clinical year (Phase 3) starts in mid-April of the second year. In Phases 1 and 2 students spend about 24 hours per week in class with 60 percent of the time spent in lectures and 40 percent in laboratory, PBL, or small group. Academic tutoring and counseling are available through the Student Affairs Office. Grading is honors/pass/fail. Student must pass USMLE 1 to begin the clinical years.

CLINICAL TRAINING

The 48 week core clinical year (Phase 3) has six eight weeks blocks: Care of the hospitalized patient; operative and perioperative care; mental health and neurologic care; women and newborn and urgent care; infant, child, and adolescent care and musculoskeletal disease; ambulatory primary care of the adult; and rural and community care. The core affiliated hospitals are University Hospital, Denver Health, the VA Hospital, Denver Children's Hospital, and the National Jewish Center for Immunology and Respiratory Medicine. Several other metro Denver hospitals—including Rose Medical Center and Presbyterian/St. Luke's Medical Center—are also used as clinical sites. All Phase 3 rotations are taken in Colorado with students encouraged to take at least one rotation outside of metro Denver. Phase 4, the advanced studies year, runs from May of the third year until graduation and includes a 4 week intensive care requirement, a capstone scientific block of 4 to 6 weeks, as well as 32 weeks of electives. Electives may be taken in Colorado or out-of-state. Approximately 40 percent of the senior class takes at least one elective overseas. Denver is a large metropolitan area of more than 2 million with access to four season outdoor activities. Evaluation during the clinical years is honors/pass/fail with narratives from all clinical rotations. There are a large number of elective opportunities for students in all four years involving the care of Denver's homeless, low-income, and uninsured populations. Passing both parts of USMLE 2 is required for graduation.

Students

Approximately 75 percent of the students are Colorado residents. Students from Montana and Wyoming are considered in-state as applicants through the WICHE program. Science and nonscience majors are equally represented. Of the 2005 entering class, 14 percent are from groups underrepresented in American medicine. The median age in the 2005 entering class was 24.5. The class size for 2006 is 156.

STUDENT LIFE

Denver is a comfortable, affordable, and student-friendly place to live. It is less than an hour from perhaps the best skiing in the country. During the summer, the hiking, swimming, climbing, and mountain biking are all outstanding. Single students live off campus in apartments and shared houses. Married students can find affordable family housing in various Denver neighborhoods. On-campus activities include student-run organizations and events having either a professional or social focus. The Office of Diversity provides support for minority students.

GRADUATES

The most popular residency programs of the 2005 graduating class were internal medicine (28 students), family medicine (17), pediatrics (14), anesthesiology (12), emergency medicine (8), ob/gyn (8), psychiatry (7), orthopedics (6), and radiology (6). More than half of the graduates entered primary care fields. Approximately half of the graduates remain in Colorado for their residencies with the remainder of the class matching across the country.

Admissions

REQUIREMENTS

Required courses are English literature and English composition or creative writing (9 hours), biology with lab (8 hours), chemistry with lab (8 hours), organic chemistry with lab (8 hours), physics with lab (8 hours), and college mathematics (6 hours). Applicants must demonstrate mathematics competency at least through college-level trigonometry, either with college courses or placement test results. The MCAT is required and, if retaken, the best scores are used.

SUGGESTIONS

In addition to required courses, a course in biochemistry is recommended. For applicants who have been out of school for a significant period of time, recent course work is suggested. Personal qualities are valued a great deal, as are extracurricular activities that involve medical research or health-related experience. As part of the generalist initiative, applicants from rural backgrounds are encouraged to apply.

PROCESS

All AMCAS applicants receive secondary applications. Of Colorado, Montana, and Wyoming residents applying, 60 percent are interviewed. Approximately 20 percent of applicants from the other 47 states are interviewed. Interviews are on campus from September through March and consist of two one-on-one interviews with members of the Admissions Committee. The Admissions Committee is made up of students, faculty, and community physicians. Notification occurs on a rolling basis. In 2006 there were more than 2,700 applicants with 570 applicants interviewed. Forty percent of the interviewed applicants received an offer of admission.

Admissions Requirements (Required)

MCAT scores, science GPA, non-science GPA, letters of recommendation, interview, state residency, essays/personal statement, extracurricular activities, exposure to medical profession.

COSTS AND AID

Tuition & Fees

In-state Tuition	$20,718
Out-of-state Tuition	$72,291
Cost of books	$1,810
Fees	$1,300

Financial Aid

% students receiving aid	94
Average grant	$5,000
Average loan	$28,000
Average debt	$92,000

University of Connecticut

School of Medicine

Medical Student Affairs, 263 Farmington Avenue, Rm AG-062, Farmington, CT 06030-1905
Admission: 860-679-3874 • Fax: 860-679-1282 • E-mail: sanford@nso1.uchc.edu • Website: www.uchc.edu

STUDENT BODY

Type	Public
Enrollment	313
% male/female	37/63
% underrepresented minorities	33
# applied (total/out)	2,685/2,105
# accepted (total/out)	193/85
# enrolled (total/out)	79/19
Average age	24

FACULTY

Total faculty (number)	539
% female	34
% minority	4
% part-time	20
Student-faculty ratio	1:1

ADMISSIONS

Average GPA and MCAT Scores

Overall GPA	3.66
MCAT Bio	10.6
MCAT Phys	10.3
MCAT Verbal	9.8
MCAT Essay	Q

Application Information

Regular application	12/15
Regular notification	10/15
Early application	6/1–8/1
Early notification	10/1
Are transfers accepted?	yes
Admissions may be deferred?	yes
Interview required?	yes
Application fee	$75

Academics

In addition to the required courses, about 75 percent of students take part in a research project while in school. Grading is strictly pass/fail, based on the notion that each student is at the top of the class with regard to some important feature or skill or ability. A combined-degree program, leading to both an MD and a PhD is pursued by about five students each year in conjunction with the following graduate programs: Cell biology, cellular and molecular pharmacology, craniofacial and oral biology, genetics and developmental biology, immunology, molecular biology and biochemistry, neuroscience, and skeletal. It is also possible for medical students to earn a MPH or MBA from the University of Connecticut's graduate program.

BASIC SCIENCES: The first two years cover the basic sciences, introduce clinical studies, and integrate behavioral and social aspects of medicine and health care. Instruction uses lectures, labs, case conferences, and problem-based learning. First-year courses are human systems, which is composed of human biology; organ systems I (neuroscience and anatomy of the head and neck); organ systems II (cardiovascular, respiratory and renal systems, anatomy of the thorax, and abdomen); and organ system III (gastrointestinal, endocrine and reproductive, genetics, and anatomy of the pelvis); electives; correlated medical problem solving; and principles of clinical medicine, which teaches history-taking, the physical examination, and general concepts related to clinical care. Second-year courses are human development and health, which encompasses ethical, social, and legal issues; mechanisms of disease, which includes concepts related to pathology; pharmacology; infectious disease; homeostasis; oncology; metabolism; nervous system; reproductive system; and skin, connective tissue, and joints; correlated medical problem solving; and clinical medicine. Facilities include modern lecture halls, classrooms for small-group discussions, the Lyman Maynard Stowe Library, and computer resources. Passing the USMLE Step 1 is a requirement for promotion to year 3.

CLINICAL TRAINING

The third year is organized into two segments, one that involves clinical training in ambulatory settings, and the other that takes place in hospitals. The ambulatory experience is composed of the following clerkships: General internal medicine (7 weeks), family medicine (7 weeks), pediatrics (5 weeks), ob/gyn (4 weeks), subspecialties (3 weeks), and psychiatry (2 weeks). The hospital, or inpatient, segment includes rotations in medicine (4 weeks); surgery (4 weeks); pediatrics (2 weeks); psychiatry (2 weeks); obstetrics (2 weeks); and beginning to end (2 weeks), in which students follow patients from their admittance to each diagnosis/service area that they visit in the hospital. The fourth year includes 20 weeks of electives, which may be taken at local or distant sites. Other fourth-year requirements are advanced inpatient experience (4 weeks); critical care experience (4 weeks); emergency/urgent experience (4 weeks); and selectives, in which students choose from rotations in research, community health, or education-related fields. Each student is paired with a faculty member of his or her choice to assist in scheduling electives and in selecting postgraduate training programs. Clinical training takes place at the University Hospital (232 beds) and at about 10 affiliated hospitals in the area. Some students gain clinical experience overseas by participating in projects in Latin America, Asia, or Africa. Passing the USMLE Step 2 is a requirement for graduation.

Students

Underrepresented minorities, mostly African American, comprise about 15 percent of the student body. The average age of incoming students is typically about 24, with ages ranging from 21 to late thirties. About 80 percent of the students are Connecticut residents, and about 10 percent graduated from the University of Connecticut undergraduate college. Approximately 80 percent of students majored in a scientific discipline in college. Class size is about 80. Dental students participate in the basic sciences classes.

STUDENT LIFE

Life outside the classroom includes theater, concerts, and restaurants in Hartford; organized team sports on campus; and numerous clubs and groups related to professional or extracurricular interests. The Department of Health Career Opportunities provides support services throughout the academic year to minority medical students. Community-service activities, such as volunteering at homeless shelters, bring students together around important projects. Facilities such as golf courses, ski slopes, and public parks are accessible to the campus. On-campus housing is not available. Students live off campus in communities surrounding the university.

GRADUATES

Of the class that graduated in 2004, the breakdown of the most prevalent specialty choices was internal medicine (22 percent), emergency medicine (13 percent), pediatrics (10 percent), and ob/gyn (9 percent). About 24 percent of graduates entered residency programs at the University of Connecticut Health Center. Other popular destinations were Massachusetts, New York, North Carolina, and California.

Admissions

REQUIREMENTS

Requirements are 1 year of biology, chemistry, organic chemistry, physics. The MCAT is required and should be no more than three years old.

SUGGESTIONS

A broad and in-depth liberal arts education that includes art, English, foreign language, history, literature, math, and political science is advised. The Admissions Committee looks very seriously at the nonacademic traits of applicants, such as their character and motivation.

PROCESS

All AMCAS applicants are sent secondary applications. About 60 percent of Connecticut applicants, and about 9 percent of out-of-state applicants are interviewed. Interviews are held from August through April and consist of two 1-hour sessions with faculty, administrators, or students. Lunch and a campus tour with medical students are provided. Some candidates are accepted shortly after their interview, while others are notified later in the year. A wait list is established in the spring. Wait-listed candidates may send supplementary information, such as transcripts.

Admissions Requirements (Required)

MCAT scores, science GPA, non-science GPA, letters of recommendation, interview, essays/personal statement, extracurricular activities, exposure to medical profession.

Admissions Requirements (Optional)

State residency.

COSTS AND AID

Tuition & Fees

In-state Tuition	$15,870
Out-of-state Tuition	$36,110
Room and board (off campus)	$18,850
Cost of books	$2,055
Fees	$6,670

Financial Aid

% students receiving aid	98
Average grant	$14,000
Average loan	$25,000
Average debt	$93,500

University of Florida

College of Medicine

PO Box 100216, J. Hillis Miller Health Center, 1600 Southwest Archer Road, Gainesville, FL 32610-0216
Admission: 352-392-4569 • Fax: 352-846-0622 • E-mail: ADMISSIONS@MAIL.MED.UFL.EDU • Website: WWW.MED.UFL.EDU

STUDENT BODY

Type	Public
Enrollment	458
% male/female	49/51
% underrepresented minorities	16
# applied (total/out)	20,079/874
# accepted (total)	197
# enrolled (total/out)	120/135
Average age	22

FACULTY

Total faculty (number)	1,020
% part-time	2

ADMISSIONS

Average GPA and MCAT Scores

Overall GPA	3.7
MCAT Bio	10.77
MCAT Phys	10.59
MCAT Verbal	9.89
MCAT Essay	P

Application Information

Regular application	12/1
Regular notification	rolling
Are transfers accepted?	yes
Admissions may be deferred?	yes
Interview required?	yes
Application fee	$30

Academics

Students may pursue their own interests with specialized institutes and centers, such as the Health Policy Institute, the Center for Mammalian Genetics, and the Brain and Cancer Institutes. Students with an interest in public health are encouraged to pursue the MPH degree in conjunction with other academic institutions. Grading uses an A–F scale, and a ranking system. Both steps of the USMLE are required for graduation.

BASIC SCIENCES: Instructional methods include lectures, labs, and small-group sessions that together occupy 25 hours per week or less. First-year basic science courses are anatomy, biochemistry, cell and tissue biology, genetics, neuroscience, physiology, and radiology. Integrated into basic sciences are behavioral sciences, ethical issues, and clinical training. Examples of first-year courses in these areas are essentials of patient care, keeping families healthy, human behavior, and the preceptor program. Second-year courses are clinical diagnosis, clinical radiology, microbiology, oncology, pathology, pharmacology, physical diagnosis, public health, and social and ethical issues in medical practice. Classrooms, labs, and the library are in one complex. A satellite library also operates in Jacksonville.

CLINICAL TRAINING

Required third-year rotations are interdisciplinary generalist clerkships (10 weeks), medicine (8 weeks), surgery (8 weeks), pediatrics (8 weeks), psychiatry (6 weeks), ob/gyn (6 weeks), and neurology (2 weeks). Fourth-year clerkships are advanced surgery (4 weeks); advanced medicine, pediatrics, or family medicine (4 weeks); clinical pharmacology (4 weeks); and electives (28 weeks). The primary teaching hospitals are Shands Hospital (576 beds), the Gainesville Veterans Affairs Medical Center (403 beds), and the University Medical Center (528 beds). Training also takes place at outpatient clinics in nearby communities and at clinical research facilities. Educational affiliations have been established in Tallahassee, Pensacola, Jacksonville, Leesburg, Broward County, and Orlando. With approval, up to 3 months of elective credits may be earned at other institutions around the country and overseas. Outside of formal rotations, students gain clinical experience through outreach projects such as camps for sick kids and care for the homeless.

Students

About 99 percent of the students are Florida residents. Underrepresented minorities account for 11 percent of the student body, and students who have taken time off after college make up at least one-fourth of each entering class. Class size is 120.

STUDENT LIFE

Popular extracurricular activities include viewing intercollegiate sports, taking part in outdoor activities made possible by the year-round temperate climate, and occasionally going out at night to restaurants, clubs, and theaters. The university has an active student union with a theater, pool tables, a bowling alley, and a cafeteria. Athletic facilities, including a student gym, are expansive and are well-used by medical students. Outside of the classroom, students get to know each other through involvement with organizations and projects. A few examples of the numerous medical student organizations are Physicians for Social Responsibility, the Christian Medical and Dental Group, and the Family Practice Student Organization. Service projects such as the School of Medicine Outreach to Rural Students (SMORS) and the Equal Access Clinic improve students' interactive skills and give them the opportunity to contribute to their community. There are numerous groups that devote time each year on medical missions to underserved countries.

GRADUATES

There are about 6,500 graduates of the College of Medicine, a number of whom are renowned for important contributions made in their respective fields. At University of Florida-affiliated hospitals there are 56 postgraduate programs. Many of the positions in these programs are filled by graduates of the College of Medicine.

Admissions

REQUIREMENTS

Requirements are biology (8 hours), physics (8 hours), chemistry (8 hours), organic chemistry (4 hours), and biochemistry (4 hours). The MCAT is required and scores must be no more than three years old from the date of expected matriculation. Generally, the best set of scores is looked at most closely.

SUGGESTIONS

Early submission, preferably by June, of the AMCAS application is advised. No undergraduate major is preferred, and science and nonscience majors are considered equally. Course work in biochemistry, genetics, and microbiology, and statistics is useful. Although there is no math requirement, there is an assumption that math up through calculus was taken as an undergraduate prerequisite for chemistry. Extracurricular activities, non-medically related community service, and health care experience and research are important as well.

PROCESS

Typically, the college receives 2,000 AMCAS applications for 120 available spaces. About 1,000 of the AMCAS applicants receive secondary applications, and about 300 of those returning secondaries are invited to interview. Interviews are held on Fridays from September through March and consist of two sessions with faculty members. On interview day, candidates also receive lunch and tours. Interview notification occurs on a rolling basis. After their interview, applicants are either accepted, rejected, or put on hold for a later decision. In April, an alternate list is established. Additional material, and updates, may be submitted by wait-listed candidates. There are the two following routes of admission to the College of Medicine: Junior honors (12 places) and regular admissions (120 places). To apply for the Junior Honors Program, students apply directly to the College of Medicine during their sophomore year of college. If accepted to the program, they complete a special series of seminars at the University of Florida during their junior year and begin medical school after the completion of their junior year. For Junior Honors, call 352-392-4569.

Admissions Requirements (Required)

MCAT scores, science GPA, non-science GPA, letters of recommendation, interview, state residency, essays/personal statement, extracurricular activities, exposure to medical profession, community service.

COSTS AND AID

Tuition & Fees

In-state Tuition	$15,666
Out-of-state Tuition	$45,092
Room and board (on campus)	$8,630
Room and board (off campus)	$9,250
Cost of books	$2,665
In-state Fees	$1,861
Out-of-state Fees	$3,332

Financial Aid

% students receiving aid	89
Average grant	$1,425
Average loan	$23,352
Average debt	$96,000

UNIVERSITY OF HAWAII
JOHN A. BURNS SCHOOL OF MEDICINE (JABSOM)

651 ILALO STREET, HONOLULU, HI 96813 • **ADMISSION:** 808-692-1000
FAX: 808-692-1251 • **E-MAIL:** MNISHIKI@HAWAII.EDU • **WEBSITE:** HTTP://JABSOM.HAWAII.EDU

STUDENT BODY

Type	Public
Enrollment	260
% male/female	40/60
% underrepresented minorities	17
# applied (total/out)	1,629/1,363
# enrolled	62
Average age	24

FACULTY

Total faculty (number)	458
% female	23
% minority	15
% part-time	51
Student-faculty ratio	1:1

ADMISSIONS

Average GPA and MCAT Scores

Overall GPA	3.6
MCAT Bio	10.0
MCAT Phys	10.0
MCAT Verbal	9.0
MCAT Essay	O

Application Information

Regular application	11/1
Regular notification	10/15
Early application	6/1–8/1
Early notification	10/1
Are transfers accepted?	yes
Admissions may be deferred?	yes
Interview required?	yes
Application fee	$50

Academics

The School of Medicine, along with the Schools of Nursing and Social Work, comprise the College of Health Sciences and Social Welfare. JABSOM offers an MD program.

BASIC SCIENCES: Throughout the first two years, instruction is entirely case-based and emphasizes self-directed learning and early clinical training. Other subjects are organized into units, each occupying 12 to 14 weeks. Unit 1 courses are health and illness and introduction to problem-based learning. Unit 2 focuses on cardiovascular, renal problems, and respiratory. Unit 3 is hematology, endocrine, and gastrointestinal problems. During the Summer following year 1, students take part in a primary care precept, which entails working with local physicians. Unit 4 is locomoter, neurologic, and behavioral problems. Unit 5 is life cycle problems in ob/gyn, pediatrics, adolescents, and geriatrics. The final three months of year 2 are used for a basic science review in preparation for the USMLE Step 1, which is required for promotion to year 3. Scheduled classes during the first two years occupy about 20 hours per week, providing ample time for independent, self-directed study. Grading is pass/fail, and students are not ranked. The Medical Education Building, where basic sciences are taught, is equipped with laboratories, audiovisual computer centers, classrooms, a library, and areas for group study and tutorials. The University Library System has the largest collection of information and research materials in the state and includes the Hamilton Library (85,000 volumes), which serves the School of Medicine.

CLINICAL TRAINING

Pre-clinical training instruction in the various basic science disciplines is integrated into the problem-based learning experience as well as provided through a basic science foundation lecture and laboratory series.

In the spring of 2005, the medical school moved to a new campus near the heart of Honolulu. This new campus provides new classrooms and study space, a biomedical sciences library, a modern educational simulation center, and a standardized patient learning and testing center. The campus includes new research laboratories that will serve as the anchor for a biotechnology park.

Clinical Training: Most students enter block rotations, referred to as Unit 6B. For these students, third-year clerkships are internal medicine (11 weeks), surgery (7 weeks), family medicine (7 weeks), ob/gyn (7 weeks), pediatrics (7 weeks), and psychiatry (7 weeks). Two weeks during year 3 are reserved for an elective. As an alternative to the standard block system, Unit 6L is a longitudinal clerkship that provides selected students an opportunity to spend half of their year in a community-based, integrated ambulatory care experience, and half of their year in hospital-based mini-blocks. Year 4, Unit 7, is reserved for electives with the exception of two required rotations in emergency medicine (4 weeks). The final month of the 4 year curriculum is for a senior seminar series, which provides an in-depth review of important topics designed specifically to help prepare graduates for their transition to residency training. Grading is honors/credit/no credit during the third year, and pass/fail during the fourth year. Students must pass the USMLE Steps 1 and 2 to graduate. Training takes place at many sites including The Queen's Medical Center, Kapiiolani Medical Center for Women and Children, St. Francis Medical Center, Tripler Army Medical Center, Hilo Family Medical Center, Hilo Medical Center, Kuakini Medical Center, Shriners Hospital, Kaiser Medical Center, Wahiawa General Hospital, Waiianae Coast Health Center, Kalihi-Palama Health Center, and the Rehabilitation Hospital of the Pacific.

Students

Hawaii's multi-ethnic population is reflected in the student body, made up of men and women of Caucasian, Chinese, Korean, Japanese, Hawaiian, Filipino, Samoan, Micronesian, and other ancestries. Class size is 62. Graduate residency programs in Hawaii include the following specialties: Family practice, internal medicine, ob/gyn, orthopedics, pathology, pediatrics, psychiatry, surgery, and transitional. Forty percent of graduates are in the military service, and 1 percent are in full-time academic positions.

STUDENT LIFE

Although the School of Medicine is relatively small and intimate, the University of Hawaii at Manoa enrolls approximately 17,000 students. Medical students take part in campus activities but are integrated into the greater community of the city of Honolulu and the island of Oahu. Almost all students live off campus. Honolulu is a city with a population of about 1 million. It is a major tourist center, offering beautiful beaches in addition to many cultural, recreational, and outdoor activities.

GRADUATES

Residency programs in Hawaii are popular with graduates and include the following specialties: Family practice, internal medicine, ob/gyn, orthopedics, pathology, pediatrics, psychiatry, surgery, and transitional.

Admissions

REQUIREMENTS

The initial screening of applicants selects those who have close ties to Hawaii and who are most likely to practice in Hawaii and in the Pacific upon completion of postgraduate study. An exception is made for applicants from Wyoming and Montana, states without medical schools that belong to WICHE (Western Interstate Commission on Higher Education). Undergraduate course requirements are physics (8 units), biology (12-semester units, including at least 4 of cell and molecular biology), chemistry (4 units), and biochemistry (3 units). All courses except biochemistry must include laboratory experience. The MCAT is required and must be no more than three years old. If the MCAT has been taken more than once, the most recent set of scores is used.

SUGGESTIONS

Additional courses in biological and social science are advised, such as anatomy, embryology, genetics, immunology, microbiology, physiology, psychology, and sociology. Previous medical experience is important, as are personal qualities that suggest the applicant will become a humanistic physician. For those who have been out of school for a significant period of time, recent course work is recommended. Each year, a post-baccalaureate program selects 10 students who are promising students for medical school. If these students complete successfully the year-long premedical training, they are offered a position in the subsequent incoming class of medical students.

PROCESS

Annually, about 15–20 percent of applicants are interviewed. Interviews are conducted from October through March and consist of two sessions with faculty members, practicing physicians, fourth-year medical students, or members of the community. Of those interviewed, about 9 percent of in-state applicants and 10 percent of out-of-state residents are accepted. Most applicants are notified of the committee's decision in late April, though a few highly qualified applicants may hear earlier. A wait list is established at this time. Wait-listed candidates are not advised to send supplementary information.

Admissions Requirements (Required)

MCAT scores, science GPA, non-science GPA, letters of recommendation, interview, essays/personal statement.

Admissions Requirements (Optional)

State residency, extracurricular activities, exposure to medical profession.

COSTS AND AID

Tuition & Fees

In-state Tuition	$18,446
Out-of-state Tuition	$35,064
Cost of books	$2,128

Financial Aid

Average grant	$6,545
Average loan	$12,561

University of Illinois at Chicago
UIC College of Medicine

808 South Wood Street, Room 165 CME, M/C 783 Chicago, IL 60612 • **Admission:** 312-996-5635
Fax: 312-996-6693 • **E-mail:** MEDADMIT@UIC.EDU • **Website:** WWW.MEDICINE.UIC.EDU

STUDENT BODY	
Type	Public
Enrollment	1,242
% male/female	59/41
% underrepresented minorities	21
# applied (total/out)	3,925/2,405
# accepted (total/out)	560/39
# enrolled (total/out)	317/20
Average age	22

ADMISSIONS

Average GPA and MCAT Scores

Overall GPA	3.5
MCAT Bio	9.6
MCAT Phys	9.4
MCAT Verbal	9
MCAT Essay	Q

Application Information

Regular application	12/31
Regular notification	6/1
Early application	6/1–8/1
Early notification	10/1
Are transfers accepted?	yes
Admissions may be deferred?	yes
Interview required?	yes
Application fee	$40

Academics

Students participate in one of the following two educational tracks: 175 students complete all four years in Chicago, while 125 spend their first year in Urbana-Champaign. After the first year in Urbana-Champaign, 50 students each complete years 2, 3, and 4 in Peoria or Rockford. The remaining 25 students in Urbana-Champaign participate in the Medical Scholars Program.

BASIC SCIENCES: The first and second years include behavioral science, biochemistry, genetics, histology, immunology, microbiology, neuroscience, pathology, pathophysiology, pharmacology, physiology, and the principles of anatomy. All students participate in a clinical medicine course. Lectures and labs are the predominant instructional modality.

CLINICAL TRAINING

Patient contact begins in the first year when students are assigned individual physician preceptors. Students sharpen their skills in diagnosis and treatment through problem solving sessions. In the third and fourth years, students focus on patient care with a series of clerkships supplemented by conferences and lectures. The 25 affiliated facilities range from rural ambulatory health care centers to major metropolitan hospitals. The diverse clinical experiences prepare UIC graduates to succeed within the nation's ever-changing health care system. Required clerkships include family medicine, internal medicine, obstetrics/gynecology, pediatrics, psychiatry, and surgery. The elective phase provides students with the opportunity to identify special interest areas and to select educational experiences most relevant to their goals. The objective of the MD/PhD program is to train students for careers in academic medicine and research. The Medical Scholars Program (MSP), located on the Urbana-Champaign campus, permits students to integrate medicine with graduate studies in both science and nonscience fields. The Independent Study Program (ISP) allows students to design their own academic programs with advice from faculty. ISP students complete an in-depth study, usually involving the basic sciences or clinical medicine. The ISP program is offered on the Chicago, Peoria, and Rockford campuses. The Rural Medical Education Program (RMED) and Rural Illinois Medical Student Assistance Program (RIMSAP) recruit students who commit to practice in medically underserved areas of Illinois.

Students

UIC is one of the most ethnically diverse medical schools in the country. Students are assigned to a faculty member who serves as an advisor. The advisor's major role is to be available to the student throughout his or her medical education for academic and personal counseling. Research interests are widely diversified and range from basic molecular biology to patient-related clinical research.

STUDENT LIFE

Students in Chicago enjoy living in one of the country's most exciting cities. In Urbana-Champaign, students benefit from a large and exciting university community. Rockford and Peoria are mid-size cities, offering all students basic urban amenities. Campus housing in Chicago includes three residence halls near the college. In Urbana-Champaign, university-certified housing includes campus and private residence halls and university apartments for family housing. In Peoria and Rockford housing is easily accessible and reasonable.

GRADUATES

UIC students undertake career specialization and training in all disciplines. Most graduates who participate in the National Residency Matching Program receive one of their top three residency choices.

Admissions

REQUIREMENTS

Only those applicants who indicate plans to obtain a baccalaureate degree prior to enrollment will be considered for admission. Major fields may be in behavioral, biological, humanities, or physical sciences. All applicants must complete: two semesters of introductory biology or the equivalent with laboratory; two semesters of general inorganic chemistry or the equivalent with laboratory; two semesters of organic chemistry with laboratory (introductory biochemistry may substitute for one semester of organic chemistry); and two semesters of general physics or the equivalent. All applicants are expected to complete three semesters of social science courses with an emphasis in the behavioral sciences. In addition, candidates are expected to take at least one of the following courses: advanced-level biology, biochemistry, comparative vertebrate anatomy, mammalian histology, molecular genetics, and physiology. All applicants must take the MCAT no later than the fall of the year prior to enrollment and no more than three years prior to application. All applicants must complete an application to the AMCAS no later than December 31 of the year prior to enrollment. All applicants must be U.S. citizens or possess a permanent resident immigrant visa at the time of application through AMCAS. On receipt of the AMCAS application, eligible applicants will be sent a UIC Supplemental Application. Materials must be postmarked by February 15 of the year prior to enrollment. A minimum of three academic letters of recommendation or one composite recommendation from a pre-professional committee must be postmarked by February 15 of the year prior to enrollment. If you are currently enrolled in a graduate or professional school, one of your three letters of recommendation must be from a faculty member at your graduate or professional school. It is advisable that letters of recommendation be sent from the institution at which the applicant had been most recently enrolled and must be completed on official university or business letterhead. Personal letters of recommendation are not acceptable.

SUGGESTIONS

At least 90 percent of UIC students are Illinois residents. Although Illinois residents are given preference, positions are open to highly qualified nonresidents. In addition to academic strength, experience, and background are considered important factors in admissions decisions.

PROCESS

About one-third of AMCAS applicants are sent a UIC Supplementary Application. Of those returning supplementals, the most highly qualified are invited to interview between September and April. The interview is a requirement and will be arranged by the Office of Medical College Admissions. Interviews are granted by invitation only. Interviews are held on all four campuses, and the interview location does not determine the campus where matriculants may attend. The interview consists of one panel interview session. Candidates have the opportunity to meet faculty members and students, receive financial aid information, tour the campus, and learn more about the College of Medicine. Interviewed candidates are accepted on a batch system. Students not immediately accepted may be put on an alternate list.

Admissions Requirements (Required)

MCAT scores, science GPA, non-science GPA, letters of recommendation, interview, state residency, essays/personal statement.

Admissions Requirements (Optional)

Extracurricular activities, exposure to medical profession.

Overlap Schools

Loyola University Chicago; Northwestern University; Rush Medical College of Rush University; Southern Illinois University—Carbondale; The University of Chicago.

COSTS AND AID

Tuition & Fees

Cost of books $1,280

UNIVERSITY OF IOWA
ROY J. AND LUCILLE A. CARVER COLLEGE OF MEDICINE

100 MEDICINE ADMINISTRATION BUILDING, IOWA CITY, IA 52242 • ADMISSION: 319-335-8052 • FAX: 319-335-8049
E-MAIL: MEDICAL-ADMISSION@UIOWA.EDU • WEBSITE: WWW.MEDICINE.UIOWA.EDU/OSAC/ADMISSIONS/

STUDENT BODY

Type	Public
Enrollment	562
% male/female	53/47
% underrepresented minorities	25
# applied (total/out)	2,513/2,176
# accepted (total/out)	300/170
# enrolled (total/out)	142/40
Average age	24

ADMISSIONS

Average GPA and MCAT Scores

Overall GPA	3.72
MCAT Bio	10.6
MCAT Phys	10.2
MCAT Verbal	9.9
MCAT Essay	P

Application Information

Regular application	11/1
Regular notification	rolling
Early application	6/1–8/1
Early notification	10/1
Are transfers accepted?	no
Admissions may be deferred?	yes
Interview required?	yes
Application fee	$50

Academics

Most students at Iowa follow a 4 year course of study, leading to the MD. About 5 percent of students are MSTP participants, earning a PhD concurrently with the MD. The doctorate degree may be earned in anatomy, biochemistry, microbiology, pharmacology, and physiology and biophysics, among other fields. Other joint-degree programs, such as those leading to a master's degree along with the MD, are also possible. Medical students are evaluated with honors/pass/fail for all courses except electives, which are pass/fail. Although the first two years are primarily devoted to basic sciences, introductory clinical training is also an important part of the curriculum. The second two years are devoted to clinical rotations.

BASIC SCIENCES: First-year courses are the following: Biochemistry; cell biology; foundations of clinical practice, which continues through the second year; gross anatomy; immunology; medical genetics; neuroscience; and structure and functions of human organ systems. Foundations of clinical practice covers topics ranging from biomedical ethics and problem-based learning to behavioral medicine, human sexuality, continuity of care, and important clinical techniques such as history-taking, the physical examination, and the doctor-patient relationship. The course structure and functions of human organ systems covers principles of histology and physiology and is organized around body/organ systems. After completing their first year, many students spend the summer working and learning in an Iowa community hospital or conducting medical research projects. Second-year courses are pathology, pharmacology, and principles of infectious diseases. Throughout the first two years, students are in lectures, discussions, labs, or tutorials for about 23 hours per week. Basic sciences are taught in the Medical Education and Research Faculty and the Bowen Science Building. The Hardin Library holds more than 200,000 volumes and nearly 3,000 periodicals and is used by students, faculty, and the medical community for research and studying. It also has a multimedia computer classroom and computer-based informational resources.

CLINICAL TRAINING

Third- and fourth-year required core clerkships are the following: Community-based primary care (6 weeks); ob/gyn (6 weeks); pediatrics (6 weeks); and surgery (6 weeks); internal medicine (inpatient, 6 weeks); internal medicine (ambulatory, 3 weeks); family practice (3 weeks). Subspecialty clerkships are neurology (4 weeks); psychiatry (weeks); two weeks of each of the following: Anesthesia, dermatology, electrocardiography and laboratory medicine, ophthalmology, orthopedics, otolaryngology, radiology and urology. Two advanced clerkships and at least 12 weeks of electives are also required. Clinical training takes place at the University Hospital (1,100 beds), the Veterans Affairs Hospital (440 beds), and various sites within the state.

Students

Each entering class has 142 students. About 70 percent of students are Iowa residents. Generally, about 30 undergraduate majors are represented in a class. Approximately percent of students are underrepresented minorities. The majority of students entered medical school one year after college graduation. The Medical Education and Research Facility opened for classes in the Fall of 2001. It also houses four learning communities to which each student is assigned.

STUDENT LIFE

Medical students are active in student organizations, ranging from groups that support minorities to professional interest groups to a medical school band. The learning communities also sponsor activities that encourage peer-to-peer support and mentoring. Each community is staffed by a faculty director and professional and support staff with leadership provided by the elected student representatives. As part of the greater University of Iowa, medical students enjoy its facilities, resources, and sponsored events, such as Big Ten athletics. The UI campus is central to Iowa City and is convenient to restaurants, clubs, theaters, shopping areas, and parks. Although the city has a population of 60,000 people, it is relatively safe and has the feeling of a friendly small town. Just outside of the city are lakes, hiking areas, and other outdoor attractions. Urban centers such as Chicago, St. Louis, Minneapolis, Omaha, and Kansas City are within a 5-hour drive. On campus housing options include coed medical fraternities with both single and double rooms and university-owned family housing. Off-campus, reasonably priced apartments are available.

GRADUATES

Graduates are successful in entering residency programs of their choice. Iowa itself offers postgraduate training programs in about 15 fields.

Admissions

REQUIREMENTS

Prerequisites are 1 year each of advanced biology (1 semester), chemistry, college-level math or statistics, general biology, organic chemistry, and physics. All science courses should include laboratory instruction. The MCAT is required, and scores must be from exams no earlier than April 2001 and no later than August 2006 for the 2007 entering class. All sets of scores are evaluated.

SUGGESTIONS

Though preference is given to Iowa residents, well-qualified nonresidents are also considered. Nonscience majors might benefit from additional science courses beyond requirements; specifically, anatomy, biochemistry, and genetics. Computer literacy, the ability to write well, strong verbal skills, and general decision-making capabilities are some of the skills sought in applicants. Also important are an applicant's personal characteristics, which are evaluated with the help of letters of reference and interviews. Some medically related experience is important.

PROCESS

Iowa participates in the AMCAS process. Most who apply through AMCAS are sent secondary applications. About one-third of Iowa residents who apply are accepted. Of the nonresident applicant pool, about 6 percent are accepted. Applicants are notified on a rolling basis and are either accepted, rejected, or wait listed. Wait-listed candidates are not encouraged to send additional information.

Admissions Requirements (Required)

MCAT scores, science GPA, non-science GPA, letters of recommendation, interview, state residency, essays/personal statement.

COSTS AND AID

Tuition & Fees

In-state Tuition	$19,736
Out-of-state Tuition	$38,942
Cost of books	$3,172

Financial Aid

Average grant	$9,936
Average loan	$23,791
Average debt	$99,812

UNIVERSITY OF KANSAS
SCHOOL OF MEDICINE

3901 RAINBOW BOULEVARD, 3040 MURPHY BUILDING, MAIL STOP 1049, KANSAS CITY, KS 66160 • ADMISSION: 913-588-5245
FAX: 913-588-5259 • E-MAIL: PREMEDINFO@KUMC.EDU • WEBSITE: WWW.KUMC.EDU/SOM/SOM.HTML

STUDENT BODY

Type	Public
Enrollment	700
% male/female	55/45
% underrepresented minorities	14
# applied (total/out)	1,585/1,168
# accepted (total/out)	229/60
# enrolled (total/out)	175/33
Average age	24

FACULTY

Total faculty (number)	658
% female	46
% minority	29
% part-time	18
Student-faculty ratio	1:1

ADMISSIONS

Average GPA and MCAT Scores

Overall GPA	3.66
MCAT Bio	9.8
MCAT Phys	9.2
MCAT Verbal	9.6
MCAT Essay	Q

Application Information

Regular application	10/15
Regular notification	3/31
Early application	7/1
	(recommended)
Early notification	10/1
Are transfers accepted?	yes
Admissions may be deferred?	yes
Interview required?	yes

Academics

In comparison to many medical schools, clinical training at the University of Kansas emphasizes rural and primary health care. Joint-MD/PhD degrees are offered in the following fields: Anatomy and cell biology, biochemistry and molecular biology, microbiology, molecular genetics and toxicology, pathology and oncology, pharmacology, and physiology. A joint-MD/MPH is also offered.

BASIC SCIENCES: Basic sciences are taught in Kansas City. The facilities are modern and fully equipped with learning tools such as computers and visual-aid equipment. The School of Medicine has recently implemented a systemic methodology for teaching basic sciences. Students take part in individual and small-group projects that require initiative and problem-solving skills. First-year students take biochemistry, cell and tissue biology, gross anatomy, introduction to clinical medicine, neuroscience, and physiology. Second-year students take introduction to clinical medicine, microbiology, pathology, and pharmacology. Tutoring is available through the Learning Resources Counseling Service. A student-operated note service, in which students share note-taking, covers regularly scheduled lectures. Students are evaluated using the following descriptions: Superior, high satisfactory, satisfactory, low satisfactory, and unsatisfactory. These marks are translated into numeric scores to determine class rank. The USMLE is required upon completion of year 2. The Dykes Library of the Health Sciences supports the educational and research demands of medical students, faculty, and the public. It contains 150,000 books and offers online informational services. In addition, the Clendening History of Medicine Library has one of the top five collections of rare medical books in the country.

CLINICAL TRAINING

Patient contact begins in year 1, when students take part in biweekly sessions with practicing physicians. Required clinical clerkships are medicine (8 weeks), neuropsychiatry (8 weeks), general surgery (8 weeks), ambulatory medicine/geriatrics (6 weeks), family medicine (6 weeks), ob/gyn (6 weeks), and pediatrics (6 weeks). Year 4 is filled primarily with electives, from which there are many to choose including preventive medicine and the history of medicine. Clinical training takes place both at the University of Kansas Hospital (464 beds), which houses nearly all the diagnostic and treatment facilities of the Medical Center and at hospitals in Wichita. Included at the Medical Center in Kansas City are the Kansas Cancer Institute, the Burnett Burn Center, the Smith Mental Retardation Center, the Center on Aging, and the Center on Environmental and Occupational Health. Patients are drawn from Kansas, Missouri, Oklahoma, Arkansas, and Nebraska. The grading scale is the same for performance in clinical rotations as it for basic science courses. In addition to formal rotations, students gain clinical experience through volunteer activities, like the Mobile Medical Unit, which brings basic prevention and care to communities in need. Many students devote free summers to volunteer in medically related activities.

Students

About 90 percent of a typical class are Kansas residents, and most students have liberal arts backgrounds. In recent years, about 13 percent of the student body have been underrepresented minorities, mostly African and Hispanic Americans. Usually, almost a quarter of matriculants in a given year are older than 25 years of age. Class size is 175.

STUDENT LIFE

Medical students from all four classes are organized into academic societies, which bring students together around academic and extracurricular activities. The Kirmayer Fitness Center is a modern facility open to all medical students. Numerous organized activities enrich the lives of medical students. Activities such as Rural Health Weekend provide opportunities for interaction with practicing physicians throughout the state. Organizations such as the Community Outreach Project provide opportunities for community service. All students live off campus.

GRADUATES

About 50 percent of graduates enter primary care fields. Graduates are successful in obtaining residency positions throughout the country. The medical school sponsors events and scholarships that encourage students and residents to consider practicing in Kansas.

Admissions

REQUIREMENTS

Required college courses are 1 year of biology with lab, chemistry with lab, organic chemistry with lab, physics with lab, 1 year of English, and 1 semester of college-level mathematics. A bachelor's degree is required. Evaluation of GPA is irrespective of where course work was completed. The MCAT is required, with the two most recent sets of scores considered. The August MCAT is acceptable.

SUGGESTIONS

Experience in a health care setting is valued, and the breadth of an applicant's undergraduate course work is important. Demonstrated interests in rural and primary care medicine are pluses. Out-of-state residents should have particularly strong qualifications. A few students each year are accepted from the University of Kansas Post-baccalaureate Program and through the Scholars in Primary Care Program.

PROCESS

All Kansas residents are sent secondary applications, while only about 10 percent of out-of-state applicants receive them. About 75 percent of Kansas residents and about 5 percent of out-of-state applicants are interviewed. Interviews are conducted in Kansas City from October through March and consist of one or two sessions each with one or two members of the interview panel. Approximately one-half of those interviewed are offered positions in the class and are notified on a rolling basis after the interview. The wait list is short, and wait-listed candidates are not encouraged to send supplementary material.

Admissions Requirements (Required)

MCAT scores, science GPA, non-science GPA, letters of recommendation, interview, essays/personal statement, extracurricular activities, exposure to medical profession, secondary app, prerequisite courses, and bachelor's degree.

Admissions Requirements (Optional)

State residency.

COSTS AND AID

Tuition & Fees

In-state Tuition	$18,920
Out-of-state Tuition	$34,674
Room and board (off campus)	$9,018
Cost of books	$3,120
Fees	$438

Financial Aid

% students receiving aid	85
Average grant	$2,500
Average loan	$27,500
Average debt	$90,600

UNIVERSITY OF KENTUCKY
COLLEGE OF MEDICINE

MN118 UKMC, 800 ROSE STREET, LEXINGTON, KY 40536-0298 • ADMISSION: 859-323-6161
FAX: 859-257-3633 • E-MAIL: KYMEDAP@UKY.EDU • WEBSITE: WWW.COMED.UKY.EDU/MEDICINE

STUDENT BODY

Type	Public
Enrollment	400
% male/female	57/43
% underrepresented minorities	6
# applied (total/out)	1,002/635
# enrolled (total/out)	103/17
Average age	23

FACULTY

Student-faculty ratio	1:1

ADMISSIONS

Average GPA and MCAT Scores

Overall GPA	3.64
MCAT Bio	9.9
MCAT Phys	9.7
MCAT Verbal	9.8
MCAT Essay	O

Application Information

Regular application	11/1
Regular notification	rolling
Early application	6/1–8/1
Early notification	10/1
Are transfers accepted?	yes
Admissions may be deferred?	yes
Interview required?	yes
Application fee	$50

Academics

The curriculum includes early patient contact and teaches lifelong learning skills, ethics, and computer-assisted learning along with traditional basic science and clinical techniques. The goal of the medical education program is to focus on principles and the organization of factual bodies of knowledge rather than on unconnected detail. Although most students complete a 4 year curriculum, a few students each year enter a combined MD/PhD program. The doctorate may be earned in anatomy, biochemistry, biophysics, cell biology, genetics, immunology, microbiology, molecular biology, neuroscience, pharmacology, or physiology. Combined MD/MPH and MD/MBA programs are also available. Medical students are evaluated with letter grades and, in some cases, with pass/fail. Passing Step 1 of the USMLE is a requirement for promotion to year 3, and passing Step 2 is a graduation requirement.

BASIC SCIENCES: During the first and second years, students are in class or other scheduled sessions for about 24 hours per week. Lectures and tutorials are the primary instructional methods. Laboratories, hands-on clinical work, and conferences are also important parts of the curriculum. The first year is devoted to basic sciences and interdisciplinary perspectives. The year is organized into blocks, each of which contains 1 or 2 courses. First-year courses are cellular structure and function/biochemistry; cellular structure and function/genetics; healthy human; human function; human structure/gross anatomy; human structure/histology; introduction to the medical profession; neuroscience; patients, physicians, and society. The second year is focused on the disease process and is also broken into blocks. These are immunity, infection, and disease; introduction to the medical profession II; and mechanisms of disease and treatment, which covers pathology and pharmacology; and patients, physicians, and society II. Students spend most of their first two years in the Medical Science Building, which houses classrooms and laboratories. Computers are important educational tools, and all incoming students are required to have their own computers. The College of Medicine has a nationally recognized program of academic computing in medical education, which provides a wide variety of services to enhance student learning. These educational support services are offered in facilities located in the College of Medicine, the Chandler Medical Center, and in the Area Health Education Centers. The library, which contains more than 150,000 volumes, is also an important resource.

CLINICAL TRAINING

Third-year required clerkships are medical and surgical care (16 weeks), principles of primary care (12 weeks), women's maternal and child health (12 weeks), and clinical neuroscience (8 weeks). The fourth year is comprised of a 1 month acting internship selected from medical specialties (family practice, internal medicine, pediatric, neurology, psychiatry, rehabilitation medicine); a 1 month acting internship selected from surgical specialties (general, subspecialty, ob/gyn); a 1 month emergency medicine clerkship; 1 month of a clinical pharmacology and anesthesiology clerkship; and 1 month of a primary care or rural medicine selective. In addition, 8 weeks of electives are required. Training takes place primarily at the University of Kentucky Hospital (473 beds), although a number of affiliated hospitals and clinics are also used.

Students

Approximately 90 percent of students are Kentucky residents. About 6 percent of students are underrepresented minorities, most of whom are African American. Generally, about 25 percent of students in each class are nontraditional, having pursued other careers or interests in between college and medical school.

STUDENT LIFE

Medical students enjoy extracurricular activities associated with the main university such as attending UK basketball games. Student groups provide additional extracurricular activities, including opportunities for involvement in community service projects. They also serve as a means of interacting outside of class. Women in Science and Medicine is a group, comprised primarily of faculty and administrators, focused on improving all aspects of life for women in medicine. Lexington is an attractive and safe city with affordable housing.

GRADUATES

Graduates enter residency programs all over the United States in both primary care and specialty fields. The University of Kentucky has postgraduate training programs in more than 20 fields.

Admissions

REQUIREMENTS

One year each of biology, English, general chemistry, organic chemistry, and physics are required. All science courses should include associated labs. The MCAT is required, and scores should be from within the past two years. For applicants who have taken the exam more than once, the most recent set of scores is weighed most heavily.

SUGGESTIONS

In addition to academic qualifications, UK seeks students who have the character, personality, values, and motivation for human service. Individual initiative and good judgment are important traits. Some medically related experience is important.

PROCESS

All AMCAS applicants who are Kentucky residents are sent secondary applications. Highly-qualified nonresidents are also sent secondaries. About 50 percent of applicants who return secondary applications are invited to interview between September and March. On interview day, candidates also tour the campus, attend group informational sessions, and have the opportunity to meet informally with current students. About 45 percent of interviewed candidates are accepted on a rolling basis. Others are rejected or wait listed. Wait-listed candidates may send additional information to update their files. The admissions process is rolling and the class is typically full by January so early completion of both the primary and the secondary application is strongly recommended.

Admissions Requirements (Required)

MCAT scores, science GPA, non-science GPA, letters of recommendation, interview, exposure to medical profession.

Admissions Requirements (Optional)

State residency, essays/personal statement, extracurricular activities.

Overlap Schools

University of Cincinnati, University of Louisville.

COSTS AND AID

Tuition & Fees

In-state Tuition	$18,342
Out-of-state Tuition	$37,316
Room and board (off campus)	$10,175
Cost of books	$2,475
Fees	$738

Financial Aid

% students receiving aid	95
Average grant	$7,605
Average loan	$28,920
Average debt	$97,170

UNIVERSITY OF LOUISVILLE
SCHOOL OF MEDICINE

ABELL ADMINISTRATION CENTER, RM 413, 323 EAST CHESTNUT STREET, LOUISVILLE, KY 40202
ADMISSION: 502-852-5193 • FAX: 502-852-0302 • E-MAIL: MEDADM@LOUISVILLE.EDU • WEBSITE: WWW.LOUISVILLE.EDU

STUDENT BODY

Type	Public
Enrollment	588
% male/female	56/44
% underrepresented minorities	16
# applied (total/out)	1,660/1,303
# accepted (total/out)	238/69
# enrolled (total/out)	149/29
Average age	23

FACULTY

Total faculty (number)	737
% female	29
% minority	24
% part-time	11

ADMISSIONS

Average GPA and MCAT Scores

Overall GPA	3.6
MCAT Bio	9.48
MCAT Phys	9.48
MCAT Verbal	9.48
MCAT Essay	0

Application Information

Regular application	10/15
Regular notification	rolling
Early application	6/1–8/1
Early notification	10/1
Are transfers accepted?	yes
Admissions may be deferred?	yes
Interview required?	yes
Application fee	$75

Academics

Although most students complete a 4 year program leading to the MD, a few earn a combined MD/PhD, which typically demands about seven years. Summer research scholarships allow first- and second-year students to participate in research projects alongside faculty mentors. Throughout all four years, students work closely with faculty advisers who assist with decisions related to academic and professional goals. Medical students are evaluated as pass/fail in both basic science and clinical courses. Passing Step 1 of the USMLE is a requirement for promotion to year 3, and passing Step 2 is a requirement for graduation.

BASIC SCIENCES: The purpose of the core curriculum, which extends over the 4 year course of study, is to provide each student with the general education and training considered essential to all physicians. It stresses understanding of concepts and general principles instead of superficial knowledge of details. It provides opportunity for correlation among the sciences so that information received in one subject can reinforce ideas and build upon concepts developed in another. The incorporation of clinical correlation into the first two years demonstrates how knowledge of the basic sciences applies directly to the solution of problems with human disease. The core curriculum, for the first 2 academic years, is divided into 4 quarters (one-half semester intervals) of 9 weeks each. Within these smaller subdivisions, it is possible to vary the balance of departmental activities to accommodate a better integrated understanding of the subject matter. The purpose of the Pre-clinical Elective Program is to allow each student to extend his/her education in certain areas of scientific knowledge. The electives make it possible to construct a program of medical education that best meets the needs, abilities, and goals of the individual student. Students also are permitted to take courses as electives in divisions of the University of Louisville other than the School of Medicine, class schedule permitting. In addition to the courses listed, students with a research interest are permitted to participate in an approved research activity for credit. Elective courses constitute an integral part of the student's total program in medical school. Second-year students take two credit hours of elective courses.

CLINICAL TRAINING

Third-year required rotations are internal medicine (10 weeks), basic surgery (8 weeks), ob/gyn (8 weeks), pediatrics (8 weeks), family medicine (6 weeks), psychiatry (6 weeks). Fourth-year requirements are inpatient medicine (4 weeks), inpatient surgery (4 weeks), neurology (4 weeks), AHEC (4 weeks), ambulatory primary care (4 weeks), ambulatory rotation (4 weeks), and perioperative medicine (2 weeks). The remaining 10 weeks in the fourth year are reserved for electives.

Students

In the entering class of 2005, 120 of 149 students were Kentucky residents. African Americans represented 7 percent of the class, and students older than 27 years old represented 7 percent of the class.

STUDENT LIFE

Students profit from the school's location in the center of Louisville. Louisville is the largest city in Kentucky, offering cultural and recreational activities such as orchestra, theater, ballet, opera, numerous restaurants and bars, and shopping areas. Louisville is the home of the Kentucky Derby. Many medical students take advantage of the university-owned medical-dental dormitory and apartment building, which is two blocks from both the School of Medicine and the University Hospital. In this residential complex, there are apartments of all sizes as well as dorm rooms.

GRADUATES

A large proportion of practicing physicians in Kentucky are Louisville School of Medicine graduates. At Louisville, at least 17 postgraduate training programs are offered.

Admissions

REQUIREMENTS

Requirements are 2 semesters each of biology, chemistry, organic chemistry, physics, and 1 semester of calculus or 2 semesters of other college-level math. All science courses must include lab work. Two semesters of English is also required. The MCAT is required, and scores should be no more than two years old. For applicants who have retaken the exam, the most recent set of scores is considered. Thus, there is no advantage in withholding scores.

SUGGESTIONS

Approximately 80 percent of positions in each class are reserved for Kentucky residents, making out-of-state admission very competitive. Premedical students should develop a strong background in the humanities, philosophy, and the arts. Communication and reading abilities are also important. The Admissions Committee values volunteer work, medically related experience, and evidence of strong interpersonal skills. Applicants are advised to take the April, rather than August, MCAT.

PROCESS

All qualified Kentucky residents and highly qualified nonresidents who submit AMCAS applications are sent secondaries. Of those returning secondary applications, about one-half of Kentucky applicants are invited to interview between September and February. Ten percent of nonresidents are invited to interview. On interview day, candidates receive two 30-minute interview sessions each with a faculty member, administrator, or medical student. In addition, interviewees have a guided campus tour, lunch, and the opportunity to meet informally with current students. About 40 percent of interviewed candidates are accepted on a rolling basis. Wait-listed candidates may send information to update their files in the spring.

UNIVERSITY OF MANITOBA

270-727 McDermot Avenue, Winnipeg, MB R3E 0W3 • Admission: 204-789-3499
Fax: 204-789-3929 • E-mail: registrar_med@umanitoba.ca • Website: www.umanitoba.ca/medicine

STUDENT BODY

Type	Public
Enrollment	362
% male/female	53/47
% underrepresented minorities	5
# applied (total/out)	703/457
# accepted (total/out)	136/39
# enrolled (total/out)	94/8
Average age	24

ADMISSIONS

Average GPA and MCAT Scores

Overall GPA	4.0
MCAT Bio	10.75
MCAT Phys	10.13
MCAT Verbal	10.04
MCAT Essay	P

Application Information

Regular application	10/2
Regular notification	5/15
Are transfers accepted?	yes
Admissions may be deferred?	yes
Interview required?	yes
Application fee	$75

Academics

Medical students complete a 4 year curriculum leading to the MD degree. Classes during the first two years are largely systems-based. Small groups are the predominant format for instruction, although lectures, labs, computer-based learning, and early clinical exposure are also important educational tools. The second two years are spent in clinical clerkships.

BASIC SCIENCES: Medicine I and Medicine II, consists of five mandatory programs: Cognitive, clinical skills, medical humanities and laboratory medicine, problem solving, plus the voluntary stress management program. The cognitive component is delivered in a variety of formats, including assigned self-study periods (A), small-group tutorials (T), traditional didactic lectures (L), small-group activities in entire class format (T1), lab practicals (LP) or demonstrations (LD), and computer-simulated labs. The Problem Solving Program attempts to integrate and reiterate important concepts presented during the cognitive component but emphasizes a symptom-based approach to your medical education. The Clinical Skills Program, which includes communication, history-taking and physical examination skills; the Medical Humanities Program, which includes human values, medical ethics, and medical history; and the Lab Medicine Program are integrated with the cognitive program as much as possible. In addition, there will be periods of unstructured, independent, self-directed learning time (SD) for the most part left blank in the weekly schedule.

CLINICAL TRAINING

Rotation through all major clinical disciplines takes place in more than a 48-week period and these are supplemented by elective periods of the students' choice. Periods are spent in family/community medicine, internal medicine, medicine and surgery selective, obstetrics/gynecology, pediatrics, psychiatry, surgery, and in a multiple clerkship rotation of anesthesia, emergency, ophthalmology, otolaryngology, and a community health sciences project. The setting for this experience includes wards and outpatient facilities of the hospitals or doctors' offices. The primary responsibility of the clerks in each of the eight 6-week rotations is the care of patients under the supervision of postgraduate students and faculty. Formal teaching of the pertinent knowledge, skills, attitudes, and behavior to the discipline is provided during the clerkships.

Students

In the entering class of 2005, approximately 50 percent of students were women. The average age of incoming students was 24 years. All students have bachelor's degrees.

STUDENT LIFE

Students are active in a number of areas, including organizing a program to help inner-city youth, coordinating an annual Medical Art Show, developing Codes of Professional Integrity, and carrying out an annual food bank drive.

Admissions

REQUIREMENTS

Applicants must have or be eligible to receive their bachelor's degree prior to admission from a university recognized by the University of Manitoba. Applicants must have completed a full course of English or French and a full course of biochemistry at the university level and received a grade of C or higher. Two full courses in humanities/social sciences are also required. The MCAT is required and should be taken within the past three years but no later than August of the year of application. Students usually prepare for the MCAT by taking university courses in biology, organic and physical chemistry, and physics.

SUGGESTIONS

Enrollment is restricted to Canadian citizens or permanent residents. Priority is given to residents of Manitoba. The most successful applicants have grade point averages between 3.8 and 4.2 on a 4.5 scale and at least an 8 on each scored section of the MCAT. In addition to academic and intellectual credentials, the Admissions Committee selects applicants who demonstrate social skills, maturity, and a sense of responsibility. The Admissions Committee selects 100 students for admission out of about 800 applicants. Typically, about nine places are offered to applicants from outside Manitoba.

PROCESS

For application materials, contact the faculty at the following e-mail: admissions@umanitoba.ca or call: 204-474-8805. Applicants who meet scholastic and MCAT requirements will be invited to interview and submit a personal statement. About 250 applicants are interviewed, and from this group the class is selected in early June. There is a special consideration category for some Manitoba residents who fall into one of the following three groups: Those who are sponsored by faculty-approved agencies, those who are from native populations of Manitoba, and those who have been employed for 2 or more years in the areas of health, social welfare, or health education.

Admissions Requirements (Required)

MCAT scores, science GPA, non-science GPA, letters of recommendation, interview, essays/personal statement, extracurricular activities, Canadian citizen or permanent resident.

Admissions Requirements (Optional)

State residency, exposure to medical profession.

COSTS AND AID

Tuition & Fees

Tuition	$7,595
Room and board (on campus)	$6,000
Room and board (off campus)	$10,000
Cost of books	$4,000

Financial Aid

% students receiving aid	35
Average grant	$750
Average loan	$10,615
Average debt	$46,000

UNIVERSITY OF MARYLAND
SCHOOL OF MEDICINE

SUITE 190, 685 WEST BALTIMORE STREET, BALTIMORE, MD 21201-1559 • ADMISSION: 410-706-7478
FAX: 410-706-0467 • E-MAIL: ADMISSIONS@SOM.UMARYLAND.EDU • WEBSITE: WWW.MEDSCHOOL.UMARYLAND.EDU

STUDENT BODY

Type	Public
Enrollment	604
% male/female	40/60
% underrepresented minorities	13
# applied (total/out)	3,713/2,965
# accepted (total/out)	311/120
# enrolled (total/out)	150/27
Average age	23

FACULTY

Total faculty (number)	1,156
% female	35
% minority	8
% part-time	18
Student-faculty ratio	2:1

ADMISSIONS

Average GPA and MCAT Scores

Overall GPA	3.66
MCAT Bio	10.4
MCAT Phys	10.0
MCAT Verbal	10.3
MCAT Essay	P

Application Information

Regular application	11/1
Regular notification	10/1
Early application	8/1
Early notification	10/1
Are transfers accepted?	yes
Admissions may be deferred?	yes
Interview required?	yes
Application fee	$70

Academics

Maryland's dynamic curriculum emphasizes independent and small-group learning, informatics, and the integration of basic and clinical science knowledge to produce outstanding clinicians and researchers. The traditional degree program takes students four years to complete. However, in selected cases, with permission of the dean, students may be granted extra time to complete the degree requirements. For students interested in a research career, the medical school offers a combined MD/PhD program in which the doctorate degree is offered in numerous disciplines such as biochemistry, biomedical engineering, genetics, molecular biology, neuroscience, and pharmacology. Grading is A–F. Students must pass Step 1 of the USMLE before beginning clinical training.

BASIC SCIENCES: The basic science curriculum is divided into integrated blocks and uses interdisciplinary teaching with both basic and clinical science instructors. Lectures and labs are limited to four hours per day; small-group and independent study are emphasized. Course work during the first year occupies 37 weeks and is organized into the following blocks: Cell and molecular biology, functional systems, informatics, neuroscience, principles of human development, and structure and development. Introduction to clinical medicine runs concurrently throughout the year, covering the doctor-patient relationship, medical ethics, population medicine, and problem-based learning. The second year is particularly rigorous. Students learn pathophysiology and therapeutics by organ system and are trained in conducting a physical examination in the introduction to clinical medicine course. Computers, not microscopes, are the laboratory tool of choice at Maryland. The multidisciplinary laboratories have the latest in educational technology and seat clusters of 10–12 students for small-group and laboratory teaching. The state-of-the-art library is among the largest and most accessible medical libraries in the United States, with at least 240,000 volumes, and is fully connected to the information superhighway. The Office of Student Affairs and Office of Medical Education closely monitor students and provide support services. In addition, a pre-matriculation summer program allows entrants to review premedical course work and preview first-year material.

CLINICAL TRAINING

Year 3 consists of seven required rotations in medicine (12 weeks), surgery (12 weeks), pediatrics (6 weeks), ob/gyn (6 weeks), psychiatry (4 weeks), family medicine (4 weeks), and neurology (4 weeks). The senior year includes a mandatory Area Health Education Center experience (8 weeks), 2 sub internships (8 weeks), and 16 weeks of elective rotations. The majority of training takes place at the University of Maryland Medical Center, a 747-bed tertiary care center adjacent to the medical school. Rotations are also spent at the Baltimore VA Medical Center, Mercy Hospital, and other community hospitals. In total, 1,400 patient beds are used for teaching. One of the most unique electives is a rotation through the R. Adams Cowley Shock Trauma Center. Shock Trauma was the first trauma center in America and continues to be a model for the rest of the world.

Students

The majority of students are Maryland residents, but the medical school attracts and accepts a significant number of out-of-state applicants. In a typical class, approximately 38 of the 150 students are from out-of-state. The student body is highly diverse with about 20 percent of students from underrepresented minority backgrounds. More than half of our students are women. Increasingly, older students are making up a higher percentage of incoming classes. At least one-third of incoming students took time off between college and medical school.

STUDENT LIFE

An extensive orientation program allows entering students to get to know fellow classmates, upperclassmen, and faculty advisors. Almost half of the incoming class attends. Other organized events, such as pot-luck suppers, community activities, and meetings of student organizations all serve to bring students together. Baltimore is a lively city, with interesting neighborhoods and real character. The harbor, the commercial district (Fells Point), the Orioles baseball stadium, Ravens football stadium, and other attractions are accessible to the campus. The university offers athletic facilities and housing in the form of dorms. Most students find affordable, private apartments off campus. While the surrounding area has undergone a renaissance in recent years, safety remains a concern, as in most large cities. The campus places a high priority on student safety and provides door-to-door transportation.

GRADUATES

About half of each year's graduates enter one of the primary care fields. Graduates, however, are competitive candidates for the entire range of specialties.

Admissions

REQUIREMENTS

Maryland requires one year each of biology, English, general chemistry, organic chemistry, and physics as prerequisite courses. A grade of C or better is mandatory in each course. While the MCAT is also required, there is no set formula for determining competitive scores. Students with a wide range of scores are accepted each year. In addition, Maryland considers the best scores for those applicants who retake the exam.

SUGGESTIONS

Maryland gives clinical experience with direct patient exposure considerable weight. Research experience and service activity are also highly valued. Letters of recommendation are very important in the selection process.

PROCESS

Maryland uses the AMCAS application. Secondary applications are sent to all applicants. Of those who complete the secondary, approximately 25 percent are interviewed beginning in October. The interview day consists of a faculty interview, a medical student interview, a casual lunch with students, and a tour of the campus. Interviewed applicants normally receive a decision within one month after the interview. Half of those interviewed are accepted, and the other half are either rejected or wait listed.

University of Massachusetts
Medical School

Associate Dean for Admissions, 55 Lake Avenue North, Worcester, MA 01655 • Admission: 508-856-2323
Fax: 506-856-3629 • E-mail: Admissions@umassmed.edu • Website: www.umassmed.edu/som/admissions/

STUDENT BODY

Type	Public
Enrollment	425
% male/female	49/51
% underrepresented minorities	7
# applied (total/out)	814/0
Average age	25

ADMISSIONS

Application Information

Regular application	11/1
Regular notification	5/15
Early application	6/1–8/1
Early notification	10/1
Are transfers accepted?	yes
Admissions may be deferred?	yes
Interview required?	yes
Application fee	$50

Academics

The 4 year program emphasizes varied educational modalities, lifelong learning, communication skills, and a generalist approach that prepares students for all medical career paths. Ethical issues are an important aspect of the education, demonstrated by the existence of an active Office of Ethics. Year-long and summer research fellowships are available, as is a joint MD/PhD program. The doctorate degree may be earned in biomedical sciences, biochemistry and molecular biology, cell biology, cellular and molecular physiology, immunology and virology, molecular genetics, microbiology, neuroscience, and pharmacology and molecular toxicology. A combined MD/MPH degree program is also offered. For pre-clinical courses, grades are honors, near honors, satisfactory, marginal, unsatisfactory, or incomplete, with the exception of a few courses that are taken as credit/no credit. During the clinical years, ratings are outstanding, above expected performance, expected performance, below expected performance, and failure.

BASIC SCIENCES: First-year courses are biochemistry/metabolism; the gene; human anatomy; cells and tissues; systems I; physiology; immunology; mind, brain, and behavior I; physician, patient, and society (PPS); and Longitudinal Preceptor Program (LPP). PPS and LPP together introduce students to medical interviewing, physician-patient relationships, physical diagnosis, medical reasoning and decision analyses, population-based medicine, ethics, epidemiology, medical informatics, and preventive medicine. Systems I covers several body/organ systems: Cardiovascular; endocrine regulation; GI/nutrition; hematology; renal and acid/base; reproduction, and respiratory. Second-year courses focus on the biology of disease. They are general pathology; general pharmacology; microbiology; mind, brain, and behavior II; neoplasia; systems II; and a continuation of PPS and LPP. In systems II, dermatology, musculoskeletal/renal, and pumps, wind, and water are among the body systems studied. Basic sciences are taught in a wing of the school's central complex. A new learning center houses amphitheaters, flexible classrooms, and a video conference facility. The Lamar Soutter Library holds more than 239,000 volumes, subscribes to 1,500 journals, and provides access to online search and database tools. The Library Computer Area contains personal computers and workstations for computer-assisted instruction, interactive programs, and educational databases.

CLINICAL TRAINING
Third-year required rotations are medicine (12 weeks), surgery (12 weeks), family and community medicine (6 weeks), ob/gyn (6 weeks), pediatrics (6 weeks), and psychiatry (6 weeks). Fourth-year requirements are neurology (4 weeks), a sub internship in medicine (4 weeks), and 24 weeks of elective study. Clinical training takes place at the UMass hospital (388 beds), a comprehensive facility with general and specialty services. Clinical specialties include the breast center, burn unit, cancer center, Level I Trauma Center, Kidney-Pancreas transplantation, Children's Medical Center, Center of Stone Disease, advanced laser technology, Cardiovascular Center, AIDS programs, and public sector psychiatry. UMass benefits from affiliations with the following hospitals in and around the Worcester area: Memorial Health Care (319 beds), Saint Vincent Hospital, and Berkshire Medical Center (330 beds).

Students

All students are Massachusetts residents. The average age of incoming students is 25, and at least half of students took some time off after college. About 60 percent of students were science majors as undergraduates. Approximately 7 percent of students are under-represented minorities. Class size is 100.

STUDENT LIFE

Recreational and athletic facilities are conveniently located in the lower level of the basic science building. Facilities include a lounge with a TV, pool and ping pong tables, study areas, and an exercise and weight room. Students are involved in organizations focused on community service, recreational interests, and professional pursuits. Worcester is a city of nearly 200,000, offering a full range of services and activities. Students live off campus, most choosing to live in the local community. Some students rely on public transportation, while others use cars.

GRADUATES

Among 1997 graduates, the most popular fields for postgraduate training were internal medicine (28 percent), family practice (25 percent), pediatrics (15 percent), emergency medicine (7 percent), ob/gyn (4 percent), and surgery (5 percent). A significant proportion entered residency programs in Massachusetts.

Admissions

REQUIREMENTS

Massachusetts residency is a requirement. Prerequisites are 1 year each of biology, English, general chemistry, organic chemistry, and physics. All science courses should include associated labs. The MCAT is required, and scores should be from within the past two years. For applicants who have taken the exam on multiple occasions, the best scores are weighed most heavily. Thus, withholding scores is not advantageous.

SUGGESTIONS

Applications should be submitted as early as possible. In addition to requirements, course work in calculus, computer psychology, science, sociology, and statistics is advised. For applicants who have been out of college for a significant period of time, some recent course work is important. Medically related experiences or research may strengthen an application.

PROCESS

All in-state AMCAS applicants are sent secondary applications. Of those returning secondaries, about half are interviewed between October and March. Interviews consist of two 30-minute sessions with faculty members and/or medical students. On interview day, candidates also have a group information session and campus tour. Approximately one-third of interviewees are accepted on a rolling basis. Wait-listed candidates may send supplementary information if it serves to update their files.

Admissions Requirements (Required)

MCAT scores, science GPA, nonscience GPA, letters of recommendation, interview, extracurricular activities, exposure to medical profession.

Admissions Requirements (Optional)

State residency, essays/personal statement.

COSTS AND AID

Tuition & Fees

In-state Tuition	$8,352
Cost of books	$460
Fees	$1,835

Financial Aid

% students receiving aid	75
Average debt	$70,068

UNIVERSITY OF MEDICINE AND DENTISTRY OF NEW JERSEY
NEW JERSEY MEDICAL SCHOOL

185 SOUTH ORANGE AVENUE, MEDICAL SCIENCE BUILDING, RM C-653, NEWARK, NJ 07103 • ADMISSION: 973-972-4631
FAX: 973-972-7986 • E-MAIL: NJMSADMISS@UMDNJ.EDU • WEBSITE: WWW.NJMS.UMDNJ.EDU

STUDENT BODY

Type	Public
Enrollment	695
% male/female	51/49
% underrepresented minorities	32
# applied (total/out)	4,047/2,948
# accepted	170
# enrolled	170

ADMISSIONS

Average GPA and MCAT Scores

Overall GPA	3.61
MCAT Bio	10.0
MCAT Phys	10.0
MCAT Verbal	9.0
MCAT Essay	P

Application Information

Regular application	6/1–12/1
Regular notification	10/15
Early application	6/1–8/1
Early notification	10/1
Are transfers accepted?	yes
Admissions may be deferred?	yes
Interview required?	yes
Application fee	$75

Academics

BASIC SCIENCES: During the first two years, small-group sessions and tutorials account for about one-third of scheduled sessions, with the remainder of class time used for lectures and labs. Students are paired with physicians in the community, working with them one afternoon each week as part of primary care preceptorships. Courses demand about 27 hours per week, in addition to individual study time. First-year courses are biochemistry and molecular biology, cell and tissue biology, genetics, gross and developmental anatomy, neuroscience, physiology, problem-based learning, psychiatry, public health, and the art of medicine. Clinical skills, which focus on the physical examination, are also part of the first year. During the second year, topics are coordinated among courses and are organized around organ systems. Courses are clinical preventive medicine and nutrition, immunology, introduction to clinical sciences, microbiology, pathology, pharmacology, and psychiatry and the clinical interview. The Medical Sciences Building, where basic sciences are taught, is connected to the University Hospital and the George F. Smith Library, the latter of which houses 70,000 volumes and more than 2,000 periodicals. The proximity of clinical facilities to classrooms and labs encourages first- and second-year students' involvement in clinical activities. The Office of Student Affairs provides services ranging from personal counseling to guidance on elective and residency selection.

CLINICAL TRAINING

Required third-year clerkships are internal medicine (12 weeks), general surgery (8 weeks), pediatrics (8 weeks), ob/gyn (8 weeks), psychiatry (6 weeks), and family medicine (6 weeks). During the fourth year, 16 weeks of electives are required in addition to neurology (4 weeks); emergency medicine (4 weeks); substance abuse (2 weeks); physical medicine and rehabilitation (2 weeks); ophthalmology, orthopedics, otolaryngology, and urology (1 week each); and an acting internship in medicine, family medicine, obstetrics, pediatrics, or surgery (4 weeks). Most clinical training takes place at the contiguous 518-bed University Hospital, which serves the needs of the immediate community and, with its specialized care units, attracts patients from around the state. Other affiliated teaching hospitals are Hackensack University Hospital, Morristown Memorial Hospital, Veterans Affairs Health Care System, East Orange, and Kessler Institute for Rehabilitation.

Students

Eighty-four percent of the NJMS entering students are New Jersey residents. Underrepresented minorities account for 19 percent of the student body. The average age of students entering the class of 2005 was 26, ranging from 19 to 41, and the matriculated class size was 170.

STUDENT LIFE

Students are involved in intramural sports and organized student events. Each entering student is assigned to a peer group of first- and second-year students. Students initiate and develop service activities such as: AMA (American Medical Association), AMSA (American Medical Students Assoc.), AMWA (American Medical Women's Association), BLHO (Boricua Latino Health Organization), Center for Humanism and Medicine, Community 2000, which conducts clinical screening and health education with local churches, Early Start Mentoring Program, Family Medicine Interest Group, New Moms, Peer Support, Project Pediatrics (Border Babies), Students Health Advocates for Resources and Education (S.H.A.R.E.), Students are actively involved in community-service projects through the SHARE Center. Student Family Health Care Center (SFHCC) (Clinic), SNMA (Student National Assoc.), STATS (Students Teaching AIDS to Students), Student Council, and Unite for Site.

NJMS is located in University Heights. Newark offers many artistic and creative activities including the performing arts, jazz clubs, and diverse neighborhoods. It is home to the Newark Bears, the NJ Symphony Orchestra, the NJ State Opera, NJ Performing Arts Center, the Newark Museum, the Ballantine House, Newark Symphony Hall, the Newark Library, the Cathedral Basilica of the Sacred Heart and the Garden State Ballet and several institutions of Higher Education. New York City is an easy train ride and serves as a convenient distraction for medical students.

GRADUATES

Each year, graduates are successful in obtaining residencies at prestigious institutions such as Massachusetts General, Columbia Presbyterian, the Children's Hospital in Washington, DC, and New Haven Hospital at Yale. The alumni association is very enthusiastic, and among its activities is the provision of scholarships and research stipends to medical students.

Admissions

REQUIREMENTS

The minimum course requirements are 8 semester hours of biology; 8 semester hours of physics, 16 semester hours chemistry (general or inorganic chemistry and organic chemistry), all with associated labs; and 6 semester hours of English. Although math is not required it is strongly recommended. The MCAT is required; scores must be no more than three years old. There is no minimum GPA or MCAT requirement but intense competition tends to favor those with stronger credentials, as the average GPA of our accepted applicants is 3.6 with an average MCAT of 30. Approximately 19 percent of the 4,047 applicants are interviewed with interviews taking place between August and April. About one-third of interviewees are accepted. Wait-listed candidates may send supplementary information to update their files.

Applicants are selected on the basis of academic excellence, leadership qualities, demonstrated compassion for others, and broad extracurricular experiences. The Admissions Committee considers related factors such as passion, motivation, perseverance, special aptitudes, and stamina (personal statement, letters of recommendation and the interview are also very important factors in evaluation). NJMS encourages nonresidents to apply but New Jersey residents will be given some preference.

SUGGESTIONS

Research or experience in a health care setting is useful. Personal traits, such as compassion, dedication, and interpersonal skills, are very important.

PROCESS

Once an application file is complete (AMCAS application, MCAT scores, letters of recommendation, supplemental application, and $75 fee) a Screening Committee reviews the applicant's file. If the Screening Committee determines that the applicant should be interviewed, the Office of Admissions notifies and formally invites the applicant for an interview. Applicants are interviewed by medical school faculty and administrators who will discuss personal and educational achievements, motivation, drive, ability, background, personality, long term goals, and extracurricular activities. Interviews vary in length but generally last about one hour.

Admissions Requirements (Required)

MCAT scores, science GPA, letters of recommendation, interview, essays/personal statement, extracurricular activities.

Admissions Requirements (Optional)

State residency, exposure to medical profession.

COSTS AND AID

Tuition & Fees

Tuition	
(in-state)	$21,390
(out-of-state)	$33,472
Fees	$810

Financial Aid

% students receiving aid	70

UNIVERSITY OF MEDICINE AND DENTISTRY OF NEW JERSEY
ROBERT WOOD JOHNSON MEDICAL SCHOOL

OFFICE OF ADMISSIONS, 675 HOES LANE, PISCATAWAY, NJ 08854 • ADMISSION: 732-235-4576
FAX: 732-235-5078 • E-MAIL: RWJAPADM@UMDNJ.EDU • WEBSITE: WWW.RWJMS.UMDNJ.EDU

STUDENT BODY

Type	Public
Enrollment	642
% male/female	47/53
% underrepresented minorities	16
# applied (total/out)	2,815/1,795
# accepted (total/out)	345/45
# enrolled (total/out)	157/2
Average age	23

FACULTY

Total faculty (number)	850
% female	35
% minority	23

ADMISSIONS

Average GPA and MCAT Scores

Overall GPA	3.62
MCAT Bio	10.6
MCAT Phys	10.2
MCAT Verbal	9.4
MCAT Essay	P

Application Information

Regular application	12/1
Regular notification	rolling
Early application	6/1–8/1
Early notification	10/1
Are transfers accepted?	yes
Admissions may be deferred?	yes
Interview required?	yes
Application fee	$75

Academics

Students are encouraged to pursue a variety of educational opportunities. In addition to the traditional 4 year medical school curriculum, students may enroll in one of the dual degree options including MD/PhD, MD/JD, MD/MPH, MD/MBA, MS/MS biomedical informatics, and MD/MS jurisprudence. A MS in clinical and translational research is planned for 2007. The flexible curriculum allows the rearranging of certain courses to enable students to pursue the dual degrees, relevant projects, personal interests, research, or employment. Student scholars may take an additional year to pursue the basic science or clinical research or off-campus community health projects. Students who complete a thesis graduate with distinction in research. A new distinction in service to the community program has been established. The grading policy uses honors/high pass/pass/low pass/fail. Steps 1 and 2 of the USMLE are required for graduation. Research facilities include the Center for Advanced Biotechnology and Medicine, Child Health Institute, The Cancer Institute of New Jersey, Environmental and Occupational Health Science Institute, Stem Cell Institute, and Cardiovascular Institute.

BASIC SCIENCES: Curricular changes in the first two years have been implemented toward the following twofold mission: Better preparation of clinicians as lifelong learners and a shift toward self-directed learning. The changes include more small-group learning, a new course in patient-centered medicine structured as small clinic groups facilitated by a mentor, problem-based approaches, a reduction in lecture time in addition to a systems-based approach in the second year. Clinical correlation is emphasized in all first-year disciplines. First-year courses include the following: Basic life support I, biological chemistry, cellular and genetic mechanisms and histology, epidemiology and biostatistics, gross and developmental anatomy, medical microbiology and immunology, medical physiology, neuroscience, patient centered medicine, principles of environmental and community medicine. Second-year courses include the following: Basic life support II, behavorial science and psychiatry, biochemical basis of nutrition, clinical pathophysiology, clinical prevention and environmental medicine, human sexuality, pathology and laboratory medicine, patient centered medicine, pharmacology, and universal precautions/venipuncture. A vast array of noncredit pre-clinical electives enriches the experience during the first and second years. Courses include alternative and complementary medicine, business in medicine elective, community and child health, emergency room elective, geriatric issues, humanities in medicine, and issues in women's health. Renovations at the Medical Science Complex bring 26 state-of-the-art multipurpose classrooms and anatomy laboratories for the educational programs.

CLINICAL TRAINING
Most clinical training takes place at the principal teaching hospitals, Robert Wood Johnson University Hospital on the New Brunswick Campus and Cooper Hospital University Medical Center on the Camden Campus. A Clinical Skills Center with a standardized patient program is used to teach and assess the clinical skills of first, second, third and fourth year medical students. During the third year of medical school, students rotate through clerkships in family medicine, medicine, neurology, obstetrics/gynecology, pediatrics, psychiatry, and surgery. Additionally, there is a significant amount of elective work during the third year. During the fourth-year students are required to take rotations in emergency medicine and critical care. A longitudinal care experience runs through the third and fourth years.

Students

Approximately 80 percent of the students apply as New Jersey residents. There is great diversity among the student body. Fifty-one percent of students describe themselves as minorities, with 14 percent from underrepresented groups. Typically between 10–20 percent of the student body took some time off between undergraduate studies and medical school. The class size is 156. One-third of the class completes their clinical training on the Camden campus.

STUDENT LIFE

New Brunswick offers the many amenities of a university city. Princeton and New York City are short train rides away. Students who complete clinical training on the Camden campus enjoy the proximity of Philadelphia. The medical school does not have on-campus housing; however, the school helps students secure accomodations in the area. Medical students have access to Rutgers University athletic facilities which include golf, swimming pools, gyms, squash, racquetball, and volleyball courts. Rutgers also offers social, cultural, and recreational activities for medical students. There are many student organizations and interest groups, including chapters of the major national medical student associations. Many students participate in volunteer organizations including the student run HIPHOP (Homeless and Indigent Persons Health Outreach Project) and UHI (Urban Health Initiatives). Honor societies include Alpha Omega Alpha and the Humanism in Medicine Honor Society.

GRADUATES

Graduates have done particularly well in securing outstanding training positions throughout the country, as well as within the school's training programs. About one-half of the class chooses internal medicine, pediatrics, or family medicine, but all specialties are represented.

Admissions

REQUIREMENTS

Two semesters of biology, general chemistry, organic chemistry, and physics, with laboratory; two semesters of English or writing intensive courses; and one semester of college-level mathematics are required. The MCAT is required and must be no more than four years old. For applicants who have taken the exam more than once, all scores are considered, but the most recent score is given the most weight.

SUGGESTIONS

Course work in the behavioral sciences and humanities is recommended. Medically related experiences, research, and community service are all valued by the Admissions Committee.

PROCESS

As a state institution, preference is given to in-state residents; however, the importance of geographic diversity is recognized and out-of-state residents are encouraged to apply. A new process allows accepted out-of-state residents to become in-state residents and hence be eligible for in-state tuition. Approximately one-half of New Jersey applicants and 5 percent of out-of-state applicants are interviewed on one of the three campuses: Piscataway, New Brunswick, or Camden. Generally students are interviewed by one faculty member. Some applicants are also interviewed by a student member of the Admissions Committee. All applicants have the opportunity to meet and tour with a current student. About one-third of those interviewed are accepted. Acceptances are offered on a rolling basis. Several alternative means of acceptance exist. There is a combined BA/MD program with Rutgers University. There is also an accelerated acceptance program for students completing post-baccalaureate studies at a number of institutions including the University of Pennsylvania, Columbia, Johns Hopkins, Rutgers, Drexel, NYU, Bryn Mawr, and LaSalle.

Admissions Requirements (Required)

MCAT scores, science GPA, non-science GPA, letters of recommendation, interview, essays/personal statement.

Admissions Requirements (Optional)

State residency, extracurricular activities, exposure to medical profession.

COSTS AND AID

Tuition & Fees

In-state Tuition	$21,390
Out-of-state Tuition	$33,472
Room and board (off campus)	$10,026
Cost of books	$1,768
Fees	$3,002

Financial Aid

% students receiving aid	78
Average grant	$5,000
Average loan	$25,000
Average debt	$102,000

UNIVERSITY OF MIAMI
MILLER SCHOOL OF MEDICINE

ADMISSIONS R-159, PO BOX 016159, MIAMI, FL 33101 • ADMISSION: 305-243-6791
FAX: 305-243-6548 • E-MAIL: MED.ADMISSIONS@MIAMI.EDU • WEBSITE: WWW.MIAMI.EDU/MEDICAL-ADMISSIONS

STUDENT BODY

Type	Private
Enrollment	615
% male/female	48/52
% underrepresented minorities	7
# applied (total/out)	3,740/2,493
# accepted (total/out)	237/86
# enrolled (total/out)	150/32
Average age	22

FACULTY

Total faculty (number)	1,085
% female	12
% minority	7

ADMISSIONS

Average GPA and MCAT Scores

Overall GPA	3.71
MCAT Bio	10.0
MCAT Phys	9.7
MCAT Verbal	9.6
MCAT Essay	Q

Application Information

Regular application	12/1
Regular notification	10/15
Are transfers accepted?	no
Admissions may be deferred?	yes
Interview required?	yes
Application fee	$65

Academics

The University of Miami Miller School of Medicine has two campuses: The original campus located close to Jackson Memorial Hospital in downtown Miami (150 students) and a new regional campus located on the campus of Florida Atlantic University in Boca Raton (64 students), about 50 miles north of Miami. The medical curricula at each campus last 4 years, but they are structured slightly differently to address the needs of the local area's population. Each year approximately 30 students enter medical school from one of the seven year Honors Medical Programs and a number of medical students participate in the MD/PhD program, earning a doctorate degree in biochemistry and molecular biology; microbiology and immunology; molecular, cell, and developmental biology; molecular and cellular pharmacology; neuroscience; or physiology and biophysics. A combined MD/MPH program is also available and an MD/MBA program is under development. Grading is done on a percentile basis, and promotion to year 3 requires a passing score on the USMLE Step 1. Step 2 of the USMLE must be taken to graduate.

BASIC SCIENCES: The first year begins with a 5 month segment of "Core Principals of a Medical Practice" and then morphs into a series of system- and organ-based modules that run almost to the end of the second year. The second year concludes with a comprehensive series of problem- and case-based sessions which enable students to integrate their knowledge and synthesize answers to complex medical questions. Patient contact begins in the first week of medical school, and students begin learning the fundamentals of physical examinations and history-taking under the tutelage of a practicing community physician. These skills are refined and broadened through interaction with clinical faculty in the student's academic society. Running throughout the first 2 years of the curriculum is a set of longitudinal themes which address topics such as alternative medicine, end of life care, ethics, geriatrics, health care delivery systems, medical economics, medical informatics, professionalism, and special population medicine. Lectures and small group sessions are the predominant instructional modalities. Competency exams occur at the end of the first and second years and assess whether the student has acquired the necessary clinical expertise to progress to the next level.

CLINICAL TRAINING

The third and fourth years of the curriculum are a continuum of electives and required clerkships. This design allows electives to be taken during the third year with a competency exam occurring at the end of that year. Required clerkships include: Family medicine, geriatrics, medicine, neurology, ob/gyn, pediatrics, primary care, psychiatry, radiology, and surgery. Part of the fourth year is devoted to selectives (which must include at least 8 weeks of direct patient care) and electives (that may be clinical or research-based). At the Miami campus, clinical training takes place at Jackson Memorial Hospital, the Veterans Affairs Medical Center, Sylvester Comprehensive Cancer Center, Ryder Trauma Center, the Diabetes Research Institute, and the Miami Project to Cure Spinal Cord Paralysis. Clinical training at the regional campus in Boca Raton is acquired at Boca Raton Community Hospital and Bethesda Community Hospital and is a collaborative, patient-centered curricular experience. Up to 3 months of the fourth year may be spent in clerkships at other institutions.

Students

A recently entering class had the following profile: Age range 19–37; 48 percent were women; 8 percent were from underrepresented minority groups; 75 percent were Florida residents; and 75 percent had been science majors. Sixty colleges and universities were represented. Class size is 150.

STUDENT LIFE

Medical students at both campuses actively participate in community service through the Department of Clinical Services (DOCS) and their academic societies. The students conduct six health fairs each year, ranging in location between Key West, Marathon, Florida City, and Del Ray Beach. Students can participate in a variety of recreational sports throughout the academic year and enjoy the good weather and multicultural environment of Miami and Boca Raton. Medical students at both campuses live off campus and usually drive to school or take Metrorail (Miami campus only).

GRADUATES

Graduates are successful in securing residency positions nationwide. A significant proportion enter programs at Jackson Memorial Hospital, or other hospitals around the state. About 90 percent get one of their top three residency choices.

Admissions

REQUIREMENTS

Prerequisites are 1 year each of biology, chemistry, English, organic chemistry, and physics. Science courses should include associated labs. The MCAT is required and scores must be from within the past three years. For applicants who have taken the exam on multiple occasions, the best set of scores is weighed most heavily.

SUGGESTIONS

Florida residents are given preference, and only highly qualified out-of-state residents (With a GPA >3.6 and a MCAT score >30) are encouraged to apply. Recommended course work includes biochemistry, cell and molecular biology, computer science, mammalian physiology, microbiology and immunology, and molecular genetics. Beyond academic credentials, the Admissions Committee highly values meaningful patient contact experiences, diversity of life experiences, interpersonal skills, maturity, motivation, and compassion.

PROCESS

About 75 percent of Florida residents and 20 percent of out-of-state residents are sent secondary applications. About 300 applicants are interviewed on campus. Interviews take place on Fridays between August and April and consist of one session with a faculty member. About 60 percent of interviewed candidates are accepted, with notification occurring on a rolling basis. Approximately 25 positions in each entering class are reserved for participants in the University of Miami Honors Program in Medicine, a 6-year BS/MD program.

Secondary applications may be sent to all US citizens and permanent residents of the United States. About 450–500 applicants are interviewed on campus. Interviews take place on Fridays and selected Mondays between August and April. About 60 percent of interviewed candidates are eventually accepted, with notification occurring on a rolling basis.

Admissions Requirements (Required)

MCAT scores, science GPA, non-science GPA, letters of recommendation, interview, essays/personal statement, extracurricular activities, exposure to medical profession.

Admissions Requirements (Optional)

State residency.

COSTS AND AID

Tuition & Fees

Tuition	
In-state	$29,298
Out-of-state	$38,504
Cost of books	$800
Fees	$550

Financial Aid

Average grant	$10,000
Average loan	$40,000

University of Michigan
Medical School

Admissions Office, M4130 Medical Science I Building, Ann Arbor, MI 48109 • Admission: 313-764-6317
Fax: 313-936-3510 • E-mail: pibs@umich.edu • Website: www.med.umich.edu/medschool

STUDENT BODY	
Type	Public
Enrollment	177
% male/female	51/49
% underrepresented minorities	15
# applied	4,931
# enrolled	177

ADMISSIONS

Average GPA and MCAT Scores

Overall GPA	3.72

Application Information

Regular application	11/15
Regular notification	rolling
Early application	6/1–8/1
Early notification	10/1
Are transfers accepted?	no
Admissions may be deferred?	yes
Interview required?	no
Application fee	$50

Academics

Most students follow a 4 year program leading to the MD, although a growing number opt for combined degrees. A combined MD/PhD curriculum allows students to pursue graduate studies in numerous departments, including anatomy and cell biology, biological chemistry, cellular and molecular biology, human genetics, microbiology and immunology, neuroscience, pharmacology, and physiology. Some MD/PhD students are MSTP participants, while others are funded through institutional sources. For students who are interested in research, but who are not interested in earning an additional degree, summer and year-long research fellowships are available. In addition, combined programs with Public Health and Business Administration are available. Passing Step 1 of the USMLE is a requirement for promotion to year 3 and passing Step 2 is a requirement for graduation.

BASIC SCIENCES: During the first year, grading is strictly satisfactory/fail. This promotes student cooperation and allows for variation in the level of scientific knowledge among incoming students. Throughout the first and second years, students take introduction to the patient, which includes interdisciplinary perspectives and the use of simulated patients; and multidisciplinary conferences, which provides clinical correlations for basic science concepts. Other first year courses are molecular and cell biology, gross anatomy, human genetics, pathology, embryology, histology, host defenses, microbiology, pharmacology, and physiology. Year 2 is organized around organ and body systems. These are cardiovascular, dermatology, endocrine, gastrointestinal, hematology, infectious diseases, musculoskeletal, neuroscience, oncology, renal, reproduction, and respiratory. The Medical School's basic science instructional facilities include recently renovated lecture halls with audiovisual and computer equipment. A Learning Resource Center is open 24 hours per day and has more than 50 computers for student use. The Taubman Medical Library is one of the largest in the United States in terms of the number of volumes, journals, and electronic resources that it holds. The Office of Academic Enrichment provides academic counseling and organizes study groups and tutoring services.

CLINICAL TRAINING

During the second, third, and fourth years, students are evaluated with honors, high pass, pass, and fail. Third-year required rotations are surgery (12 weeks), internal medicine (12 weeks), ob/gyn (6 weeks), pediatrics (6 weeks), family practice (4 weeks), neurology (4 weeks), and psychiatry (4 weeks). Students attend weekly conferences and discuss a range of topics including the ethical, social, and economic issues related to practicing medicine. Fourth-year requirements are sub internship (8 weeks); intensive care unit experience (4 weeks); advanced basic science experience (4 weeks); and electives (12–20 weeks), which are selected from more than 300 subjects. Clinical training takes place at the University Hospital (888 beds), St. Joseph Mercy Hospital (522 beds), the Veterans Affairs Hospital (486 beds), and at other affiliated institutions. With approval, students may earn elective credits at other academic or clinical sites in the United States and overseas.

Students

About 50 percent of students are Michigan residents, with the remainder of the student body coming from all regions of the country. Typically, at least 10 percent of entering students are older, having taken some time off after college. Approximately 15 percent of students are underrepresented minorities. Class size is 170.

STUDENT LIFE

Incoming medical students benefit from the support and advice of more senior medical students through a peer-counseling program called Big Sib, Little Sib. Students interact outside of the classroom through participation in organizations that focus on issues such as community service, support for minority and gay/lesbian students, and recreational and professional pursuits. The Furstenberg Student Study Center features a well-being room for information and activities related to student health, computer stations, lounges, and quiet study rooms. Expansive sports and recreation centers also enrich student life on campus. Ann Arbor is an academic and cultural center, attracting scholars from around the world. To serve the university community, the area around the campus is filled with coffee shops, bookstores, restaurants, bars, and shops. In addition to commercial districts, Ann Arbor offers parks, lakes, theaters, farmers markets, and attractive residential areas. Although some limited campus-owned housing is available to medical students, most opt to live in privately owned apartment complexes that are within walking distance of the Medical Center.

GRADUATES

Medical students consistently score above the national average on both steps of the USMLE, contributing to their success in securing top residency positions. Among graduates, popular choices for specialty areas were internal medicine (23 percent), pediatrics (12 percent), surgery (11 percent), family practice (10 percent), ob/gyn (7 percent), and emergency medicine (6 percent).

Admissions

REQUIREMENTS

Prerequisites are chemistry (8 semester hours, which includes both organic and inorganic); biology (6 semester hours); physics (6 semester hours); English composition and literature (6 semester hours); and biochemistry (3 semester hours). In addition, at least 18 semester hours must be completed in areas other than the natural sciences or math.

SUGGESTIONS

In addition to the required science courses, genetics and cell biology are considered useful preparation for medical school. Humanities and social sciences course work is also important.

PROCESS

All AMCAS applicants are sent supplementary applications. Of those returning secondaries, about 15 percent are interviewed between September and March. Interviews consist of two 30-minute sessions, each with a faculty member or medical student. Candidates are also given a group informational presentation, a campus tour, and lunch with medical students. About one-third of interviewees are accepted and are notified between November and May. Others are rejected or put on a wait list.

Admissions Requirements (Required)

MCAT scores, science GPA, non-science GPA, letters of recommendation, state residency, extracurricular activities, exposure to medical profession.

Admissions Requirements (Optional)

Interview, essays/personal statement.

COSTS AND AID

Tuition & Fees

In-state Tuition	$22,433
Out-of-state Tuition	$34,785

UNIVERSITY OF MINNESOTA—DULUTH

MEDICAL SCHOOL

180 MEDICINE, 1035 UNIVERSITY DRIVE, DULUTH, MN 55812 • ADMISSION: 218-726-8511
FAX: 218-726-7057 • E-MAIL: MEDADMIS@D.UMN.EDU • WEBSITE: WWW.MED.UMN.EDU/DULUTH/

STUDENT BODY

Type	Public
Enrollment	106
% male/female	50/50
% underrepresented minorities	6
# applied (total/out)	954/524
# accepted (total/out)	75/7
# enrolled (total/out)	55/4
Average age	24

FACULTY

Total faculty (number)	48
% female	31
% minority	4
% part-time	6
Student-faculty ratio	2:1

ADMISSIONS

Average GPA and MCAT Scores

Overall GPA	3.59
MCAT Bio	9.62
MCAT Phys	9.25
MCAT Verbal	9.05
MCAT Essay	Q

Application Information

Regular application	11/15
Regular notification	rolling
Early application	8/1
Early notification	10/1
Are transfers accepted?	no
Admissions may be deferred?	yes
Interview required?	yes
Application fee	$75

Academics

Although formal clinical rotations are not included in the 2 year UMD curriculum, early patient contact and clinical correlations are important aspects of the program. Successful completion of UMD requirements guarantees transfer after year 2 to the Twin Cities campus. Evaluation of medical student performance uses outstanding, excellent, satisfactory, incomplete, and no pass. Passing Step 1 of the USMLE is a requirement for promotion to the Medical School Twin Cities.

BASIC SCIENCES: The 2 year curriculum is a unique blend of basic medical and behavioral sciences and clinical hands-on experiences. The basic sciences, presented using an organ systems approach that begins with principles of basic science, extends to various aspects of the prevention and pathophysiology of organ system disease, and concludes with discussions of several presenting clinical symptoms and multisystems diseases. The behavioral sciences portion of the curriculum emphasizes knowledge about the psycho-social aspects of health and illness that are relevant to the clinical setting and is interwoven with the organ systems component. The clinical experience is directed by community specialists and is augmented by UMD's nationally recognized Family Practice Preceptorship program. In addition to classrooms and labs, the Learning Resource Center serves as a computer and multimedia instructional facility. It is open 24 hours per day. The Health Science Library houses 95,000 volumes, 600 current journals, and several online data bases.

CLINICAL TRAINING

In Duluth, clinical affiliates are St. Luke's Hospital and St. Mary's Medical Centers. After successfully completing year 2, students transfer to Minneapolis, where they rotate through required clerkships during their third and fourth years. These are medicine (12 weeks), ob/gyn (6 weeks), surgery (6 weeks), pediatrics (6 weeks), psychiatry (6 weeks), neurology (4 weeks), surgical specialty (4 weeks), emergency medicine (4 weeks), and ambulatory care (8 weeks). The remaining time is reserved for elective study. Clinical facilities include Abbott Northwestern Hospital, Children's Health Care, Fairview-University Medical Center, Hennepin County Medical Center, Regions Hospital, St. Luke's Hospital, St. Mary's Medical Center, and other sites. Each year, through the Rural Physician Associate Program, up to 40 third-year medical students study primary health care in a 9 month elective in Minnesota rural communities under the supervision of local physicians. Up to 12 weeks of clinical electives may be fulfilled at nonaffiliated institutions in other parts of the country or abroad.

Students

STUDENT LIFE

Small class size and students' shared interest in family medicine promotes a supportive and cohesive atmosphere. University recreational events, facilities, and activities are open to medical students, including the student center, the gym, intramural sports, and student organizations. Students also take advantage of the extracurricular opportunities afforded by the school's location. Activities such as cycling, running, skiing, hiking, and camping are easily accessible within or around Duluth. Duluth functions as a cultural center for Northern Minnesota and has a symphony, a ballet, theaters, and art museums. Affordable off-campus housing options in the immediate area are available.

GRADUATES

About 95 percent of students are Minnesota residents. About 10 percent of students are minorities, most of whom are Native American. Class size is 53. At least 70 percent of graduates enter primary care fields, and most go on to practice in rural areas.

Admissions

REQUIREMENTS

Priority consideration is given to Minnesota residents who wish to become family practice or other primary care physicians in a rural Minnesota setting or American Indian community. Applicants from other states who demonstrate a high potential and motivation for practicing medicine in rural Minnesota or an American Indian community will also be considered. Applicants must be U.S. citizens or permanent residents and must have completed all requirements for a baccalaureate degree by the time of possible matriculation. Prerequisites are 1 year each of behavioral sciences, biology, English, general chemistry, humanities/social sciences, and physics. One math course in calculus or upper-level statistics, and one biochemistry course are also required. The MCAT is required, and scores must be no more than three years old.

SUGGESTIONS

UMD looks for applicants who demonstrate interest in entering family practice and other primary care specialties and working with underserved rural or small town communities in Minnesota or American Indian communities.

PROCESS

Secondary applications are sent to all applicants who are U.S. citizens or permanent residents. Of those returning secondaries, about 30 percent are invited to interview between October and April. Interviews consist of two 1-hour sessions, each with a member of the Admissions Committee. Notification occurs on a rolling basis, and about 35 percent of interviewees are offered a place in the class.

Admissions Requirements (Required)

MCAT scores, science GPA, non-science GPA, letters of recommendation, interview, state residency, essays/personal statement.

Admissions Requirements (Optional)

Extracurricular activities, exposure to medical profession.

Overlap Schools

A.T. Still University of Health Sciences; Creighton University; Mayo Clinic College of Medicine; Medical College of Wisconsin; University of Minnesota; University of Wisconsin—Madison.

COSTS AND AID

Tuition & Fees

In-state Tuition	$26,607
Out-of-state Tuition	$33,502
Room and board (off campus)	$13,158
Cost of books	$2,534
Fees	$2,591

Financial Aid

% students receiving aid	99
Average grant	$2,000
Average loan	$43,000

University of Minnesota—Twin Cities

Medical School

Office of Admissions, PO Box 293, 420 Delaware Street, Southeast, Minneapolis, MN 55455 • Admission: 612-624-1188
Fax: 612-625-8228 • E-mail: MEDED@UMN.EDU • Website: WWW.MED.UMN.EDU

STUDENT BODY

Type	Public
Enrollment	910
# applied (total/out)	2,285/1,663
# accepted	260
# enrolled (total/out)	165/46

ADMISSIONS

Average GPA and MCAT Scores

Overall GPA	3.68
MCAT Bio	10.8
MCAT Phys	10.5
MCAT Verbal	10.2
MCAT Essay	P

Application Information

Regular application	11/15
Regular notification	rolling
Early application	6/1–8/1
Early notification	10/1
Are transfers accepted?	yes
Admissions may be deferred?	yes
Interview required?	yes
Application fee	$75

Academics

In addition to a 4 year curriculum leading to the MD degree, Minnesota offers a combined degree MSTP MD/PhD program, leading to the doctorate degree in biochemistry, biomedical engineering, biophysics, cell biology, genetics, immunology, microbiology, molecular biology, neuroscience, pharmacology, and physiology. Dual degree programs are also offered— MD/MPH, MD/MBA, MD/MHI, MD/MS [BME], JD/MD. Evaluation of medical student performance in Year 1 and Year 2 is pass/fail and honors. Evaluation of performance in the Year 3 and Year 4 curriculum uses grades of honors, excellent, satisfactory, incomplete, and fail. Passing both steps of the USMLE is a graduation requirement. Faculty members serve as advisors to medical students.

BASIC SCIENCES: Basic sciences are taught as part of an interdisciplinary curriculum that also includes behavioral, social, and ethical aspects of medicine in addition to introductory clinical instruction. On average, students are in class or other scheduled sessions for 24 hours per week. First-year courses are gross anatomy; histology; biochemistry; general pathology; general pharmacology; human behavior; human genetics; human sexuality; microbiology; molecular and cellular biology; neuroscience; nutrition; physiology; physician and society; and physician and patient, the last of which focuses on history-taking and the physical examination. Second-year curriculum is systems-based. The courses are pathology—systemic, pathophysiology, pharmacology, physician and patient, and physician and society. Second-year students participate in four 6-week tutorials in family practice, internal medicine, pediatrics, and neurology. First and second year instruction takes place in the Moos Health Tower and other buildings in the basic science complex. The Biomedical Library contains more than 428,000 volumes, 4,393 journals, 1,194 audiovisual programs, and 223 computer programs. The reference department has more than 50 computers and has access to several online databases.

CLINICAL TRAINING

Students rotate through required clerkships during their third and fourth years: Medicine (12 weeks), ambulatory care (8 weeks), ob/gyn (6 weeks), surgery (6 weeks), pediatrics (6 weeks), psychiatry (6 weeks), neurology (4 weeks), emergency medicine (6 weeks), and surgical specialty (4 weeks). The remaining time is reserved for elective study. Clinical facilities include the Fairview-University Medical Center, Variety Club Heart and Research Center, Masonic Cancer Center, Veterans of Foreign Wars Cancer Research Center, Children's Rehabilitation Center, Paul F. Dwan Cardiovascular Research Center, Hennepine County Medical Center, Regions Hospital, Abbott Northwestern Hospital, Veteran's Administration Hospital, and other hospitals and ambulatory medical facilities in the Twin Cities area. Each year, through the Rural Physician Associate Program, up to 40 third-year medical students study primary health care in Minnesota communities under the supervision of local physicians. One-fourth of clinical electives may be fulfilled at non-affiliated institutions in other parts of the country or abroad.

Students

Of the 165 students in last year's entering class, 72 percent were Minnesota residents and 25 percent were multicultural. About 17 percent were from underrepresented minority groups. Typically, the average age of incoming students is 24.

STUDENT LIFE

Some students work part-time as graduate research or teaching assistants while in medical school. These positions provide academic opportunities and a source of income or tuition reduction. The Medical Student Adytum (adytum is Greek for "innermost sanctuary") is a spacious, comfortable area reserved solely for medical students and their guests. Students use the facility for studying, socializing, eating, and relaxing. Medical students also have the opportunity to interact with other health sciences students at an alternate student center— Center for Health Interdisciplinary Participation. Organizations bring students together around common interests, allowing them to contribute to the community and providing extracurricular activities. Examples of student organizations are Healthy Moms, Happy Babies; Phillips Neighborhood Clinic; Medical Student Computer Group; CLARION; Confidential Peer Assistance Program; SNMA; Physicians for Human Rights; and Students' International Health Committee. The medical school is part of the greater university, and medical students have access to its athletic and recreational facilities. Beyond the campus, the cities of Minneapolis and St. Paul offer a wide variety of restaurants, shopping, cultural activities, and entertainment. Housing options include residence halls, medical fraternities, and privately-owned apartments that are adjacent to the medical center.

GRADUATES

In the 2005 graduating class, the most popular fields for residencies were internal medicine (22 percent), family practice (18 percent), emergency medicine (7 percent), surgery (6 percent), pediatrics (6 percent), ob/gyn (5 percent), and orthopaedic surgery (4 percent). Generally, at least half of graduates enter postgraduate programs in Minnesota.

Admissions

REQUIREMENTS

Prerequisites are biology (2 semesters/quarters), general chemistry (2 semesters/quarters), organic chemistry (2 semesters/quarters), physics (2 semesters/3 quarters), English composition and literature (2 semesters), calculus (1 course), and biochemistry (1 course). In addition, 4 semesters/6 quarters of social and behavioral sciences and humanities are required. This requirement includes one course in psychology, with remaining course work in at least two of the following areas: Anthropology, comparative studies, history, music or art, philosophy, and sociology. The MCAT is required, and scores must be no more than three years old.

SUGGESTIONS

Minnesota residents are given preference. As indicated by the social science/humanities requirement, breadth in undergraduate preparation is important. In addition to academic strength, applicants should demonstrate volunteer/community service activity, personal integrity, high ethical standards, motivation, intellectual curiosity, enthusiasm, dedication to lifelong learning, and the ability to work well with others. Consistent with the Medical Student Education Mission, the Medical School seeks to matriculate a diverse student body. Diversity benefits the education of all students and supports the Medical School's commitment to graduate physicians who will serve the health needs of a diverse society. In evaluating an applicant's potential contribution to diversity in the Medical School, disadvantaged background, race and ethnicity, evidence of outstanding leadership, creativity, unique work or service experience, community involvement, non-educational progression, and demonstrated commitment to working with diverse populations are considered.

PROCESS

Qualified applicants who submit AMCAS applications are sent secondaries. Of those returning secondaries, about 80 percent of Minnesota residents and 30 percent of out-of-state applicants are invited to interview. Interviews take place on campus from September through March and consist of one session with a faculty member. Of interviewed candidates, about 25 percent of Minnesota residents and 15 percent of out-of-state residents are offered a place in the class. Applicants are accepted on a rolling admission basis, October through April. Additional materials from wait-listed candidates are not accepted.

Admissions Requirements (Required)

MCAT scores, science GPA, non-science GPA, letters of recommendation, interview, essays/personal statement, extracurricular activities, exposure to medical profession.

Admissions Requirements (Optional)

Research.

COSTS AND AID

Tuition & Fees

In-state Tuition	$24,389
Out-of-state Tuition	$30,709
Room and board (on campus)	$9,242
Room and board (off campus)	$12,342
Cost of books	$1,400
Fees	$2,046

Financial Aid

% students receiving aid	93
Average grant	$2,000
Average loan	$38,000
Average debt	$133,000

UNIVERSITY OF MISSISSIPPI
MEDICAL CENTER

2500 NORTH STATE STREET, JACKSON, MS 39216 • ADMISSION: 601-984-5010
FAX: 601-984-5008 • E-MAIL: ADMITMD@SOM.UMSMED.EDU • WEBSITE: WWW.SOM.UMC.EDU

STUDENT BODY

Type	Public
Enrollment	519
% male/female	59/41
% underrepresented minorities	14
# applied (total/out)	236/0
# accepted (total/out)	118/0
# enrolled (total/out)	106/0
Average age	24

FACULTY

Total faculty (number)	590
% female	24
% minority	14
% part-time	19
Student-faculty ratio	1:1

ADMISSIONS

Average GPA and MCAT Scores

Overall GPA	3.7
MCAT Bio	9.6
MCAT Phys	9.0
MCAT Verbal	9.68
MCAT Essay	0

Application Information

Regular application	10/15
Regular notification	3/15
Early application	8/1
Early notification	10/1
Are transfers accepted?	yes
Admissions may be deferred?	yes
Interview required?	yes

Academics

While most medical students follow a 4 year curriculum leading to the MD, some take advantage of other schools within the Medical Center and pursue joint-degree programs such as the combined MD/PhD curriculum, which leads to the doctorate in anatomy, biochemistry, microbiology, neuroscience, pathology, and pharmacology. Medical students receive percent scores and a class rank and may be awarded honors at the time of graduation. To be eligible for promotion, a student must achieve at least a 70 in each course, have a weighted average of 75 or higher, and attend 80 percent of the lectures and classes. Passing the USMLE Step 1 is a requirement for promotion to year 3, and passing Step 2 is a requirement for graduation.

BASIC SCIENCES: The basic sciences are integrated with clinical science courses and are taught through a combination of lectures, small groups, labs, and hands-on clinical experiences. Students are in class or other scheduled activity for about 22 hours per week. First-year courses are behavioral science and psychiatry, biochemistry, cardiopulmonary resuscitation, gross anatomy, histology, neurobiology, and medical physiology. Second-year courses are biostatistics, clinical psychiatry, general and systemic pathology, introduction to clinical medicine (ICM), medical genetics, medical microbiology, pharmacology, and preventive medicine and public health. In the ICM course students learn history-taking, examination, and diagnosis skills through classroom presentations and small-group sessions. The ICM experience helps prepare students for the clinical phase of the curriculum. Basic-science instruction facilities are central to the campus and include the Holmes Learning Resources Center, which houses the Rowland Medical Library. The library is impressive, with more than 160,000 volumes and 2,500 periodicals.

CLINICAL TRAINING

Required third-year rotations are medicine/neurology (12 weeks), surgery (12 weeks), ob/gyn (6 weeks), family medicine (6 weeks), psychiatry (6 weeks), and pediatrics (6 weeks). The fourth year is organized into 8 month-long blocks of selectives. Students choose specialty areas from within internal medicine, ob/gyn, pediatrics, and surgery. In addition, three blocks of selectives in an ambulatory setting and two blocks in inpatient settings are required. Throughout the fourth year, students participate in a senior seminar, which provides a forum for interdisciplinary instruction and discussion of issues relevant to modern medical practice. Clinical training takes place at the University Hospital (593 beds), Blair E. Batson Hospital for Children, the Veterans Administration Hospital, McBryde Rehabilitation Center for the Blind, Jackson Medical Mall Ambulatory Clinic, and State Health Department offices.

Students

In recent years all students have been Mississippi residents. Approximately 10 percent of students are underrepresented minorities, most of whom are African Americans. The average age of incoming students is generally around 24. Class size is 100.

STUDENT LIFE

Medical students use the resources and facilities of the university in addition to those of the greater community. As the state capital of Mississippi, Jackson offers numerous cultural and recreational attractions. Beyond clinical-care provision, the Medical School contributes directly to the community through activities such as the Base-Pair Mentorship Program, which pairs Medical School researchers and high school students and encourages them to jointly pursue academic projects. On-campus housing options include a residence hall for female students and an apartment complex with 1-, 2-, and 3-bedroom units.

GRADUATES

Graduates are successful in securing positions in a range of specialty areas. At the University Hospital in Jackson, there are more then 20 residency programs into which a number of graduates enter each year.

Admissions

REQUIREMENTS

Due to high competition in the admissions process, state residency is virtually a requirement. Required science courses are eight semester hours each of biology, chemistry, organic chemistry, and physics, all with associated labs. Three semester hours of college-level algebra and three of college-level trigonometry, or three semester hours of calculus, satisfies the math requirement. Six semester hours of English is an additional prerequisite. The MCAT is required, and scores for the class entering in 2006 must be from tests taken after 2001.

SUGGESTIONS

The April, rather than August, MCAT is advised. Beyond requirements, some advanced science course work in areas such as advanced physics, anatomy, biochemistry, embryology, genetics, histology, or physical chemistry is recommended. Other suggested courses are advanced English, fine arts, computer science, foreign language, geography, history, philosophy, psychology, and sociology. Math and science courses designed for non-science majors are not counted toward minimum requirements.

PROCESS

All Mississippi residents who submit AMCAS applications are sent secondaries. About half of those returning secondary applications are interviewed between August and January. Candidates have three interview sessions, each with a faculty member or administrator. In addition, a tour of the campus and the opportunity to have lunch with a current medical student is provided. Among interviewees, about half are accepted with notification occurring throughout the application cycle. Wait-listed candidates may send additional information to update their files.

Admissions Requirements (Required)

MCAT scores, science GPA, non-science GPA, letters of recommendation, interview, state residency, essays/personal statement, extracurricular activities, exposure to medical profession.

COSTS AND AID

Tuition & Fees

In-state Tuition	$7,649
Out-of-state Tuition	$14,327
Room and board (off campus)	$11,000
Cost of books	$4,000

Financial Aid

% students receiving aid	95
Average grant	$7,000
Average loan	$18,500
Average debt	$66,000

UNIVERSITY OF MISSOURI—COLUMBIA
SCHOOL OF MEDICINE

MA215 MEDICAL SCIENCES BUILDING, COLUMBIA, MO 65212 • ADMISSION: 573-882-9219
FAX: 573-884-2988 • E-MAIL: NOLKEJ@HEALTH.MISSOURI.EDU • WEBSITE: WWW.MUHEALTH.ORG/~MEDICINE

STUDENT BODY

Type	Public
Enrollment	375
% male/female	51/49
% underrepresented minorities	7
# applied (total/out)	959/557
# accepted	155
# enrolled (total/out)	96/12

FACULTY

Total faculty (number)	542
% female	30
% minority	14
% part-time	16
Student-faculty ratio	1:1

ADMISSIONS

Average GPA and MCAT Scores

Overall GPA	3.75
MCAT Bio	10.23
MCAT Phys	9.57
MCAT Verbal	10.05
MCAT Essay	P

Application Information

Regular application	11/1
Regular notification	3/15
Early application	8/1
Early notification	10/1
Are transfers accepted?	yes
Admissions may be deferred?	yes
Interview required?	yes
Application fee	$75

Academics

Although most students complete the MD curriculum in 4 years, some follow an extended program, leading to the MS or PhD along with the MD. Doctoral programs are available in diverse areas.

BASIC SCIENCES: Missouri is one of the leaders in the movement toward problem-based learning. Students learn in small groups and, with fewer than 20 hours per week in scheduled sessions, have ample time for self-study or individualized projects. The first two years are organized into eight 10-week blocks, each of which consists of 8 weeks of instruction followed by 1 week of evaluation and 1 week of vacation. Each block is divided into two general instructional components, problem-based learning and introduction to patient care. Block 1 is devoted to the structure and function of the human body, covering anatomy, biochemistry, embryology, histology, and molecular biology and genetics. Blocks 2, 3, and 4 each focus on a set of body/organ systems, which include the following: Cardiovascular, endocrine, gastrointestinal, hematology, immune response and pharmacokinetics, reproductive, liver, metabolism, neuroscience, pulmonary, renal, and respiratory. Year 2 is comprised of blocks 5–8, which concentrate on pathophysiology and clinical management. One of the main objectives of the second year is to prepare students for clinical rotations. Grading for the first year is satisfactory/unsatisfactory and for the second year is honors/satisfactory/unsatisfactory. The medical library and computer facilities are comprehensive and serve as educational resources for faculty, students, and the medical community.

CLINICAL TRAINING

Year 3 is divided into 7 blocks of required clerkships, which are the following: Child health, family medicine, internal medicine, ob/gyn, psychiatry, neurology, and surgery. A separate rural track offers up to 6 months of clinical experience in a rural community during the third year in lieu of some of the required rotations. Year 4 consists of 16 weeks of general electives and three 4-week advanced clinical selectives—one must be in a core medical specialty, and another must be in a core surgical specialty. Finally, fourth-year students must complete 4 weeks of advanced basic science selectives. The majority of clinical training is conducted at University Hospital and Clinics, a 288-bed tertiary care facility that draws patients from throughout central Missouri. Other training sites include Children's Hospital, Ellis Fischel Cancer Center, Columbia Regional Hospital, Truman VA Hospital, and the Rusk Rehabilitation Center. In total, clinical training sites encompass more than 1,000 patient beds. Grading for both of the clinical years is honors/letters of commendation/satisfactory/unsatisfactory. Students must pass Step 1 of the USMLE to be promoted to year 4 and Step 2-CK and 2-CS to graduate.

Students

The University of Missouri—Columbia is a state school, and the vast majority of the 96 entering students are Missouri residents. A large percentage attended the various public undergraduate colleges and universities throughout the state. Among students in the 2005 entering class, 76 percent were science majors as undergraduates. Approximately 7 percent of medical students are underrepresented minorities. The average age of incoming students is usually 24.

STUDENT LIFE

The School of Medicine is located in the heart of the University of Missouri's main campus, allowing students to take advantage of its recreational, athletic, and entertainment facilities. The curriculum gives students flexibility within their schedules, allowing them to explore both their academic and nonacademic interests. Student organizations are active, including Medical Student Activities Council (MSAC) and the local chapter of American Medical Student Association (AMSA), which coordinate academic, social, and cultural events and sponsor community-service projects. Columbia is located within a few hours of both Kansas City and St. Louis. Most medical students live in privately-owned apartments, generally a short distance from campus.

GRADUATES

About half of the graduates enter residencies in one of the primary care fields. A limited number of students seeking primary care careers are selected for a program that integrates the senior year of medical school with residency training in family medicine, internal medicine, pediatrics, or psychiatry.

Admissions

REQUIREMENTS

The School of Medicine requires 8 credit hours each of the following courses, all of which must be taken with associated labs: Biology, general chemistry, general physics, and organic chemistry. In addition to the traditional premedical courses, one semester of math and two semesters of English composition are also prerequisites. The MCAT is required. If a student has taken the MCAT more than once, the highest total set of MCAT scores is considered.

SUGGESTIONS

Course work in biology and chemistry beyond requirements and biochemistry is strongly recommended. In addition, applicants are encouraged to study humanities and social sciences while in college.

PROCESS

All Missouri residents (and some residents of other states) who submit an AMCAS application receive a secondary, which should be submitted as soon as possible. Almost 50 percent of the Missouri-resident applicants and at least 50 out-of-state applicants are invited to interview between October and April. Students are interviewed one-on-one by two members of the Admissions Committee. Current medical students give a short tour of the facilities and host a lunch. About one month after interviewing, applicants may be notified of the Committee's decision. Approximately 40 percent of interviewed candidates are accepted. Wait-listed candidates are not encouraged to send supplementary information.

Admissions Requirements (Required)

MCAT scores, science GPA, non-science GPA, letters of recommendation, interview, essays/personal statement, extracurricular activities, exposure to medical profession.

Admissions Requirements (Optional)

State residency, required course work from an accredited college.

COSTS AND AID

Tuition & Fees

In-state Tuition	$21,895
Out-of-state Tuition	$43,620
Room and board (on campus)	$8,433
Cost of books	$2,226

Financial Aid

% students receiving aid	94
Average grant	$3,495
Average loan	$33,495
Average debt	$119,666

UNIVERSITY OF MISSOURI—KANSAS CITY

SCHOOL OF MEDICINE

COUNCIL ON SELECTION, 2411 HOLMES, KANSAS CITY, MO 64108-2792 • ADMISSION: 816-235-1870
FAX: 816-235-6579 • E-MAIL: MORGENEGGM@UMKC.EDU • WEBSITE: WWW.UMKC.EDU/MED

STUDENT BODY	
Type	Public
Enrollment	630
% male/female	40/60
% underrepresented minorities	9
# applied (total/out)	476/199
# accepted (total/out)	176/44
# enrolled (total/out)	118/21
Average age	18

FACULTY	
Total faculty (number)	484
% female	32
% minority	14

ADMISSIONS

Average GPA and MCAT Scores

MCAT Essay	M

Application Information

Regular application	11/15
Regular notification	4/1
Are transfers accepted?	no
Admissions may be deferred?	no
Interview required?	yes
Application fee (in/out)	$35/$50

Academics

Rather than distinguishing premedical course work, pre-clinical medical course work, and clinical instruction, the curriculum integrates liberal arts, didactic medical sciences, and clinical training. Grading is letter grade, honors/credit/no credit, and narrative, and students must pass both Steps of the USMLE to graduate.

BASIC SCIENCES: During the first two years, students focus most of their efforts on working toward a baccalaureate degree through arts and science course work. Seventy-five percent of classroom hours are devoted to liberal arts studies and 25 percent to introductory medical course work. Year 1 (35 weeks) consists of undergraduate-level courses in biology, general chemistry, introduction to medicine, psychology, and sociology. The introduction to medicine course gives special attention to the effects of illness on the patient, family, and community. Students become acclimated to the hospital environment and are introduced to the medical vocabulary and to basic clinical skills such as patient interviews and simple data gathering. The second year (44 weeks) includes biostatistics, human biochemistry, life cycles, medical physiology, organic chemistry, and ongoing introductory clinical experiences. In years 3 and 4 (both 48 weeks), students take courses in anatomy, microbiology, pathology, and pharmacology and participate in clinical rotations, including a weekly continuing care clinic and family medicine preceptorship. Throughout the first four years, additional liberal arts courses are included in the curriculum that are considered part of the BA. To assist with clinical training, a physician-scholar (or docent) instructs and advises groups of 11 or 12 students. The docent acts as a mentor, guide, and preceptor throughout the entire six years.

CLINICAL TRAINING

Students enter fifth- and sixth-year clerkships having already had significant clinical exposure. They continue their weekly continuing care clinic experience. Year 5 (48 weeks) is comprised of rotations in ob/gyn (2 months), pediatrics (2 months), surgery (2 months), internal medicine (2 months), community medicine/family practice (1 month), and psychiatry (1 month). One month is reserved for electives. The sixth year (48 weeks) gives students ample opportunity to explore their specific areas of interest with 6 months of elective rotations. Required rotations include internal medicine (2 months) and emergency medicine (1 month). During the fifth or sixth year, students also take 1 month of liberal arts courses. Most training takes place at Truman Medical Center, one of the clinical facilities associated with UMKC.

Students

Approximately 80 percent of students are Missouri residents. Others come from high schools in neighboring states and other regions of the country. Underrepresented minorities account for about 6 percent of the student body. As a result of the structure of the program, students within a class are all roughly the same age.

STUDENT LIFE

For the most part, classes run year-round. Although the atmosphere is intense, students are committed and supportive of one another particularly because of the junior-senior partnership program. Students enjoy the resources of both the undergraduate campus and Kansas City. All students live on campus during the first year, but most choose to live off campus for the remainder of their studies.

GRADUATES

Graduates are successful in securing residency positions in all fields. Approximately 25 percent enter programs affiliated with UMKC.

Admissions

REQUIREMENTS

Applicants for admission at the freshman level must take the American College Test (ACT) or the SAT (out-of-state applicants only). Applicants should have completed 4 years of high school English; 4 years of math; 3 years of science, including 1 year each of biology and chemistry; 3 years of social studies; 1 year of foreign language; and 1 year in the fine arts. In addition, 1 year of physics and 1 semester of computer science are highly recommended by the medical school. If Advanced Placement (AP) courses are available, these are recommended as well. A limited number of positions are available at the year 3 level. Applicants to year 3 must have completed the standard premedical requirements of 1 year each of biology, chemistry, and organic chemistry as well as other requirements. The MCAT is required of these applicants, and scores must be from within the past 3 years.

SUGGESTIONS

For applicants to the BA/MD program and for those applying after college, some medically related experience is considered useful. High school students are encouraged to volunteer or work in a hospital or other health care environment.

PROCESS

UMKC is not a part of AMCAS. Applications may be obtained from the address above and are due by November 15. Interviews take place between December and mid-March and consist of two sessions, each of which is one-on-one. In addition to the interview, students and their parents attend group orientation sessions that cover a range of topics including financial aid. Applicants tour the campus and have the opportunity to meet with current students. All candidates are notified of the Admissions Committee's decision on April 1. Some are accepted from a wait list later in the spring.

Admissions Requirements (Required)

Letters of recommendation, interview, essays/personal statement, performance on the Toledo Chemistry Assessment.

Admissions Requirements (Optional)

MCAT scores, science GPA, non-science GPA, state residency, extracurricular activities, exposure to medical profession.

COSTS AND AID

Tuition & Fees

In-state Tuition	$28,102
Out-of-state Tuition	$53,398
Room and board (on campus)	$7,390
Cost of books	$800

Financial Aid

Average loan	$27,000

UNIVERSITY OF MONTREAL
FACULTÉ DE MEDÉCINE

CP 6128, SUCCURSALE CENTRE-VILLE, MONTREAL, QC H3C 3J7 • ADMISSION: 514-343-6265
E-MAIL: FACMED@MEDDIR.UMONTREAL.CA • WEBSITE: WWW.MED.UMONTREAL.CA

STUDENT BODY

Type	Public
# applied (total/out)	1,859/270

ADMISSIONS

Application Information

Regular application	3/1
Regular notification	3/31
Admissions may be deferred?	no
Interview required?	yes
Application fee	$45

Academics

Instruction is solely in French. Some students enter a 1 year premedical program that leads into the 4 year MD curriculum, while others who qualify enter the medical curriculum directly. Although clinical exposure begins during the first year of premedical or medical training, intensive clinical training begins in the third year. The premedical program is taught through lectures. On the other hand, the majority of instruction for medical students takes place in a small-group setting. In addition to the 4 year MD curriculum, graduate degree programs are offered in all major medical science fields. Affiliated with the School of Medicine are other health science programs in areas such as health administration, public health, social and preventive medicine, nutrition, rehabilitation, and speech language therapy.

BASIC SCIENCES: Students who enter the premedical program take courses in basic concepts in ethics, biostatistics, cell biology and general histology, cell and molecular biology, cell physiology and pharmacology, clinical immersion, genetics and embryology, general microbiology and virology, introduction to clinical anatomy, introduction to physiology, introduction to sociology, nutrition and metabolism, psychology and human behavior, and an elective. First-year medical school courses are introduction to medical studies; growth, development, and aging; general pathology and immunology; infectious diseases; hematology; neurological sciences; mind; musculoskeletal system; introduction to clinical medicine; history of medicine; epidemiology; and an elective. Second-year studies are largely organized by anatomical systems. These are cardiovascular, digestion, endocrinology, multisystem, respiratory, and kidney. Second-year students also take an elective and continue with introduction to clinical medicine.

CLINICAL TRAINING

For clinical training, students complete a series of required clerkships that provide hands-on experience in the major medical disciplines. During the third year, required clerkships are medicine (8 weeks), surgery (8 weeks), pediatrics (8 weeks), psychiatry (8 weeks), ob/gyn (8 weeks), and family medicine (4 weeks). Third-year students also have the opportunity for a 4 week clinical elective. Fourth-year clerkships are radiology (4 weeks), geriatrics (4 weeks), community medicine (4 weeks), anesthesiology (2 weeks), ophthalmology (2 weeks), and an elective (4 weeks). Selectives are chosen from medical or pediatric subspecialties (8 weeks) and from surgical subspecialties (4 weeks). Clinical training takes place at more than 15 affiliated hospitals including Hôpital Maisonneuve-Rosemont, Hôpital Notre-Dame, Hôpital Riviere-des-Prairies, Hôpital du Sacre-Coeur de Montréal, Hôpital Louis-H Lafontaine, Hôpital Sainte-Justine, Hôpital Saint-Luc, Hotel-Dieu de Montréal, Institute de Cardiologie de Montréal, Institut de Readaptation de Montréal, Centre Hospitalier de Verdun, Cite de la Sante de Laval, Institue de Recherches Clinique de Montréal, Institut Philippe-Pinel de Montréal, and Centre Hospitalier Cote des-Neiges.

Students

Entering class size is 143. In a recent class, all but four students were from the province of Quebec. About 60 percent of the students are women.

STUDENT LIFE

Medical students enjoy a good quality of life. The School of Medicine is committed to its students, providing academic and nonacademic support services. Outside of the classroom, medical students interact through student groups and organized social activities. The resources of the greater university, including athletic and recreational facilities, are available to medical students as well. Finally, the city of Montreal is an internationally recognized cultural center with a wealth of activities accessible to students.

GRADUATES

Graduates enter both academic and clinical medicine. At hospitals affiliated with the University of Montreal, postgraduate medical training is available in anesthesiology, family medicine, medicine, ob/gyn, ophthalmology, pediatrics, psychiatry, radiology, surgery, and many other postgraduate programs.

Admissions

REQUIREMENTS

Only Canadian citizens, landed immigrants, and highly-qualified French-speaking applicants from the United States are considered for admission. Fluency in French is a requirement. Two years of college is the minimum requirement for admission to the School of Medicine. Prerequisites are behavioral sciences, biology, English, French, general chemistry, mathematics (through trigonometry), organic chemistry, philosophy, physics, social sciences.

SUGGESTIONS

Strong preference is given to applicants from the province of Quebec. Selection is based on both records of academic performance and interviews.

PROCESS

The absolute deadline for applications is March 1. About one-third of all applicants are asked to interview, with invitations based on the candidate's academic record. The strongest candidates are then selected from those interviewed. Admissions decisions are made in the spring, with the first acceptance notices given in May. Accepted applicants have 2 weeks in which to confirm their place in the entering class.

Admissions Requirements (Required)

Interview.

COSTS AND AID

Tuition & Fees

In-state Tuition	$2,575
Out-of-state Tuition	$12,836
Fees	$30

UNIVERSITY OF NEBRASKA MEDICAL CENTER

COLLEGE OF MEDICINE

986585 NEBRASKA MEDICAL CENTER, OMAHA, NE 68198-6585 • ADMISSION: 402-559-6140
FAX: 402-559-6840 • E-MAIL: GRROGERS@UNMC.EDU • WEBSITE: WWW.UNMC.EDU/UNCOM/

STUDENT BODY

Type	Public
Enrollment	475
% male/female	59/41
% underrepresented minorities	10
# applied (total/out)	1,101/807
# accepted (total/out)	169/35
# enrolled (total/out)	122/17

FACULTY

Total faculty (number)	579
% part-time	20

ADMISSIONS

Average GPA and MCAT Scores

Overall GPA	3.75
MCAT Bio	10
MCAT Phys	9.5
MCAT Verbal	9.6
MCAT Essay	O

Application Information

Regular application	11/1
Regular notification	rolling
Early application	8/1
Early notification	10/1
Are transfers accepted?	yes
Admissions may be deferred?	no
Interview required?	yes
Application fee	$45

Academics

Most medical students complete the MD curriculum in 4 years, although some may take one additional year for research projects or other activities. A combined MD/PhD program is offered to qualified students, leading to the doctorate degree in a number of fields, including biochemistry and molecular biology, cell biology and anatomy, physiology and biophysics, pathology and microbiology, and pharmacology. For medical students interested in discrete research projects, summer research stipends are available on a competitive basis. Passing the USMLE Step 1 is a requirement for promotion to year 3, and all students must record a score on Step 2 to graduate.

BASIC SCIENCES: Throughout the first two years, basic sciences are integrated with introductory clinical instruction and topics are organized into blocks, referred to as cores. Students are in class for about 32 hours per week, most of which is spent in lectures, small groups, or labs. During the first year, these are cellular processes, function of the human body, neuroscience, and structure and development of the human body. Throughout the first and second years, integrated clinical experience (ICE) covers behavioral sciences, ethics, history and physical examination, health care policy, health care services research, interviewing skills, and preventive medicine. Through ICE, students have the opportunity to work alongside primary care physicians in a longitudinal clinical experience and a summer preceptorship. Also spanning both years is problem-based learning, in which students work in small groups and apply basic science concepts to clinical case studies. Second-year cores are cardiology/pulmonary/endocrinology/ear, nose, and throat; dermatology and infectious disease; genitourinary/gastroenterology; hematology/oncology/musculoskeletal; introduction to disease processes; and neurology, ophthalmology, and psychiatry. Instruction takes place in the Durham Research Center and in Wittson Hall, which also houses administrative offices, laboratories, and audiovisual resources. The Leon S. McGoogan Library of Medicine holds more than 200,000 volumes and 2,100 current journals. Multimedia materials for computer-assisted learning and self-instruction are available, as are online informational systems.

CLINICAL TRAINING

Required third-year clerkships are internal medicine (12 weeks), surgery (10 weeks), pediatrics (8 weeks), community preceptorship (8 weeks), psychiatry (6 weeks), ob/gyn (6 weeks), basic science selective (4 weeks), and a mini-clerkship in an area of choice (4 weeks). During the fourth year, a basic science selective in addition to 28 weeks of electives are required. Clinical facilities at UNMC are Nebraska Health System (650 beds); University Medical Associates, which operates more than 60 primary care and subspecialty clinics throughout the greater Omaha metropolitan area; Meyer Rehabilitation Institute; Omaha Veterans Affairs Medical Center; Children's Hospital; Immanuel Hospital; and Methodist Hospital.

Students

Most students in each class are Nebraska residents. Class size is 120.

STUDENT LIFE

Medical students are active in student organizations ranging from the Student Alliance for Global Health to the Family Practice Club to a group focused on alternative medicine. The local chapter of the American Medical Student Association is particularly active, organizing volunteer projects, film series, and opportunities for enhanced clinical exposure. Omaha is a city of 800,000, offering a symphony, theaters, art museums, shopping, restaurants, and parks, among other attractions. Students live off campus in the surrounding communities, where, for an urban area, housing is relatively inexpensive.

GRADUATES

Students are successful at securing residencies in both primary care and specialty areas. A significant percentage of graduates enter postgraduate programs at UNMC, which oversees 18 residency programs. In recent years, at least 60 percent of graduates have gone on to practice in the state of Nebraska.

Admissions

REQUIREMENTS

Prerequisites are humanities and/or social sciences (12 hours), biology (8 semester hours), general chemistry (8 hours), organic chemistry (8 hours), physics (8 hours), English composition (3 hours), calculus or statistics (3 credits), biochemistry (3 hours), and genetics (3 hours). All science courses must include associated labs. The MCAT is required, and scores cannot be more than three years old.

SUGGESTIONS

State residents are given preference, but other highly-qualified candidates are considered, particularly if they have ties to Nebraska and are interested in practicing in underserved communities in the state. Beyond required courses, the following are recommended: Communications, ethics, and personnel management; molecular biology; immunology; and microbiology.

PROCESS

All Nebraska residents who apply through AMCAS, and a small percentage of out-of-state applicants, are asked to submit supplementary materials and are interviewed. Interviews are conducted between October and February and consist of a 30-minute session with a faculty member. On interview day, there is also a group information session and a campus tour. Typically, about 50 percent of Nebraska residents are accepted, with notification beginning in December. Wait-listed candidates may send additional information to update their files.

Admissions Requirements (Required)

MCAT scores, science GPA, non-science GPA, letters of recommendation, interview, state residency, essays/personal statement, extracurricular activities, exposure to medical profession.

COSTS AND AID

Tuition & Fees

In-state Tuition	$19,568
Out-of-state Tuition	$47,198
Room and board (on campus)	$13,500
Cost of books	$1,800
Fees	$1,907

Financial Aid

% students receiving aid	92
Average debt	$100,875

University of Nevada
School of Medicine

Office of Admissions, Reno, NV 89557 • Admission: 702-784-6063
Fax: 702-784-6194 • E-mail: ASA@SCS.UNR.EDU • Website: WWW.UNR.EDU/UNR/MED.HTML

STUDENT BODY

Type	Public
Enrollment	208
% male/female	61/39
% underrepresented minorities	5
# applied	871
# accepted (total/out)	52/5
# enrolled (out-of-state)	5

ADMISSIONS

Average GPA and MCAT Scores

Overall GPA	3.6

Application Information

Regular application	11/1
Early application	6/1–8/1
Early notification	10/1
Are transfers accepted?	yes
Admissions may be deferred?	yes
Interview required?	yes
Application fee	$45

Academics

The first 2 years provide a foundation in basic clinical sciences, significant pre-clinical training, and clerkships that take place statewide in community clinics as well as hospital settings. The School of Medicine applicants or current medical students may apply to jointly pursue a MD/PhD program in several areas including cell and molecular biology, pharmacology, and physiology. For students interested in research without undertaking a PhD, projects can be arranged with faculty members.

BASIC SCIENCES: The first 2 years at Nevada focus not only on the basic sciences but also give considerable attention to community health and social issues. Additional scientific material is presented through lectures, labs, and small-group formats at the Reno campus. Students apply scientific principles to clinical challenges through problem-solving courses using case study methods. This approach promotes the development of problem-solving skills in medical students. Concurrent with basic and behavioral science courses, students learn fundamental skills in doctor-patient relationship and physical exams through weekly sessions that are supervised by physicians and senior medical students. In this way, students learn not only from full-time faculty but also from knowledgeable and experienced clinical faculty physicians throughout the state. First-year course work includes clinical problem solving, embryology, human biochemistry, human anatomy, histology, neuroanatomy, human behavior, introduction to patient care, medical cell biology, neurosciences, nutrition, and systems physiology. Year 2 courses include clinical problem solving II, community medicine, human genetics, introduction to patient care II, laboratory medicine, medical ethics, medical mircobiology, medical pharmacology, pathology, and psychiatric medicine. Most courses are graded on a letter grade from A–F, and students must receive at least a C to be promoted. Students are evaluated on both cognitive and noncognitive factors. The two following major medical libraries serve the medical students: The Savitt Medical Library on the Reno campus, containing more than 40,000 volumes, and the University Medical Center Library in Las Vegas, both of which maintain computer labs that feature an assortment of general and curriculum-based software. Additional learning resource labs are available in Las Vegas in the ambulatory care centers. Students have electronic access to all of Nevada's university and community college collections through terminals located throughout the teaching sites in the state. Students are issued computer accounts for e-mail and Internet access. In addition, passing the USMLE Step 1 is required for promotion to year 3.

CLINICAL TRAINING

Training takes place at affiliated hospitals, clinics, and ambulatory care centers throughout the state. Most students have required rotations including the practice of medicine, which is a 24-week integrated clerkship experience that includes internal medicine (12 weeks), family medicine (6 weeks), and pediatrics (6 weeks). The practice of medicine also includes a core curriculum that runs throughout the state via distance education facilities. Medical students also complete required specialty rotations of surgery (12 weeks), ob/gyn (6 weeks), and psychiatry (6 weeks). There is an increased emphasis in all of the rotations to blend ambulatory and hospital-based practice to give the students a balanced educational experience. During the fourth year, students rotate through 32 weeks of elective clerkships and 4 weeks of a required rural clerkship. Elective study can take place in Reno, Las Vegas, rural Nevada, other states, or abroad. Although the obvi ous emphasis and strength of the program is primary care and rural medicine, hospitals in Reno and Las Vegas treat urban and often international populations. Evaluation of clinical performance is honors/pass/fail. In addition, special awards and honors are granted to students who have made unique and outstanding achievements in clinical areas. Passing the USMLE Step 2 is required for graduation.

Students

Eighty-five percent of students majored in a science-related discipline in college. About 5 percent are underrepresented minorities, most of whom are Mexican or Native American. Almost all students are Nevada residents, although many attended college in other states. About one-fourth of each class took some time off between college and medical school.

STUDENT LIFE

Small class size promotes cohesion among students. A designated lounge on campus gives medical students a place to relax and interact. The following athletic facilities are available: Students in the Reno area use the Lombardi Recreational Facility and, in Las Vegas, the McDermott Physical Education Facility. Student organizations include AMWA and OSR medical specialty interest groups; the Significant Others Group for Partners of Medical Students; and the University of Nevada Student Outreach Clinic, through which medical students, with supervision, volunteer to treat patients from underserved areas. Beyond campus, Lake Tahoe is just 1 hour from Reno and offers outstanding outdoor activities all year. Virtually all medical students live off campus, where housing is affordable and comfortable.

GRADUATES

The majority of graduates enter residency programs outside the state. Almost all graduates ultimately become practicing clinical physicians.

Admissions

REQUIREMENTS

Required course work includes biology (12 semester hours), chemistry (8 hours), organic chemistry (8 hours), physics (8 hours), and behavioral science (6 hours). The biology and behavioral science requirements specify that at least 3 semester hours be upper-division credit. GPA is used, along with MCAT scores, to screen for interview invitations. The most recent MCAT scores are used, and the exam must have been taken within the past 3 years.

SUGGESTIONS

Only applicants from Nevada, Wyoming, Alaska, Montana, and Idaho, and those who have close ties to Nevada are considered for admission. Nevada residents are given preference. Community-focused work and health care experience are considered important.

PROCESS

Interviews are held from September through January. The interview is composed of two 50-minute sessions, which may be with faculty or medical students. Of interviewed candidates, about 25 percent of Nevada residents are offered a place in the class, and about 10 percent of out-of-state applicants are accepted. The first acceptances are sent in January. Wait-listed candidates are ranked.

Admissions Requirements (Required)

MCAT scores, science GPA, non-science GPA, letters of recommendation, interview, state residency, essays/personal statement, extracurricular activities, exposure to medical profession.

COSTS AND AID

Tuition & Fees

In-state Tuition	$9,232
Out-of-state Tuition	$26,810
Fees	$2,375

Financial Aid

% students receiving aid	80

UNIVERSITY OF NEW MEXICO
SCHOOL OF MEDICINE

MSC 08 4690, BMSB ROOM 106, ALBUQUERQUE, NM 87131 • ADMISSION: 505-272-4766
FAX: 505-272-8239 • E-MAIL: SOMADMISSIONS@SALUD.UNM.EDU • WEBSITE: WWW.HSC.UNM.EDU/SOM/

STUDENT BODY

Type	Public
Enrollment	324
% male/female	43/57
% underrepresented minorities	43
# applied (total/out)	994/760
# accepted (total/out)	92/4
# enrolled (total/out)	75/4
Average age	28

FACULTY

Total faculty (number)	715
% part-time	14
Student-faculty ratio	2:1

ADMISSIONS

Average GPA and MCAT Scores

Overall GPA	3.59
MCAT Bio	9.8
MCAT Phys	9.1
MCAT Verbal	9.5

Application Information

Regular application	11/15
Regular notification	3/15
Early application	8/1
Early notification	10/1
Are transfers accepted?	yes
Admissions may be deferred?	yes
Interview required?	yes
Application fee	$50

Academics

The 4 year curriculum is organized into 3 phases, all of which involve at least some basic science instruction and clinical training. In addition, all students conduct research projects under the guidance of a faculty mentor. The complete project consists of research, presentation, and a written paper. Applicants interested in pursuing a combined MD/PhD may apply to the graduate committee at the School of Medicine in addition to completing medical school admissions requirements. Medical students are evaluated as outstanding, good, satisfactory, marginal, and unsatisfactory. The USMLE Step 1 must be passed prior to graduation, and Step 2 must be taken to graduate.

BASIC SCIENCES: The first year and a half (phase I) is organized into discrete segments, most of which focus on an organ system. First-year subjects are cardiovascular/pulmonary, foundations, GI/nutrition/metabolism, musculoskeletal, neuroscience, and renal/endocrine. During the summer following year 1, students take part in a 3 month practical immersion experience that involves hands-on clinical work in either a rural or urban setting. Phase I continues in the first semester of year 2 with human sex and reproduction, infectious disease, neoplasma, and molecular genetics. A range of learning methodologies are used, including lectures, labs, discussions, tutorials, and seminars. Concurrent to basic science instruction are weekly clinical experiences in both inpatient and ambulatory settings. Here, students learn interviewing and examination techniques, and are able to improve communication and personal interaction skills. Much of phase I and II take place in the Basic Medical Sciences Building. The nearby Health Sciences Center Library supports educational, research, and clinical activities. It houses 150,000 volumes in addition to audiovisuals, online search services, and computer software.

CLINICAL TRAINING

Phase II begins midway through year 2 with a 3-week pharmacology block and orientation to the hospital. Clinical rotations are accompanied by ongoing small-group sessions focused on problem solving and integrating information. Students rotate through required clerkships throughout the spring and summer of the second year and the fall and winter of the third year. Requirements are internal medicine (8 weeks), surgery (8 weeks), neurology/psychiatry (8 weeks), family medicine ambulatory (8 weeks), pediatrics ambulatory/inpatient (8 weeks), and ob/gyn ambulatory/inpatient (8 weeks). Phase III begins in the spring of year 3 and is comprised entirely of selectives and electives. A one month-long, community-based preceptorship, in which students work alongside a primary care physician who serves as a mentor, is also required. Clinical training takes place at the University Hospital (370 beds) and at several affiliated sites, namely: Regional Federal Medical Center (429 beds); UNM Cancer Center; UNM Mental Health Center; UNM Children's Psychiatric Hospital (73 beds); and the Carrie Tingley Hospital for Children.

Students

About 25 percent of students are underrepresented minorities, most of whom are Mexican Americans. At least 90 percent of students are New Mexico residents, and about half of each class graduated from UNM's undergraduate college. In a recent class, the average age of entering students was 25, and around one-third of students took time off after college. Class size is 73.

STUDENT LIFE

The medical school is located on the North campus of UNM, allowing students access to the resources and facilities of the university. The city also provides an outlet for students who need a break from studying. The greater Albuquerque metropolitan area is home to nearly one-third of the state's population and offers numerous cultural and recreational opportunities. Although no on-campus housing is available, off-campus options are convenient and comfortable.

GRADUATES

About 35 percent of graduates enter residencies at UNM, which offers programs in 12 different departments. The majority of graduates enter primary care fields.

Admissions

REQUIREMENTS

Prerequisites are general biology (8 semester hours), general chemistry (8 semester hours), organic chemistry (8 semester hours), physics (6 semester hours), and biochemistry (3 semester hours). Competency in English and the MCAT are additional requirements.

SUGGESTIONS

Knowledge of Spanish or a Native American language is an advantage. Course work in the humanities and social sciences is important. The April, rather than August, MCAT is advised. Students are selected on the basis of academic achievement, motivation for the study of medicine, problem-solving ability, self-appraisal, ability to relate to people, maturity, breadth of interest and achievements, professional goals, and the likelihood of serving the health care needs of the state following postgraduate training.

PROCESS

All New Mexico AMCAS applicants receive secondary applications and are invited to interview. Qualified WICHE and other out-of-state applicants who apply for early decision are also sent secondary materials and invited to interview. Interviews are conducted from June through March and consist of two sessions with members of the Admissions Committee, who are either full-time faculty members or community physicians. On interview day, lunch and a tour of the facilities are provided. Of interviewed candidates, about 20–25 percent are accepted. Wait-listed candidates are ranked and notified of their position on the list.

Admissions Requirements (Required)

MCAT scores, letters of recommendation, interview, state residency, essays/personal statement, extracurricular activities, exposure to medical profession.

Admissions Requirements (Optional)

Science GPA, nonscience GPA.

COSTS AND AID

Tuition & Fees

In-state Tuition	$12,893
Out-of-state Tuition	$37,032
Room and board	
(off campus)	$9,976
Cost of books	$1,546
Fees	$1,749

Financial Aid

% students receiving aid	89
Average grant	$3,700
Average loan	$23,000
Average debt	$91,461

UNIVERSITY OF NORTH CAROLINA SCHOOL OF MEDICINE AT CHAPEL HILL
UNC SCHOOL OF MEDICINE

121 MACNIDER BUILDING, CB #9500, CHAPEL HILL, NC 27599 • ADMISSION: 919-962-8331
FAX: 919-966-9930 • E-MAIL: ADMISSIONS@MED.UNC.EDU • WEBSITE: WWW.MED.UNC.EDU

STUDENT BODY

Type	Public

ADMISSIONS

Average GPA and MCAT Scores

Overall GPA	3.7
MCAT Bio	10.57
MCAT Phys	10.48
MCAT Verbal	10.25

Academics

The core curriculum gives students the required comprehensive education needed before they embark on the next stage of their careers. In addition, many students pursue focused research training in the clinic or at the bench. Research stipends are available through training grants or individual research grants. Students with a particular interest in research may apply for the MSTP-supported MD/PhD program at UNC. Other students take the opportunity to combine an advanced degree in business, law, or public health with their medical studies. Grades of honors, pass, and fail are used to evaluate medical students in the first two years. Students must pass the USMLE Step 1 examination before promotion to the third year and pass Step 2 before graduation.

BASIC SCIENCES: The first 2 years are devoted primarily to studying the scientific basis of clinical practice, with emphasis on demonstrating clinical implications and correlation. Clinical instruction begins early in the first year with the 2 year course introduction to clinical medicine (ICM), in which students have the opportunity to develop the clinical skills (such as history-taking, physical examination) and problem-solving abilities needed for the clinical years. ICM also serves as a forum for discussion of a wide range of cross-cutting topics such as substance abuse, domestic violence, and computing in medicine. Three months of both the first and second years are spent in a community working with a physician tutor. Other first-year courses are biochemistry, cell biology, gross anatomy, histology, immunology, introduction to pathology, medical embryology, medical physiology, medicine and society, microbiology, and neurobiology. Many of the courses in the second year are organized around the pathophysiology of particular organ systems such as cardiovascular, endocrine, gastrointestinal, hematology/oncology, musculoskeletal, neurology and special senses, reproductive biology, respiratory, skin, and urinary. Closely integrated with the study of particular organ systems are courses in genetics, humanities, pathology, psychiatry, and social sciences. Throughout the first and second years, students participate in small group discussions, lectures, labs, clinical practice sessions, and real clinical experiences. The needs of the curriculum are well served by continuous training in information technology coupled with the requirement that each student have a laptop computer. The Health Sciences Library serves the Schools of Dentistry, Medicine, Nursing, Pharmacy, and Public Health and the UNC Hospitals. The library has approximately 300,000 volumes, 4,000 serial titles, and 9,000 audiovisual and microcomputer software programs.

CLINICAL TRAINING
Students rotate through 6 major clinical disciplines during their third year. These are medicine (12 weeks), pediatrics (8 weeks), surgery (8 weeks), family medicine (6 weeks), psychiatry (6 weeks), and obstetrics/gynecology (6 weeks). An additional requirement is life support skills (1 week). The purpose of the fourth-year program is to offer a flexible educational experience that can be tailored to the career goals and intellectual interests of each student. Requirements are an ambulatory care selective (4 weeks), an acting internship (4 weeks), a neuroscience selective (4 weeks), and a critical care/surgery selective. A total of 28 weeks of electives is required, some of which may be completed at other universities or clinical settings, either in the United States or overseas.

Students

Approximately 90 percent of students are North Carolina residents. The School of Medicine is committed to admitting students who are representative of the diversity of the population of North Carolina. About one-third of entering students have pursued other interests or careers before applying to medical school.

STUDENT LIFE

The School of Medicine is responsive to students' needs and provides a range of support services. Faculty advisors are assigned to entering students and serve as mentors and academic counselors throughout all four years. The School of Medicine has 26 student organizations, including the student body government, student chapters of national medical professional organizations, community service groups, and special interest groups. Students are particularly active in outreach efforts such as Habitat for Humanity, the Domestic Violence Coalition, Physicians for Social Responsibility, and manage two community clinics. During the academic year, scheduled events bring faculty, students, families, and the community together. The university offers single room accommodations for some graduate students in a building near the medical center. Other students live off campus in surrounding neighborhoods.

GRADUATES

Among 2,000 graduates, 53 percent entered primary care fields, and 30.6 percent chose postgraduate training programs within North Carolina. Eighty-four percent of the class of 2000 matched with one of their top three choices for residency training.

Admissions

REQUIREMENTS

Prerequisites are under review and may be changed. Current prerequisites are 8 semester hours of biology, at least 4 hours of which must be accompanied by a lab. Students are strongly encouraged to have taken at least one course in molecular and cell biology. Eight semester hours of general chemistry, organic chemistry, and physics, all with lab, are also required, in addition to 6 semester hours of English. The MCAT is required.

SUGGESTIONS

Preference is given to residents of North Carolina. Thus, successful applicants who are not residents of North Carolina typically have outstanding qualifications.

PROCESS

Approximately 50 percent of AMCAS applicants who are North Carolina residents, and fewer than 10 percent of nonresidents, are sent secondary applications and are invited to interview. Interviews take place between August and March and consist of two sessions with faculty members and one member of the Admissions Committee. On interview day, candidates also have lunch with currently enrolled medical students and go on tours of the campus.

COSTS AND AID	
Tuition & Fees	
In-state Tuition	$8,188
Out-of-state Tuition	$33,656
Room and board	
(on campus)	$12,128
Cost of books	$1,050

UNIVERSITY OF NORTH DAKOTA
SCHOOL OF MEDICINE AND HEALTH SCIENCES

501 NORTH COLUMBIA ROAD, PO BOX 9037, GRAND FORKS, ND 58202-9037 • ADMISSION: 701-777-4221
FAX: 701-777-4942 • E-MAIL: JDHEIT@MEDICINE.NODAK.EDU • WEBSITE: WWW.MED.UND.NODAK.EDU

STUDENT BODY

Type	Public
Enrollment	236
% male/female	48/52
% underrepresented minorities	12
# applied (total/out)	250/122
# accepted (total/out)	84/28
# enrolled (total/out)	61/17
Average age	24

FACULTY

Total faculty (number)	1,442
% female	39
% part-time	90
Student-faculty ratio	2:1

ADMISSIONS

Average GPA and MCAT Scores

Overall GPA	3.7
MCAT Bio	9.7
MCAT Phys	8.85
MCAT Verbal	8.85
MCAT Essay	0

Application Information

Regular application	11/1
Regular notification	1/15
Are transfers accepted?	no
Admissions may be deferred?	yes
Interview required?	yes
Application fee	$50

Academics

Pre-clinical instruction takes place at the University of North Dakota campus in Grand Forks, and clinical training takes place throughout the state. After students have been admitted to the MD program, they may apply to pursue a joint-MD/PhD program in anatomy and cell biology, biochemistry and molecular biology, microbiology and immunology, physiology, pharmacology, and therapeutics. Evaluation of students is with ratings of satisfactory or unsatisfactory during the first year and honors, satisfactory, or unsatisfactory for the final three years. Step 1 and 2 of the USMLE must be passed to graduate.

BASIC SCIENCES: The basic sciences are taught through a combination of lectures, labs, and small-group sessions. The curriculum puts significant emphasis on active student participation and early clinical experience. Social science courses that address topics such as statistics, human behavioral patterns, and social issues that are relevant in North Dakota and other rural areas are integrated into the basic science and clinical curriculum throughout the first and second years. The first-year courses are organized into blocks, namely functional biology of cells and tissues, biology of organ systems I, biology of organ systems II, and biology of the nervous system. These blocks are offered in the morning. The afternoons are reserved for self-study, or introduction to patient care (IPC), which is the clinical component and is also organized into blocks, such as IPC block I—interviewing and professionalism. The same format continues into the second year. Second-year blocks include the following: Introduction to pathobiology and pathobiology I, II, and III. The IPC component again is covered during afternoon sessions. Students also complete their first clinical rotation and introduction to inpatient and ambulatory practice of medicine (3 weeks). Most instruction takes place in the Medical Sciences Building, which houses administrative offices, classrooms, labs, and the library. The Harley E. French Library of the Health Sciences has more than 80,000 books, periodicals, and audiovisual programs. It is fully automated and offers computers for informational and research purposes. The proximity of basic science instructional facilities to the clinical and research facilities promotes an integrated-learning experience during the first 2 years.

CLINICAL TRAINING

Third-year, required clerkships are medicine (8 weeks); surgery (8 weeks); pediatrics (8 weeks); ob/gyn (8 weeks); psychiatry (8 weeks); family medicine (8 weeks); and clinical epidemiology, which is taken throughout the year. Students are assigned to the Bismarck, Fargo, or Grand Forks campuses for the third year, or they may participate in the ROME (Rural Opportunities in Medical Education) Program. ROME students are assigned to a rural practice site for 7 months of the third year and to their home campus for the balance of the year. During the fourth year, students train at regional sites in Bismarck, Fargo, Minot, and Grand Forks. Each campus is affiliated with as many as 10–22 hospitals and provides health care services to anywhere from 9–18 counties. The fourth year includes acting internships and electives. Clinical students train at sites throughout the state, including community hospitals, clinics that are part of the Indian Health Service, and physicians' offices. The University of North Dakota's Center for Rural Health focuses on policy analysis and research on rural health care delivery at the state, regional, and national level.

Students

Most students are North Dakota residents, although up to 11 students in each class may be from Minnesota, Montana, and Wyoming. Up to seven students in each class (admitted as part of INMED) are Native American. In total, underrepresented minorities account for about 17 percent of the student body. About 20–25 percent of an entering class is composed of older students who took time off between college and medical school. Class size is 62.

STUDENT LIFE

Grand Forks is a community of 50,000 people, located in the Red River Valley on the border between North Dakota and Minnesota. The city is affordable and safe and offers the services that students need. Students have access to the facilities of the greater university and are encouraged to participate in student organizations, including the local chapters of national medical student organizations. On-campus housing is available, although many students opt to live off campus. Since clinical training takes place around the state, students will experience a variety of living situations throughout their 4 years.

GRADUATES

About one-half of the graduates enter residency programs in primary care fields, and a significant number go on to practice in North Dakota. Postgraduate training programs are offered at all the regional training sites.

Admissions

REQUIREMENTS

State residency is a requirement, with the exception of applicants certified by the Western Interstate Commission for Higher Education (WICHE) and Native Americans, admitted through the INMED Program, who must be enrolled members of a federally recognized tribe. Minnesota residents also are given some consideration. Prerequisite course work is general chemistry (8 hours), organic/biochemistry (8 hours), biology (8 hours), physics (8 hours), language arts (6 hours), psychology/sociology (3 hours), and college algebra (3 hours). All science course work must be completed with the appropriate laboratory sessions. A minimum GPA of 3.0 is expected. The MCAT is required, and scores must be no more than 3 years old. For applicants who have retaken the test, the most recent set of scores is considered.

SUGGESTIONS

Preference is given to students who are broadly educated in the sciences and humanities. For students who have been out of college for a period of time, some recent course work is suggested. Computer literacy is also advised.

PROCESS

North Dakota does not participate in AMCAS. Applicants may apply either online or using the traditional paper application. Applications should be requested from the address listed above or at www.med.und.nodak.edu. About 40 percent of applicants are invited to interview in December or January. The committee consists of faculty, administrators, practicing physicians, and medical students. After interviewing, candidates are notified of the committee's decision within 4–6 weeks. About 40 percent of interviewees are accepted. Wait-listed candidates are not encouraged to send supplementary information.

Admissions Requirements (Required)

MCAT scores, science GPA, non-science GPA, letters of recommendation, interview, state residency, essays/personal statement, extracurricular activities, exposure to medical profession.

COSTS AND AID

Tuition & Fees

In-state Tuition	$18,908
Out-of-state Tuition	$50,482
Room and board (on campus)	$8,704
Cost of books	$2,250
Fees	$1,262

Financial Aid

% students receiving aid	98
Average grant	$1,250
Average loan	$35,380
Average debt	$123,520

UNIVERSITY OF OKLAHOMA
COLLEGE OF MEDICINE

PO BOX 26901, OKLAHOMA CITY, OK 73190 • ADMISSION: 405-271-2331
FAX: 405-271-3032 • E-MAIL: ADMINMED@OUHSC.EDU • WEBSITE: WWW.MEDICINE.OUHSC.EDU/ADMISSIONS

STUDENT BODY

Type	Public
Enrollment	575
% male/female	61/39
% underrepresented minorities	27
# applied (total/out)	1,012/633
# accepted (total/out)	198/31
# enrolled (total/out)	152/15
Average age	23

FACULTY

Total faculty (number)	801
% female	32
% part-time	15
Student-faculty ratio	1:1

ADMISSIONS

Average GPA and MCAT Scores

Overall GPA	3.68
MCAT Bio	9.74
MCAT Phys	9.49
MCAT Verbal	9.7
MCAT Essay	O

Application Information

Regular application	10/15
Are transfers accepted?	yes
Admissions may be deferred?	no
Interview required?	yes
Application fee	$65

Academics

All students spend their first two years on the Oklahoma City campus. On completion of year 2, about 25 percent of the class enter clinical rotations at sites affiliated with the University of Oklahoma's Tulsa campus. Tulsa is particularly well-equipped for primary care and community-based medical instruction. Qualified students may pursue the joint MD/PhD degree from any graduate department. OUHSC also offers a joint-MD/MPH. Medical students are evaluated on an A–F scale. They must pass Step 1 of the USMLE to be promoted to year 3, and graduates must take, but not necessarily pass, Step 2 to earn their diploma.

BASIC SCIENCES: Basic sciences are taught through lectures, labs, computer-assisted instruction, problem-based learning, and small-group discussions. During the first two years, students are in class or other scheduled sessions for 20–25 hours per week, allowing ample time for self-directed study. First-year courses are biochemistry/molecular biology, embryology, gross anatomy, histology, human behavior I, integrated medical problem solving, medical statistics, neuroscience, principles of clinical medicine I, and physiology. Second-year courses are human behavior II, integrated medical problem solving, introduction to human illness, microbiology and immunology, principles of clinical medicine II, pharmacology, and professional ethics and professionalism. Basic sciences are taught in the Basic Sciences Education Building, which, in addition to classrooms and labs, houses a study area. The Robert Bird Library contains more than 250,000 books, journals, and audiovisuals and has two special collections—the Indian Health Collection and the Rare Book Collection. Students can access a number of online catalogs and databases from the library.

CLINICAL TRAINING

Third-year rotations are medicine (8 weeks), surgery (8 weeks), ob/gyn (6 weeks), psychiatry (6 weeks), pediatrics (6 weeks), family medicine (4 weeks), geriatrics (4 weeks), specialty selectives (6 weeks), and neuroscience (2 weeks). Fourth-year clerkships are specialty selectives (6 weeks), adult ambulatory medicine (4 weeks), a rural preceptorship (4 weeks), and clinical electives (24 weeks). Clinical affiliates and training sites are OU Medical Center, Department of Veterans Affairs Medical Center, Oklahoma Medical Research Foundation, Oklahoma City Clinic, Oklahoma Allergy Clinic, Dean A. McGee Eye Institute, Oklahoma Blood Institute, State Medical Examiner's Office, Department of Mental Health, and Oklahoma State Department of Health. Students may also do training at the Baptist Medical Center, St. Anthony Hospital, and Mercy Health Center in Oklahoma City. At the Tulsa campus, clinical facilities contain more than 2,000 patient beds, and additional rural training sites are currently being developed. The Oklahoma Telemedicine Network is among the largest medical communications systems in the world, successfully bringing information and expertise to rural physicians, clinics, and hospitals.

Students

At least 85 percent of students must be Oklahoma residents, but generally only five or ten students are from out of state. There is a wide age range among incoming students, and students older than 35 are not unusual. About 26 percent of students are underrepresented minorities, most of whom are Native Americans. Class size is 162.

STUDENT LIFE

Students are cohesive, both inside and outside of the classroom. A student-run note service is one example of cooperation among students. The OUHSC Student Center facilitates both social and academic interaction. It features an exercise room, study areas, computers, a food service court, and common rooms. For a fee, medical students also have access to the recreational center at the nearby Healthy Living Center. Medical students are active in student organizations that offer support and focus on recreational pursuits, professional goals, and community service. Medical students are also involved in coed intramural football, basketball, and soccer. Students are eligible for intercollegiate athletic tickets and other university-wide events. Affordable and comfortable university-owned housing for married and single students is available on the Norman campus. Downtown Oklahoma City is one mile from the OUHSC campus and offers a range of activities and attractions.

GRADUATES

Typically, about half of graduates enter residencies in Oklahoma. Others are successful in securing positions nationwide. There are seven OUHSC-affiliated postgraduate programs in Tulsa and more than 25 in Oklahoma City.

Admissions

REQUIREMENTS

Prerequisites are general zoology/biology with lab (1 semester); embryology, genetics, anatomy, cellular biology, or histology (1 semester); inorganic chemistry (1 year); organic chemistry (1 year); general physics (1 year); English (3 semesters); any combination of sociology, psychology, anthropology, humanities, philosophy, or foreign language (3 semesters). The MCAT is required. For applicants who have retaken the exam, the most recent set of scores is considered. Basic computer skills are required.

SUGGESTIONS

Strong preference is given to Oklahoma residents, making competition intense for out-of-state residents. Applicants are encouraged to take additional courses in computer sciences, English, fine arts, humanities, and social sciences. In addition to academic achievement, a candidate's personality, maturity, and character are evaluated. Admissions decisions are made with recognition of the importance of social and cultural diversity.

PROCESS

All AMCAS applicants receive secondary applications. Of those returning secondaries, about 20 percent are interviewed. Interviews are conducted between September and February, and consist of one session with a panel of three members of the Admissions Committee. On interview day, applicants tour the campus and have the opportunity to meet informally with current students. Of interviewed candidates, about 80 percent (not including wait-listed candidates) are accepted on a rolling basis. Wait-listed candidates may send updated transcripts.

Admissions Requirements (Required)

MCAT scores, science GPA, non-science GPA, letters of recommendation, interview, essays/personal statement, extracurricular activities, exposure to medical profession.

Admissions Requirements (Optional)

State residency.

COSTS AND AID

Tuition & Fees

In-state Tuition	$12,959
Out-of-state Tuition	$35,047
Cost of books	$7,500
Fees	$2,181

Financial Aid

Average grant	$5,500
Average loan	$32,800

UNIVERSITY OF OTTAWA

451 SMYTH ROAD, ROOM 2046, OTTAWA, ON K1H 8M5 • **ADMISSION:** 613-562-5409 • **FAX:** 613-562-5651
E-MAIL: ADMISSMD@UOTTAWA.CA • **WEBSITE:** WWW.MEDICINE.UOTTAWA.CA/ENG/UNDERGRADUATE.HTML

STUDENT BODY

Type	Public
# applied	2,440
# accepted	191
# enrolled	136

ADMISSIONS

Average GPA Scores

Overall GPA	3.65

Application Information

Regular application	10/15
Regular notification	5/31
Are transfers accepted?	yes
Admissions may be deferred?	yes
Interview required?	yes
Application fee	$175

Academics

During the 4 year MD program, students acquire the knowledge, skills, and attitudes they need to apply effective, efficient strategies for the prevention and management of health problems ranging from the most common to the most severe. The program integrates the basic and clinical sciences throughout the 4 years. It also emphasizes health promotion and disease prevention and is responsive to individual needs and abilities and to the changes occurring in society and the health care system. Instruction is available in both French and English. In addition to the MD, master's, and PhD, programs are offered in biochemistry, epidemiology and cellular and molecular medicine, microbiology and immunology, and neuroscience.

The program is scheduled over four calendar years and is divided into two stages. The first stage includes 70 weeks of study of essential biomedical principles and consists of 14 multidisciplinary blocks. Students learn communication and clinical skills in an integrated fashion with the study of body systems. The second stage lasts for two calendar years and is devoted to clinical clerkships; an extended period of 14 weeks is available for elective study. For more information on the undergraduate MD program at the University of Ottawa, visit the program website at www.medicine.uottawa.ca/eng/undergraduate.html.

Students

For the 2004–2005 academic year there were 123 year 1 positions available. Additionally, there were eight positions made available through the "Centre national de formation en sante" program, and five positions available through the Canadian Department of National Defense. Typically, all but a few are residents of the province of Ontario. About 50 percent of members of the student body are women.

STUDENT LIFE

Medical students benefit from the resources and activities of a large university and an urban environment. Student clubs and organizations exist within the medical school and the greater university. Support services, such as counseling, child care, health care, and academic assistance are available to medical students. On-campus housing is offered.

GRADUATES

Graduates enter both clinical medicine and research-oriented careers. Graduate-level medical training is offered at Ottawa in most clinical fields.

Admissions

REQUIREMENTS

To be eligible for admissions, applicants must have successfully completed 3 years of full-time university studies in any undergraduate program leading to a bachelor's degree, including 1 year of general biology (with laboratory session); 1 year of humanities or social sciences; and 2 years of some combination of biochemistry, general chemistry, and organic chemistry (with laboratory sessions). Because the University of Ottawa does not require the submission of MCAT scores, an applicant's academic records will likely meet with increased scrutiny during the review process. Only Canadian citizens or permanent residents are accepted, with the exception of eligible children of the University of Ottawa alumni.

SUGGESTIONS

The Admissions Committee primarily considers those eligible candidates who have maintained a weighted average of at least a B+ in the last 3 years of their undergraduate university studies. Priority is given in order to Franco-Ontarians, Aboriginal applicants, residents of underserviced areas, bona fide residents of the Ottawa-Outaouais region, Ontario residents, and residents of other provinces. In recent entering classes, about 8 percent of applicants were accepted.

PROCESS

After a written application is submitted, supporting materials and an interview will be requested of applicants with acceptable academic records. The interview is used to further screen applicants. Documents for application to the first year of medicine are available through the Faculty or through OMSAS (Ontario Medical School Application Service). Kits are available in July of the preceding year from: OMSAS, PO Box 1328, 650 Woodlawn Road, West, Block C, Guelph, Ontario N1H 7P4. Applications must be completed and returned by October 15.

Admissions Requirements (Required)

Interview.

COSTS AND AID

Tuition & Fees

In-state Tuition	$14,000
Fees	$552

UNIVERSITY OF PENNSYLVANIA
SCHOOL OF MEDICINE

DIRECTOR OF ADMISSIONS, EDWARD J. STEMMLER HALL, SUITE 100, PHILADELPHIA, PA 19104 • ADMISSION: 215-898-8001
FAX: 215-573-6645 • E-MAIL: ADMISS@MAIL.MED.UPENN.EDU • WEBSITE: WWW.MED.UPENN.EDU

STUDENT BODY

Type	Private
Enrollment	720
% male/female	51/49
% underrepresented minorities	17
# applied (total/out)	5,586/4,956
# accepted (total/out)	147/110
Average age	24

ADMISSIONS

Application Information

Regular application	10/15
Regular notification	3/15
Are transfers accepted?	no
Admissions may be deferred?	yes
Interview required?	yes
Application fee	$80

Academics

The 4 year curriculum is organized into five modules, some of which overlap. Patient contact begins on day 1, and clinical rotations begin midway through the second year. Research and scholarly projects are encouraged, and may be pursued in a wide range of areas including biomedical science, clinical medicine, behavioral science, and public-health related fields. For qualified students, combined MD/PhD, and MD/master's degree programs are available. Among other disciplines, graduate degrees may be earned in bioengineering, cell and molecular biology, chemical/structural biology and biophysics, epidemiology, health care systems, history and sociology of science, immunology, neuroscience, pharmacological sciences, philosophy, psychology, and public policy and management. Another option is a joint MD/MBA in conjunction with the Wharton School of Business. Grading is pass/fail during module 1 and honors/high pass/pass/fail during the remaining modules.

BASIC SCIENCES: Basic sciences are taught primarily through an integrated organ/disease system model, correlated with clinical examples and hands-on experiences. Module 1 occupies the first semester and is devoted to core principles. Courses are cellular physiology, metabolism, and pharmacological processes; developmental and molecular biology; human body structure and function; host defenses; and pharmacological responses. Module 2 spans the second semester of the first year and the first semester of the second year. It is entitled integrative systems and disease and is organized around body or organ systems. These are brain and behavior, cardiology/pulmonary, endocrinology and reproduction, gastrointestinal and nutrition, skin/connective tissue/musculoskeletal/hematology/oncology. Throughout the entire first year and a half, students are introduced to clinical medicine in Module 3, the technology, art, and practice of medicine. In addition to providing training in basic clinical techniques, Module 3 addresses ethics, technological issues, population-based medicine, public health, and humanistic perspectives. Classroom instruction is enhanced by various academic resources, including multimedia, video, and computerized instructional programs. The Biomedical Science Library houses more than 100,000 volumes and receives more than 2,000 periodicals.

CLINICAL TRAINING

Students rotate through required clerkships during Module 4, which covers the second semester of year 2 and the first semester of year 3. These are internal medicine (9 weeks), surgery/anesthesia (9 weeks), ob/gyn (6 weeks), pediatrics (6 weeks), psychiatry/substance abuse (6 weeks), emergency medicine (3 weeks), family medicine (3 weeks), neurology (3 weeks), and clinical specialists (3 weeks). Module 5 begins in the second semester of year 3 and continues until graduation at the end of year 4. It includes a sub internship, advanced electives, and a required 3 month scholarly or research experience. A large portion of clinical training takes place at the Hospital of the University of Pennsylvania and also at the site of research institutions and labs. Other training sites are Children's Hospital of Philadelphia, Veterans Affairs of Philadelphia Hospitals, Phoenixville Hospital, Penn Medicine at Radnor, Chestnut Hill Health Care, Chester County Hospital, Friends Hospital, Holy Redeemer Health System, and the Presbyterian-University of Pennsylvania Medical Center.

Students

The student body at U. Penn is nationally represented. About 16 percent of students are underrepresented minorities, and about 20 percent of students took significant time off after college. Class size is 150.

STUDENT LIFE

Pass/fail grading in the first semester contributes to the high degree of cooperation among students. U. Penn, a comprehensive private university, offers a wide range of extracurricular activities on and around campus, and students are involved in both school and community organizations. Medical students have access to all recreational facilities, including athletic centers. Philadelphia is an important urban center and is also the home of a very large number of universities. The student community is vast, and the city serves the student community well. Other metropolitan areas such as New York, Baltimore, and Washington, DC, are easily accessible by train, and mountains and beaches are a short drive. The Graduate Towers and High Rise North is a university-owned graduate student apartment complex available to medical students. However, most students choose to live off campus.

GRADUATES

During a recent 3-year period, the most prevalent residency programs selected by graduates were primary care disciplines (37 percent), which included medicine (22 percent) and pediatrics (13 percent); surgical specialties (19 percent), which included ophthalmology (6 percent), orthopedics (6 percent), and neurosurgery (2 percent); radiology (8 percent); surgery (7 percent); psychiatry (5 percent); emergency medicine (4 percent); and ob/gyn (2 percent).

Admissions

REQUIREMENTS

Applicants must complete a course of study leading to a baccalaureate degree at an accredited college or university. No prerequisites are specified, although the MCAT is required, suggesting a comprehensive science preparation. Penn recommends that applicants submit MCAT scores from the spring, but no later than the summer, of the calendar year prior to entrance.

SUGGESTIONS

Recommended undergraduate preparation includes courses in anthropology, biology, chemistry, economics, ethics, history, math, organic chemistry, physics, philosophy, and political science. For applicants who have taken time off after college, some recent course work is advised. Experience in hospitals, clinics, or community service projects is important.

PROCESS

All AMCAS applicants receive secondary applications. Of those returning secondaries, about 20 percent are interviewed between October and February. Interviews consist of two sessions, one with a student and one with a faculty member. On interview day, candidates tour the campus, attend group informational sessions, and have the opportunity to meet informally with students. Of interviewed candidates, about 20 percent are accepted. Wait-listed candidates may send additional information to update their files.

Admissions Requirements (Required)

MCAT scores, science GPA, non-science GPA, letters of recommendation, extracurricular activities, exposure to medical profession.

COSTS AND AID

Tuition & Fees

Tuition	$38,308
Room and board (on campus)	$12,925
Cost of books	$800
Fees	$2,855

Financial Aid

% students receiving aid	80
Average debt	$108,000

University of Pittsburgh
School of Medicine

Office of Admissions, 518 Scaife Hall, Pittsburgh, PA 15261 • Admission: 412-648-9891
Fax: 412-648-8768 • E-mail: ADMISSIONS@MEDSCHOOL.PITT.EDU • Website: WWW.MEDSCHOOL.PITT.EDU

STUDENT BODY

Type	Public
Enrollment	592
% male/female	52/48
% underrepresented minorities	9
# applied (total/out)	4,722/3,745

FACULTY

Total faculty (number)	1,400
Student-faculty ratio	3:1

ADMISSIONS

Application Information

Regular application	12/1
Regular notification	10/15
	until filled
Early application	6/1–8/1
Early notification	10/1
Are transfers accepted?	yes
Admissions may be deferred?	yes
Interview required?	no
Application fee	$75

Academics

The 4 year curriculum encourages personal interaction among students, between faculty and students, and between patients and students. Students can obtain joint master's degrees in medical ethics and public health with nearby Carnegie-Mellon University. The MSTP-funded MD/PhD is offered in conjunction with Carnegie-Mellon University.

BASIC SCIENCES: During the first two years, students take classes that are grouped into blocks. Year 1 has the following four blocks: The patient-doctor block, which covers ethical, behavioral, and sociological issues related to medicine; the basic science block, which covers the biological elements of medicine; the organ systems block, which includes host defenses and the musculoskeletal system; and the introduction to patient care block, which encompasses physical diagnosis. The blocks are synchronized so that single topics are approached in an interdisciplinary way. The blocks in year 2 are patient-doctor relationship, patient care, and organ systems, which includes the following systems: Dermatology; digestion; endocrine; homeostasis; neuroscience; and reproductive. As in year 1, the blocks are planned to complement each other. The final segment of year 2 integrates all the organ systems and, while doing so, reviews important points of the previous two years. Lectures, small-group sessions, conferences, labs, and tutorials are the instructional methods used during the first two years, and students are in a structured learning environment for about 28 hours per week. Problem-based learning is used with most instructional methods. With the exception of clinical work, instruction is given in Scaife Hall, a renovated building with classrooms, labs, and a library, which has 220,000 volumes and subscribes to the major online medical informational services. Grades during the first two years are honors/pass/fail. The USMLE Steps 1 and 2 are required for graduation.

CLINICAL TRAINING

Patient contact begins in year 1 during the patient care block. Third-year rotations begin in July immediately following year 2. These are pediatrics (8 weeks); ambulatory sub-specialties (6 weeks—includes dermatology, neurosurgery, ophthalmology, orthopedics, otolaryngology, pediatric surgery, plastic surgery, and urology); ob/gyn (6 weeks); psychiatry (6 weeks); surgery (6 weeks); family medicine (4 weeks); and an elective (4 weeks). The fourth year is made up solely of selectives and electives. Clinical training takes place at the University Health Center, which is composed of the following five major hospitals: The Presbyterian University Hospital, Montefiore Hospital, the Eye and Ear Institute, the Western Psychiatric Institute, and the University of Pittsburgh Cancer Institute. The passing rate for students at the University of Pittsburgh on both parts of the USMLE is higher than that for medical schools nationally, and for the past 2 years 100 percent of all students passed both Step 1 and 2.

Students

About 9 percent of students are underrepresented minorities, most of whom are African Americans. Approximately half of the students in each class are Pennsylvania residents. There is a large age range within the student body, and many students took some time off before entering medical school. Class size is 148.

STUDENT LIFE

The structure of the curriculum promotes student interaction and collegiality. In addition, medical students get to know each other through involvement in organizations and extracurricular activities. Some of the many student groups on campus are Pitt Women in Medicine, the Christian Medical Society, and the History of Medicine Society. Medical students have access to all facilities of the University of Pittsburgh, including athletic facilities. Pittsburgh is an accessible and exciting city, and, although on-campus housing is available, most medical students choose to live off campus.

GRADUATES

Graduates are successful in gaining admittance to some of most prestigious residency programs in the country. Seventy-eight percent of the graduating class obtained one of their top three choices in the National Residency Matching Program. About 50 percent of graduates enter primary care fields.

Admissions

REQUIREMENTS

Requirements are 1 year each of biology, chemistry, organic chemistry, and physics, all with associated labs, and English. In assessing grades, consideration is given to the undergraduate institution attended and the course load taken. The MCAT is required and must be no more than three years old.

SUGGESTIONS

Competence in math is valued as is evidence of success in social science and humanities courses. The University of Pittsburgh looks for interpersonal skills and commitment to community service in applicants. For applicants who graduated college several years ago, some recent course work is advised.

PROCESS

Secondary applications are sent selectively to AMCAS applicants. About 20 percent of Pennsylvania residents, and 10 percent of out-of-state residents, are interviewed. Interviews are conducted from September through April and consist of two sessions, one with a faculty member and one with a medical student. Notification occurs toward the end of February. Wait-listed candidates may send additional information to strengthen their applications and to indicate interest in the school.

Admissions Requirements (Required)

MCAT scores, state residency, essays/personal statement, exposure to medical profession.

Admissions Requirements (Optional)

Science GPA, nonscience GPA, letters of recommendation, interview, extracurricular activities.

COSTS AND AID

Tuition & Fees

In-state Tuition	$30,084
Out-of-state Tuition	$35,876
Cost of books	$2,000
Fees	$600

Financial Aid

% students receiving aid	26
Average grant	$6,626
Average loan	$3,000
Average debt	$74,952

University of Puerto Rico

Medical Sciences Campus

A-878 Main Building, PO Box 365067, San Juan, PR 00936-5067 • Admission: 787-758-2525 ext. 1800
Fax: 787-756-8475 • E-mail: MARRIVERA@RCM.UPR.EDU • Website: WWW.RCM.UPR.EDU

STUDENT BODY	
Type	Public
Enrollment	1,716

FACULTY	
Total faculty	189
Student-faculty ratio	9:1

ADMISSIONS

Application Information

Regular application	12/1
Regular notification	rolling
Early application	6/1
Early notification	rolling
Application fee	$15

Academics

Medical training is accomplished through a variety of educational experiences, both in the classroom and at multiple service settings in the public and private sectors of Puerto Rico. Medical students benefit from the resources of other health professional schools and from interaction with students at other schools. Through the Center for International Health, medical students gain exposure to the research and policy issues surrounding global health. Grading for all courses is on an A–F scale.

BASIC SCIENCES: Basic sciences are taught using a combination of lectures, small group discussions, labs, and exposure to clinical correlates. Required first-year courses are behavioral sciences, human development I, human physiology, introduction to biochemistry, introduction to clinical diagnosis, integration seminar I, medical embryology, medical gross anatomy, medical histology, medical neuroscience, and public health and preventive medicine I. Second-year courses consist of basic clinical clerkship, fundamentals of clinical diagnosis, human development II, infectious diseases, integration seminar II, mechanisms of disease, medical pharmacology, pathobiology—introduction to laboratory medicine, public health and preventive medicine II, and psychopathology. Outside of the classroom, students learn in the Learning Resources Center, the Standardized Patient Laboratory, and the Clinical Learning Laboratory.

CLINICAL TRAINING

The third year is comprised of clinical rotations. These are medicine (12 weeks), pediatrics (10 weeks), surgery (10 weeks), ob/gyn (6 weeks), psychiatry (4 weeks), family medicine (4 weeks), and radiology (2 weeks). During year 4, clerkships are public health (3 weeks); dermatology (1 week); physical medicine and rehabilitation (1 week); legal, ethical, and administrative aspects in medicine (1 week); and selective clerkships (8 weeks). In addition, 18 weeks are open for clinical and research electives. Clinical education uses a variety of settings including University Hospital, University Pediatric Hospital, San Juan City Hospital, Veterans Administration Hospital, and the Oncology Hospital. In addition, the school uses certain private hospitals, clinics, and public health facilities. Some electives may be taken at institutions other than those affiliated with the University of Puerto Rico, such as hospitals in other regions of Puerto Rico and in other countries.

Students

Each entering class has about 100 students. Students come from foreign countries and the mainland United States as well as Puerto Rico. Fifty percent of students are women.

STUDENT LIFE

Recreational facilities on campus include the sports and gym center. The medical school promotes student health through its exercise/wellness program and by sponsoring a range of student activities and events. When they have free time, medical students enjoy the city of San Juan and its surroundings.

GRADUATES

The University of Puerto Rico and its affiliated hospitals offer residency programs in most major medical fields.

Admissions

REQUIREMENTS

With few exceptions, entering students must have completed their bachelor's degree. Prerequisite courses are 1 year each of biology, general chemistry, organic chemistry, and physics. The MCAT is required, and August in the year prior to admission is the latest acceptable test date.

SUGGESTIONS

Both residents of Puerto Rico and nonresidents are considered for admission. Grade point average and MCAT scores are important in admissions decisions. In addition to academic credentials, the University of Puerto Rico looks for integrity and motivation in its students.

PROCESS

All applicants are encouraged to visit the campus. Candidates for the MD program must submit an application by December 1. Those who qualify are invited to interview after their applications are reviewed. Final decisions and notifications are made throughout the year and are completed in the spring.

Admissions Requirements (Required)

MCAT scores, letters of recommendation, science GPA.

Admissions Requirements (Optional)

State residency.

COSTS AND AID

Tuition & Fees

In-state Tuition	$5,000
Fees	$870
Room and board (on campus)	$4,840
Books and expenses	$7,893

UNIVERSITY OF ROCHESTER
SCHOOL OF MEDICINE AND DENTISTRY

MEDICAL CENTER, PO BOX 601A, ROCHESTER, NY 14642 • ADMISSION: 585-275-4539 • FAX: 585-756-5479
E-MAIL: MDADMISH@URMC.ROCHESTER.EDU • WEBSITE: WWW.URMC.ROCHESTER.EDU/SMD/ADMISS

STUDENT BODY

Type	Private
Enrollment	433
% male/female	45/55
% underrepresented minorities	14
# applied (total/out)	3,496/2,598
# accepted (total/out)	260/170
# enrolled (total/out)	100/63
Average age	24

FACULTY

Total faculty (number)	1,317
% female	33
% minority	3
% part-time	10
Student-faculty ratio	3:1

ADMISSIONS

Average GPA and MCAT Scores

Overall GPA	3.68
MCAT Bio	11.0
MCAT Phys	10.8
MCAT Verbal	10.5
MCAT Essay	P

Application Information

Regular application	10/15
Regular notification	11/1
Are transfers accepted?	no
Admissions may be deferred?	yes
Interview required?	yes
Application fee	$75

Academics

Special emphasis is placed on skills acquisition and use, with a commitment to lifelong learning. Sensitivity to the world of the patient is encompassed in the biopsychosocial integration of the curriculum and the learning experience, with mechanisms in place for continuous curricular improvement through the collaboration of students and faculty. By ensuring adequate and early electivity for students to enhance their special interests, along with rigorous training and assessment of all of the competencies demanded by modern medical practice, the curriculum generates a knowledge base characterized by depth, breadth, rigor, and flexibility. Students interested in careers in medical science may participate in the fully funded Medical Scientist Training Program (MD/PhD), or joint-degree programs including the MPH/MD and MBA/MD program in Health Care Management in conjunction with the William E. Simon Graduate School of Business Administration. Vacation and full-year fellowships facilitate student research or international medicine experiences. Evaluation of student performance uses satisfactory/fail, except in the required clerkships, where honors/high pass/pass/fail grades are used. Passing the USMLE is not required for promotion to the third year.

BASIC SCIENCES: An introductory module at the beginning of year 1 prepares students in the acquisition, management, and presentation of medical information. Students learn how to meet the challenges of active and independent learning by becoming competent in data management, information technology, and critical evaluation of the medical literature. Every course is interdisciplinary; basic sciences are integrated with one another and basic and clinical sciences are woven together as the strands of the Double Helix Curriculum throughout the 4 years. Clinical skills training from day 1 leads not to shadowing or preceptor experiences in clinics but to real clinical work as part of the health care team while still in the first year. Not just paper cases, but students' actual clinical cases drive the learning of science through the school-wide use of multidisciplinary Problem-Based Learning (PBL) cases. Three 2-hour PBL tutorials per week and an average of about 14 hours of lecture per week, with adequate time for self-study, and the use of labs, conferences, seminars, and computer-assisted learning—all these things characterize the classroom setting of the curriculum. Electives are available during all four years, including electives in medical humanities, international medicine, and community outreach programs. The Edward G. Miner Library holds more than 225,000 volumes and a modern, computer-based learning resource center.

CLINICAL TRAINING

Beginning in year 1, students complete their introduction to clinical medicine in the fall and then participate in an Ambulatory Clerkship Experience beginning in the spring. This experience, unlike any other in the country, includes all the ambulatory components of ambulatory surgery, family medicine, internal medicine, pediatrics, psychiatry, and women's health, and is completed by the end of the second year. Inpatient clerkships are completed by December of the fourth year and focus on acute illness experiences in adult medicine, women's and children's health, mind/brain/behavior, and urgent/emergent care. Strong Memorial Hospital (700 beds) is the principal site for clinical teaching, along with a newly completed ambulatory care center and four affiliated hospitals (2,000 beds), covering acute and chronic care.

Students

Students come from all regions of the country. About 14 percent are underrepresented minorities. The average age of incoming students is 24; one-third have majored in areas outside the sciences, and 100 students are accepted each year.

STUDENT LIFE

Most medical students have active lives outside of the classroom. Many participate in community outreach programs, international medicine electives, and student organizations and events. Students have access to resources of the university campus and athletic facilities in the medical center. Located on the southern shore of Lake Ontario in the Finger Lakes wine-producing region of upstate New York, Rochester is a progressive, metropolitan community of more than 1 million people. Rochester has a rich cultural life and is an affordable and friendly city. It is a haven for boaters and other outdoor enthusiasts.

GRADUATES

Among the 2006 graduates, the most popular residencies were internal medicine (21 percent), pediatrics (13 percent), surgery (9 percent), neurology (7 percent), radiology (7 percent), med-peds (6 percent), emergency medicine (5 percent), anesthesiology (4 percent), ob/gyn (4 percent), orthopedics (4 percent), and psychiatry (4 percent).

Admissions

REQUIREMENTS

Prerequisite science courses are 1 year of biology, general chemistry, organic chemistry, and physics, all associated with labs. One semester of biochemistry may be substituted for one semester of organic. One year of English or expository writing is also required. Rochester belongs to AMCAS, and the MCAT exam is required; scores should be from the past 3 years. The best set of scores is considered.

SUGGESTIONS

In addition to required science courses, 12–16 credit hours in the humanities and/or social sciences are required. Experiences in research, clinical settings, and the community are strongly recommended. Rochester looks for evidence of leadership, excellent interpersonal skills, a love of learning, appreciation of diversity, and outstanding scholarship.

PROCESS

Rochester is an AMCAS school. About 19 percent of applicants are interviewed between September and February. Interviews consist of two sessions with faculty, and applicants have a tour, lunch with current students, and a financial aid presentation. About 40 percent of the interviewed applicants are offered acceptance, with notification beginning in November and continuing through May. About 15 positions in each class are reserved for students from several programs, such as the Rochester Early Medical Scholar Program and the Bryn Mawr or Johns Hopkins post-baccalaureate program.

Admissions Requirements (Required)

MCAT scores, science GPA, non-science GPA, letters of recommendation, interview, essays/personal statement, extracurricular activities, exposure to medical profession, exposure to research.

Admissions Requirements (Optional)

State residency.

Overlap Schools

Boston University, Case Western Reserve University, Cornell University, Dartmouth College, Harvard University, Mt. Sinai School of Medicine, New York University, Tufts University, University of Pittsburgh, University of Virginia.

COSTS AND AID

Tuition & Fees

Tuition	$35,800
Room and board (off campus)	$9,500
Cost of books	$2,000
Fees	$1,885

Financial Aid

% students receiving aid	92
Average grant	$17,217
Average loan	$26,866
Average debt	$134,367

University of Saskatchewan
College of Medicine

A204 Health Science Building, 107 Wiggins Road, Saskatoon, SK Canada • Admission: 306-966-8554
Fax: 306-966-2601 • E-mail: MED.ADMISSIONS@USASK.CA • Website: WWW.USASK.CA/MEDICINE

STUDENT BODY

Type	Public
Enrollment	60
% male/female	52/48
% underrepresented minorities	5
# applied	463
# accepted (total/out)	60/6
# enrolled (total/out)	60/6
Average age	23

FACULTY

Total faculty (number)	245
% female	30

ADMISSIONS

Average GPA and MCAT Scores

MCAT Bio	9.77
MCAT Phys	9.73
MCAT Verbal	9.4
MCAT Essay	P

Application Information

Regular application	12/1
Regular notification	5/16
Are transfers accepted?	no
Admissions may be deferred?	yes
Interview required?	yes
Application fee	$40

Academics

The goal of the College of Medicine is to enable medical students to develop the knowledge, skills, values, and attitudes that will serve as a foundation for subsequent education in primary and specialty patient care and research. In its curriculum, the college promotes the integration of basic and clinical sciences. Independent learning, problem-solving, and early patient interaction are emphasized. The curriculum is divided into 4 phases. For the most part, basic science instruction occurs during the first 3 phases. However, basic science and clinical training are integrated throughout the 4 year curriculum.

BASIC SCIENCES: Phase A (1 year) comprises 33 weeks and includes the introductory study of basic sciences, the history of medicine, professional skills (includes 2 week community experience), and life cycle and humanities. Instruction in basic sciences is interdisciplinary, covering fundamental principles of anatomy, biochemistry, microbiology, and physiology. Instruction in the basic sciences continues into phase B (1 year), which lasts 33 weeks. Subjects include microbiology, pathology, and pharmacology. Also included in phase B is clinical sciences, genetics, and systems. Phase C is only 15 weeks and is a continuation of clinical sciences and systems. It also includes the community health and epidemiology, linking courses, and microbiology.

CLINICAL TRAINING

Phase D (16 months) is a discipline-based rotation clerkship that builds on the clinical training and offers students the opportunity to study clinical electives (12 weeks) and specialty fields. Teaching Hospitals are Royal University Hospital, St. Paul's Hospital, Saskatoon City Hospital, Regina General Hospital, and Pasqua Hospital.

Students

The maximum size of entering classes is 60. Typically, 90 percent of students are from the province of Saskatchewan. In general, about 50 percent of students are women.

STUDENT LIFE

With a relatively small student body and a curriculum that encourages interaction, students are generally cohesive. Between the medical school and the greater university, a wide range of extracurricular activities and events are offered. Medical students live both on and off campus.

GRADUATES

Although research is an increasingly important activity for the College of Medicine, a large number of graduates become practicing clinical physicians in the province of Saskatchewan.

Admissions

REQUIREMENTS

A minimum of 2 years of undergraduate work is required. In general, prerequisites are biochemistry, biology, chemistry, English, humanities, organic chemistry, physics, and social sciences. Incoming students should also have an academic average of 70 percent in prerequisite courses to be considered for admission. Overall academic averages must be at least 78 percent. The MCAT must be taken and a minimum score of 8 in all sections is required.

SUGGESTIONS

Criteria for selection are academic performance and personal qualities. Academic performance is based on applicants' two best full undergraduate years of study. Personal qualities are assessed primarily by interview. Realistically, to be competitive academically, an overall 2 year average of over 80 percent is required.

PROCESS

Application forms may be obtained from the Admissions Secretary after July 1 or from the Internet at the address above. Applications must be postmarked no later than December 1. Interviews are approximately 45 minutes and occur during a weekend in March. The applicant is interviewed by a team of four, including a medical doctor, a faculty member, a medical student, and a community member. Three letters of reference are also considered. All candidates are notified of their acceptance by the end of June.

Admissions Requirements (Required)

MCAT scores, science GPA, non-science GPA, letters of recommendation, interview, state residency.

Admissions Requirements (Optional)

Essays/personal statement, extracurricular activities, exposure to medical profession.

Overlap Schools

University of Alberta, University of Calgary.

COSTS AND AID

Tuition & Fees

Tuition	$11,390
Room and board (on campus)	$4,832
Cost of books	$1,700

UNIVERSITY OF SHERBROOKE

2500 BOULEVARD DE L'UNIVERSITÉ, SHERBROOKE, QC J1K 2R1 • **ADMISSION:** 819-821-7686
E-MAIL: STIC-MED@USHERBROOKE.CA • **WEBSITE:** WWW.USHERBROOKE.CA/MEDECINE/

STUDENT BODY

Type	Public

ADMISSIONS

Application Information

Regular application	3/1
Regular notification	rolling
Admissions may be deferred?	no
Application fee	$30

Academics

Sherbrooke offers a 4 year curriculum leading to the MD degree. Educational methodology is based on small group discussions, case studies, audiovisual and computer-assisted learning, and hands-on clinical experiences. Combined degree programs, such as the MD/MSc program are open to highly qualified students who have an interest in research.

BASIC SCIENCES: The first academic period begins in late August and spans 39 weeks. In general, students are in class or other scheduled session for approximately 30 hours per week. Courses are introduction to MD program, biological medicine I and II, clinical immersion, growth development and aging, locomoter system, nervous system, psycho-social sciences, preventive medicine and community health, integration, and clinical skills. The second year is organized into blocks based on anatomical/physiological systems. These are cardiovascular system, endocrine system, gastrointestinal system, hemato-immunologic system, human sexuality, infectious disease, respiratory system, reproductive system, and urinary system. In addition, students take part in a rotation in community hospitals and a course in clinical skills.

CLINICAL TRAINING

The third and fourth years are organized into several components. These are required courses, required primary clerkships, rotations in community, elective programs, integration period, and final exam. Required courses are clinical skills, interdisciplinary concepts, and introduction to clerkships. The required primary clerkships are medicine (10.5 weeks); surgery (7 weeks); pediatrics (7 weeks); psychiatry (7 weeks); ob/gyn (7 weeks); and multidisciplinary (3.5 weeks). Rotations in community include family medicine and emergency (7 weeks) and community health (4 weeks). The elective program lasts 12 weeks, followed by the integration period (6 weeks) and the final exam period (1 week). Teaching hospitals are Cuse Fleurimont, Cuse Bowen, Hôpital Charles Le Moyne, and Hôpital Sainte-Croix.

Students

Each entering class has approximately 105 students. About 80 percent of students are from the Province of Quebec. Women account for 60 percent of students.

STUDENT LIFE

The University of Sherbrooke is a large university with many social, recreational, and other extracurricular activities for medical students. Medical students have both on-campus and off-campus housing options.

GRADUATES

Many graduates enter one of the residency programs offered at hospitals affiliated with Sherbrooke.

Admissions

REQUIREMENTS

Fluency in French is required. The minimum requirement for admissions is 2 years of university or a BA degree. Prerequisites are general biology (1 year), general chemistry (1 year), organic chemistry (1 year), physics (3 semesters), and mathematics through calculus. The MCAT is not required.

SUGGESTIONS

In addition to prerequisite courses, students should complete course work in the humanities and in the social sciences. Priority is given to residents of Quebec, and 86 positions in each entering class are reserved for this group of applicants. Fifteen additional places are reserved for applicants from New Brunswick, one place is reserved for an applicant from Prince Edward Island, one from Nova Scotia, and two places are available for qualified foreign applicants. Overall, about 5 percent of applicants are admitted each year.

PROCESS

Applications are available from the Admissions Office at the address above. Following review of applications, qualified candidates are invited to a learning-skills test (THAMUS).

COSTS AND AID	
Tuition & Fees	
In-state Tuition	$3,127
Out-of-state Tuition	$15,127

UNIVERSITY OF SOUTH ALABAMA

COLLEGE OF MEDICINE

OFFICE OF ADMISSIONS, 241 CSAB, MOBILE, AL 36688 • ADMISSION: 251-460-7176
FAX: 251-460-6278 • E-MAIL: MSCOTT@USOUTHAL.EDU • WEBSITE: WWW.USOUTHAL.EDU/USA/DEPS-GRD.HTML

STUDENT BODY

Type	Public
Enrollment	280
% male/female	49/51
% underrepresented minorities	11
# applied (total/out)	809/449
# accepted (total/out)	116/20
# enrolled (total/out)	70/8
Average age	24

FACULTY

Total faculty (number)	300
% female	30
% minority	10
% part-time	9
Student-faculty ratio	1:1

ADMISSIONS

Average GPA and MCAT Scores

Overall GPA	3.7
MCAT Bio	11.0
MCAT Phys	10.0
MCAT Verbal	10.0
MCAT Essay	O

Application Information

Regular application	11/15
Regular notification	rolling
Early application	6/1–8/1
Early notification	10/1
Are transfers accepted?	yes
Admissions may be deferred?	yes
Interview required?	yes
Application fee	$75

Academics

The curriculum is semi-traditional and uses a lecture format for most of the pre-clinical instruction. Although some early clinical exposure is offered, during the first 2 years, the program focuses on ensuring a solid understanding of the basic sciences. Combining medical and doctorate studies is possible if pursuing a PhD degree in a medically related discipline. About 10 percent of the class enters the School of Medicine via a combined undergraduate-medical school program that is open to both Alabama and out-of-state high school seniors.

BASIC SCIENCES: The school operates on a quarter system. During the first year, lecture courses are biochemistry, developmental anatomy, gross anatomy, histology, neuroanatomy, and physiology. Generally, students are in lecture for about 25 hours per week. The course medical ethics is taught by using both lecture and small-group format. Medical practice and society and physical diagnosis use lectures and a case-based approach. During the second year, traditional lecture/lab courses include genetics, microbiology, pharmacology, and pathology. Introduction to behavioral sciences and a course covering principles of public health are also part of the curriculum. In addition, students take part in weekly sessions in clinical settings, as part of an introductory course in clinical medicine. Basic sciences are taught in the Medical Sciences Building, which contains administrative offices, classrooms, and laboratories. The Biomedical Library houses 65,000 volumes and offers computer and online services. Grading is A–F for most courses, and promotions are based not only on grades but also on faculty evaluation of students' ethical and personal maturity. Medical students are involved in the schools' administrative affairs through an elected student governing body, which also participates in issues relating to the greater university. The schedule for the first two years is relatively firm, and students are encouraged to focus on their studies, rather than pursue employment or other activities during this period. The USMLE Step 1 is required following the basic-science portion of study.

CLINICAL TRAINING

Year 3 is composed entirely of required clerkships: Medicine (12 weeks), surgery (8 weeks), psychiatry/neurology (8 weeks), pediatrics (8 weeks), ob/gyn (6 weeks), and family practice (6 weeks). The fourth year is also 48 weeks but is composed of elective rather than required rotations. Students must select a 1 month rotation from each broad field: Ambulatory care, neuroscience, surgical subspecialties, primary care, and in-house elective. Students train at university-affiliated hospitals that together constitute the largest medical complex along the Gulf Coast and that contain a total of 880 beds. All levels of trauma care and surgery are available, and patients come not only from around the state but from neighboring states as well. In downtown Mobile, the Children's and Women's Hospital offers clinical rotations in pediatric services and neonatal care. The hospital system serves managed care clients, among others, ensuring a client base. Cancer research and treatment, organic transplant, aeromedical transport, and preventative care are a few of the noteworthy services available through the university network. Students receive grades of A–F for clinical performance during required rotations and honors/pass/fail during elective rotations. The USMLE Step 2 is required for graduation. A large percentage of students take part in rotations at out-of-state institutions or overseas.

Students

At least 80 percent of medical students must be Alabama residents. Reflecting the state's demographics, about 9 percent are underrepresented minorities, most of whom are African American. Each year, about 15 students enter who have taken time off after college. The student body is diverse in terms of undergraduate majors, and class size is relatively small, about 74 students.

STUDENT LIFE

Students take advantage of the university campus, with its recreational facilities and activities. Students also use nearby municipal recreational facilities, which include a golf course. The School of Medicine provides opportunities for students to participate in medically related projects and events, such as volunteer activities and special seminars. The majority of students live in a variety of apartment complexes that are in close proximity to the campus. Many students find buying a house a very viable option.

GRADUATES

Of the graduating class of 70, 50 percent chose primary care specialties, 20 percent went into internal medicine, 5 percent into family medicine, and 2 percent chose medicine/pediatrics. Ob/Gyn, pathology, radiology, and surgery were also popular choices.

Admissions

REQUIREMENTS

Requirements are 1 year each of biology, general chemistry, organic chemistry, and physics, all with associated labs; and 1 year each of English, math, and humanities. In total, 90 semester hours of undergraduate course work are required. The quality of the undergraduate institution is considered in evaluating GPA. Generally, courses taken abroad are not counted. The MCAT is required and should be no more than 3 years old. The most recent score is considered, and there is no preference for the April or August MCAT.

SUGGESTIONS

Preferably, the math requirement should be fulfilled with calculus. Nontraditional students who have taken time off after college are advised to demonstrate recent course work, particularly in the sciences. The goal of the Admissions Committee is to select candidates who have the potential to address the wide spectrum of needs faced by the medical profession, suggesting that diverse backgrounds are valued in addition to medically related experience. Because spots are few, out-of state candidates should be competitive on a national level.

PROCESS

All Alabama residents receive a secondary application, which is sent upon receipt of the AMCAS application. About one-fourth of out-of-state residents receive a secondary. The secondary application is due on November 15, but the School of Medicine advises applicants to submit it as soon as possible. Fifty percent of Alabama residents and about 10 percent of out-of-state residents are interviewed. Interviews are held on campus from September through March. Students receive three half-hour interviews, which may vary in format. The interview day provides applicants and faculty an opportunity to become acquainted and is considered a two-way process. Of those interviewed, about 30 percent are accepted and 20 percent are placed on a ranked wait list. Candidates are accepted on a weekly basis, beginning in December.

COSTS AND AID

Tuition & Fees

In-state Tuition	$15,077
Out-of-state Tuition	$26,117
Cost of books	$2,500
Fees	$2,028

Financial Aid

% students receiving aid	90
Average grant	$5,000
Average loan	$22,000
Average debt	$83,762

UNIVERSITY OF SOUTH CAROLINA
SCHOOL OF MEDICINE

ADMISSIONS OFFICE, COLUMBIA, SC 29208 • ADMISSION: 803-733-3325
FAX: 803-733-3328 • E-MAIL: MILLS@GW.MED.SC.EDU • WEBSITE: WWW.MED.SC.EDU

STUDENT BODY

Type	Public
Enrollment	297
% male/female	53/47
% underrepresented minorities	20
# applied (total/out)	1,047/715
# accepted (total/out)	133/19
# enrolled (total/out)	80/10
Average age	23

FACULTY

Student-faculty ratio	1:1

ADMISSIONS

Average GPA and MCAT Scores

Overall GPA	3.5
MCAT Bio	9.0
MCAT Phys	8.0
MCAT Verbal	9.0
MCAT Essay	0

Application Information

Regular application	12/1
Regular notification	10/15
Early application	6/1–8/1
Early notification	10/1
Are transfers accepted?	yes
Admissions may be deferred?	yes
Interview required?	yes
Application fee	$45

Academics

In addition to the MD, the School of Medicine offers the MS and PhD degrees in biomedical science with specialization in anatomy, cell biology, experimental pathology, microbiology and immunology, pharmacology, and physiology. For qualified students, a combined MD/PhD program is possible. A combined MD/MPH program, offered in conjunction with the School of Public Health at USC, is available. Also offered is the MS in genetics counseling and biomedical science, with specialization in nurse anesthesia and rehabilitation counseling. The MD curriculum stresses psychological and social perspectives along with biological principles. Elective opportunities are available throughout all four years to assist students in pursuing individual interests and career goals. Medical students are evaluated with an A–F scale. Passing Step 1 of the USMLE is a requirement for promotion to year 3, and passing Step 2 is a graduation requirement.

BASIC SCIENCES: Throughout the first 2 years, clinical case studies are correlated with basic-science material. The 2 year introduction to clinical practice course emphasizes active, independent, and cooperative learning and uses a small-group format. Other first-year courses are biochemistry, gross anatomy, microscopic anatomy, neuroanatomy, and physiology. Second-year courses are microbiology, pathology/pathophysiology, and pharmacology. An important resource is the USCSM Library, which has a collection of more than 90,0000 volumes. Medical students also use the USC Thomas Cooper Library, which has more than 2.5 million bound volumes.

CLINICAL TRAINING

Clerkship experiences in the third year include 8 week rotations in family medicine, medicine, ob/gyn, surgery, pediatrics, and psychiatry. During the fourth year, required clerkships are 4 weeks each in neurology, surgery, and medicine, and a 4-week acting internship. A 4-week multidisciplinary rotation concludes undergraduate clinical training and prepares students for the transition to residency and clinical practice. The remainder of the year is reserved for electives and selectives, many of which may be completed at locations around the state, at other medical schools, with federal and state agencies, and through an international elective program. While the majority of students complete core clinical training at the five affiliated hospitals in Columbia, about 15 students in each class train at the Greenville Hospital System in Greenville, South Carolina. In the Columbia area, teaching hospitals include Palmetto Richland Memorial Hospital (649 beds), Dorn Veterans Hospital (447 beds), and the William S. Hall Psychiatric Institute (270 beds).

Students

Approximately 98 percent of students are South Carolina residents. About 10 percent of students are underrepresented minorities, most of whom are African American. Typically, about 20 percent of students in each entering class are nontraditional, having taken time off or pursued other careers or interests after college.

STUDENT LIFE

Because the School of Medicine is an important component of a comprehensive research university, medical students have many opportunities for interaction with students in other disciplines and can take advantage of the numerous student organizations, intramural sporting events, and social opportunities of the main university. Medical student organizations include chapters of the AMSA and the American Medical Women's Association, in addition to professionally focused groups such as the emergency medicine, family practice, internal medicine, and pediatrics clubs and the psychiatry/behavioral science society. Medical students have initiated a number of community service activities, including participation in the Columbia Free Medical Clinic, tutoring and social events at area children's homes, and the Health Education Leadership Program for primary school students. The School of Medicine has its own fitness center, but medical students also have access to all athletic facilities of the main campus. Columbia is a city with a population of almost 500,000, providing a wide variety of recreational and cultural activities. Both the ocean and the Great Smoky Mountains are within a few hours drive. On-campus housing is available for married couples, although most students live off campus in the area adjacent to the USC campus.

GRADUATES

Two-thirds of USCSM graduates go on to practice in primary care fields, making the School of Medicine a leader among U.S. medical schools in the percentage of graduates entering primary care. Although many graduates do enter primary care, USCSM grads match in all specialties all over the United States.

Admissions

REQUIREMENTS

Prerequisites are 8 semester hours each of general biology or zoology, inorganic chemistry, organic chemistry, and general physics, all with associated labs. In addition, 6 semester hours of college-level English and math are required. The MCAT is required, and scores must be no more than 5 years old. For applicants who have taken the exam more than once, the most recent set of scores is weighed most heavily.

SUGGESTIONS

A maximum of 6–8 positions in each class are open to residents of states other than South Carolina. Thus, nonresident applicants should be highly qualified. USCSM looks for applicants who are interested in primary care and who are likely to serve within the state.

PROCESS

All competitive AMCAS applicants who are South Carolina residents are sent secondary applications. About 40 percent of nonresident AMCAS applicants are sent secondaries. Of those returning secondaries, about 25 percent are interviewed between August and April. Interviews consist of two sessions, each with a member of the Admissions Committee. Candidates also have lunch with medical students and attend informational presentations. Notification of the Committee's decision occurs on a rolling basis, beginning in October. Approximately one-third of interviewed candidates are accepted. Others are rejected or put on hold and possibly accepted later in the year.

Admissions Requirements (Required)

MCAT scores, science GPA, non-science GPA, letters of recommendation, interview, essays/personal statement, extracurricular activities, exposure to medical profession.

Admissions Requirements (Optional)

State residency.

Overlap Schools

Medical University of South Carolina.

COSTS AND AID

Tuition & Fees

In-state Tuition	$16,900
Out-of-state Tuition	$48,870
Room and board (on campus)	$10,050
Cost of books	$7,000
Fees	$50

Financial Aid

% students receiving aid	95
Average grant	$3,000
Average loan	$25,000
Average debt	$71,352

The University of South Dakota
Sanford School of Medicine

Office of Medical Student Affairs, 414 East Clark Street, Vermillion, SD 57069 • Admission: 605-677-6886
Fax: 605-677-5109 • E-mail: usdsmsa@usd.edu • Website: www.usd.edu/med/md

STUDENT BODY

Type	Public
Enrollment	206
% male/female	52/48
% underrepresented minorities	5
# applied (total/out)	717/573
# accepted (total/out)	66/4
# enrolled (total/out)	50/2
Average age	24

FACULTY

Total faculty (number)	942
% part-time	74

ADMISSIONS

Average GPA and MCAT Scores

Overall GPA	3.66
MCAT Bio	9.71
MCAT Phys	8.93
MCAT Verbal	9.42
MCAT Essay	0

Application Information

Regular application	11/15
Regular notification	rolling
Are transfers accepted?	yes
Admissions may be deferred?	yes
Interview required?	yes
Application fee	$35

Academics

Students complete 167 credits during their 4 year MD program. They are evaluated with letter and numerical grades. Students must pass USMLE Step 1, Step 2-CK, and a school administered OSCE. They must also take USMLE Step 2-CS to graduate. During the break between years 1 and 2, medical students have the opportunity to undertake clinical or basic science research projects, arranged through the Summer Research Program. This program teams qualified students with physician/faculty mentors and offers fellowship support.

BASIC SCIENCES: Basic biomedical sciences are taught in the Lee Memorial Medical Science Building on the USD campus in Vermillion. The Lommen Health Sciences Library is also on the Vermillion campus. The basic biomedical sciences are taught by lecture, lab, small-group discussions, and case-based presentations, all with an emphasis on clinical correlation. Students are in class or other scheduled sessions for about 30 hours per week. First-year courses are biochemistry, gross anatomy with embryology, histology with physiology, neuroscience, and introduction to clinical medicine (ICM). The ICM course is an interdisciplinary sequence that continues into the second year. During the first year, the course is titled introduction to the patient: personal and professional issues. The focus is on integrating biological, social, and psychological models and introducing the patient in all stages of the life cycle. Students also learn doctor/patient communication skills. Second-year courses are advanced behavorial science, ICM, laboratory medicine, microbiology, and pharmacology. During year 2, ICM provides students with experiences in performing comprehensive history and physical examinations on patients in a clinical setting. At the end of year 2, students travel to a rural community within the state to take a 4-week preceptorship with a family practice physician.

CLINICAL TRAINING

During the third and fourth years, students rotate through hospitals and clinics in Sioux Falls, Rapid City, or Yankton. All students participate in 3 weeks of clinical colloquium. For the Sioux Falls and Rapid City campuses, the third year consists of six clerkships, which are taken two at a time during three blocks of 16 weeks. The clerkships are family medicine paired with general internal medicine, pediatrics and adolescent medicine paired with obstetrics and gynecology, and general surgery paired with psychiatry and neurology. In addition, students take radiology and participate in a weekly primary care ambulatory clinic throughout the year. Alternatively, third-year students may enter a unique, primary care curriculum at the Yankton campus that emphasizes community involvement and self-directed learning. The entire 12 months is based in a multidisciplinary clinic, and students follow patients in each of the six specialties throughout the year. Fourth-year required clerkships for all students are surgical specialties (7 weeks), family medicine (4 weeks), and emergency room (4 weeks). An additional 23 weeks are reserved for electives. As a community-based medical school, the School of Medicine neither owns nor operates the clinical facilities utilized for teaching. Rather, the school maintains strong affiliations with a range of health care providers throughout the state, including Rapid City Regional Hospital; Sioux Valley Hospital-University of South Dakota Medical Center in Sioux Falls, Avera McKennan Hospital, and University Health Center in Sioux Falls; Avera Sacred Heart Hospital and the Yankton Medical Clinic in Yankton; and Veterans Affairs Hospitals in Sioux Falls, Fort Meade, and Hot Springs.

Students

All admitted students are either South Dakota residents or have significant personal ties to South Dakota. About 5 percent of students are underrepresented minorities, most of whom are Native Americans. The average age of incoming students is about 24. Class size is 50.

STUDENT LIFE

The small class size encourages cohesion and interaction among students, as well as between faculty and students. Several student organizations give the students an opportunity to become involved in a variety of service and support activities. During years 1 and 2, students have access to the recreational and athletic facilities of the University of South Dakota as well as on-campus residence halls. During years 3 and 4, students have varied options, depending on where their clinical training takes place.

GRADUATES

Graduates are successful in securing residencies nationwide and typically choose 10–14 different specialties. Approximately one-third of graduates enter primary care fields.

Admissions

REQUIREMENTS

Prerequisites are 1 year each of biology, chemistry, organic chemistry, physics, and college-level math. Advanced Placement and CLEP courses may count for meeting prerequisites, if granted on premedical transcript, and there is other evidence of appropriate knowledge in the subject area. The MCAT is required, and scores must be no more than 3 years old. For applicants who have retaken the exam, the most recent set of scores is compared to previous scores.

SUGGESTIONS

Residents of South Dakota, nonresidents with strong personal ties to the state (for example, they graduated from high school in South Dakota or their parents live in-state), and applicants of Native American descent who can demonstrate enrollment in federally recognized tribes in South Dakota or in border states are invited to submit secondary applications. Beyond academic credentials, exposure to the medical profession, volunteer activities, and interest in practicing primary care medicine and working with underserved communities are all valued.

PROCESS

Qualified AMCAS applicants who meet residency criteria are sent secondary applications. These applicants are invited to interview with the Admissions Committee between October and February. Interviews consist of two one-to-one interviews with a faculty member who serves on the Admissions Committee. Of interviewed candidates, about 30 percent are accepted, with notification beginning in December. Several students are placed on an alternate list and are given a rank order for admission if vacancies occur. All accepted applicants must pass background checks prior to matriculation. Sanford School of Medicine does not consider applications for transfer with advanced standing from students at non-LCME–accredited medical schools.

Admissions Requirements (Required)

MCAT scores, science GPA, non-science GPA, letters of recommendation, interview, supplemental application.

Admissions Requirements (Optional)

State residency, essays/personal statement, extracurricular activities, exposure to medical profession.

Overlap Schools

Creighton University, Mayo Clinic College of Medicine, The University of Iowa, University of Minnesota, University of Nebraska Medical Center.

COSTS AND AID

Tuition & Fees

In-state Tuition	$13,234
Out-of-state Tuition	$31,700
Room and board (on campus)	$17,725
Cost of books	$1,650
Fees	$3,497

Financial Aid

% students receiving aid	96
Average grant	$3,921
Average loan	$31,947
Average debt	$113,984

UNIVERSITY OF SOUTH FLORIDA
COLLEGE OF MEDICINE

12901 Bruce B Downs Boulevard, MDC-3, Tampa, FL 33612 • **Admission:** 813-974-2229 • **Fax:** 813-974-4990
E-mail: MD-ADMISSIONS@LYRIS.HSC.USF.EDU • **Website:** WWW.HSC.USF.EDU/MEDICINE/MDADMISSIONS

STUDENT BODY

Type	Public
Enrollment	458
% male/female	47/53
% underrepresented minorities	37
# applied (total/out)	1,822/531
# accepted (total/out)	120/5
# enrolled (total/out)	120/5
Average age	25

ADMISSIONS

Average GPA and MCAT Scores

Overall GPA	3.68
MCAT Bio	9.9
MCAT Phys	9.7
MCAT Verbal	9.4
MCAT Essay	O

Application Information

Regular application	12/1
Regular notification	10/15
Early application	8/15
Early notification	10/1
Are transfers accepted?	yes
Admissions may be deferred?	yes
Interview required?	yes
Application fee	$30

Academics

The 4 year curriculum is designed to permit the student to learn the fundamental principles of medicine, to acquire skills of critical judgment based on evidence and experience, and to develop an ability to use principles and skills wisely in solving problems of health and disease. Medical students interested in careers in research may pursue a combined MD/PhD program, earning the doctorate in a number of biomedical fields. For students interested in public and community health issues, a combined MD/MPH program is offered in conjunction with the College of Public Health. A combined MD/MBA is available to students interested in the Business of Medicine. Medical students are evaluated with honors, pass with commendation, pass, and fail. Passing Step 1 of the USMLE is a requirement for promotion to year 3, and passing Step 2 Clinical Knowledge and Clinical Skills exams is a graduation requirement.

BASIC SCIENCES: First-year students focus mainly on basic sciences and are instructed in a variety of ways including lectures, labs, small-group conferences, and interdisciplinary methods. Computers are also an important educational resource. In addition to science courses, first-year students investigate ethical and behavioral aspects of medicine in the courses behavioral medicine and medical ethics. In the second semester, they begin to learn patient interaction skills through a physical diagnosis course that extends into the second year. Other first-year courses are biochemistry, gross anatomy, human embryology, medical neuroscience, microscopic anatomy, molecular biology and human genetics, and physiology. The second year is a continuation of basic sciences with increased emphasis on clinical correlation. The remainder of physical diagnosis and introduction to clinical medicine further develop patient examination and evaluation skills and prepare students for the clinical phase of the curriculum. Other second-year courses are clinical correlation, medical microbiology and immunology, pathology and laboratory medicine, and pharmacology. Students are in class or other scheduled sessions for about 25 hours per week. In between the first and second year, there are opportunities for involvement in research.

CLINICAL TRAINING

Third-year required clinical rotations are arranged in five clinical areas including outpatient primary care/special populations (16 weeks), surgical care (8 weeks), inpatient medicine/pediatrics (8 weeks), neuropsychiatry (8 weeks), emergency medicine/urgent care (4 weeks) and maternal/newborn (4 weeks). The fourth year is divided between 4 required clerkship blocks (2 in critical care, 1 oncology, 1 dermatology/musculosketal) and 5 electives, a portion of which may be taken at other academic or clinical institutions or locations around the state, country, or overseas. Most clinical training takes place at Tampa General Hospital (1,000 beds); H. Lee Moffitt Cancer Center and Research Institute (162 beds); James A. Haley Veterans Hospital (577 beds); the USF Psychiatry Center, USF Medical Clinic; All Children's Hospital (168 beds); USF Eye Institute; University Diagnostic Institute; Shriners Hospital for Crippled Children; Bayfront Medical Center (518 beds); and Bay Pines Veterans Medical Center (520 beds). A number of community based clinics are also used as clinical training.

PRE-CLINICAL TRAINING

First-year students focus mainly on basic sciences and are instructed in a variety of ways including lectures, labs, small-group conferences, and interdisciplinary methods. Computers are an important educational resource. Students begin year 1 with an introduction to medicine in the profession of medicine course (3 weeks) before transitioning to science courses, required as first-year students investigate ethical and behavioral aspects of medicine in the courses behavioral medicine and medical ethics. They begin to learn patient interaction skills through physical diagnosis and longitudinal clinical experience (LCE) courses that extend into the second year. Other first-year courses are human anatomy, molecular medicine, medical neuroscience, and physiology. The second year is an integrated presentation of basic and clinical sciences with year-long courses in evidence based medicine; immunology and infectious diseases; pathology and laboratory medicine; pharmacology; clinical diagnosis and reasoning; principles of microbiology; and a problem-based learning course, clinical problem solving. Students are in class or other scheduled sessions for about 32 hours per week. In between the first and second year, there are opportunities for involvement in research. The pre-clinical curriculum provides a solid foundation for the transition to Clinical Medicine.

Students

Most students are Florida residents. A significant percentage of students are from those ethnic groups underrepresented in medicine, representing only a portion of the diverse cultures found among students. Although most students enter shortly after college graduation, there is a wide age range in each class. Class size is 120.

STUDENT LIFE

Students are cooperative, often studying together and interacting outside of the academic setting. The Medical School sponsors student events and organizations, and has a strong emphasis on involvement in school and community activities. The Medical School is located on the main USF campus, giving students access to the amenities of a large university. Tampa has many cultural and recreational opportunities and is generally a popular city among students. Most students live off campus where housing is relatively affordable and comfortable.

GRADUATES

Graduates are successful in securing residency positions in all specialty areas. At USF, postgraduate training programs are offered in more than 10 fields.

Admissions

REQUIREMENTS

Science requirements include 1 year each of basic introductory courses and laboratories in biological science, general chemistry, organic chemistry, and physics. One year of both English and mathematics is also required. The MCAT is required, and at least one score must be from within the past 3 years. For applicants who have taken the exam more than once, the best set of scores is weighed most heavily. Thus, there is no advantage in withholding scores.

SUGGESTIONS

State residency is given preference. Courses that are recommended, but not required, include biochemistry, cell biology, comparative anatomy, embryology, genetics, logic, physical or biological chemistry, rhetoric, and statistics. Knowledge of calculus, computer science, and statistics is useful. Consideration is given to a student's participation in honors courses, independent study, and scientific research. All applicants are advised to apply as early as possible because the application process is rolling. Noncognitive experiences (shadowing, health care experience—voluntary or paid—community service, leadership roles, and research) enhance an applicant's understanding of careers in medicine.

PROCESS

All AMCAS applicants who meet minimum standards are sent secondary applications. About 15 percent of those who return secondary applications are invited to interview between September and April. Interviews are one-on-one with two faculty members or a fourth-year medical student. On interview day, candidates have the opportunity to tour the campus and to meet informally with current medical students. About 50 percent of interviewees are accepted with notification occurring on a rolling basis. Others are rejected or wait listed.

Admissions Requirements (Required)

MCAT scores, science GPA, non-science GPA, letters of recommendation, interview, essays/personal statement, extracurricular activities, exposure to medical profession.

Admissions Requirements (Optional)

State residency.

Overlap Schools

University of Florida, University of Miami.

COSTS AND AID

Tuition & Fees

In-state Tuition	$16,499
Out-of-state Tuition	$48,533
Room and board (off campus)	$9,420
Cost of books	$1,913
Fees	$1,982

Financial Aid

% students receiving aid	85
Average grant	$5,000
Average loan	$20,500
Average debt	$104,000

University of Southern California

Keck School of Medicine

1975 Zonal Avenue, KAM 100-C, Los Angeles, CA 90089-9021 • Admission: 323-442-2552
Fax: 323-442-2433 • E-mail: MEDADMIT@HSC.USC.EDU • Website: WWW.USC.EDU/MEDICINE/

STUDENT BODY

Type	Private
Enrollment	659
% male/female	52/48
% underrepresented minorities	17
# applied (total/out)	5,445/2,087
# accepted (total/out)	334/54
# enrolled (total/out)	161/26
Average age	24

FACULTY

Total faculty (number)	206
% female	26
% minority	19
% part-time	3

ADMISSIONS

Average GPA and MCAT Scores

Overall GPA	3.6
MCAT Bio	10.56
MCAT Phys	10.48
MCAT Verbal	9.66
MCAT Essay	R

Application Information

Regular application	10/1
Regular notification	4/2
Early application	8/1
Early notification	10/1
Are transfers accepted?	yes
Admissions may be deferred?	yes
Interview required?	yes
Application fee	$90

Academics

While the majority of students earn their MD in 4 years, USC offers a variety of joint degree programs. The MD/PhD program is administered by the USC Graduate School and the School of Medicine, allowing students to earn the doctorate in anatomy, biochemistry, biomedical engineering, biophysics, cell biology, genetics, immunology, microbiology, molecular biology, neuroscience, pathology, pharmacology, and physiology. For those interested in more discrete research projects, the Research Scholar Program allows students to spend 1 year involved in research at USC or another approved institution. Students also have the option of entering a combined MD/MPH program.

BASIC SCIENCES: Lectures, labs, and periodic small-group discussions are the instructional modalities used during the first 2 years. Currently, the faculty and students are working together to design a revised curriculum, which may depend more on small-group sessions and problem-based learning. The first year (38 weeks) begins with an introductory review course entitled human biology, which is followed by a sequence of courses based on organ systems. They are cardiovascular, endocrine/reproduction, gastrointestinal/liver, renal/respiratory/skin, neuroscience, and blood. Students benefit from patient contact from the very beginning in introduction to clinical medicine. The second year (37 weeks) is also organized around body/organ systems and is dedicated to studying the mechanisms of disease. USC's library is comprehensive and has an ample supply of computers. Computers with course material, online resources, and other study aids are also available in individually assigned laboratory spaces, which serve as student study areas. Grading for the first 2 years is honors/satisfactory/unsatisfactory. Students must pass Step 1 of the USMLE to be promoted to year 3.

CLINICAL TRAINING

The clinical years are the hallmark of USC's education. The majority of teaching takes place in L.A. County and USC Medical Center. It is among the major public hospitals for Los Angeles and receives patients with every imaginable illness and injury. Students are allowed extensive patient contact. The curriculum of required courses and electives is continuous over the third and fourth years and is individually designed. Required clerkships are family medicine (6 weeks), pediatrics (6 weeks), ob/gyn (6 weeks), general surgery (6 weeks), psychiatry (6 weeks), neurology (4 weeks), internal medicine (two of 6 weeks each), specialized surgery (2–3 weeks), and a basic or clinical sciences clerkship (4 weeks). An additional 12 weeks of selectives are required. Students may take up to 16 weeks of electives at approved institutions throughout the nation. In addition to LAC and USC Medical Center, clinical facilities include Children's Hospital Los Angeles, USC University Hospital, and USC/Norris Comprehensive Cancer Center. Grading during the clinical years is honors/near honors/satisfactory/unsatisfactory. Students must record a score on the USMLE Step 2 to graduate.

Students

Of the 150 students in each class, almost 80 percent are California residents. About 16 percent of students are underrepresented minorities. The average age of incoming students is about 24, with a wide age range including significant numbers of students in their thirties.

STUDENT LIFE

The Medical School campus is not situated in an ideal residential area, and the majority of students commute to school from surrounding communities. Nonetheless, USC has a cohesive and cooperative student body. Many first-year students attend a camping retreat prior to the beginning of classes, during which they are introduced to each other and to returning students. During the academic year, students typically study in groups, and spend time together outside of school. The School of Medicine offers a wide range of extracurricular activities, including volunteer programs, intramural sports, and student clubs and organizations. USC's main campus is easily accessible by car, and medical students regularly use its extensive recreational facilities. University-sponsored activities, such as intercollegiate sporting events, films, and parties, are also popular with medical students.

GRADUATES

Graduates are successful in securing positions nationwide, in both specialty and primary care fields. Most enter residency programs in California.

Admissions

REQUIREMENTS

Prerequisites are 2 semesters each, with associated labs, in biology, general chemistry, organic chemistry, and physics. In addition, applicants must have completed a course in basic molecular biology and an additional 30 semester hours in a combination of English composition, humanities, and social sciences. The MCAT is required, and scores must be from within the previous 2 years.

SUGGESTIONS

The Admissions Committee looks very favorably upon hospital or other medical experience that involves patient care and demonstrates a commitment to service. Research experience is also helpful. USC strongly recommends additional course work in statistics and higher mathematics.

PROCESS

All AMCAS applicants are asked to submit a supplemental application. Of those students who return supplemental applications, approximately 800 are invited for interviews. The interview day consists of a tour, lunch with medical students, and one or two hour-long interviews with faculty and/or medical students. Initial acceptances are sent at the beginning of January, but most students are placed in a hold category, with the majority of acceptances offered in May. About 40 percent of interviewed candidates are accepted. Wait-listed candidates may send additional information to update or strengthen their files.

Admissions Requirements (Required)

MCAT scores, science GPA, non-science GPA, letters of recommendation, interview, essays/personal statement, extracurricular activities, exposure to medical profession.

Admissions Requirements (Optional)

State residency.

COSTS AND AID

Tuition & Fees

Tuition	$35,052
Room and board (on campus)	$9,802
Cost of books	$2,200
Fees	$1,013

Financial Aid

% students receiving aid	75
Average grant	$10,000
Average loan	$29,800
Average debt	$93,000

UNIVERSITY OF TENNESSEE—MEMPHIS

COLLEGE OF MEDICINE

ADMISSIONS OFFICE, 790 MADISON AVENUE, ROOM 307, MEMPHIS, TN 38163 • ADMISSION: 901-448-5559
FAX: 901-448-1740 • WEBSITE: WWW.UTMEM.EDU/MEDICINE

STUDENT BODY

Type	Public
Enrollment	686
% male/female	61/39
% underrepresented minorities	15
# applied (total/out)	1,700/1,054
Average age	24

FACULTY

Total faculty (number)	1,711
% female	17
% minority	10
% part-time	3
Student-faculty ratio	2:1

ADMISSIONS

Application Information

Regular application	11/15
Regular notification	10/15–4/1
Are transfers accepted?	yes
Admissions may be deferred?	yes
Interview required?	no
Application fee	$50

Academics

Most students follow a 4 year curriculum, leading to the MD. The Optional Expanded Academic Program allows students to expand the first 2 years into 3. The Clinical Scholars Program provides special educational and financial assistance to entering students interested in careers in family medicine, general internal medicine, general pediatrics, medicine and pediatrics (med-peds), or ob/gyn. Students are encouraged to pursue research, either during the summer following year 1 or as ongoing projects. For students interested in intensive research, an MD/PhD program is available. Medical students generally receive percentage scores on exams and are evaluated with an A–F scale. Examinations in some courses are administered by computer. Passing both steps of the USMLE is a requirement for graduation.

BASIC SCIENCES: The basic sciences are taught during the first 2 years primarily through lectures and lab work. Students are in class or other scheduled sessions for about 23 hours per week. First-year science courses are the following: Biochemistry; fundamentals of cellular and molecular biology, medical genetics, gross anatomy, histology, neuroanatomy, and physiology. Other first-year courses are behavioral sciences and preventive medicine, both of which involve small-group discussions. Throughout the first and second years, students take introduction to clinical skills, which correlates basic science concepts with actual medical cases and teaches students introductory clinical techniques. Students also participate in a longitudinal, community-based clinical program. Second-year courses are microbiology, neuroscience, nutrition, pathology, pathophysiology, and pharmacology. Most of the first 2 years is spent in the Cecil C. Humphreys General Education Building that houses classrooms, labs, and a computer center. A 3 year longitudinal community program incorporates content of five current courses including behavioral science, preventive medicine, nutrition, ICS, and longitudinal community-based clinical program. An important educational resource is the Plane Tree Center with multimedia software technologies for learning anatomy, embryology, histology, EKG readings, and lung and heart sounds. Plane Tree also provides health-oriented books, audiovisuals, and Internet connections. The Health Sciences Library is used by students both for research purposes and for studying. It is fully computerized, subscribes to approximately 1,550 current periodicals, and contains a total volume count of more than 170,000.

CLINICAL TRAINING

Third-year required clerkships are 2 months each of the following: Family medicine, medicine, ob/gyn, pediatrics, psychiatry, and surgery. The fourth year is composed of five 1-month clerkships and 3 months of electives that provide students the opportunity to select the clinical or basic science experiences to best meet their particular career goals. Electives allow for increased responsibility in patient care as well as the opportunity to pursue areas of individual interest. Fourth-year required clerkships are ambulatory care medicine, neurology, and a senior clerkship in medicine and surgical subspecialties. As part of a selective requirement, 1 month of either family medicine, medicine, pediatrics ob/gyn, psychiatry, or surgery is also required. All students must spend a minimum of 10 months of clerkship and elective time on the Memphis campus. This requirement allows a maximum of 10 months (excluding option months) to be spent at Knoxville Chattanooga, and/or Nashville. Two of the 10 months away from the Memphis campus may be taken at another institution, either in the United States or overseas.

Students

At least 90 percent of students are Tennessee residents. Others are usually from the eight states contiguous to Tennessee. These are Mississippi, Arkansas, Missouri, Kentucky, Virginia, North Carolina, Georgia, and Alabama. The average age of incoming students is typically about 24 with a wide age range among students. Underrepresented minorities account for about 12 percent of students. Class size is 165.

STUDENT LIFE

Medical students are cohesive and supportive of one another. As part of the Big Sib Program, incoming medical students are assigned to senior students as mentors. Typically, the Big Sibs will pass along their class notes to the new students to use as a guide during basic science lectures. Medical students are part of a larger community that includes students of all professional schools and programs. The Student Alumni Center (SAC) is the focal point of campus life, providing meeting areas, a restaurant, lounges, a television room, shopping areas, and other services. More than 35 campus-wide organizations are open to medical students. Students enjoy a fitness center that houses a multi-purpose gym, a swimming pool, spa, racketball courts, and a weight room. An outdoor complex has playing fields, volleyball courts, tennis courts, golf-practice facilities, and a track. Intramural sports are popular, as is the Outdoor Adventures Program, which leads canoeing, hiking, rafting, and camping trips. Memphis is a festive city, renowned for its music scene. Other attractions include riverside areas, parks, restaurants, a lively arts community, and quiet residential neighborhoods. UT Memphis offers both residence halls and apartment-style facilities for single students. The university assists married students with finding housing in the city.

GRADUATES

Among 1999 graduates, the most popular fields for residencies were the following: Internal medicine (31 percent), pediatrics (10 percent), family practice (21 percent), ob/gyn (21 percent), surgery (12 percent), radiology (6 percent), and medicine/pediatrics (8 percent). A significant proportion of graduates remains in Tennessee for postgraduate training.

Admissions

REQUIREMENTS

Prerequisite course work is 8 semester hours each of biology, general chemistry, general physics, and organic chemistry, all taken with associated labs. In addition, 6 hours of English is required. The MCAT is required and scores must be no more than 5 years old. For applicants who have taken the exam more than once, all sets of scores are considered.

SUGGESTIONS

Residents of Tennessee are given preference. Children of UT alumni are also considered, regardless of their state of residence. As a state-supported institution, no more than 10 percent of students may be nonresidents. Thus, nonresident applicants should be highly qualified. Students are encouraged to take courses in the humanities, fine arts, and social sciences. Demonstration of analytic ability and independent thinking is important.

PROCESS

All AMCAS applicants who are considered competitive are sent supplemental applications. Of those returning supplementals, approximately 400 applicants are invited to interview between October and March. The interview gives insights into the applicant's character and how well he or she has formulated plans for the study of medicine. Interviews consist of two sessions, each with a faculty member or current medical student. On interview day, applicants have lunch, attend group informational sessions, sit in on classes, and tour the campus. Of interviewed candidates, about 60 percent are accepted on a rolling basis. Others are either rejected or placed on a wait list.

Admissions Requirements (Required)

MCAT scores, state residency, extracurricular activities, exposure to medical profession.

Admissions Requirements (Optional)

Science GPA, nonscience GPA, letters of recommendation, interview, essays/personal statement.

COSTS AND AID

Tuition & Fees

In-state Tuition	$9,256
Out-of-state Tuition	$17,920
Room and board (on campus)	$1,400
Room and board (off campus)	$3,600
Cost of books	$1,600
Fees	$213

Financial Aid

% students receiving aid	80
Average grant	$8,695
Average loan	$15,700
Average debt	$63,000

UNIVERSITY OF TEXAS
MEDICAL BRANCH AT GALVESTON SCHOOL OF MEDICINE

OFFICE OF ADMISSIONS, G-210, ASHBEL SMITH BUILDING, GALVESTON, TX 77555-1317 • ADMISSION: 409-772-3517
FAX: 409-772-5753 • E-MAIL: PWYLIE@MSPO4.MED.EDU • WEBSITE: WWW.UTMB.EDU

STUDENT BODY

Type	Public
Enrollment	821
% male/female	59/41
% underrepresented minorities	15
# applied (total/out)	2,772/485
# accepted (total/out)	37/15
# enrolled (out-of-state)	12

ADMISSIONS

Application Information

Regular application	10/15
Regular notification	1/15
	until filled
Are transfers accepted?	no
Admissions may be deferred?	yes
Interview required?	no
Application fee	$45

Academics

In addition to the standard 4 year MD curriculum, UTMB offers a combined MD/PhD program for students interested in training for a career in biomedical research. Generally, about five students enter this program each year and receive full funding for the duration of their studies. Summer and year-long research projects are also open to medical students. As an alternative to the primarily lecture-based basic-science curriculum, 24 incoming students each year enter an interactive learning track, which relies on small-group instruction.

BASIC SCIENCES: First-year courses are the following: Biochemistry, cells, and genes; community continuity experience; gross anatomy and developmental anatomy; introduction to patient evaluation; medical ethics; microanatomy; neuroscience; and physiology and biophysics. Second-year courses are community continuity experience, endocrinology, microbiology, pathology, pharmacology and toxicology, immunology, introduction to clinical medicine, and introduction to patient evaluation. During the first and second years, students are in class or other scheduled sessions for about 30 hours per week. In addition to teaching basic-science principles, the pre-clinical curriculum involves practical problem-solving experiences and case studies that demonstrate the interrelationship between the basic and clinical sciences. The community continuity experience gives first- and second-year students the opportunity to work with primary care physicians, interact with patients, and apply and expand knowledge and skills gained in the classroom. Educational support services include academic counseling, peer tutorials, study skills workshops, and stress-management workshops. An educational support center provides medical students with computer-assisted educational support. For research purposes, and as a place to study, students use the Moody Medical Library, which is the oldest medical library in Texas and one of the largest medical research centers in the Southwest. Collections include nearly 250,000 volumes in addition to computerized informational services.

CLINICAL TRAINING

Third-year required clerkships include a multidisciplinary ambulatory clerkship (12 weeks), internal medicine (8 weeks), surgery (8 weeks), ob/gyn (6 weeks), psychiatry (6 weeks), family medicine (6 weeks), and pediatrics (4 weeks). Lectures in anesthesiology, medical jurisprudence, ophthalmology, and otolaryngology are also part of the third-year curriculum. Fourth-year required clerkships are neurology (4 weeks), surgery (4 weeks), emergency medicine (4 weeks), an acting internship selective (4 weeks), radiology (2 weeks), and dermatology (2 weeks). At least 20 weeks are reserved for elective study. Clinical training takes place primarily at UTMB hospitals and clinics. Some electives may be taken at other institutions.

Students

At least 90 percent of students are Texas residents. Typically, about 10 percent of entering students are a bit older, having taken significant time off after college. Approximately 15 percent of students are underrepresented minorities. Class size is 200.

STUDENT LIFE

Students benefit from the resources and facilities of a large, modernized campus. The Lee Hage Jamail Student Center serves as a meeting place for medical students. It has a cafeteria, meeting rooms, study areas, and recreational facilities. Coed medical fraternities located close to campus offer housing, meals, and social opportunities to medical students. The UTMB Alumni Fields House features a variety of indoor and outdoor facilities, including tennis courts, baseball diamonds, volleyball courts, an outdoor basketball court, racquetball courts, fitness centers, spa facilities, an outdoor track, and an Olympic size pool. UTMB has more than 50 student organizations that range from support groups for minority students to community service-oriented groups to professional organizations. The university operates both dormitories and apartments for single students.

GRADUATES

Graduates are successful in securing residencies at top institutions nationwide.

Admissions

REQUIREMENTS

A grade of at least a C must be earned in all of the prerequisite courses. These are biology (two years), English (1 year), math (1 semester of college-level), physics (1 year), chemistry (1 year), and organic chemistry (1 year). All science courses must include laboratory work. The MCAT is required, and scores should be from within the past year. For applicants who have taken the exam on multiple occasions, the most recent set of scores is considered.

SUGGESTIONS

As a state-supported institution, UTMB gives preference to Texas residents. Applicants are encouraged to take the spring MCAT because late receipt of scores from the fall cycle may delay application processing. Medical experience, volunteer activities, and research are all helpful.

PROCESS

The University of Texas does not participate in the AMCAS system. Applications may be obtained from The University of Texas System, Medical/Dental Application Center, Suite 6400, 702 Colorado Street, Austin, TX, 78701, phone: 512-499-4785. Applications must be submitted between May 15 and October 15. About 1,000 applicants are invited to interview during November and December. Candidates receive two interviews, each with a faculty member. On interview day, there are also orientation sessions, a campus tour, and several opportunities to meet informally with current medical students. About 20 percent of interviewed candidates are accepted. Others are rejected or placed on a wait list and possibly accepted later in the year.

Admissions Requirements (Required)

MCAT scores, science GPA, non-science GPA, letters of recommendation, state residency, extracurricular activities, exposure to medical profession.

Admissions Requirements (Optional)

Interview, essays/personal statement.

COSTS AND AID

Tuition & Fees

Tuition	$1,000
Cost of books	$2,000
Fees	$1,000
Average grant	$10
Average loan	$125,141

University of Texas Health Science Center at Houston
Medical School at Houston

Office of Admissions, MSB G420, Houston, TX 77030 • Admission: 713-500-5116
Fax: 713-500-0604 • E-mail: MSADMISSIONS@UTH.TMC.EDU • Website: WWW.MED.UTH.TMC.EDU

STUDENT BODY

Type	Public
Enrollment	848
% male/female	52/48
% underrepresented minorities	27
# applied (total/out)	3,245/459
# accepted (total/out)	256/28
# enrolled (total/out)	210/18
Average age	23

FACULTY

Total faculty (number)	910
% female	37
% minority	31
% part-time	12
Student-faculty ratio	1:1

ADMISSIONS

Average GPA and MCAT Scores

Overall GPA	3.66
MCAT Bio	10
MCAT Phys	9.3
MCAT Verbal	9.3
MCAT Essay	P

Application Information

Regular application	10/15
Regular notification	2/1
Are transfers accepted?	no
Admissions may be deferred?	no
Interview required?	yes
Application fee	$55

Academics

Although most medical students complete studies in 4 years, some follow an alternate pathway curriculum, which extends first-year courses more than a 2 year period and leads to the MD degree in 5 years. Others follow a 7 year program, leading to both the MD and the PhD degrees, while others earn a MPH along with the MD in 5 years. Summer research opportunities are available, most of which are paid. Medical students are evaluated with honors, high pass, pass, marginal performance, and fail. All students must take the USMLE Steps 1 and 2.

BASIC SCIENCES: First-year courses are biochemistry, gross anatomy, developmental anatomy, histology, immunology, introduction to clinical medicine (ICM), microbiology, neuroscience, and physiology. The ICM course introduces students to interviewing, history-taking, and physical-examination skills. Instructional methods used during the first year include lectures, small-group sessions, tutorials, and labs. A problem-based learning curriculum links basic and clinical sciences and allows second-year students to begin addressing complex medical problems. Problem-based learning is an important part of the second-year curriculum, serving to integrate the various courses and provide clinical skills. Second-year courses are behavioral science, genetics, fundamentals of clinical medicine, pathology, pharmacology, physical diagnosis, and reproductive biology. During the first 2 years, students are in class or other scheduled sessions for about 22 hours per week. The Learning Resource Center has textbooks, audiovisuals, anatomical models, audiotapes and videotapes of lectures, computers, files of past exams, USMLE review materials, and other instructional aids. Networked computers with free access to computer-based services and instructional materials are also provided.

CLINICAL TRAINING

Third-year required rotations are medicine (12 weeks), surgery (8 weeks), ob/gyn (8 weeks), pediatrics (8 weeks), psychiatry (8 weeks), family medicine (4 weeks), and radiology (1 week). During the fourth year, required rotations are family practice (1 month), medicine (1 month), neurology (1 month), and surgery (1 month). Third and fourth-year students receive advanced technical skills training. Clinical training takes place primarily at the numerous hospitals, clinics, and care centers associated with the Texas Medical Center in Houston and in a city/county hospital in northeast Houston. There is flexibility in terms of where elective credits may be earned, and some students opt to study elsewhere in the country or at one of several international programs.

Students

At least 90 percent of students are Texas residents. Most students are recent college graduates, although there is typically a wide age range among incoming students. In terms of ethnic backgrounds, students represent the diverse population of the state.

STUDENT LIFE

There are numerous student organizations, focusing on areas such as public service projects, professional interests, religious and ethnic interests, athletics, and recreation. Houston is an exciting city for students, with a wide range of entertainment, recreational attractions, restaurants, shopping areas, and facilities for outdoor activities. The university offers apartments a short distance from school and a free shuttle runs throughout the week.

GRADUATES

Of approximately 4,200 UT Houston Medical School graduates, about 59 percent go on to practice in Texas. Among the 2005 graduates, the most popular fields for residencies were internal medicine (19.5 percent), family practice (9 percent), anesthesiology (8 percent), ob/gyn (8 percent), surgery (8 percent), pediatrics (7.5 percent), pathology (7 percent), emergency medicine (4 percent), and surgery preliminary (4 percent).

Admissions

REQUIREMENTS

Prerequisites are 1 year of English, 1 semester of college-level calculus, 1 year of physics with lab, 2 years of biology with lab, 1 year of general chemistry with lab, and 1 year of organic chemistry with lab. The MCAT is required, and scores should be from within the past 5 years. For applicants who have retaken the exam, the last three scores will be reviewed.

SUGGESTIONS

No more than 10 percent of students may be nonresidents; thus, admission is very competitive for nonresidents. A liberal arts background is important and, as long as science requirements are fulfilled, students are encouraged to pursue a major in their area of interest while in college. Technological, vocational engineering, or business courses of study are not viewed as favorably as those providing a broad educational background. Important traits include intellectual capacity, interpersonal, and communication skills, breadth and depth of premedical educational experience, potential for service to the State of Texas, motivation, and integrity.

PROCESS

The University of Texas does not participate in the AMCAS system. Applications may only be made online at the Texas Medical and Dental Schools Application Service website, www.utsystem.edu/tmdsas. Applications must be submitted between May 1 and October 15. Additional information about the admissions process may be obtained from Texas Medical and Dental Schools, Application Service, 702 Colorado Street, Suite 6400, Austin, TX 78701, Phone: 512-499-4785. About 1,250 applicants are interviewed at UT Houston between August and January. Applicants generally receive two one-on-one interviews, each with a faculty member. On interview day, candidates also have lunch with medical students, tour the campus, and attend group orientation sessions. About one-fifth of interviewees are accepted, with notification occurring via the TMDSAS website on February 1. Some wait-listed candidates are accepted later in the spring and summer.

Admissions Requirements (Required)

MCAT scores, science GPA, non-science GPA, letters of recommendation, interview, essays/personal statement, extracurricular activities, exposure to medical profession.

Admissions Requirements (Optional)

State residency.

Overlap Schools

Baylor College of Medicine; Texas A&M University—College Station; Texas Tech University; University of North Texas; University of Texas Health Science Center at San Antonio; University of Texas Southwestern Medical Center; University of Texas.

COSTS AND AID

Tuition & Fees

In-state Tuition	$9,025
Out-of-state Tuition	$22,875
Room and board (off campus)	$12,410
Cost of books	$2,000
In-state Fees	$1,730
Out-of-state Fees	$1,833

Financial Aid

% students receiving aid	98
Average grant	$2,539
Average loan	$10,012
Average debt	$98,345

UNIVERSITY OF TEXAS HEALTH SCIENCE CENTER AT SAN ANTONIO
MEDICAL SCHOOL AT SAN ANTONIO

MEDICAL SCHOOL ADMISSIONS OFFICE, 7703 FLOYD CURL DRIVE, SAN ANTONIO, TX 78229 • ADMISSION: 210-567-2665
FAX: 210-567-2685 • E-MAIL: CHAPAB@UTHSCSA.EDU • WEBSITE: WWW.UTHSCSA.EDU

STUDENT BODY

Type	Public
Enrollment	814
% male/female	58/42
% underrepresented minorities	16
# applied (total/out)	2,795/525
Average age	24

FACULTY

Total faculty (number)	678
% female	28
% part-time	5

ADMISSIONS

Application Information

Regular application	10/1
Regular notification	1/15
	until filled
Are transfers accepted?	yes
Admissions may be deferred?	no
Interview required?	no
Application fee	$45

Academics

Almost all medical students follow a 4 year curriculum leading to the MD. A few students enter combined MD/PhD programs after their first year of medical school. Grading for most courses uses an A–F system. All students must pass Step 1 of the USMLE for promotion to year 3.

BASIC SCIENCES: Basic sciences are primarily covered during the first two years, although introductory clinical training also begins in year 1. San Antonio operates on a semester system, with a break scheduled around Christmas. First-year, first semester courses are the biochemistry, clinical integration course, gross anatomy and embryology, microscopic anatomy, and microbiology. Second semester courses are neuroscience and physiology. Other first-year courses use a combination of lectures, labs, and small-group sessions. Students are in class or other scheduled sessions for about 21 hours per week during year 1. During the second year, the curriculum is increasingly clinically oriented. First semester courses are behavioral sciences, pathology, and pharmacology. Second semester courses are pathology and psychopathology. During year 2, students are in class for about 19 hours per week, providing ample study time. An important resource for students, faculty, and the community is the Dolph Briscoe Library, which houses more than 200,000 books and journals.

CLINICAL TRAINING

The clinical integration course is an interdisciplinary program that starts with the first month of medical school and extends through the second year. Students learn basic clinical skills in the initial month of the program, spend time with community physicians, rotate with third-year students, and assume patient responsibilities to gain experience in continuity of care. The third and fourth years are devoted primarily to clinical clerkships. However, didactic instruction is also an important part of the curriculum. Topics covered are advanced cardiopulmonary resuscitation, basic cardiac life support, clinical orientation, clinical pathology, emergency medicine, epidemiology, genetics, infectious disease, medical humanities, medical jurisprudence, patient rehabilitation, and radiology. Third-year required rotations are medicine (12 weeks), surgery (12 weeks), pediatrics (6 weeks), psychiatry (6 weeks), ob/gyn (6 weeks), and family practice (6 weeks). Fourth-year requirements are medicine (8 weeks); surgery (4 weeks); a choice of pediatrics, ob/gyn, psychiatry, or family practice (4 weeks); and other selectives (16 weeks). An additional 8 weeks are reserved for electives. The primary teaching hospital is the University Hospital, which has 547 beds. Training also takes place at the facilities of the South Texas Veterans Health Care System and at other affiliates. University-affiliated patient care covers a geographical area from San Antonio to the Rio Grande Valley and is delivered in clinics, hospitals, traveling vans, as well as in sites in schools and churches. The Health Science Center serves the entire South Texas/Border region.

Students

At least 90 percent of students are Texas residents. Underrepresented minorities account for 16 percent of the student population. Mexican Americans are particularly well represented. The student body is slightly older than at many other medical schools. The average age of incoming students is usually about 24, and about 15 percent of students in each class are in their thirties or older.

STUDENT LIFE

Medical students enjoy a collegial environment and appreciate the diversity within the student body. Mentoring and peer-support programs help incoming students with the transition to medical school, and special programs are available to assist underrepresented minority students. Students are very active in community service programs and events. Activities range from volunteering at clinics to participating in health education programs in schools. All students live off campus. San Antonio offers affordable housing accessible to the Medical Center by public transportation.

GRADUATES

More than half of graduates enter primary care fields, and a significant number go on to practice in Texas.

Admissions

REQUIREMENTS

Required courses are 2 years of biology (1 of which may be biochemistry); 2 years of chemistry, which should include both organic and inorganic chemistry; 1 semester of calculus; and 1 year each of English and physics. The MCAT is required. For applicants who have taken the exam more than once, the best set of scores is weighed most heavily. Thus, there is no advantage in withholding scores.

SUGGESTIONS

In addition to academic requirements, personal traits and an applicant's background are considered. Some type of medically related experience or research is required.

PROCESS

The University of Texas medical schools do not participate in AMCAS. Rather, applications may be obtained from The Texas Medical and Dental Application Service, 702 Colorado, Suite 6400 Austin, Texas 78701. Applications must be completed by October 15. About one-third of applicants are interviewed between August and December. Interviews consist of two half-hour sessions with Admissions Committee members who may be faculty or senior students. On interview day, candidates also have lunch with students, attend group-orientation sessions, and tour the campus. The initial group of accepted candidates are notified in January. Others are notified later in the spring. An alternate pool of applicants is established and candidates are admitted as positions become available.

Admissions Requirements (Required)

MCAT scores, state residency, essays/personal statement, extracurricular activities, likelihood of serving in most urgently needed types of primary care.

Admissions Requirements (Optional)

Science GPA, nonscience GPA, letters of recommendation, interview, exposure to medical profession.

UNIVERSITY OF TEXAS SOUTHWESTERN
MEDICAL SCHOOL AT DALLAS

5323 HARRY HINES BOULEVARD, DALLAS, TX 75390-9162 • ADMISSION: 214-648-5617
FAX: 214-648-3289 • E-MAIL: ADMISSIONS@UTSOUTHWESTERN.EDU • WEBSITE: WWW.UTSOUTHWESTERN.EDU

STUDENT BODY

Type	Public
Enrollment	904
% male/female	56/44
% underrepresented minorities	20
# applied (total/out)	3,268/678
# accepted (total/out)	434/61
# enrolled (total/out)	229/36
Average age	25

FACULTY

Total faculty (number)	1,587
% female	25
% minority	16
% part-time	14
Student-faculty ratio	1:1

ADMISSIONS

Average GPA and MCAT Scores

Overall GPA	3.78
MCAT Bio	11.4
MCAT Phys	11.3
MCAT Verbal	10.3
MCAT Essay	P

Application Information

Regular application	10/15
Regular notification	11/15
Are transfers accepted?	yes
Admissions may be deferred?	yes
Interview required?	yes
Application fee	$65

Academics

The vast majority of students follow a 4 year path leading to the MD degree. A small number of students each year enter a joint MD/PhD program in conjunction with the Southwestern Graduate School of Biomedical Sciences. For the most part, students are evaluated using an A–F scale in which a C is required to pass. Fourth year courses are taken pass/fail.

BASIC SCIENCES: During the first 2 years, a variety of teaching/learning formats are used, including lectures, small-group, problem-based learning, computerized curriculum, and standardized patient interviews. First year courses include biology of cells and tissues, endocrinology and human reproduction, human anatomy and embryology, human behavior, integrative human biology, and medical biochemistry. In addition, clinical ethics in medicine exposes first-year students to the ethical, behavioral, and clinical perspectives of medicine in a problem-based learning format. During the 10-week period between the first and second years, numerous clinical and research opportunities are available for students who wish to participate. Clinical exposure continues in the second year through clinical medicine as follows: Principles and practice when students learn about the physical examination and experience direct, one-on-one, patient contact. Second year courses also include anatomic and clinical pathology, immunology and medical microbiology, medical pharmacology, and psychopathology. On average, students are in scheduled sessions for 25–30 hours per week. The campus where pre-clinical instruction takes place is also part of a large medical complex that includes several hospitals, research centers, and the medical school library, which holds more than 229,000 volumes and currently subscribes to almost 2,000 journals. Passing the USMLE Step 1 is required to graduate.

CLINICAL TRAINING

Building upon the clinical experiences in the first 2 years, the third and fourth years offer intense clinical experiences involving medical students in direct patient care. Third year required clinical rotations are internal medicine (12 weeks), surgery (8 weeks), pediatrics (8 weeks), obstetrics and gynecology (6 weeks), psychiatry (6 weeks), and family practice (4 weeks). The fourth year is organized into 4-week periods filled with electives, selectives, and a few remaining required rotations. Requirements include neurology (4 weeks), internal medicine (4 weeks of a sub internship and 4 weeks of ambulatory care), and women's health care (4 weeks). Four 4-week periods remain, two of which are for selectives and two of which are reserved for electives. Clinical training takes place at university sites and affiliated institutions, including Parkland Memorial Hospital, the James Aston Ambulatory Care Center, Zale Lipshy University Hospital, Children's Medical Center, Dallas Veterans Affairs Medical Center, Southwestern Institute of Forensic Sciences, Baylor University Medical Center, Presbyterian Hospital of Dallas, Methodist Hospitals of Dallas, St. Paul Medical Center, Texas Scottish Rite Hospital for Children, and John Peter Smith Hospital in Fort Worth. Students may fulfill many of their senior rotations at academic or medical institutions in other parts of the state, the country, or the world.

Students

At least 90 percent of the student body are Texas residents. Underrepresented minorities account for about 10 percent of the population. The average age of incoming students is usually 24; the range of ages is typically 20–45. Incoming class size at UT Southwestern is 230 students.

STUDENT LIFE

The Bryan Williams, MD Student Center has exercise and recreational facilities and offers students a convenient place to relax and socialize. Dynamic campus activity programming includes intramural sports, special-interest organizations, recreational and cultural events, and parties. Students also join groups based on professional and academic interests or participate in community service projects. Dallas is an exciting city with a diverse population and many kinds of cultural, recreational, and entertainment activities. All students live off campus, and most students own cars.

GRADUATES

Graduates are successful in securing residencies at prestigious institutions all over the country. The majority of graduates go on to become practicing physicians, typically with a large percentage choosing primary care specialties. Some go into academic medicine or research.

Admissions

REQUIREMENTS

Prerequisite courses include 4 semesters of biology (two of which should be with lab and one of which may be biochemistry); and 4 semesters of chemistry with lab, which should be equally divided between organic and inorganic chemistry; 2 semesters of English; 2 semesters of physics with lab; and 1 semester of calculus or statistics. The MCAT is required, and scores must be no more than 5 years old. For applicants who have retaken the exam, the best set of scores is used.

SUGGESTIONS

Admission for out-of-state applicants is highly competitive, as Texas law requires that no more than 10 percent of each class be nonresidents. In addition to academic credentials (GPA, MCAT score, relative rigor of the undergraduate curriculum, letters of recommendation), the Admissions Committee considers extracurricular activities, socioeconomic background, any time spent in outside employment, personal integrity and compassion for others, race/ethnicity, the ability to communicate in English, motivation for a career in medicine, and other personal qualities and individual factors such as leadership, insightful self-appraisal, determination, social/family support, and maturity/coping capabilities. Applicants are also evaluated for the demonstration of significant interest and experiences that parallel the mission of UT Southwestern.

PROCESS

UT Southwestern does not participate in the AMCAS system. A common application is available for the University of Texas System medical schools (Southwestern at Dallas, Galveston, Houston, and San Antonio), Texas A&M University College of Medicine, and Texas Tech University School of Medicine. An online application is available at http://dpweb1.dp.utexas.edu/mdac/homepage.htm. Applications must be submitted between May 1 and October 15. About one-fourth of the applicants are invited to interview, with interviews taking place between August and December. Interviews consist of two sessions with individual faculty members. About 40 percent of interviewed candidates are accepted, with notification beginning on November 15.

Admissions Requirements (Required)

MCAT scores, science GPA, non-science GPA, letters of recommendation, interview, essays/personal statement, extracurricular activities, exposure to medical profession.

Admissions Requirements (Optional)

State residency.

Overlap Schools

Baylor College of Medicine; Duke University; Texas A&M University—College Station; Texas Tech University; The University of Texas HSC at Houston; University of Texas Health Science Center at San Antonio; Vanderbilt University.

COSTS AND AID

Tuition & Fees

In-state Tuition	$9,325
Out-of-state Tuition	$22,425
Cost of books	$1,940
Fees	$1,307

Financial Aid

% students receiving aid	82
Average grant	$4,500
Average loan	$18,700
Average debt	$74,000

UNIVERSITY OF TORONTO
FACULTY OF MEDICINE

315 BLOOR STREET, WEST TORONTO, ON M5S1A3 • ADMISSION: 416-978-2190
FAX: 416-978-7022 • WEBSITE: WWW.UTORONTO.CA

STUDENT BODY	
Type	Public
# applied	1,731

ADMISSIONS

Application Information

Regular application	10/15
Regular notification	5/31
Are transfers accepted?	no
Admissions may be deferred?	yes
Interview required?	yes
Application fee	$75

Academics

The curriculum is based on four guidelines: Patient-centered learning, integrated and multidisciplinary content, student-motivated learning, and structured problem-based learning. In addition to the 4 year program leading to an MD, a 6 year MD/PhD program is offered jointly by the Faculty of Medicine and the School of Graduate Studies.

BASIC SCIENCES: The initial phase of the undergraduate medical program spans approximately 82 weeks. The curriculum consists of the following sequential blocks or units, which focus on principles of medicine: Art and science of clinical medicine, brain and behavior, foundations of medical practice, metabolism and nutrition, determination of community health, pathobiology of disease, and structure and function. Students meet actual as well as simulated patients and are introduced to clinical medicine by faculty members in teaching hospitals. The emphasis is on student-centered, self-directed work, and small group tutorials. Students are in scheduled sessions for approximately 35 hours per week. Most learning takes place in small group settings. Independent study is also important.

CLINICAL TRAINING

The third and fourth academic periods are comprised mainly of 6-week clinical clerkships. These are ambulatory and community experience, emergency medicine and anesthesia, family and community medicine, medicine, ob/gyn, pediatrics, psychiatry, specialty medicine, specialty surgery, surgery, and three electives. Training takes place at a network of teaching hospitals and community-based health agencies. Affiliated hospitals include Baycrest Centre for Geriatric Care, Centre for Addiction and Mental Health (formerly Addiction Research Foundation and the Clarke Institute of Psychiatry), The Hospital for Sick Children, Mount Sinai Hospital, St. Michael's Hospital, Toronto Rehabilitation Institute (formerly Hillcrest Hospital and Queen Elizabeth Hospital), Sunnybrook and Women's College Health Science Centre, The Toronto Hospital (formerly the Toronto Hospital and the Ontario Cancer Institute/Princess Margaret Hospital). Students are also able to learn in the community through participation in settings such as teaching health units and physicians' offices.

Students

About 15 percent of students are from outside of the province. Approximately 40 percent of students are women. Class size is 177.

STUDENT LIFE

One of the advantages of attending medical school at the University of Toronto is the city itself. The university campus is located within easy walking distance of the attractions and facilities of Toronto. Students enjoy clubs, concerts, museums, major league sporting events, and shopping. Just outside of the city, skiing and other outdoor sports are readily accessible. On-campus activities include pubs, concerts, special lectures, theaters, intramural sports, student government, special interest clubs, and the Medical Journal. Medical students benefit from the large campus of 55,000 students and its resources. Student support includes health services and a housing office that coordinates both on- and off-campus housing. Residence halls with meal plans are one of many housing options.

GRADUATES

A key aspect of the program is that it provides exposure to all medical career options. Graduates enter primary care fields, specialties, academic medicine, research, and leadership positions.

Admissions

REQUIREMENTS

Academic achievement is measured by grades and MCAT results. Prerequisite courses are at least two full course equivalents in life sciences and at least one full course equivalent in humanities, social sciences, or languages. These courses should provide applicants with an understanding of the basic principles and vocabulary of physics, chemistry, and biology, a working knowledge of statistics, and the ability to gather, interpret, and present information from complex texts both in writing and orally. Students must be in their third year or higher of university to be considered for admission.

SUGGESTIONS

Students from social sciences, humanities, and physical and life sciences are encouraged to apply. Demonstrated high-level proficiency in oral and written English is considered essential for success in the curriculum and in practice, and applicants are encouraged to have completed at least two full equivalents in a course that required expository writing. Generally, minimum requirements are an average grade point average of 3.6/4.0 and a minimum of 8 on each section of the MCAT. Desired personal characteristics include a perceptive nature, strong commitment, high personal standards, and a history of academic and personal achievement.

PROCESS

Applications for admission to the medical school must be submitted by October 15 to OMSAS, Ontario Universities Application Center, PO Box 1328, Guelph, Ontario N1H 7P4. The faculty will invite selected applicants for an interview. Notices of acceptance are sent to students in the spring or summer prior to the proposed date of enrollment.

Admissions Requirements (Required)

Interview.

COSTS AND AID

Tuition & Fees

In-state Tuition	$14,000
Out-of-state Tuition	$23,750
In-state Fees	$919
Out-of-state Fees	$1,498

UNIVERSITY OF UTAH
SCHOOL OF MEDICINE

OFFICE OF ADMISSIONS, 30 NORTH, 1900 EAST #1C029, SALT LAKE CITY, UT 84132-2101 • ADMISSION: 801-581-7498
FAX: 801-581-2931 • E-MAIL: DEANS.ADMISSIONS@HSC.UTAH.EDU • WEBSITE: HTTP://UUHSC.UTAH.EDU/SOM

STUDENT BODY	
Type	Public
Enrollment	409
% male/female	63/37
% underrepresented minorities	12
# applied (total/out)	1,065/637
# accepted (total/out)	102/27
# enrolled (out-of-state)	27
Average age	26

ADMISSIONS

Average GPA and MCAT Scores

Overall GPA	3.6
MCAT Bio	10.0
MCAT Phys	9.0
MCAT Verbal	9.0

Application Information

Regular application	11/1
Are transfers accepted?	yes
Admissions may be deferred?	yes
Interview required?	yes
Application fee	$100

Academics

The University of Utah School of Medicine implemented a new curriculum during the 1997–1998 academic year that emphasizes active learning approaches, critical thinking skills, and information management techniques. The new curriculum builds upon the strengths of the traditional one and, in addition, explores areas of study opened up by the explosion of biomedical knowledge and the transformation of America's health care delivery system. The goal of the curriculum is to produce highly skilled physicians who are technically proficient, caring and compassionate, and flexible enough to adapt to the changing demands they will face in the 21st century medical environment. In the first two years of medical school, students will receive a solid foundation in the sciences basic to medicine, including biochemistry, embryology, genetics, gross anatomy, histology, immunology, microbiology, organ system pathophysiology, pharmacology, pathology, physiology, and psychiatry. Courses cover such topics as biostatistics, community and public health, epidemiology, health care financing and delivery, research methodology, and medical literature analysis. The critical skills of communicating with, examining, and diagnosing patients are also covered in depth. The third year of the curriculum centers on clinical clerkships in family practice, internal medicine, neurology, obstetrics and gynecology, pediatrics, psychiatry, and surgery. During the fourth year a preceptorship in primary care medicine gives students a broader perspective on the health care issues facing medically underserved rural and urban areas; students generally live in the underserved area during the 6-week preceptorship. Ample elective time is available for students to pursue areas of particular interest. Finally, a required sub internship will serve as a transition to residency. Students, with the help of faculty advisors, will apply to various postgraduate residency-training programs through the National Resident Matching Program.

Students

Almost all students are from Utah or neighboring states. About 9 percent of entering students are typically from underrepresented ethnic groups. The age range of entering students is typically from 19–40. A significant number of medical students at Utah are married by the fourth year. Class size is 100.

STUDENT LIFE

Medical students take advantage of the campus and the surrounding areas. The University of Utah is situated on a 1,500-acre campus that offers indoor and outdoor recreational activities. Salt Lake City is at the base of spectacular mountains and is only a short drive from excellent skiing or hiking, depending on the season. Several national parks are accessible to the city. The city is relatively safe and student-friendly, with cultural activities as well as the basic amenities, such as malls, movie theaters, and restaurants. On-campus housing is available for married couples and single parents in the University Village, for all students in the Medical Plaza Towers (apartments and townhouses), and for single students in University Residence Halls. There are organizations that unite medical students around common interests or that promote interaction with students from medical schools in neighboring states.

GRADUATES

Graduates are usually successful at obtaining their first choice of residencies. Typically, more than half of graduates enter primary care fields.

Admissions

REQUIREMENTS

The MCAT is required and must be taken within three years of application. The Admissions Committee is eager to admit students with a broad perspective of life. The school believes that a true physician is not only skilled in medicine and the allied sciences but also is a person of culture and broad intelligence. In addition to a bachelor's degree, the applicant must have subject matter competence in the following course work: two years of chemistry, the general chemistry series including quantitative and qualitative analysis (AP credit accepted if at a level 4 or 5), and the organic series (AP credit not accepted), both with a laboratory; 1 year of physics with a laboratory (AP credit not accepted); 1 year of English writing/speech courses that must fulfill the institution writing/composition classification (AP credit not accepted); 2 college courses of biology, 1 in cellular biology or biochemistry (no substitutions, AP credit not accepted); a college course in social science (AP credit not accepted); and a college course in humanities (AP credit not accepted). With the exception of Advanced Placement credit for general chemistry at a level of 4 or 5, CLEP, advanced placement, and home-study credit will not be accepted for completion of required course work. All premedical courses must be completed at an accredited college or university in the United States or Canada. Completion of four years of college work and a bachelor's degree are required before entering the School of Medicine. Only those students who have completed most of their undergraduate training in a U.S. or Canadian school will be considered.

SUGGESTIONS

Taking on independent research projects while in college is encouraged. Demonstration of writing skills and computer literacy is also important. Applicants should have participated in both health-related and volunteer work. For applicants who graduated college several years ago, some recent course work is required.

PROCESS

Many Utah residents are asked to submit secondary applications, and 50 percent of those who submit them are invited to interview. Approximately one-third of Utah interviewees are accepted. About one-third of out-of-state applicants are sent secondary applications, and of those who submit them, 30 percent are invited to interview. Fifty percent of out-of-state interviewees are accepted. Interviews take place from September through February and consist of two 1-hour sessions with members of the faculty or administration, or with students. Candidates are notified on a rolling basis after they interview. A ranked wait list is created.

Admissions Requirements (Required)

MCAT scores, science GPA, non-science GPA, letters of recommendation, state residency, extracurricular activities, exposure to medical profession.

COSTS AND AID

Tuition & Fees

In-state Tuition	$17,647
Out-of-state Tuition	$32,806
Fees	$673

University of Vermont
College of Medicine

89 Beaumont Avenue, E215 Given Building, Burlington, VT 05405 • **Admission:** 802-656-2154
Fax: 802-656-9663 • **E-mail:** MedAdmissions@uvm.edu • **Website:** www.med.uvm.edu

STUDENT BODY	
Type	Public
Enrollment	400
% male/female	41/59
% underrepresented minorities	20
# applied (total/out)	5,119/5,005
# accepted (total/out)	202/142
# enrolled (total/out)	101/58
Average age	24

FACULTY	
Total faculty (number)	1,806
% female	30
% minority	10
% part-time	10

ADMISSIONS

Average GPA and MCAT Scores

Overall GPA	3.5
MCAT Bio	9.6
MCAT Phys	9.0
MCAT Verbal	9.6
MCAT Essay	Q

Application Information

Regular application	11/1
Regular notification	10/15
Early application	8/1
Early notification	10/1
Are transfers accepted?	yes
Admissions may be deferred?	yes
Interview required?	yes
Application fee	$85

Academics

The new integrated curriculum, fully launched in Fall 2003, progresses through 3 levels of increasing competency. Block courses in level I/foundations provide students with a fundamental understanding of the basic biology of health and illness within systems ranging from genes to organs to individuals to populations. A comprehensive assessment of integrated knowledge and skills takes place at the end of the first year and again at the completion of the level midway through the second year of school. Level II/clinical clerkships focuses on the student's development of clinical skills, decision-making skills, and application of foundational sciences. It consists of seven clerkships with a longitudinal bridge curriculum of advanced sciences and clinical skills over a period of 13 months. Clinical training takes place primarily at adjacent teaching hospital Fletcher Allen Health Care, an integrated health care delivery system located in Burlington, which serves the State of Vermont and beyond, attracting patients from New York and around New England. Students also have the opportunity to do some clerkship rotations at Maine Medical Center, located in Portland. The patient population is largely rural, and rural medicine is considered a strength of UVM. Students advance to level III/advanced integration after successful achievement on a clinical competency exam. During the final 15 months of advanced integration, the student gains an understanding of the impact of economic, social, and political systems on the health care environment. This level includes acting internships, an emergency medicine rotation, a teaching practicum, and scholarly project. During this section, there is flexibility in how students may earn elective credit. Many rotate to hospitals outside of the state, some work on Indian reservations, and others head overseas. Throughout the college's curriculum, complementary curricular themes aim to teach the student to take an integrated approach to patient care and responsibility for their own professional development. Student leadership groups provide the student with an opportunity to collaborate with classmates, a faculty facilitator, and various family faculty members from the community. These groups, which begin the first week and continue through the curriculum, support such efforts as public health research projects, individual scholarly projects, and teaching requirements and statewide health education and health delivery programs. The MD/PhD program is designed to train future physician-scientists through a curriculum that integrates clinical care with basic research. The MD-PhD degree is awarded by the joint efforts of The College of Medicine and the Graduate College. Award of the MD degree requires completion of the entire medical curriculum. Award of the PhD degree requires fulfillment of the requirements of any of the basic science graduate programs, which include anatomy and neurobiology, biochemistry, microbiology and molecular genetics, molecular physiology and biophysics, and pharmacology, or those of the multidisciplinary program in cell and molecular biology. It is anticipated that a period of seven years will be necessary to complete the combined program. Four students are chosen yearly for this program. Students enrolled in the program will receive financial support that includes full medical and graduate school tuition remission, as well as a stipend consistent with National Institutes of Health guidelines. A new ambulatory center opened adjacent to the campus in Fall 2005. A student assessment center, built in 2002, is home to a well-established standardized patient program. The Academic Medical Center, along with the rest of the University of Vermont campus, is located in picturesque Burlington. The city is safe, affordable, and comfortable.

Students

Approximately 40 percent of students are residents of Vermont, 10 percent are from Maine, and the remainder come from out of area. In the class entering in 2005, the average age was 24. Students came from 64 different universities, 6 countries, and a variety of academic backgrounds. Class size is 105.

STUDENT LIFE

Students have access to all of the university's athletic facilities. In addition, Burlington and the surrounding area offer excellent skiing, hiking, and mountain biking. The campus is integrated into the city, which is safe, friendly, and student-oriented. Housing options on- and off-campus are good. On-campus choices include UVM's married-student housing, about 4 miles from campus, and nearby apartments and residence halls. Group houses or shared apartments in walking or biking distance from school are popular off-campus choices. Student organizations are numerous and include Cyberdocs, a medical computer interest group, and The Diversity in Medicine Committee, a group that works to promote awareness of many types of diversity (ethnic, religious, age, gender, sexual orientation) in student life, medical education, and patient care.

GRADUATES

Graduates are successful in obtaining residencies at strong programs nationwide. In 2005, about half of the graduates entered primary care residencies. Favored specialties include internal medicine (23 percent), emergency medicine (12 percent), pediatrics (16 percent), and anesthesiology (10 percent).

Admissions

REQUIREMENTS

One year each of biology, chemistry, organic chemistry and physics, all with associated labs, are required. The MCAT is required, and all sets of scores are considered.

SUGGESTIONS

We recommend one course in biochemistry or molecular genetics be taken. We recommend that the MCAT be taken no later than April of the application year to facilitate timely review of the entire application file. We encourage students who have a broad and balanced educational background during their undergraduate years. In addition to prerequisite courses in the sciences, recommended areas of study include literature, mathematics, behavioral sciences, history, philosophy, and the arts. College work must demonstrate intellectual drive, independent thinking, curiosity, and self-discipline. A career in medicine calls for excellent oral and written communication skills. Applicants should seek out opportunities to develop such skills during their college years. Successful applicants often have a history of service to community. We encourage students who have a broad and balanced educational background during their undergraduate years. In addition to prerequisite courses in the sciences, recommended areas of study include behavioral sciences, history, literature, mathematics, philosophy and the arts. College work must demonstrate intellectual drive, independent thinking, curiosity, and self-discipline.

PROCESS

All AMCAS applicants receive a supplemental application. All well-qualified VT residents who apply are interviewed. Approximately 10 percent of out-of-state applicants are interviewed. Interviews take place from September through March and consist of a meeting with a faculty member of the admission committee. Decisions are made on a rolling basis, and applicants are notified of their status—accept, reject, or wait list—shortly after the interview. Wait-listed candidates should indicate if UVM is their first choice.

Admissions Requirements (Required)

MCAT scores, science GPA, non-science GPA, letters of recommendation, interview, essays/personal statement, extracurricular activities, exposure to medical profession.

Admissions Requirements (Optional)

State residency.

Overlap Schools

Albany Law School, Dartmouth College, Thomas Jefferson University, Tufts University, University of Rochester.

COSTS AND AID

Tuition & Fees

In-state Tuition	$23,080
Out-of-state Tuition	$40,390
Room and board (on campus)	$9,392
Cost of books	$8,000
Fees	$1,287

Financial Aid

% students receiving aid	91
Average grant	$15,272
Average loan	$37,576
Average debt	$130,914

UNIVERSITY OF VIRGINIA
SCHOOL OF MEDICINE

PO Box 800725, CHARLOTTESVILLE, VA 22908 • ADMISSION: 804-924-5571
FAX: 804-982-2586 • E-MAIL: BAB7G@VIRGINIA.EDU • WEBSITE: WWW.MED.VIRGINIA.EDU/HOME.HTML

STUDENT BODY

Type	Public
Enrollment	556
% male/female	50/50
% underrepresented minorities	8
# applied (total/out)	3,604/2,892
# accepted (total/out)	141/48
# enrolled (total/out)	141/48
Average age	24

FACULTY

Total faculty (number)	800
Student-faculty ratio	1:1

ADMISSIONS

Average GPA and MCAT Scores

Overall GPA	3.74
MCAT Bio	10.96
MCAT Phys	10.88
MCAT Verbal	10.39
MCAT Essay	P

Application Information

Regular application	11/1
Regular notification	10/15
Are transfers accepted?	yes
Admissions may be deferred?	yes
Interview required?	yes
Application fee	$75

Academics

Most medical students follow a 4 year, highly integrated curriculum leading to the MD. Each year 6 students enter a combined MD/PhD curriculum. Training for the PhD degree is usually in one of the biomedical science programs, which include anatomy, biochemistry, biophysics, microbiology, neuroscience, pharmacology, and physiology. A Generalist Scholars Program supplements the medical education of students with special opportunities in the area of primary care. Students who participate in this program work closely with a faculty mentor and complete a thesis as part of their graduation requirements. Medical students are evaluated in a variety of ways including both pass/fail and letter grades.

BASIC SCIENCES: First-year courses are biochemistry; cell and tissue structure; genetics; gross anatomy; human behavior; medical ethics; neuroscience; physiology; physical diagnosis; and the practice of medicine, in which topics such as human behavior and medical ethics are discussed. Basic clinical skills such as the patient interview are also introduced. Second-year courses are clinical epidemiology, community preceptorship, introduction to clinical medicine (ICM), microbiology, pathology, pharmacology, psychiatric medicine, and psychopathology. Basic-science concepts are coordinated with the ICM course, which involves discussion of clinical cases in small-group tutorials. In the spring of the second year, each student completes a 1 month community medicine preceptorship that provides hands-on primary care experience and serves as a transition to third-year clinical rotations. Instruction takes place at the Harvey E. Jordan Hall, a 7-story structure that houses lecture halls and laboratories. First- and second-year students also use the School of Medicine Learning Center, which contains conference rooms, tutorial rooms, and a student lounge. The Claude Moore Health Sciences Library is a modern, fully computerized facility with almost 79,000 books, 3,000 periodicals, and 4,000 audiovisual titles.

CLINICAL TRAINING

Third-year required rotations are medicine (12 weeks), surgery (12 weeks), pediatrics (8 weeks), obstetrics (6 weeks), psychiatry (6 weeks), family medicine (4 weeks), and neurology (4 weeks). Clinical training takes place primarily at the University of Virginia Medical Center University Hospital (552 beds), Kluge Children's Rehabilitation Center, and at 40 outpatient clinics associated with the Medical Center. Students also train at affiliated hospitals, which include The Community Hospital of Roanoke Valley (400 beds), Roanoke Memorial Hospital (677 beds), and the Veterans Affairs Medical Center (750 beds). Electives may be taken at other academic or clinical institutions in other parts of the country or abroad.

Students

About 90 of the 139 students in each class are Virginia residents. Underrepresented minorities account for approximately 10 percent of the student body. There is typically a wide age range among incoming students, with at least a few students in their thirties.

STUDENT LIFE

Students are highly active in on-campus activities and events. Many are involved in community activities such as Service, Humanity, Action, Responsibility, Education (SHARE), which initiates health education projects and other service-oriented activities. Support groups for minority students are available, as are clubs focused on professional interests and recreational pursuits, such as singing. UVA also has local chapters of national medical student organizations. Medical students enjoy Charlottesville, a thriving tourist and cultural center located at the foot of the Blue Ridge Mountains and close to the Shenandoah Valley. The city of Richmond, Virginia, is a 1 hour drive, and Washington, DC, is just 2 hours away.

GRADUATES

Graduates are successful in securing top residency positions in all regions of the country. A significant number stay on to do postgraduate training at UVA-affiliated hospitals.

Admissions

REQUIREMENTS

Prerequisites are 1 year each of biology, general chemistry, organic chemistry, and physics, all with associated labs. The MCAT is required, and scores must be no more than 3 years old at the time of matriculation. For applicants who have taken the exam more than once, the best scores are considered. Thus, there is no advantage to withholding scores.

SUGGESTIONS

State residency is a factor in admissions decisions as about 65 percent of positions in a class are reserved for Virginia resident applicants. The Admissions Committee looks for students who will make significant contributions to society as members of the medical profession. Factors such as depth of motivation and commitment to medicine are evaluated. Some medically related experience that involves patient contact is considered important.

PROCESS

AMCAS applicants are sent secondary applications. About 25–30 percent of Virginia resident applicants are interviewed, while only about 10 percent of nonresidents make it to the interview stage. On interview day, applicants have two interviews, each with a member of the Admissions Committee. Candidates also attend a group orientation session, have the opportunity to tour the campus, and eat lunch with current medical students. Notification begins after October 15 and continues on a rolling basis until the class is filled. Wait-listed candidates may send additional information to update their files.

Admissions Requirements (Required)

MCAT scores, science GPA, non-science GPA, letters of recommendation, interview, essays/personal statement, extracurricular activities, exposure to medical profession.

Admissions Requirements (Optional)

State residency.

Overlap Schools

Duke University, Johns Hopkins University, Vanderbilt University.

COSTS AND AID

Tuition & Fees

In-state Tuition	$28,700
Out-of-state Tuition	$38,700
Room and board (off campus)	$12,000
Cost of books	$1,000

Financial Aid

% students receiving aid	85
Average grant	$12,000
Average loan	$18,000
Average debt	$82,000

UNIVERSITY OF WASHINGTON
SCHOOL OF MEDICINE

ADMISSIONS OFFICE, A-300 HEALTH SCIENCES, PO BOX 356340, SEATTLE, WA 98195 • ADMISSION: 206-543-7212
FAX: 206-616-3341 • E-MAIL: ASKUWSOM@U.WASHINGTON.EDU • WEBSITE: WWW.WASHINGTON.EDU/MEDICINE/SOM/

STUDENT BODY

Type	Public
Enrollment	734
% male/female	52/48
% underrepresented minorities	10
# applied (total/out)	3,124/2,203
# accepted (total/out)	229/39
# enrolled (total/out)	176/12

ADMISSIONS

Average GPA and MCAT Scores

Overall GPA	3.7
MCAT Bio	11.2
MCAT Phys	10.7
MCAT Verbal	10.3
MCAT Essay	Q

Application Information

Regular application	11/1
Regular notification	11/1
Are transfers accepted?	yes
Admissions may be deferred?	yes
Interview required?	yes
Application fee	$35

Academics

Students who enter UW as residents of Wyoming, Alaska, Montana, and Idaho spend their first year at the university site in their home state. Twenty Washington students begin medical studies at Washington State University in Pullman and then transfer to the UW campus after completion of their first year. Other students complete a 4 year program based in Seattle. From 8–10 students each year enter the MSTP MD/PhD program. The doctorate degree may be earned in biochemistry, bioengineering, biomathematics/biostatistics, biological structure, epidemiology, environmental health, genetics, immunology, microbiology, molecular biotechnology, pathology, pharmacology, physiology, biophysics, and zoology. Medical students are evaluated with honors, satisfactory, and not satisfactory. Passing Step 1 of the USMLE is a requirement for promotion to year 3 and passing Step 2 is a requirement for graduation.

BASIC SCIENCES: First-year courses at the UW campus are biochemistry; cell and tissue response to injury; epidemiology; gross anatomy and embryology; introduction to immunology; mechanisms in cell physiology; microscopic anatomy; natural history of infectious diseases and chemotherapy; nervous system; and systems of human behavior, head, neck, ear, nose and throat. Most second-year topics are organized around body/organ systems, which are cardiovascular, complementary medicine, endocrine, gastrointestinal, genetics, hematology, musculoskeletal, nutrition, pharmacology, reproduction, respiratory, skin, systemic pathology, and urinary. Other courses are introduction to clinical medicine and medicine, health, and society. The Rural/Underserved Opportunities Program enables first-year medical students to work with practicing physicians in small towns or inner-city neighborhoods and to learn first-hand about working with underserved communities.

CLINICAL TRAINING

The clinical curriculum covers the third and fourth years and includes clerkships in medicine (12 weeks), ob/gyn (6 weeks), pediatrics (6 weeks), psychiatry (6 weeks), surgery (6 weeks), family medicine (6 weeks), emergency medicine (4 weeks), and rehabilitation (2 weeks). An additional 24 weeks of electives are required. Selected third-year students participate in an alternate, rural training program, which involves 6 months in a rural, primary care practice. In its teaching, patient care, and research programs, the School of Medicine is affiliated with Children's Hospital, Harborview Hospital (411 beds), UW Medical Center (450 beds), Seattle Veterans Affairs Hospital, Fred Hutchinson Cancer Research Center, Boise Veterans Affairs Hospital, Providence Hospital, Swedish Hospital, Madigan Hospital, and the Group Health Cooperative. Additional affiliations across the Pacific Northwest enable medical students to train in more than 75 communities in Washington, Alaska, Montana, and Idaho. The International Medical Education Office organizes a range of activities including exchange programs that allow UW medical students to participate in clinical electives overseas.

Students

About 93 percent of the 176 students in each class are residents of Washington, Alaska, Montana, Wyoming, or Idaho. Out-of-region students, which includes a total of about 10 percent of the student body, are MD/PhD students. There is a wide age range among medical students, with significant numbers of entrants in their late twenties and thirties.

STUDENT LIFE

UW offers countless extracurricular opportunities and attractions, including cultural programs, student groups, intercollegiate sporting events, and social functions. Medical students take advantage of these opportunities and the tremendous resources afforded by UW and its student community. Seattle is an ideal city for students, offering outstanding daytime and outdoor activities and an excellent nightlife. Around the city are beautiful areas suitable for hiking, camping, mountain climbing, running, biking, swimming, and skiing. Most students live off campus.

GRADUATES

Of the roughly 5,000 UW School of Medicine alumni, about 50 percent are practicing or training in fields designated as physician-shortage specialties, which include family physicians, general internists, general pediatricians, psychiatrists, general surgeons, and general practitioners.

Admissions

REQUIREMENTS

Prerequisites are chemistry (12 semester hours, which can be satisfied by any combination of inorganic, organic, biochemistry, or molecular biology courses), biology (8 semester hours), and physics (4 semester hours). In addition, the understanding of basic biochemistry molecular biology concepts is required. An additional 8 semester hours of unspecified science course work is required. This requirement can be met by taking other courses in any of the above three categories. The MCAT is required, and scores must be from within three years of application.

SUGGESTIONS

Preference is given to legal residents of Washington, Wyoming, Alaska, Montana, and Idaho. Applicants from disadvantaged backgrounds or who are willing to serve the underserved are also considered. Candidates should be proficient in the use of the English language and in basic mathematics and are expected to have an understanding of personal computing and information technologies. Some biochemistry or molecular biology is also recommended.

PROCESS

All Washington residents and a limited number of highly qualified nonresidents are sent secondary applications and invited to interview. Interviews take place between October and April and consist of one session with a panel of interviewers. Also on interview day, candidates have the opportunity to meet with current students and tour the campus. About 30 percent of interviewed candidates are accepted. Others are rejected or put in a hold category.

Admissions Requirements (Required)

MCAT scores, letters of recommendation, interview, state residency, essays/personal statement.

Admissions Requirements (Optional)

Science GPA, nonscience GPA, extracurricular activities, exposure to medical profession.

COSTS AND AID

Tuition & Fees

In-state Tuition	$12,450
Out-of-state Tuition	$29,391

Financial Aid

% students receiving aid	83

University of Western Ontario

Admissions and Student Affairs

Health Sciences Building, London, Ontario N6A 5C1 • Admission: 519-661-3744
Fax: 519-661-3797 • E-mail: ADMISSIONS@SCHULICH.UWO.CA • Website: WWW.SCHULICH.UWO.CA

STUDENT BODY

Type	Public
Enrollment	534
% male/female	55/45
# applied	1,872
# accepted	133
# enrolled	133
Average age	23

ADMISSIONS

Average GPA and MCAT Scores

Overall GPA	3.7
MCAT Bio	10.0
MCAT Phys	9.0
MCAT Verbal	10.0
MCAT Essay	P

Application Information

Regular application	10/15
Regular notification	5/15
Are transfers accepted?	no
Admissions may be deferred?	no
Interview required?	yes
Application fee	$175

Academics

The Faculty of Medicine and Dentistry, along with the Faculty of Graduate Studies, has established a combined MD-PhD program in which the research curriculum of the graduate program is integrated into the MD program. Applicants must be accepted to the medical school as MD candidates before entering the combined program.

BASIC SCIENCES: During the third year integrated clerkship, the student will become an active member of clinical care teams in the following medical disciplines: Family medicine, medicine, obstetrics and gynaecology, pediatrics, psychiatry, and surgery. Under the supervision of faculty and more senior house staff, clerks will be given graded responsibility in the investigation, diagnosis, and management of patients in hospital and outpatient settings. The clerkship year incorporates rural experiences throughout Southwestern Ontario. Some students will be placed outside London for the entire clerkship year.

Beginning in year 4, clinical electives will be arranged by the student in any area of medicine, at UWO or other approved centers. For students wishing to arrange electives in developing countries, we have a medical electives overseas officer who advises and assists students in making their arrangements. After completion of the clinical electives, students will return to the UWO in February for the transition period, which includes advanced basic sciences (e.g., surgical anatomy, medical physiology); advanced communication skills; general review; and health care systems. This will permit students to further integrate the basic and clinical aspects of medicine in light of their clinical experience.

CLINICAL TRAINING

The first 2 years of the new curriculum will provide students with a solid grounding in the basic and clinical sciences. These 2 years are each divided into a series of 6 blocks. Within each block various subject areas are presented which integrate the basic and clinical sciences. The blocks are digestive systems and nutrition, endocrine and metabolism, eye and ear, genito-urinary system, heart and circulation, immunology and skin, introduction to medicine, life cycle, musculoskeletal, neurosciences, psychiatry and behavioral sciences, reproduction, and respiration and airways.

During each week or block, the case of a single patient will be discussed. A facilitator will help students determine the biological, behavorial, and population issues that are pertinent to the patient, and the objectives for the week's instruction will be described. Students will then receive instruction throughout the week relevant to the patient's case using a variety of teaching methods such as lectures, small-group sessions, and labs. Students will also be expected to obtain information pertinent to the case objectives. The faculty has excellent library and resource facilities to support self study. In the middle of the week, students will meet to review the instruction to date and relate it to the patient case. At the end of the week, the students will meet in a plenary session to discuss the case of the week. A particular strength of our program will be the opportunity for early patient contact. Patient-centered care recognizes the need to see the health concerns of a patient through the patient's eyes. The illness experience differs markedly from the traditional teaching in medical schools in which the emphasis has been on teaching about the disease only and not on the experiences of the patient with that disease. In the patient-centered approach, the emphasis is on defining the unique illness experience of the patient and his or her relation to family and community in economic, social, and environmental dimensions. The first 2 years of the program provide a variety of opportunities for students to better understand the relationship between health care and the community.

Students

Class size is 133.

STUDENT LIFE

The University of Western Ontario offers students a rich lifestyle. School-sponsored events and countless clubs and organizations are offered on campus. London is a small city of about 300,000 with a range of cultural and recreational activities. Both on- and off-campus housing is available.

GRADUATES

The curriculum is designed to allow graduates to enter any clinical or medical research field. A significant portion of graduates enter residency programs at hospitals affiliated with the University of Western Ontario.

Admissions

REQUIREMENTS

Enrollment is limited to Canadian citizens and permanent residents of Canada. Those who are in the third year or have successfully completed 3 full years of study in any degree program at a recognized university are eligible to apply. A minimum of 5 full or equivalent courses must be included in the final undergraduate year (September to April only). Science prerequisites are 1 full course in biology, 1 full course in organic chemistry, and 1 additional full science course. Nonscience prerequisites are 2 full nonscience courses from different disciplines and 1 senior-level course in one of these 2 subjects. Interested applicants should contact the faculty for more detailed course requirements. The MCAT is required. The latest date that applicants should take the exam is August in the year of application. Only applicants who have achieved a certain GPA and MCAT scores will be considered for admission. Typically, the minimum GPA is 3.50 and minimum MCAT scores are a 9 on biological sciences, an 8 on physical sciences, a 9 on verbal reasoning, and a Q on the writing sample. English proficiency is a requirement.

SUGGESTIONS

For entrance in the Fall of 2005, there were 1,872 applicants for 133 positions. Thus, admission is competitive. Apart from science prerequisites, there is no prescribed premed program. Students at Western Ontario come from a variety of undergraduate programs and a wide range of disciplines. For those who have taken the MCAT more than once, only the most recent scores are used.

PROCESS

The deadline for application is October 15 for matriculation the following September. Applicants now apply online at: www.ouac.on.ca/omsas. Those applicants who satisfy the course load, GPA, and MCAT requirements will generally be invited for an interview. Letters indicating admissions decisions are sent to applicants beginning in the end of May and continuing until the class is full.

Admissions Requirements (Required)

MCAT scores, science GPA, non-science GPA, letters of recommendation, interview, state residency.

Admissions Requirements (Optional)

Essays/personal statement, extracurricular activities, exposure to medical profession.

COSTS AND AID

Tuition & Fees

Tuition	$14,566
Room and board (off campus)	$13,000
Cost of books	$2,200
Fees	$863

University of Wisconsin—Madison

School of Medicine and Public Health

2130 Health Sciences Learning Center, 750 Highland Avenue, Madison, WI 53705 • Admission: 608-263-4925
Fax: 608-262-4226 • E-mail: lwall@wisc.edu • Website: www.med.wisc.edu

STUDENT BODY

Type	Public
Enrollment	607
% male/female	48/52
% underrepresented minorities	8
# applied (total/out)	935/389
# accepted (total/out)	277/80
# enrolled (total/out)	163/24
Average age	24

ADMISSIONS

Average GPA and MCAT Scores

Overall GPA	3.7
MCAT Bio	10.7
MCAT Phys	10.4
MCAT Verbal	10.1
MCAT Essay	P

Application Information

Regular application	11/1
Regular notification	rolling
Early application	8/1 and 9/1
Early notification	10/1
Are transfers accepted?	yes
Admissions may be deferred?	yes
Interview required?	yes
Application fee	$45

Academics

The UW School of Medicine and Public Health offers an MD degree and a dual degree (MD and PhD) option. In addition, flexibility exists to allow for combining training for the MD degree with earning a MPH. Medical students are evaluated with letter grades. Students must pass Step 1 of the USMLE for promotion to year 3, and Step 2 and 3 must be taken to graduate.

BASIC SCIENCES: The revised curriculum features fewer lectures and more small-group discussions, practical laboratories, multimedia computer programs and videos, and significant opportunities to learn through real-life clinical examples. An important component of the new curriculum is the Generalist Partners Program (GPP), which matches first-year medical students with primary care physicians who practice in the community and who serve as teachers and mentors to students. Through GPP, students learn first-hand about generalist medicine, and enjoy early patient care opportunities. Also during the first and second years, students take an interdisciplinary course that addresses practicing medicine in a variety of modern-day environments. Other first-year courses are biomolecular chemistry, genetics, integrated medical anatomy, neuroscience, pathology, physiology, and psychiatry. The second-year pathophysiology courses are organized around body/organ systems, including cardiovascular, endocrine, gastrointestinal, hematology, hepatic, neoplastic disease, renal, and respiratory. Other courses are infection and immunity and pharmacology. The Ebling Medical Library is used by students for research and for studying. It houses more than 330,000 volumes and 3,000 publications.

CLINICAL TRAINING

The third- and fourth-year clerkships expose students to a wide variety of clinical settings (outpatient, inpatient, community-based, rural, and inner city). Training takes place at the university and other hospitals in Madison as well as in affiliated sites in Milwaukee, La Crosse, and Marshfield. Third-year required clerkships are medicine (8 weeks), primary care (8 weeks), surgery (8 weeks), pediatrics (6 weeks), ob/gyn (6 weeks), neuroscience (6 weeks), psychiatry (4 weeks), anesthesia (2 weeks), and radiology (2 weeks). During the fourth year, students complete a preceptorship (6 weeks), an acting internship in medicine (4 weeks), an advanced surgery clerkship (4 weeks), and 18 weeks of electives. A portion of electives may be taken at other academic and clinical institutions, both in the United States and overseas. The UW International Health Exchange is an affiliated nonprofit foundation that increases awareness of international health issues through a range of activities including promoting overseas clinical experiences for students.

Students

Each class is comprised of 150 students. Approximately 80 percent of students are Wisconsin residents, and during the past 4 years, about 50 percent of students attended UW for their undergraduate education. About 12 percent of students are underrepresented minorities. About 10 or more students in each class are in their late twenties or thirties.

STUDENT LIFE

The Medical School benefits from the resources of one of the nation's top public universities. Medical students have access to the facilities of the large campus and enjoy the lively environment of a popular college city. Students are active in community service projects such as volunteering at homeless shelters and clinics and organizing AIDS or other education projects. On-campus housing, including married-student facilities, is available. However, most students prefer to live in shared apartments off campus. Madison is a medium-sized city, organized around three lakes, which provide many opportunities for outdoor recreation.

GRADUATES

Graduates are successful in securing residency positions at prestigious institutions nationwide.

Admissions

REQUIREMENTS

Minimum science requirements are mathematics (2 semesters), general biology with lab (1 semester), advanced biology/zoology with lab (1 semester), biochemistry (1 semester), general chemistry with lab (1 year), organic chemistry with lab (1 year), and general physics with lab (1 year). The MCAT is required, and for the 2007 entering class, scores must be from 2003 or later. Where more than one MCAT has been taken, the higher values of the two most recent scores are used.

SUGGESTIONS

UW gives preference to residents of Wisconsin. Each incoming class consists of 15-20 percent nonresidents. A sound liberal arts education, including both humanities and social sciences, is considered important. While specific courses are not required, the applicant's preparation should include courses in those areas that prepare for the social, psychological, and economic aspects of medical practice. The Admissions Committee members rely heavily on the applicants' essays, letters of recommendation, and the personal interviews to assess motivation and personal character.

PROCESS

Upon receipt of the AMCAS application, the UW Secondary Application is sent to selected Wisconsin residents who meet the minimal academic thresholds (GPA, 2.80 and MCATS, 7.78) and to highly-qualified nonresidents. Selected applicants are invited to interview. Interviews take place between August and March and consist of one session with a faculty member and one session with a small group of medical students and applicants. Interview-day activities include group informational sessions, a tour, and lunch with medical students.

Admissions Requirements (Required)

MCAT scores, science GPA, non-science GPA, letters of recommendation, interview, essays/personal statement, extracurricular activities, exposure to medical profession, volunteer experience.

Admissions Requirements (Optional)

State residency.

Overlap Schools

Medical College of Wisconsin; Stanford University; University of California—San Francisco; University of Michigan—Ann Arbor; University of Pittsburgh; University of Washington; Washington University.

COSTS AND AID

Tuition & Fees

In-state Tuition	$21,152
Out-of-state Tuition	$32,276
Room and board (on campus)	$11,064
Room and board (off campus)	$9,624
Cost of books	$2,000
Fees	$666

Financial Aid

% students receiving aid	70
Average grant	$6,533
Average loan	$33,943
Average debt	$130,000

Vanderbilt University
School of Medicine

215 Light Hall, Nashville, TN 37232-0685 • Admission: 615-322-2145 • Fax: 615-343-8397
E-mail: hal.helderman@vanderbilt.edu • Website: www.mc.vanderbilt.edu/medschool/admissions/index.php

STUDENT BODY

Type	Private
Enrollment	432
% male/female	53/47
% underrepresented minorities	9
# applied (total/out)	4,369/4,052
# accepted (total/out)	291/270
# enrolled (total/out)	105/88
Average age	23

FACULTY

Total faculty (number)	1,626
% female	31
% minority	19
% part-time	4

ADMISSIONS

Average GPA and MCAT Scores

Overall GPA	3.73
MCAT Bio	11.65
MCAT Phys	11.54
MCAT Verbal	10.62
MCAT Essay	Q

Application Information

Regular application	11/15
Regular notification	rolling
Early application	6/1–8/1
Early notification	10/1
Are transfers accepted?	yes
Admissions may be deferred?	yes
Interview required?	yes
Application fee	$50

Academics

Most students complete a 4 year curriculum leading to an MD degree. Some students opt to take an additional year for research or independent projects. A few students each year enter one of a series of combined degrees including MD/PhD, MD/JD, and MD/MBA. Grading is entirely pass/fail in the VMS I year. For students in the VMS II-IV years, an honors grade is also possible for those with exemplary performance in a particular course/clerkship. Students may also receive a high pass grade in the VMS III-IV year.

BASIC SCIENCES: During the first year, students focus on the basic sciences, which are taught primarily through small-group sessions, tutorials, individualized study, labs, and some lectures. Courses are behavioral science, biochemistry, cell and tissue biology, gross anatomy, introduction to biomedical research, microbiology, and physiology. Several afternoons each week are reserved for electives, many of which are problem-based. During the second year, introductory clinical training is integrated into basic science instruction, and small-group discussions complement the lecture/lab format. Second-year courses are neurobiology, laboratory diagnosis, pathology, pharmacology, physical diagnosis, preventive medicine, psychiatry, and radiology. During the first two years, students are in class or other scheduled sessions for about 34 hours per week. Additionally, all students participate in the Emphasis Program, which allows a student an opportunity to conduct independent study/research in any 1 of 9 different subject areas. Students are paired with a faculty mentor and have protected time throughout both the first and second years of medical school in order to conduct their work. The Emphasis Program is designed to encourage student scholarship and to provide students with the freedom to explore an area of interest in great depth. Most instruction takes place in Light Hall, which is connected by tunnels to clinical and research facilities. For research and study purposes, students and faculty use the Eskind Biomedical Library, which houses more than 200,000 volumes and 2,000 periodicals, in addition to computer-based informational resources. The Vanderbilt University Computer Center provides a full range of computing services and resources to faculty, staff, and students.

CLINICAL TRAINING

Required third-year clerkships are medicine (10 weeks), surgery (10 weeks), pediatrics (8 weeks), psychiatry-neurology (8 weeks), and ob/gyn (8 weeks). During their fourth year, students must also complete advanced clerkships selected from medical, surgical, primary care, and emergency medicine fields. Sixteen weeks of electives are also required. Most clinical training takes place at the Vanderbilt University Hospital (660 beds), and other VUMC institutions, and at clinical affiliates such as Veterans Administration Medical Center (439 beds); Howard Hughes Medical Institute; Saint Thomas Hospital; Baptist Hospital; and Middle Tennessee Mental Health Institute. With permission, some elective requirements may be fulfilled at other academic or clinical institutions.

Students

The 2005 entering class came from 33 states and 6 foreign countries. Sixty undergraduate institutions were represented. The age range was 21–30, 12 percent of students were underrepresented minorities, and 45 percent were females.

STUDENT LIFE

Vanderbilt's attractive campus provides a focal point for student life and promotes cohesiveness within the student body. Students interact in common areas, such as dining halls, cafes, study areas, and the student center. Athletic facilities include fitness centers, indoor and outdoor tracks, a tennis center, playing fields, a swimming pool, basketball, racquetball and squash courts, and a rock-climbing wall. Medical students join other graduate and professional students for intramural sports, fitness classes, and recreational clubs. In addition to being a world-renowned hub for live music, Nashville offers many attractions including a historic riverfront district, many restaurants, brew pubs, coffeehouses, nightclubs, bookstores, seasonal street fairs, farmers markets, museums, and a large performing arts center. Nashville is also an academic center and is home to more than a dozen colleges and universities. Conveniently located, university-owned apartments are available to single and partnered students and to students with larger families. In addition, off-campus housing is readily available.

GRADUATES

Students perform exceptionally well on the USMLE, contributing to their success in securing residency positions at prestigious institutions nationwide.

Admissions

REQUIREMENTS

Prerequisites are 8 semester hours each (with labs) of biology, chemistry, organic chemistry, and physics. Six semester hours of English are also required. The MCAT is required, and scores should be from within the past three years. For applicants who have taken the exam on multiple occasions, the most recent set of scores is considered. Thus, there is no real advantage in withholding scores. No AP credit nor pass/fail or CLEP credit is accepted for any required course.

SUGGESTIONS

Students with strong backgrounds in both the sciences and liberal arts are sought. The Spring, rather than Fall, MCAT is advised. Extracurricular activities, particularly those that involve hospital and medical exposure, are important.

PROCESS

Secondary applications will be sent only to those granted an interview. Interviews are conducted between September and March and consist of one session with a faculty member or administrator. On interview day, applicants also take part in a group orientation session, lunch with students, and a tour of the campus. About 25 percent of interviewees are accepted with notification occurring on a rolling basis. Wait-listed candidates may send supplementary information to update their files.

Admissions Requirements (Required)

MCAT scores, science GPA, non-science GPA, letters of recommendation, interview, essays/personal statement.

Admissions Requirements (Optional)

State residency, extracurricular activities, exposure to medical profession.

Overlap Schools

Duke University, Harvard University, Johns Hopkins University, University of Pennsylvania, Washington University.

COSTS AND AID

Tuition & Fees

Tuition	$33,200
Room and board (on campus)	$8,640
Cost of books	$4,979
Fees	$2,801

Financial Aid

% students receiving aid	86
Average grant	$28,300
Average loan	$31,900
Average debt	$108,500

VIRGINIA COMMONWEALTH UNIVERSITY

SCHOOL OF MEDICINE

PO BOX 980565, RICHMOND, VA 23298 • **ADMISSION:** 804-828-9629
FAX: 804-828-1246 • **E-MAIL:** SOMUME@HSC.VCU.EDU • **WEBSITE:** WWW.MEDSCHOOL.VCU.EDU

STUDENT BODY

Type	Public
Enrollment	698
% male/female	51/49
% underrepresented minorities	7
# applied (total/out)	3,471/2,750
# accepted (total/out)	394/201
# enrolled (total/out)	184/69
Average age	23

FACULTY

Total faculty (number)	982
% female	33
% minority	4
% part-time	26
Student-faculty ratio	1:1

ADMISSIONS

Average GPA and MCAT Scores

Overall GPA	3.5
MCAT Bio	9.9
MCAT Phys	9.6
MCAT Verbal	9.3
MCAT Essay	O

Application Information

Regular application	11/15
Regular notification	10/15
Early application	6/1–8/1
Early notification	10/1
Are transfers accepted?	yes
Admissions may be deferred?	yes
Interview required?	yes
Application fee	$80

Academics

The MD degree program is 4 years in length. A combined MD/PhD program is also offered and generally takes 7 years to complete. Medical students interested in public health can earn an MPH concurrently with the MD degree. A fellowship program gives medical students the opportunity to participate in research projects, either during summers or throughout the school year. Medical students are graded with honors, high pass, pass, marginal, and fail.

BASIC SCIENCES: Although the emphasis is on the basic sciences, behavioral science, preventive medicine, epidemiology, and public health are also taught during the first two years. Laboratory and classroom time is supplemented by a longitudinal experience designed to give students early clinical exposure. First-year courses are the following: anatomical sciences; behavioral sciences; biochemistry; cell biology; ethics; human genetics; immunology; neuroscience; physiology; population medicine/biostatistics; pathogenesis; and foundations of clinical medicine, which meets two half-days per week, uses community physicians as mentors, and teaches the basics of patient interviewing and physical diagnosis. The second-year curriculum is organized largely by body/organ systems. Courses are the following: Autonomic pharmacology, behavioral science, cardiovascular, central nervous system, endocrine, gastroenterology, hematology/oncology, microbiology/infectious diseases, musculoskeletal/dermatology, preventive medicine, renal, reproduction, respiratory, and continuation of foundations of clinical medicine. Two libraries, the University Library and the Tompkins-McCaw Library, support the research needs of students and faculty. Another important educational resource is the computer-based instructional laboratory, which features computer workstations and audiovisual equipment.

CLINICAL TRAINING

Third-year required clerkships are the following: Medicine (12 weeks); surgery (8 weeks), psychiatry (6 weeks), ob/gyn (6 weeks), pediatrics (8 weeks), family practice (4 weeks) and neurology (4 weeks). An additional requirement is 1 week of a workshop that covers topics such as nutrition, ethics, legal medicine, health economics, and clinical pharmacology. Fourth-year requirements are an acting internship, a board review course, clinical update course, and 24 weeks of electives. For training purposes, medical students have access to more than 1,050 beds at MCV hospitals. A level I trauma center, a transplant center, and one of the nation's most prominent head injury centers are among MCV's clinical facilities. Students also have contact with outpatients at McGuire Veterans Administration Medical Center.

Students

Approximately 70 percent of students are Virginia residents. The average age of incoming students is usually 23, and each year about 30 students in their late twenties and thirties enter VCU. Underrepresented minorities account for about 10 percent of the student body. Class size is 184.

STUDENT LIFE

VCU has at least 20 student organizations. These include groups focused on professional pursuits, community service, and religious interests. A variety of facilities, services, and programs designed to meet the leisure and health needs of students are coordinated by the recreational sports staff. The Cary Street Recreation complex and the main VCU gym offer fitness facilities including a pool, weight rooms, areas for fitness classes and squash, tennis, and basketball courts. Students have the opportunity to interact outside of class in the new student lounge and in other common areas. Richmond offers many recreational attractions such as parks, museums, historical centers, and shopping areas. While some medical students live in campus residence halls, most live in nearby restored neighborhoods or in surrounding suburban areas.

GRADUATES

MCV students score above the national average on the USMLE, contributing to their success in obtaining postgraduate positions. About 25 percent of each graduating class enters residency programs administered by MCV Hospitals, while others are successful at securing positions in other parts of the state and country. VCU alumni sponsor a unique bed-and-breakfast program, whereby members of the alumni host medical students when they travel for residency interviews.

Admissions

REQUIREMENTS

Prerequisites are 8 semester hours each of biology, chemistry, organic chemistry, and physics all with associated labs. Two semesters of English and two semesters of college-level math are also required. The MCAT is required and must have been taken within three years of application. For applicants who have taken the exam more than once, the best set of scores is considered.

SUGGESTIONS

Students are encouraged to pursue their own intellectual interests in college. VCU recognizes that studying medicine requires commitment, strong analytical abilities, good judgment, and sound communication skills. In addition to academic abilities, the Admissions Committee looks for important attributes of character and personality.

PROCESS

About 75 percent of AMCAS applicants who are Virginia residents are sent secondary applications, and about 40 percent of nonresidents are sent secondaries. Applicants returning secondary applications are further screened, and some are invited to interview on campus. Interviews take place between August and March, and consist of one session with a faculty member, medical student, or administrator. On interview day, students also attend group informational sessions, have lunch with current medical students, and tour the campus. Notification occurs on October 15, in mid-December, and in mid-March.

Admissions Requirements (Required)

MCAT scores, science GPA, non-science GPA, letters of recommendation, interview, essays/personal statement, extracurricular activities, exposure to medical profession.

Admissions Requirements (Optional)

State residency.

Overlap Schools

Duke University, Eastern Virginia Medical School, Emory University, Georgetown University, Johns Hopkins University, The George Washington University, University of Virginia.

COSTS AND AID

Tuition & Fees

In-state Tuition	$12,025
Out-of-state Tuition	$30,350
Room and board (on campus)	$8,630
Cost of books	$1,480
Fees	$1,306

Financial Aid

Average grant	$4,069
Average loan	$27,338
Average debt	$94,681

WAKE FOREST UNIVERSITY
SCHOOL OF MEDICINE

OFFICE OF ADMISSIONS, MEDICAL CENTER BOULEVARD, WINSTON-SALEM, NC 27157-1090 • **ADMISSION:** 336-716-4264
FAX: 910-716-9593 • **E-MAIL:** MEDADMIT@WFUBMC.EDU • **WEBSITE:** WWW.WFUBMC.EDU

STUDENT BODY

Type	Private
Enrollment	431
% male/female	56/44
% underrepresented minorities	30
# applied (total/out)	5,983/5,356
# accepted (total/out)	280/202
# enrolled (total/out)	108/67
Average age	23

FACULTY

Total faculty (number)	1,443
% female	26
% minority	13
% part-time	41
Student-faculty ratio	1:1

ADMISSIONS

Average GPA and MCAT Scores

Overall GPA	3.63
MCAT Bio	10.1
MCAT Phys	10.1
MCAT Verbal	10.1
MCAT Essay	P

Application Information

Regular application	11/1
Regular notification	rolling
Early application	6/1–8/1
Early notification	10/1
Are transfers accepted?	yes
Admissions may be deferred?	yes
Interview required?	yes
Application fee	$55

Academics

The curriculum combines features of traditional and problem-based learning methodologies. For details about the curriculum, contact the Admissions Office. Joint-degree programs include the MD/MBA in conjunction with The Babcock Graduate School of Management; the MD/MS in Health Sciences Research; and the MD/PhD in conjuction with the Graduate School. The PhD degree is offered in the following fields: Anatomy, biochemistry, genetics, immunology, microbiology, molecular biology, neuroscience, pathology, pharmacology, and physiology. Students are evaluated using a 0–3 scale, and both steps of the USMLE are required for graduation.

BASIC SCIENCES: The pre-clinical curriculum emphasizes self-directed and lifelong learning skills, core biomedical science knowledge, problem solving/reasoning, interviewing and communication skills, information management, and professional attitudes and behavior. The course foundations of clinical medicine is taken throughout year 1 and 2 and provides instruction in interviewing and physical examination skills. First-year courses provide a foundation in the core biomedical sciences and second-year courses are organized around body/organ systems. The course, being a physician, is an interdisciplinary course that touches on a range of issues related to the practice of medicine. Most pre-clinical instruction takes place in the Hanes Research Building. The James A Gray Building houses the library, which contains more than 150,000 volumes and 2,300 medical and scientific journals, in addition to audiovisual and computer-based educational aids.

CLINICAL TRAINING

Third-year required rotations are: Inpatient medicine (8 weeks), surgery (8 weeks), ob/gyn (6 weeks), pediatrics (8 weeks), neurology/rehabilitation medicine (4 weeks), anesthesiology (1 week), and radiology (1 week). Required outpatient clerkships are ob/gyn and women's health (6 weeks), internal medicine (4 weeks), and family medicine (4 weeks). During the fourth year, students fullfill the remaining requirements, which are emergency medicine (4 weeks), intensive care (4 weeks), 8 weeks of required advancement patient management clerkships, and electives (24 weeks). Training takes place at North Carolina Baptist Hospital (806 beds), which includes a children's hospital and a rehabilitation unit, among other specialty facilities. Other sites used for instruction, located in both rural and urban areas, include Forsyth Memorial Hospital and the Downtown Health Plaza.

Students

Approximately 30–40 percent of each class is made up of North Carolina residents, and about 10 percent are from Wake Forest's undergraduate program. The remainder represent up to 100 different colleges. About 14 percent of students are underrepresented minorities, most of whom are African American. Class size is 108.

STUDENT LIFE

A Student Life and Fitness Center gives students the opportunity to work out, study, gather, or simply relax. The fitness center includes Nautilis equipment, free weights, showers, and a steam room. Other features are a quiet, 24-hour study area, vending machines, a TV lounge, and rooms suitable for small-group discussions. The School of Medicine is located on the Bowman Gray campus, about 4 miles from the Reynolda campus of Wake Forest, where many academic and cultural events take place. Two state parks are within a 1-hour drive of Wake Forest, and the Carolina beaches are about 4 hours away. There is no campus housing, but apartments and rooms are readily available in the surrounding area.

GRADUATES

Wake Forest's reputation, coupled with its students' above-average scores on national boards, allows graduates to enter competitive residency programs all over the country.

Admissions

REQUIREMENTS

Ninety semester hours (3 years) of undergraduate course work, including 8 semester hours each of biology, chemistry, organic chemistry, and physics. The MCAT is required and scores must be no more than three years old. For applicants who have retaken the exam, the best set of scores is considered.

SUGGESTIONS

A well-rounded academic experience, including courses in the humanities, is strongly advised. For students who have taken significant time off after college, recent course work is suggested. The April, rather than August, MCAT is recommended, as it allows applicants to retake the exam if necessary. Medically related or community-service experiences are considered valuable. Most entering students have 4 year degrees.

PROCESS

Approximately a third of AMCAS applicants are sent secondary application materials. About 10 percent of those returning secondary applications are invited to interview sometime between September and March. Interviews are one-on-one, and consist of three 15–20 minute sessions with faculty and/or Admissions Committee members. On interview day, candidates also receive a tour and a group orientation. Notification occurs on a rolling basis, the possible outcomes being accept, reject, or wait list. Wait-listed candidates are generally not encouraged to submit supplementary materials. An alternate path to admissions is through an early assurance program, which accepts competitive college juniors without the MCAT. If successful, these students complete their senior year knowing that they have been admitted to medical school for the year following college graduation.

Admissions Requirements (Required)

MCAT scores, science GPA, non-science GPA, letters of recommendation, interview, essays/personal statement, extracurricular activities, exposure to medical profession.

Admissions Requirements (Optional)

State residency.

Overlap Schools

Duke University, Emory University, University of North Carolina at Chapel Hill, Vanderbilt University, Virginia Commonwealth University.

COSTS AND AID

Tuition & Fees

Tuition	$34,006
Room and board (off campus)	$15,040
Cost of books	$1,536

Financial Aid

% students receiving aid	85
Average grant	$13,177
Average loan	$35,437
Average debt	$119,475

WASHINGTON UNIVERSITY IN ST. LOUIS
SCHOOL OF MEDICINE

OFFICE OF ADMISSIONS, BOX 8107, 660 SOUTH EUCLID STREET, ST. LOUIS, MO 63110 • ADMISSION: 314-362-6848
FAX: 314-362-4658 • E-MAIL: WUMSCOA@MSNOTES.WUSTL.EDU • WEBSITE: WWW.MEDSCHOOL.WUSTL.EDU / ADMISSIONS

STUDENT BODY

Type	Private
Enrollment	578
% male/female	55/45
% underrepresented minorities	40
# applied	3,733
# accepted	337
# enrolled	122
Average age	23

FACULTY

Total faculty (number)	2,787
% female	26
% minority	10
% part-time	41
Student-faculty ratio	2:1

ADMISSIONS

Average GPA and MCAT Scores

Overall GPA	3.8
MCAT Bio	12.5
MCAT Phys	12.6
MCAT Verbal	11.3
MCAT Essay	Q

Application Information

Regular application	12/1
Regular notification	rolling
Are transfers accepted?	yes
Admissions may be deferred?	yes
Interview required?	yes
Application fee	$50

Academics

In addition to the 4 year MD program, students may apply for a 5 year combined MA/MD program, which involves a year of funded research and the completion of a thesis. The MSTP-sponsored MD/PhD program is one of the largest in the country, with up to 23 positions available each year. During the first year, students are graded using a pass/fail system, but grades of honors/high pass/pass/fail are used from the second year onward.

BASIC SCIENCES: During the first 2 years, students are in class for about 20 hours per week. Scheduled sessions are divided among lectures, labs, and problem-based sessions conducted in small groups. Topics covered in lectures are documented by a transcript service, to which most students subscribe. Most first-year courses address normal human structure and function. They are anatomy, cell and organ systems biology, genetics, immunology, neuroscience, and the molecular foundations of medicine. The course physicians, patients, and society offers first-year students a multidisciplinary perspective on practicing medicine and continues into the second year. Patient contact begins in the first year, in introduction to clinical medicine. Second-year courses focus on the effects of disease and are organized into blocks, most of which are defined by body systems or physiological concepts. These are cardiovascular, clinical epidemiology, dermatology, ENT, endocrinology and metabolism, nervous system, gastrointestinal and liver disease/nutrition, hematology and oncology, infectious disease, nervous system, ob/gyn, ophthalmology, pathology, pediatrics, pulmonary, renal and genitourinary, and rheumatology. Clinical experience is expanded and integrated into pathology, pathophysiology, and pharmacology. Students have significant input in curriculum development and revision. The library is extensive, housing about 300,000 volumes and equipped with computer and Internet facilities. The gross anatomy lab is particularly renowned.

CLINICAL TRAINING

The third year is reserved for core, required clerkships, which are combined ob/gyn and pediatrics (12 weeks); ambulatory care, which involves emergency medicine, family practice, and psychiatric consultation (12 weeks); medicine (12 weeks); surgery (12 weeks); neurology (4 weeks); and psychiatry (4 weeks). The fourth year (44 weeks) is reserved entirely for electives, which may be in clinical and/or basic science departments. Students are permitted to fulfill up to 12 weeks of clinical clerkships at nonaffiliated institutions. While many other academic health care institutions are struggling, Washington University's Medical Center and their other Barnes-Jewish associated hospitals and clinics are thriving and expanding. Children's Hospital ranks as one of the premier pediatric hospitals in the country. In total, affiliated hospitals provide more than 2,000 patient beds. Students are exposed to a local population in need of basic care and to patients who have come from around the world for the most advanced treatments. The School of Medicine expects students to play important roles in the provision of patient care

Students

The current student body represents 43 states and 21 foreign countries. Although most are recent college graduates with degrees in one of the hard sciences, there is tremendous diversity in terms of age and undergraduate background. Class size is 120.

STUDENT LIFE

Since most students come from out-of-state (and country), they are eager to get to know each other and tend to form a coherent group quickly. An extensive orientation session at the beginning of the year aids in this process. Student groups are extremely active and range from those that focus on community service projects, such as operating a free clinic on weekends to intramural sports clubs to Hot Docs (a musical group). Well-used, on-campus facilities include the Hilltop Campus Athletic Facility, which is a comprehensive gym and sports center. Social life often centers on the restaurants and bars of the Central West End and the tree-lined paths of Forest Park. Campus housing is available adjacent to the Medical School, but many students prefer to live in the surrounding areas, where housing is affordable and attractive.

GRADUATES

Graduates gain acceptance to the nation's most competitive residency programs. About half enter a primary care field.

Admissions

REQUIREMENTS

Washington University expects applicants to have completed 1 year each of biology, general chemistry, organic chemistry, and physics, in addition to math through the calculus level. The MCAT is required, and scores must be no more than three years old.

SUGGESTIONS

The Admissions Committee looks favorably on those who have pursued in-depth study of a particular subject, whether in the natural sciences, social sciences, or humanities. Successful applicants also demonstrate commitment and leadership through their extracurricular activities. Since the medical school offers rolling admissions beginning October 15, applicants should make every attempt to complete materials early.

PROCESS

About 20 percent of AMCAS applicants are interviewed, with interviews taking place between September and March. Interviews consist of one session with a member of the school's faculty or administration. Notification occurs on a rolling basis, and about one-third of interviewees are accepted. Wait-listed candidates are not ranked and are generally not encouraged to send supplementary material.

Admissions Requirements (Required)

MCAT scores, science GPA, non-science GPA, letters of recommendation, interview, essays/personal statement.

Admissions Requirements (Optional)

State residency, extracurricular activities, exposure to medical profession.

COSTS AND AID

Tuition & Fees

Tuition	$37,032
Cost of books	$1,613

Financial Aid

% students receiving aid	72
Average grant	$27,192
Average loan	$25,264
Average debt	$49,905

WAYNE STATE UNIVERSITY
SCHOOL OF MEDICINE

ADMISSIONS, 540 EAST CANFIELD, SUITE 1310, DETROIT, MI 48201 • ADMISSION: 313-577-1466
FAX: 313-577-9420 • E-MAIL: ADMISSIONS@MED.WAYNE.EDU • WEBSITE: WWW.MED.WAYNE.EDU/ADMISSIONS

STUDENT BODY

Type	Public
% male/female	100/0
# applied (total/out)	2,722/1,640
# accepted (total/out)	504/102
# enrolled (total/out)	257/30
Average age	24

ADMISSIONS

Average GPA and MCAT Scores

Overall GPA	3.5
MCAT Bio	9.8
MCAT Phys	9.5
MCAT Verbal	8.8
MCAT Essay	0

Application Information

Regular application	12/15
Regular notification	10/15
Early application	6/1–8/1
Early notification	10/1
Are transfers accepted?	yes
Admissions may be deferred?	yes
Interview required?	yes
Application fee	$50

Academics

The School of Medicine administers academic programs leading to the MD, MS, and PhD. Some medical students pursue a combined MD/PhD, leading to the doctorate degree in anatomy and cell biology, cellular and clinical neurobiology, immunology/microbiology, medical physics, molecular biology and genetics, pathology, pharmacology, and physiology. Other students earn an MS in biomedical or behavioral sciences along with the MD. The standard medical curriculum consists of 2 years of basic sciences, a year of clinical clerkships, and a year of clinical electives. Evaluation of medical student performance uses honors, pass, and fail. Promotion to year 3 requires passing Step 1 of the USMLE. To graduate, all students must record a score on Step 2 of the USMLE.

BASIC SCIENCES: Basic-science courses are taught primarily in a lecture/lab format, with some use of small-group sessions. Students are in class for about 20 hours per week. This schedule gives students the time they need to study, pursue independent projects, and take part in community service or other extracurricular activities. During year 1, students learn about the normal functions of the human body. Courses are anatomy, behavioral medicine, biochemistry, clinical nutrition, embryology, evidence based medicine, genetics, histology, introduction to the patient, human sexuality, neuroscience, and physiology. Second-year courses focus on the effects of disease and the principles of drug action and therapy. The pathophysiology course is organized by body/organ systems, which are connective tissue, cardiovascular, endocrine, gastrointestinal, hematology, neuroscience, pulmonary, and renal. Other courses are human sexuality, introduction to the patient, medical ethics, microbiology, pathology, pharmacology, physical diagnosis/interviewing, psychiatry, and public health and preventive medicine. The majority of first- and second-year classes are conducted in Scott Hall, a modern building that houses laboratories, lecture halls, and faculty offices. The Shiffman Medical Library has more than 150,000 volumes, computer facilities, and ample space for studying. Students can view recorded lectures and take advantage of other audiovisual study aids in the Self-Instruction Center.

CLINICAL TRAINING

During the third year, students complete 8-week, required clerkships in internal medicine, ob/gyn, pediatrics, and surgery. There are also 4-week clerkships in family medicine, neurology, and psychiatry. During the fourth year, selectives in ambulatory medicine (4 weeks) and emergency medicine (4 weeks), in addition to a sub internship (4 weeks), are required. Five months of electives are also required, a significant portion of which may be taken at other institutions. Clinical training takes place at the Detroit Medical Center (DMC), which is comprised of numerous hospitals, institutes, and care centers and has, in total, more than 2,400 beds. DMC includes Harper Hospital, Grace Hospital, Hutzel Hospital, Children's Hospital of Michigan, Rehabilitation Institute of Michigan, Detroit Receiving Hospital/University Health Center, Gershenson Radiation Oncology Center, Kresge Eye Institute, and Huron Valley Hospital. Medical students also rotate to affiliated hospitals in suburban areas.

Students

About 90 percent of the 256 students in each class are Michigan residents. Approximately 12 percent of students are underrepresented minorities, most of whom are African American. Although a few students are older or nontraditional, most entering students are in their early twenties.

STUDENT LIFE

Medical students are involved in chapters of national organizations, such as the American Medical Student Association; professionally oriented groups, such as the Family Medicine Interest Group; production of a student newspaper; and numerous community-service projects. Volunteer activities involve working with the city's youth, elderly, and under- and noninsured populations. Medical students also enjoy the extensive extracurricular offerings of Wayne State University, as well as the diverse culture of Detroit. Students live off campus, usually in apartments in the Detroit metropolitan area or in surrounding suburbs. Parking is available on campus, and most students own cars.

GRADUATES

About 65 percent of graduates chose residency programs in Michigan hospitals, with more than 50 percent staying in the Detroit area. In recent years, more than half of graduates entered primary care fields.

Admissions

REQUIREMENTS

One year each of biology, chemistry, organic chemistry, and physics, all with associated labs, is required. The MCAT is required, and scores should be from the spring or fall of the year prior to entrance. For applicants who have retaken the exam, the most recent set of scores is weighed most heavily. Thus, there is no advantage in withholding scores.

SUGGESTIONS

Although most positions are reserved for Michigan residents, well-qualified nonresidents are also considered. In addition to academic credentials, the Admissions Committee is interested in extracurricular activities and work. Health-related volunteer work and research are valuable.

PROCESS

About 50 percent of AMCAS applicants are sent secondary applications. Of those returning secondaries, about 20 percent are interviewed between September and April. The interview consists of one session with a member of the Admissions Committee. Candidates also receive a tour and have the opportunity to meet with current students. About one-third of interviewed candidates are accepted and are notified shortly after the interview. Wait-listed candidates are generally not encouraged to send additional information.

Admissions Requirements (Required)

MCAT scores, science GPA, non-science GPA, letters of recommendation, interview, essays/personal statement, extracurricular activities, exposure to medical profession.

Admissions Requirements (Optional)

State residency.

Overlap Schools

Michigan State University; University of Michigan—Ann Arbor.

COSTS AND AID

Tuition & Fees

In-state Tuition	$14,204
Out-of-state Tuition	$29,556
Cost of books	$1,000

Financial Aid

% students receiving aid	83
Average grant	$5,452
Average loan	$22,649
Average debt	$62,468

WEST VIRGINIA UNIVERSITY
SCHOOL OF MEDICINE

ROBERT C. BYRD HEALTH SCIENCES CENTER, PO BOX 9111, MORGANTOWN, WV 26506 • **ADMISSION:** 304-293-2408
FAX: 304-293-7814 • **E-MAIL:** MEDADMISSIONS@HSC.WVU.EDU • **WEBSITE:** WWW.HSC.WVU.EDU/SOM

STUDENT BODY

Type	Public
Enrollment	404
% male/female	60/40
% underrepresented minorities	2
# applied (total/out)	1,054/865
# accepted (total/out)	110/50
# enrolled (total/out)	110/36
Average age	22

FACULTY

Total faculty (number)	611
% female	32
% minority	17
% part-time	16
Student-faculty ratio	1:1

ADMISSIONS

Average GPA and MCAT Scores

Overall GPA	3.66
MCAT Bio	9.2
MCAT Phys	8.7
MCAT Verbal	8.9
MCAT Essay	P

Application Information

Regular application	11/15
Regular notification	rolling
Early application	8/1
Early notification	10/1
Are transfers accepted?	yes
Admissions may be deferred?	yes
Interview required?	yes
Application fee	$100

Academics

While most medical students follow a 4 year curriculum and earn the MD degree, about two medical students each year pursue joint MD/PhD degrees, leading to the doctorate in anatomy, biochemistry, medical technology, microbiology, pathology, pharmacology and toxicology, and physiology. Medical students are graded with honors, satisfactory, or unsatisfactory for all courses and clerkships. All students must pass Step 1 of the USMLE to be promoted to year 3.

BASIC SCIENCES: First-year courses are gross anatomy; biochemistry; embryology; genetics; histology; microanatomy; physiology; and problem-based learning, which integrates clinical correlation to the basic sciences. Second-year courses are behavioral medicine and psychiatry, community medicine, genetics, introduction to clinical medicine (ICM), microbiology, pathology, and pharmacology and toxicology. The ICM courses uses faculty mentors as teachers and trains students in basic clinical techniques, such as the physical examination and patient interview. Instructional aids include computer-assisted learning programs. For research purposes and for studying, students use the Health Sciences Library, which has a collection of more than 205,000 volumes, in addition to extensive holdings of audiovisual equipment.

CLINICAL TRAINING

Third-year, required clerkships are 8 weeks each of behavioral medicine and psychiatry; medicine; ob/gyn; pediatrics; surgery; and family medicine, which includes a rural rotation. Fourth-year requirements include 1 month of a sub internship in internal medicine, pediatrics, or family medicine; a 1 month critical care clerkship, an additional 1 month surgery clerkship; and 2 months of a rural primary care experience. Half of the fourth year is reserved for electives. Five months of fourth-year clerkships must be taken at WVU sites, leaving ample opportunity for students to rotate to other academic and clinical institutions. Clinical training takes place primarily at the Ruby Memorial Hospital (376 beds), which is part of the West Virginia University Robert C. Byrd Health Sciences Center Complex. The complex also includes the Physicians Office Center, the Mary Babb Randolph Cancer Center, Chestnut Ridge Psychiatric Hospital (70 beds), Southview Regional Rehabilitation Hospital (60 beds), and the National Institute of Occupational Safety and Health (NIOSH). About one-third of third-year students enter a clinical training program at university-affiliated hospitals in Charleston. All students also have the opportunity to rotate to facilities that are part of a large network of hospitals and physicians in rural areas of the state.

Students

At least 95 percent of students are West Virginia residents, and more than one-third attended WVU for undergraduate studies. About 40 other undergraduate institutions are represented in a typical class. Approximately 68 percent of students were biology or chemistry majors in college. In a recently admitted class of 88 students, 25 were 20 or 21 years of age, 56 were 22 or 23, and 7 were 24 or older.

STUDENT LIFE

With more than 1,700 students enrolled in programs at the Health Sciences Center, a camaraderie exists among WVU students. The small class size of the medical school also promotes class cohesion and cooperation. Student organizations include local chapters of national medical student organizations, community service-based groups, and clubs focused on professional interests. University-owned housing is available to medical and graduate students.

GRADUATES

About one-third of the practicing physicians in the state of West Virginia are graduates of WVU. At least half of graduates enter primary care fields, such as family medicine, internal medicine, pediatrics, and ob/gyn.

Admissions

REQUIREMENTS

All science courses should include lab work. The MCAT is required and is used, along with undergraduate transcripts, to assess academic achievement. For applicants who have taken the exam on multiple occasions, all scores are considered.

SUGGESTIONS

State residents are given strong preference in admission. However, a limited number of highly-qualified nonresidents may also be admitted. Beyond required course work, recommended courses are biochemistry, calculus, and cell and molecular biology. The Admissions Committee expects strength in the sciences but gives no preference to any particular major. Demonstration of an understanding of the medical profession is important.

PROCESS

All qualified West Virginia resident applicants and highly-qualified nonresidents are sent secondary applications. Of those returning secondaries, about 50 percent of residents and 10 percent of nonresidents are interviewed between September and February. Interviews generally consist of one two-on-one session, usually with medical school faculty, fourth-year students, or administrators. On interview day, students also have the opportunity to tour the campus and meet current students. Approximately one-third of interviewed candidates are accepted on a rolling basis. Others are either rejected or wait listed. West Virginia residents on the wait list have a reasonable chance of being accepted later in the spring.

Admissions Requirements (Required)

MCAT scores, science GPA, non-science GPA, letters of recommendation, interview, essays/personal statement, extracurricular activities, exposure to medical profession, computer literacy.

Admissions Requirements (Optional)

State residency.

Overlap Schools

Marshall University, University of Sherbrooke, West Virginia School of Osteopathic Medicine.

COSTS AND AID

Tuition & Fees

In-state Tuition	$15,456
Out-of-state Tuition	$35,858
Room and board (off campus)	$10,194
Cost of books	$4,650

Financial Aid

% students receiving aid	92
Average grant	$8,348
Average loan	$26,225
Average debt	$90,403

WRIGHT STATE UNIVERSITY
BOONSHOFT SCHOOL OF MEDICINE

OFFICE OF STUDENT AFFAIRS/ADMISSIONS, PO BOX 1751, DAYTON, OH 45401-1751 • **ADMISSION:** 937-775-2934
FAX: 937-775-3322 • **E-MAIL:** SOM_SAA@DESIRE.WRIGHT.EDU • **WEBSITE:** WWW.MED.WRIGHT.EDU

STUDENT BODY

Type	Public
Enrollment	375
% male/female	44/56
% underrepresented minorities	23
# applied (total/out)	2,710/1,860
# accepted (total/out)	225/39
# enrolled (total/out)	100/14
Average age	23

FACULTY

Total faculty (number)	1,500
% female	25
Student-faculty ratio	4:1

ADMISSIONS

Average GPA and MCAT Scores

Overall GPA	3.58
MCAT Bio	9.28
MCAT Phys	8.61
MCAT Verbal	9.11
MCAT Essay	0

Application Information

Regular application	11/15
Regular notification	10/15
Early application	8/1
Early notification	10/1
Are transfers accepted?	yes
Admissions may be deferred?	yes
Interview required?	yes
Application fee	$45

Academics

Although most students complete the MD curriculum in 4 years, a few enter the MD/PhD program, which requires additional course work. Graduate degrees are offered in most biomedical sciences, including anatomy, biochemistry, pathology, pharmacology, and physiology. Medical students are evaluated with percentile scores and ratings of pass/fail. Students take the USMLE Step 1 after completion of year 2 and Step 2 after the completion of year 3.

BASIC SCIENCES: Basic-science instruction includes use of small groups, clinical case studies, team-based learning, and computer-aided instruction. First-year courses are human structure, human development, introduction to clinical medicine I (ICM I), molecular basis of medicine, cellular, and tissue biology; social and ethical issues in medicine; principles of disease; and evidence-based medicine. The second year is organized around organ/body systems. These are pathobiology and therapeutics, blood, cardiology, endocrine, GI, integument, musculoskeletal, neuroscience, renal, reproductive, and respiratory. Students also learn about infectious diseases and continue clinical training in ICM II. The ICM course provides clinical contact from the very first week of class. In this series, students learn to take medical histories, conduct physical exams, and identify common diseases. Three 2-week elective periods during the first 2 years give students the opportunity to pursue intensive research or clinical projects. Students are also encouraged to participate in faculty-guided research during the summer in between the first and second years. The Fordham Health Sciences Library is fully computerized and provides 106,000 volumes, in addition to journals and special collections. Students also study in the student lounge and the main university's libraries. The Interdisciplinary Teaching Laboratory enhances learning through the use of audiovisual equipment, hard-wired labs, and medical software. Video streaming and PowerPoint slides from lectures are available from a password-protected website.

CLINICAL TRAINING

Third-year required rotations are: Internal medicine (12 weeks), women's health (8 weeks), surgery (8 weeks), pediatrics (8 weeks), psychiatry (6 weeks), and family medicine (6 weeks). Fourth-year requirements are emergency medicine (4 weeks), neurology (4 weeks), and a variety of electives (6 months). Training takes place at Children's Medical Center (155 beds), Dayton Veterans Affairs Medical Center, Good Samaritan Hospital and Health Center (560 beds), Green Memorial Hospital (210 beds), Kettering Medical Center (486 beds), Miami Valley Hospital (811 beds), and Wright-Patterson Air Force Base Medical Center (301 beds). Some students rotate overseas as part of individually-designed or faculty-led experiences.

Students

About 90 percent of entering students are Ohio residents. From 20–25 percent of entering students are typically minorities. Typically, about 10 percent of entering students took significant time off between college and medical school. The class size is 100.

STUDENT LIFE

Medical students have active extracurricular lives, taking advantage of the offerings of the medical school, the main university, and the greater community. Students are involved in community service organizations and projects such as the Center for Healthy Communities, which provides health education services to the Dayton community. Other student organizations are chapters of state and national medical organizations, honor societies, support groups, and clubs focused on professional or recreational interests. Athletic facilities on campus include racquetball, squash, basketball and tennis courts, indoor and outdoor tracks, and several fitness centers. The university's 200 acres of woods are used for walking and jogging. The university is located 12 miles northeast of Dayton, a city of nearly 1 million residents. Students live in privately-owned apartments, condominiums, and homes, which are generally affordable and conveniently located.

GRADUATES

Typically about 55 percent enter primary care residencies, which include family medicine, internal medicine, and pediatrics. About 50 percent typically choose residency programs in Ohio.

Admissions

REQUIREMENTS

Prerequisites are 1 year each of biology, chemistry, organic chemistry, and physics, all with associated labs. In addition, 1 year each of English and mathematics are required. The MCAT is required, and scores should be from within the past three years. For applicants who have retaken the exam, all scores are considered.

SUGGESTIONS

Ohio residents are given strong preference, making admission for nonresidents very competitive. In addition to academic strength, selection is based on dedication to human concerns, communication skills, maturity, and motivation. Some hospital or other medically related experience is recommended.

PROCESS

All AMCAS applicants receive secondary applications. About 10 percent of those returning secondaries are invited to interview between September and March. Interviews consist of two sessions, each with a member of the Admissions Committee. On interview day, students also attend group information presentations, have lunch with students, and tour the campus. About 45 percent of interviewed candidates are accepted on a rolling basis. Others are rejected or put on a wait list. Wait-listed candidates are not encouraged to send additional information.

Admissions Requirements (Required)

MCAT scores, science GPA, non-science GPA, letters of recommendation, interview, essays/personal statement, extracurricular activities, exposure to medical profession.

Admissions Requirements (Optional)

State residency.

COSTS AND AID

Tuition & Fees

In-state Tuition	$20,988
Out-of-state Tuition	$29,712
Room and board (off campus)	$10,560
Cost of books	$1,757
Fees	$1,400

Financial Aid

% students receiving aid	92
Average grant	$5,670
Average loan	$33,618
Average debt	$121,615

YALE UNIVERSITY
SCHOOL OF MEDICINE

OFFICE OF ADMISSIONS, 367 CEDAR STREET, NEW HAVEN, CT 06510 • ADMISSION: 203-785-2643
FAX: 203-785-3234 • E-MAIL: MEDICALSCHOOL.ADMISSIONS@QUICKMAIL.YALE.EDU
WEBSITE: WWW.INFO.MED.YALE.EDU/EDUCATION/ADMISSIONS/INDEX.HTML

STUDENT BODY

Type	Private
Enrollment	479
% male/female	51/49
% underrepresented minorities	18
# applied (total/out)	3,093/3,472
Average age	24

ADMISSIONS

Application Information

Regular application	10/15
Regular notification	3/15
	until filled
Early application	6/1–8/1
Early notification	10/1
Are transfers accepted?	yes
Admissions may be deferred?	yes
Interview required?	no
Application fee	$60

Academics

Although most students complete courses, clerkships, and a thesis in 4 years, about 30–50 percent of students extend their studies over a 5 year period at no extra cost. Some students take an extra year to earn a MPH along with the MD. Other combined degree programs offered are the MD/JD, MD/MDiv, and MD/PhD. Entering students are assigned a clinical tutor who serves as a mentor during all 4 years. Also throughout all 4 years, students take a series of lectures, workshops, and clinical discussion under the broad topic of medicine, society, and public health. Evaluation of students is strictly pass/fail. Passing Steps 1 and 2 of the USMLE is a graduation requirement.

BASIC SCIENCES: The first 2 years are spent building a foundation in the basic sciences, as well as learning skills and techniques for training in clinical responsibilities. Year 1 is devoted to understanding normal relevant biological form and function. Year 2 concentrates on the study of disease. Formats include lecture, small-group discussion, laboratories, demonstrations, and individual tutorials; many of these involve patients, both at the bedside and in the classroom. First-year students must pass the following courses: Aspects of child and adolescent development, biological basis of behavior, cellular and physiologic basis of medicine (physiology and cell biology), human genetics, human anatomy and development, molecular foundations of medicine (biochemistry), neurobiology, and psychological basis of medical practice. In addition there is an umbrella course called medicine, society, and public health that includes related but distinct subcourses: Biostatistics, history of medicine, professional responsibility, and health policy. Pre-clinical training is included in the course: the doctor/patient encounter. The major, second-year course is called mechanisms of disease and is organized into two segments. The initial offering, called basic principles, includes immunobiology, laboratory medicine, pathology, pharmacology, microbiology, and basics of diagnostic radiology. The second segment is called mechanisms of disease: organs/systems. Each integrated module, organized around body systems or organs, includes diagnostic radiology, laboratory medicine, pathology, pharmacology, pathophysiology, and prevention. The modules are blood/hematology; cardiovascular system; clinical neuroscience; digestive system; endocrine systems; female reproductive system; musculoskeletal system; neoplasias/oncology; psychiatry; renal, urinary tract and male reproductive system; respiratory system; and skin. Medicine, society, and public health continues, offering epidemiology and public health in the first semester and relevant prevention during the modules. The doctor/patient encounter course also continues, building as it progresses.

CLINICAL TRAINING

There are seven required clerkships in the third year, one of which may be completed early in the fourth year. These are internal medicine (12 weeks), general surgery/surgical subspecialties (12 weeks), pediatrics (8 weeks), psychiatry (6 weeks), ob/gyn (6 weeks), and clinical neuroscience (4 weeks). During the fourth year, an integrated clinical medicine clerkship (3 weeks) and a primary care clerkship (4 weeks) are required. The primary care clerkship takes place in a variety of community- and practice-based sites. Most clinical rotations are completed at the Yale New Haven Hospital and the West Haven Veteran's Administration Hospital. Other affiliated hospitals are Bridgeport Hospital, Danbury Hospital, Greenwich Hospital, Griffin Hospital in Derby, Hospital of Saint Raphael, Lawrence and Memorial Hospital, Norwalk Hospital, Saint Mary's

Hospital in Waterbury, Saint Vincent's Medical Center in Bridgeport, and Waterbury Hospital. Several clinics and mental health centers are also used for training. Although some students begin working on their thesis early in medical school, the majority of research and writing takes from 4–7 months and is completed in the fourth year. Some students publish their work, while others continue developing their research post-graduation.

Students

Yale attracts students from all regions of the country. Approximately 15–20 percent of entering students are underrepresented minorities. Class size is 100.

STUDENT LIFE

The School of Medicine is a short walk from the university's main campus. This gives medical students access to athletic facilities, student meeting areas, libraries, and university-sponsored events. Medical students participate in intramural sports, competing against other graduate and professional school teams. About three-quarters of medical students are involved in community service activities such as STATS (Students Teaching AIDS to Students), the Prenatal Care Project, and ASAP (the Adolescent Substance Abuse Prevention Project). The Office for Women in Medicine is the oldest of its kind in the nation and provides support, guidance, and special programs of interest for women medical students. The Office for Multicultural Affairs recruits and supports minority students, serves as a link between the school and its surrounding community, and sponsors various cultural events and centers. The Edward S. Harkness Memorial Hall is a residence hall for medical, physician associate, nursing, public health, and other graduate students. Both dormitory-style rooms and apartments are available.

GRADUATES

Among graduates, the most popular areas for residency training were internal medicine (40 percent), pediatrics (12 percent), orthopedics (8 percent), surgery (5 percent), otolaryngology (5 percent), plastic surgery (4 percent), dermatology (3 percent), and diagnostic radiology (1 percent).

Admissions

REQUIREMENTS

Prerequisites are 1 year each of general biology or zoology, general chemistry, organic chemistry, and general physics, all taken with associated labs. The MCAT is required, and scores should be from within the past 4 years. For applicants who have retaken the exam, the best set of scores is considered.

SUGGESTIONS

In addition to academic credentials, the Admissions Committee looks for intelligent, mature, and highly motivated students who possess integrity, common sense, personal stability, dedication to service, and the ability to inspire and maintain confidence.

PROCESS

Yale does not participate in AMCAS. Applications should be requested from the address above, or downloaded from info.med.yale.edu/medadmit. About 25 percent of applicants are interviewed between October and February. Interviews consist of two sessions, each with a faculty member or medical student committee member. Candidates attend group information sessions and have the opportunity to eat lunch and tour the campus with current medical students. About 15 percent of interviewed candidates are accepted. Notification occurs in mid-March.

Admissions Requirements (Required)

MCAT scores, state residency, essays/personal statement, extracurricular activities, exposure to medical profession.

Admissions Requirements (Optional)

Science GPA, nonscience GPA, letters of recommendation, interview.

COSTS

Tuition & Fees

Tuition	$33,800
Room and board (on campus)	$9,650
Cost of books	$1,700
Fees	$300

Yeshiva University

Albert Einstein College of Medicine

1300 Morris Park Avenue, 1300 Morris Park Avenue, Bronx, NY 10461 • Admission: 718-430-2106
Fax: 718-430-8825 • E-mail: ADMISSIONS@AECOM.YU.EDU • Website: WWW.AECOM.YU.EDU

STUDENT BODY

Type	Private
Enrollment	724
% male/female	51/49
% underrepresented minorities	7
# applied (total/out)	5,943/4,522
# accepted (total/out)	521/336
# enrolled (total/out)	180/92
Average age	23

FACULTY

Total faculty (number)	3,510
% female	35
% part-time	42
Student-faculty ratio	1:1

ADMISSIONS

Average GPA and MCAT Scores

Overall GPA	3.6
MCAT Bio	10.6
MCAT Phys	10.5
MCAT Verbal	9.4
MCAT Essay	P

Application Information

Regular application	12/31
Regular notification	1/15
Early application	8/1
Early notification	10/1
Are transfers accepted?	no
Admissions may be deferred?	yes
Interview required?	yes
Application fee	$90

Academics

In addition to the requirements described below, all students conduct research projects through the Independent Scholars Program. Such research often leads to publication or to distinction at the time of graduation. Projects involve a faculty mentor and can be in traditional or nontraditional medical science fields. Students may apply for joint-PhD/MD programs at the time of initial application or while enrolled in the MD program. Those accepted into this program receive stipends, either through the MSTP program or from institutional sources. The PhD may be earned in the following fields: Anatomy, biochemistry, biophysics, cell biology, genetics, immunology, microbiology, molecular biology, neuroscience, pathology, pharmacology, and physiology. Evaluation of student performance uses honors, pass, and fail. Passing the USMLE Steps 1 and 2 is a requirement for graduation.

BASIC SCIENCES: Throughout the first and second years, introduction to clinical medicine complements the basic science curriculum by addressing practical and personal issues related to the patient interview and examination. About 40 entering students participate in a Generalist Mentorship Program, which involves shadowing a primary care physician. First-year courses, taught primarily with lectures and labs, are anatomy, cardiovascular physiology, disease mechanisms, histology, and principles of pharmacology. The course molecular and cellular foundations of medicine uses both lectures and small-group sessions. During the second part of year 1, and throughout all of year 2, instruction is organ-based, is carried out in small groups, and uses a case-based approach. Courses are cardiovascular system, endocrine system, gastrointestinal system and liver, hematology, nervous system and behavior, renal physiology and pathobiology, reproductive system and human sexuality, respiratory system, and rheumatologic and orthopedic disease. Other second-year courses are microbiology and infectious disease and parasitology. On average, students spend about 20 hours per week in class. A Cognitive Skills Program offers reviews for the USMLE and tutoring for students who will benefit from it. Basic science instruction takes place in the Arthur B. and Diane Belfer Educational Center for Sciences, which is open 24 hours a day and contains classrooms, laboratories, study areas, a student bookstore, and computer rooms. The D. Samuel Gottesman Library has 250,000 volumes, 2,400 journal subscriptions, computer databases, and other informational technology. Electronic search mechanisms allow easy access to several large collections in the New York area.

CLINICAL TRAINING

Third-year required clerkships are medicine (11 weeks), pediatrics (7 weeks), psychiatry (6 weeks), ob/gyn (6 weeks), surgery (8 weeks), family medicine (6 weeks), geriatrics (2 weeks), and neurology (2 weeks). During the fourth year, 2 months of a sub internship in either medicine or pediatrics is required, as are 2 months in an ambulatory care program. For clinical training, Einstein students have access to six prominent hospitals in New York, comprising a total of 6,988 beds. These are Jacobi Medical Center (537 beds), Montefiore Medical Center (745 beds), Long Island Jewish Medical Center (829 beds), Beth Israel Medical Center (212 beds), and the Bronx-Lebanon Medical Center (two centers with 540 beds). Training also takes place at mental health facilities and long-term care centers primarily for older populations. Several nationally recognized research institutes are part of Einstein's resources and provide further opportunities for students.

Fellowships are available for up to 20 fourth-year students, enabling them to fulfill elective requirements overseas. Numerous organized exchange programs also exist, with countries such as Germany, Sweden, Israel, France, Japan, and Cuba.

Students

Students come from around the country. Undergraduate institutions that are particularly well represented are Yeshiva, State Universities of New York, private northeastern colleges and universities, and public universities in California. In a typical entering class, about 9 percent of students are minorities, most of whom are African American. Students who have taken time off after college account for about one-third of entering classes, and those over 30 years old account for about 5–10 percent. Class size is 180.

STUDENT LIFE

Central meeting areas, such as the Lubin Student Lounge and the Max and Sadie Friedman Lounge, feature music, food, television, and an opportunity for interaction outside of the academic environment. There are full athletic facilities for student use. School-sponsored activities include class parties, clubs focused on films or the outdoors, and organizations based on cultural, religious, or ethnic affiliations. Einstein has its own symphony orchestra. The beaches of Long Island and the culture, entertainment, and excitement of Manhattan are easily accessible by car or public transportation. Most students live on campus, in the Eastchester Road or Rhinelander Residences, where studios and 1- and 2-bedroom apartments are available.

GRADUATES

Among graduates, the predominant residency choices were internal medicine (45 percent), pediatrics (12 percent), surgery or general surgery (10 percent), ob/gyn (6 percent), emergency medicine (6 percent), psychiatry (5 percent), family practice (4 percent), and ophthalmology (3 percent). Einstein has the largest postgraduate training program in the country and is the destination of about 40 percent of Einstein School of Medicine graduates. Programs at other New York institutions, in the Philadelphia area, and in California are also popular choices.

Admissions

REQUIREMENTS

Requirements are biology (8 hours), chemistry (8 hours), English (8 hours), organic chemistry (8 hours), physics (8 hours), and college math (6 hours). The MCAT is required and should be no more than three years old. For those who have retaken the MCAT, the best score is counted. Thus, there is no advantage to withholding scores.

SUGGESTIONS

College students should pursue studies in their area of interest, as no particular major is considered more appropriate than the next. Course work in the humanities and social sciences is important. Statistics is useful, and computer literacy is necessary. Einstein looks closely at the personal interaction skills of its applicants and at their ability to work with people from diverse backgrounds.

PROCESS

All AMCAS applicants are sent secondary applications. Of those returning secondaries, about 20 percent are invited to interview. Interviews with faculty members last for about 1 hour and take place between August and May. On interview day, there is a tour of the campus and a lunch period with current Einstein students. Notification begins in January, during which applicants are accepted, wait listed, or rejected. Wait-listed candidates may submit additional material.

Admissions Requirements (Required)

MCAT scores, science GPA, non-science GPA, letters of recommendation, interview, essays/personal statement, extracurricular activities, exposure to medical profession.

Admissions Requirements (Optional)

State residency.

Overlap Schools

New York University, Stony Brook University, SUNY Downstate Medical Center, UMDNJ.

COSTS AND AID

Tuition & Fees

Tuition	$35,925
Room and board (on campus)	$4,000
Room and board (off campus)	$7,000
Cost of books	$1,600
Fees	$1,600

Financial Aid

% students receiving aid	75
Average grant	$8,500
Average loan	$20,000
Average debt	$65,000

8 Naturopathic Profiles

BASTYR UNIVERSITY
SCHOOL OF NATUROPATHIC MEDICINE

14500 JUANITA DRIVE NORTHEAST, KENMORE, WA 98028 • ADMISSION: 425-602-3330 • FAX: 425-602-3090
E-MAIL: ADMISSIONS@BASTYR.EDU • INTERNET: WWW.BASTYR.EDU

STUDENT BODY	
Type	Private
Enrollment	477
% male/female	28/72
% underrepresented minorities	6
# applied (total/out)	260/202
# accepted (total/out)	195/140
# enrolled (total/out)	118/98
Average age	28

FACULTY	
Total faculty (number)	28
% female	60
% part-time	64

ADMISSIONS

Average GPA and MCAT Scores

Overall GPA	3.3

Application Information

Regular application	2/1
Regular notification	4/15
Early application	11/1
Early notification	2/1
Are transfers accepted?	yes
Admissions may be deferred?	yes
Interview required?	yes
Application fee	$75

Academics

Bastyr's naturopathic doctoral (ND) program educates future physicians in the tradition of medical science and the art of natural healing. The school does this by providing a comprehensive understanding of the basic medical sciences, accurate diagnostic skills and the ability to apply the natural and minimally invasive methods of whole-person health care characteristic of naturopathic medicine.

Bastyr's mission is as follows: We educate future leaders in the natural health sciences that integrate mind, body, spirit, and nature. Through natural health education, research and clinical services, we improve the health and well being of the human community.

Original research is conducted regularly through NIH grants and other funding and a research fellowship has been funded. The university has established an AIDS Research Center with funding from the NIH Office of Complementary and Alternative Medicine. Students are engaged in primary clinical research at the teaching clinic. The university maintains a library with current journals; special collections in alternative medicine, acupuncture, nutrition, midwifery, and naturopathic medicine; and audiovisual aids. Students also have access to the nearby University of Washington Health Sciences Libraries.

BASIC SCIENCES: During the first two years of the program, students receive a thorough foundation in the basic medical sciences along with instruction in naturopathic medicine, clinical and laboratory diagnosis, nutrition, and counseling. Basic science courses within the ND program emphasize anatomy, physiology, and biochemistry as the foundation for further basic science and all chemical courses. Further courses include pathology, immunology, infectious diseases, embryology, and research methods. Problem-solving, clinical cases, and examples are an integral part of the basic science curriculum.

CLINICAL TRAINING

The second two years of education at Bastyr University focus on clinical diagnosis and therapeutics, including clinical studies in nutrition, botanical medicine, homeopathy, obstetrics, pediatrics, geriatrics, and other specialty areas.

Students receive their clinical education through supervised internships at the university's own teaching clinic, Bastyr Center for Natural Health (BCNH), as well as at various off-site clinic placements. A paid residency position at BCNH is another practical way to strengthen clinical skills.

Students in the ND/Acupuncture and Oriental Medicine (AOM) dual program are eligible to participate in clinical internships in China—at either Chengdu University of TCM or Shanghai University of TCM. Chengdu University has been Bastyr's sister college since 1993 and is 1 of the 4 colleges approved by the State Council in 1956.

Students

Bastyr University's natural health science campus is located in Kenmore, just north of Seattle in the beautiful Pacific Northwest. The 186,000 square foot facility rests on fifty acres of fields and woodlands on the northeast shore of Lake Washington. Built in 1959 as a Catholic seminary, this building houses the university's classrooms and other facilities such as laboratories and research facilities, library and reading room, university bookstore, conference and seminar space, administrative offices, vegetarian cafeteria, chapel, and dormitory space on campus. A variety of off-campus apartments and rental homes are available in the Juanita, Mountlake Terrace, Bothell, and Kenmore areas.

The Bastyr campus setting is uniquely suited for the study of natural health sciences. The grounds, well-watered by the Pacific Northwest rainfall, stay green most of the year. The burgeoning herb and culinary garden draws students to learn, get their fingers in the dirt, or just admire the aesthetic beauty of nature's medicinal plants.

Adjacent to the university's own playfields and gardens are miles of wooded trails winding through 316-acre St. Edward State Park to the shore of Lake Washington. The park has a secluded beach and a natural habitat where coyotes, eagles, and spotted owls find refuge. The park also manages a swimming pool, outdoor volleyball courts, tennis courts, and playfields available to Bastyr students, faculty, and staff.

STUDENT LIFE

Bastyr students find a wide variety of activities on campus to keep them busy. Students are involved in the governance system of the university through student and university councils, and board of trustees memberships. Other activities include service in the medicinal and culinary herb garden and various clubs and committees, including the Bastyr Environmental Action Team (BEAT), Herbal Ways, Nutrition Advisory Committee, American Psychological Association, Aikido, African American Support Group, Student Dietetics Association, Supper Club, Student Chapter of Physicians for Social Responsibility, Natural Products Student Reps, various spiritual groups, and various athletic groups.

Various special events help create a sense of school identity and a feeling of community. Bastyr students are involved in making the surrounding community a "well" place to live.

GRADUATES

Graduates of Bastyr's ND program are qualified primary health care practitioners who, as they diagnose and treat disease, are focused on treating the whole person and promoting optimal health. Their scope of practice includes all aspects of family care, from pediatrics to geriatrics, and relies on a broad spectrum of modalities, including botanical medicine, nutrition, homeopathy, hydrotherapy, naturopathic manipulation, and psychological counseling.

Graduates leave Bastyr University qualified to pass professional licensure exams and prepared to set up and maintain private practices or work in integrative medical clinics.

Admissions

REQUIREMENTS

Credentials to be submitted are all official transcripts, two letters of recommendation, a completed application form, and a $75 application fee. While a bachelor's degree is strongly recommended, exceptions are made for outstanding students who have completed at least 135 quarter credits or 90 semester credits (must include at least 45 quarter or 30 semester credits of upper-division course work). In recent years, more than 97 percent of entrants have held a bachelor's degree. Required minimum course work includes 1 course in college-level algebra or precalculus, 4 courses in chemistry (including a two-term sequence of organic with lab), 3 quarters or 2 semesters of biology with labs (must include work in cell biology and genetics), at least 1 course in physics (must include mechanics, optics, electricity, and magnetism), and 1 course in psychology, 2 courses in English, and 2 courses in humanities. Courses earning a C-minus or below are not accepted for prerequisite consideration. Required chemistry and biology courses not taken within 7 years of matriculation into the program are subject to review by the Admissions Committee. Additional course work may be required. Applicants who meet the basic admission standards may be invited to an interview.

SUGGESTIONS

For priority consideration, applications should be received by February 1 for admission the following Fall, although late applications are considered on a space-available basis. When requesting an application or program information, please be sure to indicate the specific program of interest and what materials you would like sent.

PROCESS

Admission is based on academic achievement, personal and social development, relevant experience, financial planning, and demonstrated humanistic qualities.

Admissions Requirements (Required)

Science GPA, nonscience GPA, letters of recommendation, interview, essays/personal statement, exposure to medical profession.

Admissions Requirements (Optional)

MCAT scores, state residency, extracurricular activities, Experience with CAM desired.

COSTS AND AID

Tuition & Fees

Tuition	$21,919
Room and board (off campus)	$9,200
Cost of books	$1,938

Financial Aid

% students receiving aid	80
Average grant	$3,000
Average loan	$28,500
Average debt	$100,000

BOUCHER INSTITUTE OF NATUROPATHIC MEDICINE

300-435 COLUMBIA STREET, NEW WESTMINSTER, BC V3L 5N8 • ADMISSION: 604-777-9981 • FAX: 604-777-9982
E-MAIL: SSPARLIN@BINM.ORG • INTERNET: WWW.BINM.ORG

STUDENT BODY

Type	Private
Enrollment	80
# applied	64
# accepted	32
# enrolled	32
Average age	30

FACULTY

Total faculty (number)	28
% female	50

ADMISSIONS

Application Information

Regular application	11/30
Are transfers accepted?	yes
Admissions may be deferred?	no
Interview required?	yes
Application fee	$100

Academics

The academic philosophy as evidenced by the Institute's curriculum design strives to incorporate principles of both proven conventional academic wisdom and a mentorship program. BINM's commitment to small class size allows maximum flexibility in the incorporation of various educational methodologies including hands-on situational learning. Thirty-five hundred hours of instruction are divided among the five basic categories of courses which constitute the Naturopathic Medical Program academic curriculum. They include the following: Clinical science, clinical practice and integration, health sciences, naturopathic therapeutic modalities, professional development.

BASIC SCIENCES: Anatomy, biochemistry, diagnostic imaging, differential diagnosis, infectious disease, laboratory diagnosis, neuroanatomy, oncology, pathology, physical clinical diagnosis, physiology.

CLINICAL TRAINING

Twelve-hundred hours are spent on the clinical component of the education, with an additional 300 preceptorship hours spent in the offices of practicing physicians.

The Boucher Institute of Naturopathic Medicine recently acquired the 46,000 square-foot Columbia Centre building located at 435 Columbia Street in New Westminster, which also provides access to the Columbia Street Sky Train Station. This acquisition enabled the institute to expand its campus by occupying about half the building to accommodate its growing enrollment of approximately 85 naturopathic medical students expected for the 2005–2006 academic year. Established in 2001, the Boucher Institute is Western Canada's only initially approved college of naturopathic medicine, offering a four-year, 5,000 hour program of post-graduate training culminating in a Doctor of Naturopathic Medicine diploma. This new campus will provide the institute with over 20,000 square feet of contiguous, newly renovated space for modern classrooms, expanded library facilities, teaching labs, an expanded teaching clinic, administrative offices, and student activities.

Admissions

REQUIREMENTS

A university degree (BSC) is preferred but not required. Applicants must have completed a minimum of 3 years of course work (90 credit hours, 15 full-year courses, or 30 half-year courses) at a recognized Canadian University or the equivalent (as listed by the Canadian Information Centre for International Credentials at www.cicic.ca or as listed by the U.S. Department of Education at ope.ed.gov/accreditation). For international applicants from outside the United States and Canada, a credentials evaluation must be completed from ICES (www.bcit.ca/ices) or any other approved credentials evaluation service. At least 30 credit hours (5 full-year courses or 10 half-year courses) must be upper division (i.e. third or fourth year level at a four-year institution). The following specific courses are required prerequisites: 1 full year of biology (6 credit hours). This may be fulfilled by 1 year of general biology or 1 semester of cell biology, plus 1 semester of an appropriate biology such as botany, genetics, zoology, anatomy, microbiology. One-half full year of biochemistry (3 credit hours). One full year of English/humanities (6 credit hours). This must include an essay component. (Note: Applicants may be required to write a short essay at the time of the interview.) One full year of general chemistry (6 credit hours). One-half full year of organic chemistry (3 credit hours). One-half full year of psychology (3 credit hours).

In addition, prospective students would benefit by completing additional courses in some or all of the following areas: Anatomy, cell biology, genetics, human physiology, microbiology, physics, sociology, and statistics.

A passing mark of 60 percent is the absolute minimum grade required for all prerequisites. It is recommended that an overall cumulative grade point average of 3.0 on a 4-point scale (i.e., 75 percent) be attained for the applicant to be competitive for the limited seats available.

BINM is developing and endorses a Prior Learning Assessment Policy for our prerequisite courses only. For more information, contact the Registrar's office.

Credit may not be given for courses completed more than 10 years prior to application for admission.

PROCESS

The Boucher Institute of Naturopathic Medicine evaluates all applicants in accordance with the constitutional guidelines that protect the rights of individuals. The primary objective of the applicant screening process is to assure that applicants accepted into the program have made an informed commitment to naturopathic medicine as a career and that there is a good match between the applicant's goals and expectations and what the Boucher's unique program has to offer. Applicants must be temperamentally and morally suited to the profession and must also have a reasonable probability of successfully completing the program and becoming licensed to practice in a regulated jurisdiction.

The successful applicant is expected to have the following: A demonstrated reasonable academic ability in previous educational endeavors and knowledge of and realistic attitudes toward health, healing, and naturopathic medicine in particular. He or she must also understand the importance of self-care and holistic health care and be able to discuss the role of the healer in the natural self-healing process. The applicant should have some knowledge of and personal experience in naturopathic medicine; be able to recognize the ongoing responsibilities inherent in a life of service to the community as a naturopathic physician; understand that naturopathic medicine is a rapidly advancing field in which there is a continuing need to update skills and knowledge by keeping up on current information with journals and continuing education; have realistic expectations regarding the income potential of naturopathic physicians, be aware of the potential for mental and emotional stress involved in this occupation, and have an understanding of the relationship of naturopathic medicine to other health care professions; have devoted sufficient time and energy to researching the naturopathic medicine profession and, considering personal goals and expectations, to be confident in this career choice; have an appreciation of the importance of diversity in society and show evidence of the maturity, emotional stability, and physical ability necessary to engage in the activities required for naturopathic training and practice. The applicant must also be able to demonstrate an ability for critical thinking, have good communication skills, be able to discuss professionalism as it applies to the provision of health care, provide references supporting his or her character and ability, and demonstrate adequate financial resources to become a full-time student.

Applicants who have satisfied the above criteria, as evidenced through their application, essay, and interview, are eligible for admission to the institute at the discretion of the Admissions Committee.

Admissions Requirements (Required)

Letters of recommendation, interview, essays/personal statement, exposure to medical profession, BINM credit and science prerequisites.

Overlap Schools

Bastyr University, Canadian College of Naturopathic Medicine, National College of Naturopathic Medicine.

COSTS AND AID

Tuition & Fees

Tuition	$15,850
Room and board (off campus)	$5,000
Cost of books	$1,000
Fees	$300

Financial Aid

Average loan	$12,000

THE CANADIAN COLLEGE OF NATUROPATHIC MEDICINE

1255 SHEPPARD AVENUE, TORONTO, ON M2K 1E2 • ADMISSION: 416-498-1255, EXT. 245 • FAX: 416-498-3197
E-MAIL: INFO@CCNM.EDU • INTERNET: WWW.CCNM.EDU

STUDENT BODY

Type	Private
Enrollment	485
% male/female	25/75
# applied	164
# enrolled	97
Average age	27

ADMISSIONS

Average GPA and MCAT Scores

Overall GPA	3.35

Application Information

Are transfers accepted?	yes
Admissions may be deferred?	yes
Interview required?	yes
Application fee	$150

Academics

The Canadian College of Naturopathic Medicine's four-year accredited professional program in naturopathic medicine provides more than 4,200 hours of classroom training and clinical experience. It is composed of a number of subdisciplines that are taught in a series of sequential courses.

BASIC SCIENCES: This area of the program consists of courses in anatomy, biochemistry, histopathology, immunology, microbiology, and physiology. Development of problem-solving skills in applied basic life sciences is done through lecture, case discussion, tutorial groups, and clinical simulations. Some of these courses include a laboratory component. Laboratory facilities include diagnostic test kits, diagnostic laboratory, and access to pro-sected human cadavers for gross anatomy study. A variety of audiovisual resources are also available.

CLINICAL TRAINING

Clinical disciplines under diagnostic medicine include the following: Advanced imaging, differential and laboratory diagnosis, health psychology, physical assessment, physical and clinical diagnosis, and primary care and pathology. The principles and philosophy of naturopathic medicine form the bridgework between the academic and clinical parts of the college curriculum.

Students

Campus facilities include a student lounge, which is a spacious common area for student use. It is located on the second level and contains satellite TV, a game room, a meditation room, a piano room, as well as the student newspaper, extracurricular clubs, and naturopathic students' association. The indoor fitness center is fully-equipped and features change rooms with saunas. It is available for student use and is located on the lower level. A tennis/basketball court is located behind the building on the northwest corner. Each year a variety of campus and intramural sports teams are organized by students. Students, staff, and faculty are encouraged to visit the courtyard for group meetings, studying, or just relaxing. The Paracelsus Herb Garden, brick barbecues, and picnic tables are also available for student use. Funding for the Paracelsus Herb Garden was made possible by a generous donation from Wayne Steinke, ND, and his parents Herb and Shirley through Select Oilfield Services Ltd. and Cherway Holdings Ltd. It offers a relaxing oasis for reflection and meditation and is used as a teaching garden for CCNM students and visitors. The Green Life Café is the school cafeteria, which offers healthy, organic foods at reasonable prices in a pleasant atmosphere. The Green Life Café, adjacent to the courtyard, is generally open Monday to Friday from 7:30 A.M. to 6:00 P.M. during the regular academic year (September through April), excluding holidays. During the summer and College reading weeks it operates on a limited basis.

Housekeeping, grounds keeping, and a resident compost caretaker implement the college's waste reduction program. Cans, bottles, and paper are collected throughout the campus. Food waste is collected in the student residence kitchens, staff and student lounges, and in the cafeteria. Used household batteries are also collected. A comprehensive composting program is coordinated by property operations and development. In addition to yard waste, food waste is recycled into compost that is used on campus lawns and gardens.

STUDENT LIFE

There are a limited number of parking spaces available at the front of the college by entering on Sheppard Avenue East or Old Leslie Street. The current rate is $80 for monthly parking and the maximum daily rate is $12. Monthly permits are issued on a first-come, first-served basis, available at the front desk through an application process. Discounted public transit passes are also available.

Lockers are available to students. They may rent a locker and combination lock through the student services office at a charge of $10 for their academic period.

The Body Mind Science (BMS) Resources is CCNM's on-campus textbook and medical supply store. BMS Resources provides students with discounted textbooks, software, and medical equipment. Over the last few years, BMS Resources has become a comprehensive supply store serving complementary health-care professionals, carrying a complete line of clinic sundry supplies.

Admissions

REQUIREMENTS

There are six major naturopathic disciplines that define the areas of naturopathic practice. Each discipline is a distinct area of practice and includes both diagnostic principles and practices as well as therapeutic skills and techniques. These disciplines are integrated to effectively meet the individual needs of each patient, which is the objective of the ND program. Any of these disciplines may be ultimately developed by a naturopathic doctor as a clinical specialty.

The Canadian College of Naturopathic Medicine is committed to excellence in naturopathic education and to the success of the college's graduates. All candidates for admission are evaluated based on their academic history, their motivation for becoming a naturopathic doctor, leadership skills, problem-solving and critical-thinking skills, and specific personal qualities and characteristics.

To be considered for admission to the ND program, applicants must have completed a minimum of 3 years (equivalent to 15 full courses or 90 credit hours) toward a baccalaureate degree. For September admission, courses must be completed by August 31 of the year of application. For January admission, courses must be completed by December 31 of the year of application.

Competitive applications should have a cumulative grade point average of at least 3.3 on a 4-point scale (equivalent to B-plus). A lower grade point average may be acceptable, depending on the applicant's academic history, interview, essay, references, and autobiographical sketch.

Credit will not be given for the completion of prerequisites unless a grade of C-minus (60 percent) or better is earned. Required courses include the following: Biochemistry (3 credit hours), general biology (6 credit hours), general chemistry with lab (6 credit hours), humanities (6 credit hours), introductory psychology (6 credit hours), and organic chemistry with lab (3 credit hours).

Admissions Requirements (Required)

Science GPA, letters of recommendation, interview, essays/personal statement.

Admissions Requirements (Optional)

Nonscience GPA, state residency, extracurricular activities, exposure to medical profession.

Overlap Schools

Bastyr University, Boucher Institute of Naturopathic Medicine, National College of Naturopathic Medicine, Southwest College of Natural Medicine, University of Bridgeport, College of Naturopathic Medicine.

COSTS AND AID

Tuition & Fees

Tuition	$16,819
Room and board (on campus, per month)	$385
Cost of books	$1,500
Fees	$665

NATIONAL COLLEGE OF NATUROPATHIC MEDICINE

049 SOUTHWEST PORTER STREET, PORTLAND, OR 97201 • ADMISSION: 503-552-1660 • FAX: 503-499-0027
E-MAIL: ADMISSIONS@NCNM.EDU • INTERNET: NCNM.EDU

STUDENT BODY

Type	Private
Enrollment	351
% male/female	21/79
% underrepresented minorities	12
# applied (total/out)	195
# accepted (total/out)	165
# enrolled (total/out)	89
Average age	29

FACULTY

Total faculty (number)	84
% female	45
% minority	15
% part-time	63
Student-faculty ratio	9:1

ADMISSIONS

Average GPA and MCAT Scores

Overall GPA	3.36

Application Information

Are transfers accepted?	yes
Admissions may be deferred?	yes
Interview required?	yes
Application fee	$75

Academics

Naturopathic medicine is a patient-centered primary care approach that uses natural means to restore and optimize health. It is a distinct system of health care—an art, science, philosophy, and practice of diagnosing, treating, and preventing disease. Naturopathic medicine is heir to the vitalistic tradition of medicine in the Western world and emphasizes the treatment of disease through the stimulation, enhancement, and support of the inherent healing power of the body. Methods of treatment are chosen that respect the natural healing process. Graduates will have attained competency in the following areas: Incorporation of the principles of naturopathic medicine in diagnosis and treatment, completion of a medical history and physical examination, utilization of medical diagnostic procedures, integration of clinical data and therapeutic intervention, education of patients in disease prevention and therapeutic needs, communication with medical peers and practice management, development of ongoing learning skills and professional development, principles of evidence-based medicine.

BASIC SCIENCES: The basic science courses involve an in-depth study of the human body's structure and function, from the gross anatomical to the microscopic and molecular levels.

CLINICAL TRAINING

These courses in naturopathic clinical sciences present the naturopathic perspective on diagnosis and prevention and treatment of disease by system and region. They integrate multiple treatment forms with the principles of naturopathic philosophy into case management, along with criteria for referral.

In addition to two college-owned teaching clinics, NCNM, in conjunction with other agencies and as a member of the Coalition of Community Clinics, offers free and low-cost naturopathic and Chinese medicine health care at many sites around the Portland metropolitan area. These community clinics offer natural health care to underserved populations and provide NCNM faculty and students the opportunity to work with a broad range of medical conditions.

Students

Life in Portland, Oregon: Situated in the northernmost part of the Willamette Valley, Portland is nestled between the Cascade mountain range to the east and the coast range to the west. Prominent peaks—Mount Hood, Mount St. Helens, Mount Adams, and even Mount Rainier—can be seen on clear days. Mount Hood is a playground for outdoor enthusiasts offering hiking trails, ski areas, and campgrounds. To the northeast, and 30 minutes from downtown, is the Columbia River Gorge National Scenic Area. The Scenic Highway provides access to hiking trails, river beaches, inspiring views, and dramatic waterfalls—the 620-foot Multnomah Falls is the second highest year-round waterfall in the nation.

The Pacific coast, with its rugged rocky headlands and lush forests, is a 90-minute drive from Portland. Sprinkled along 300 miles of public beach, coastal communities are small and inviting, providing a treasure of local art, food, and lodging.

In Wine Country, the valley farmlands, which extend into southern Oregon, are home to a growing number of organic farms and orchards, flower fields, and dozens of small, nationally acclaimed wineries. Oregon provides ideal conditions for pinot noir grapes and produces spectacular wines.

The Portland metropolitan area is home to nearly 2 million residents. Divided by the Willamette River and bordered to the north by the Columbia River, Portland abounds in parks (10 percent of all city land), including the 5,100-acre Forest Park. The city offers an array of restaurants from gourmet to bistros to organic and vegetarian. Coffee houses, clubs, galleries, and a wide range of event venues support a rich and diverse nightlife. Many varied residential areas for renters or homeowners surround the NCNM campus allowing easy access by foot, bike, or public transportation.

Known for its extended, bloom-filled spring, the Portland area enjoys a mild turn of the four seasons. While it has a reputation for rain, on average 37 inches a year, other large cities, such as Atlanta, get more rainfall. Summer temperatures average in the mid 70s with little precipitation. A benefit of the mountain rain is an abundant water supply—among the purest in the nation.

Perennial attractions include the acclaimed Oregon Zoo, Portland Art Museum, Oregon Museum of Science and Industry (OMSI), Japanese Garden, Classical Chinese Garden, Portland's Saturday Market (the largest weekend open-air crafts market in the nation), and Powell's City of Books (one of the largest bookstores in the nation).

The Portland metro area leads the country in light-rail development and boasts the best transit system in the country. MAX (Metropolitan Area Express) light-rail trains link downtown Portland with outlying areas and the Portland International Airport.

STUDENT LIFE

Although on-campus housing is not available, NCNM is located near residential areas with ample rentals at reasonable rates. Students may contact the Student Affairs Office for additional information.

GRADUATES

The college is alma mater to over 1,500 alumni who practice in nearly every state and Canadian province as well as in many foreign countries. More than 50 percent of the licensed naturopathic physicians who practice in the United States are graduates of NCNM.

Admissions

ADMISIONS REQUIREMENTS

All candidates must possess a bachelor's degree or higher from a regionally accredited college or university, or the equivalent (as determined by NCNM), from an institution outside the United States.

Historically, many great physicians have had skills and creative abilities reaching far beyond the scope of science and medicine. Well-rounded people with backgrounds in the humanities, arts, and social sciences are often excellent candidates for medical professions. At NCNM, we value and encourage a broad range of life experiences, along with the development of multiple talents. There is no advantage to holding a BS rather than a BA, as long as you have completed the program's prerequisites.

Criteria for selecting applicants for admission to NCNM's programs include motivation, intellect, and character essential to becoming a physician or practitioner of natural medicine. Applicants are considered on the basis of academic performance, maturity, and demonstrated humanitarian qualities. Work and/or volunteer experience in health care, coupled with an awareness of the field of natural medicine, is strongly recommended.

Admissions Requirements (Required)

Science GPA, nonscience GPA, letters of recommendation, interview, essays/personal statement.

Overlap Schools

Bastyr University, Canadian College of Naturopathic Medicine.

COSTS AND AID

Tuition & Fees

Room and board	
(off campus)	$11,925
Cost of books	$1,500

Financial Aid

% students receiving aid	85
Average grant	$1,500
Average loan	$38,500
Average debt	$115,000

SOUTHWEST COLLEGE OF NATUROPATHIC MEDICINE

2140 EAST BROADWAY ROAD, TEMPE, AZ 85282 • ADMISSION: 888-882-7266 • FAX: 480-858-9116
E-MAIL: ADMISSIONS@SCNM.EDU • INTERNET: WWW.SCNM.EDU

STUDENT BODY

Type	Private
Enrollment	347
% male/female	31/69
% underrepresented minorities	35
# applied	202
# accepted	103
# enrolled	79
Average age	31

FACULTY

Total faculty (number)	21
% female	25
% part-time	65
Student-faculty ratio	14:1

ADMISSIONS

Average GPA and MCAT Scores

Overall GPA	3.46

Application Information

Are transfers accepted?	yes
Admissions may be deferred?	yes
Interview required?	yes
Application fee	$65

Academics

Founded in 1992, SCNM offers a four-year professional medical degree in Naturopathic Medicine accredited by the Council on Naturopathic Medical Education (CNME) and The Higher Learning Commission of the North Central Association of Colleges and Schools. Students are educated in the same basic sciences as MDs, including natural therapeutics and nontoxic approaches to therapy with an emphasis on disease prevention and optimizing wellness. Naturopathic physicians are primary care practitioners, trained as specialists in preventative medicine and natural therapies. We combine and individualize a wide variety of therapies based on a philosophy which acknowledge and encourage patients to be active participates in their own health care as well treat and deal with physical, psychological, and emotional aspects and barriers. Graduates are trained in the use of natural therapies such as nutrition, botanical medicine, homeopathy, acupuncture, oriental medicine, counseling, and hydrotherapy to treat disease, and combine these therapies with conventional medical treatments when appropriate.

BASIC SCIENCES: SCNM's curriculum features several required courses in every naturopathic modality. Students are educated in all modalities and methods of treatment, including botanical medicine and homeopathic medicine, nutrition, acupuncture, physical manipulation, and mind/body medicine. Therefore, a student is educated to be a manager of total integrated naturopathic medical care.

CLINICAL TRAINING

The clinical training program at SCNM is a key part of your medical education. As students under the supervision of attending physicians, they apply the scientific knowledge acquired in the academies study to real-life clinical cases and develop the skills and confidences necessary to deliver patient oriented care. Clinical rotations with NDs, MDs and DOs are available through the College's Medical Center or affiliated extended and offsite clinics and treatment centers. This combination of clinical training opportunities makes the clinical education at SCNM a unique experience—one which is committed to excellence in clinical education leading to superior healthcare which empowers the individual and the community.

Students

The campus is set on 15 acres in the college town of Tempe, Arizona, home to Arizona State University. Campus grounds offer students beautiful and tranquil outdoor spaces to study, relax, and play; all of course in the generously sunny and warm climate of Arizona.

STUDENT LIFE

The Southwest College campus culture is easy to sense, yet difficult to describe in words. Once you walk onto our campus, you'll feel the energy. This is a place for meaningful discovery, academic challenge, real-life experience, and lasting friendships. Students enroll at Southwest College and quickly realize they share a common bond in their passion for naturopathic medicine and a unified goal in making an impact in medicine and health care. More than 15 student clubs and organizations provide unlimited leadership, educational, social and cultural opportunities, as well as terrific resume-building material and networking opportunities for students. SCNM encourages student involvement in professional and community organizations which can range in variation. Here are just a few of the organization that are here on campus.

SGA is the official voice of the SCNM student body. SGA representatives work closely with students and College administrators to work on policies and identify ways to best serve the campus and its students. SGA also sponsors several services and events, such as New Student Welcome Dinners, student activities, and student club/organizations.

The American Association of Naturopathic Physicians (AANP) is the national professional society representing naturopathic physicians who are licensed or eligible for licensing as primary care providers.

The Arizona Naturopathic Medical Association is the state professional society representing naturopathic physicians who are silenced or eligible for licensure in the state of Arizona.

Homeopathic Society: The purpose of the Homeopathic Society is to broaden and strengthen knowledge of homeopathy through readings and discussions of the Origin of Medicine, Materia Medica, and guest lectures.

Imhotep Circle's mission is to encourage and develop programs that promote unity and contribute to the education, welfare, and growth of underserved communities and the students of SCNM. This organization's goals are to raise funds for local programs, volunteer our time to benefit the underserved communities, and establish programs within the SCNM community that promote our mission.

The Naturopathic Public Awareness Campaign is dedicated to furthering and supporting current and future public awareness efforts for naturopathic medicine in the United States and Canada. In coordination with the AANP and the accredited naturopathic medical schools, we strive to expand public awareness of naturopathic medicine as a viable, affordable option for quality health care. As a strong naturopathic student organization, NPAC is an extremely effective vehicle for public health education and community outreach.

Naturopathic Society International provides educational opportunities and resources concerning Naturopathic Philosophy for physicians and students of naturopathic medicine.

Admissions

REQUIREMENTS

Application, application fee, professional essay, 3 letters of reference, official transcripts, professional resume, and an in-personal interview.

SUGGESTIONS

Visit our website for more information on our program and admission requirements. Please do not hesitate to contact us by phone: 480-858-9100, toll-free: 1-888-882-SCNM (7266), or by e-mail at admissions@scnm.edu with any questions you may have regarding application, naturopathic medicine, relocation, naturopathic career opportunities, etc.

PROCESS

Two intakes a year (spring and fall). Application deadlines: February 1 for the fall intake; December 1 for the spring intake.

Admissions Requirements (Required)

Science GPA, nonscience GPA, letters of recommendation, interview, essays/personal statement, professional resume.

Admissions Requirements (Optional)

MCAT scores, state residency, extracurricular activities, exposure to medical profession.

Overlap Schools

Bastyr University, National College of Naturopathic Medicine.

COSTS AND AID

Tuition & Fees

Tuition	$20,984
Room and board (off campus)	$8,400
Cost of books	$1,940

Financial Aid

% students receiving aid	92
Average grant	$1,000
Average loan	$40,000
Average debt	$120,000

UNIVERSITY OF BRIDGEPORT
COLLEGE OF NATUROPATHIC MEDICINE

126 PARK AVENUE, BRIDGEPORT, CT 06604 • ADMISSION: 203-576-4108 • FAX: 203-576-4941
E-MAIL: NATMED@BRIDGEPORT.EDU • INTERNET: WWW.BRIDGEPORT.EDU

STUDENT BODY

Type	Private
Enrollment	126
% male/female	30/70
# applied	96
# accepted	58
# enrolled	40
Average age	31

FACULTY

Total faculty (number)	32
% female	38
% part-time	78
Student-faculty ratio	4:1

ADMISSIONS

Average GPA

Overall GPA	3.16

Application Information

Are transfers accepted?	yes
Admissions may be deferred?	yes
Interview required?	yes
Application fee	$75

Academics

University of Bridgeport College of Naturopathic Medicine provides an educational program for the training of generalist naturopathic physicians able to competently provide comprehensive natural health care. The college's mission is to provide appropriate educational experiences to prepare candidates to become doctors of naturopathic medicine. UBCNM's mission is to train the next generation of physicians as competent and caring clinicians; as insightful scholars and researchers; and as courageous leaders in the integration of natural medicine into the health care system. The school provides comprehensive natural health care through the Integrated Health Science Center and in conjunction with a variety of community agencies. Students are involved with the research department, which conducts basic and clinical research on natural and alternative therapeutics. Joint degree programs such as ND/MS in Acupuncture and ND/MS in Nutrition are offered. The University of Bridgeport library supports student/faculty research with over 272,000 volumes of classified books and bound journals/indexes, over 1,128,000 microforms, and subscriptions to more than 1,100 periodicals.

BASIC SCIENCES: The first two years of the program focus on basic science courses such as anatomy, physiology, biochemistry, histology, microbiology, embryology, pathology, research methods, public health, clinical and laboratory diagnosis, counseling, nutrition, and history and philosophy of naturopathic medicine. These basic science courses are the foundation of clinical education and training at UBCNM.

CLINICAL TRAINING

The third and fourth year of ND education at UBCNM focuses on clinical education the focus of which is diagnosis and therapeutics which includes botanical medicine, homeopathy, clinical nutrition, physical medicine, obstetrics and gynecology, pediatrics, geriatrics, cardiology, gastroenterology, eye & ENT, diagnostic imaging, pharmacology, environmental medicine, endocrinology, neurology, urology/proctology, oncology, dermatology, and hydrotherapy. Students receive their clinical training at the university's own Health Science Center and at various off-site clinics through supervised internships.

Students

University of Bridgeport was founded in 1927 as the Junior College of Connecticut—the first junior college chartered by any legislature in the Northeastern states. The Junior College of Connecticut became the University of Bridgeport in 1947. The university is located on the 86-acre, picturesque Long Island Sound 50 miles north of New York City. The architectural diversity of UB's 75 buildings, from stately homes as well as newer structures of modern design, reflects the origins and progress of the university and also embodies its twofold commitment to solidity and change. University of Bridgeport offers a wide range of opportunities for students to learn about other cultures and to understand American culture. Students from approximately 80 countries attend the university. The College of Naturopathic Medicine was founded in 1997, and is an integral part of the University of Bridgeport. It is the only college of naturopathic medicine in the Eastern United States. The main Magnus Wahlstrom Library occupies five floors in the centrally located Wahlstrom Building, and supports student/faculty research with over 272,000 volumes of classified books. UB has a large dining hall, café, and recreation center. The university supports a wide range of clubs, organizations, and special interest groups that expand and cultivate the academic, professional, and cultural interests of the students.

STUDENT LIFE

Being a part of the large university, naturopathic students at the University of Bridgeport are always involved in activities with other programs within UB or within the Division of Health Sciences programs which includes naturopathic medicine, chiropractic, the Acupuncture Institute, human nutrition, and dental hygiene. Students are involved in the decision-making process of the university as well as that of the College of Naturopathic Medicine through various committees. The Naturopathic Student Government Association and college administration work very closely.

GRADUATES

Graduates of University of Bridgeport College of Naturopathic Medicine are trained and qualified primary health care professionals who are qualified to pass professional licensure exams and are prepared to set up and maintain private practices. Some of UB's graduates have joined group practices and are part of research teams in various medical universities. Depending on the state laws, their scope of practice varies but includes all aspects of family care.

Admissions

REQUIREMENTS

Applicants must submit a completed application with $75 application fee, personal statement, three letters of recommendation—one must be from a health care provider—and official transcripts from all colleges/universities attended. A bachelors degree is required with 6 semester hours of biology with lab (2 courses), 6 semester hours of general chemistry with lab, 6 semester hours of organic chemistry with lab, 3 semester hours of physics with lab, 3 semester hours of psychology, 6 semester hours (2 courses) of communication/language skills, 3 semester hours of social science, 3 semester hours of humanities, and 9 semester hours of elective courses. Earned grades of C-minus or below are not accepted. All science courses must be completed within the last seven years. Applicants meeting all the requirements are invited for an interview.

SUGGESTIONS

For the fall semester, applications should be received by February 1. The school does have rolling admissions, but it is better to apply early. Late applications are considered on a space available basis.

PROCESS

Acceptance decision is made by the admission committee and is based on academic achievement, relevant experience, knowledge of naturopathic philosophy, personal standard of ethics, financial planning, demonstrated verbal communication ability, and personal attitude.

Admissions Requirements (Required)

Science GPA, nonscience GPA, letters of recommendation, interview, essays/personal statement.

Admissions Requirements (Optional)

State residency, extracurricular activities, exposure to medical profession.

COSTS AND AID

Tuition & Fees

Tuition	$18,000

9 Osteopathic Profiles

A.T. Still University of Health Sciences

Kirksville College of Osteopathic Medicine

800 West Jefferson, Kirksville, MO 63501 • Admission: 660-626-2237 • Fax: 660-626-2969
E-mail: ADMISSIONS@ATSU.EDU • Website: WWW.ATSU.EDU

STUDENT BODY

Type	Private
Enrollment	670
% male/female	60/40
% underrepresented minorities	1
# applied (total/out)	2,634/2,516
# accepted (total/out)	388/348
# enrolled (total/out)	172/144
Average age	25

FACULTY

Total faculty (number)	92
Student-faculty ratio	3:1

ADMISSIONS

Average GPA and MCAT Scores

Overall GPA	3.50
MCAT Bio	8.80
MCAT Phys	8.20
MCAT Verbal	8.23
MCAT Essay	O

Application Information

Regular application	2/1
Regular notification	rolling
Early application	8/1
Early notification	10/15
Are transfers accepted?	yes
Admissions may be deferred?	yes
Interview required?	yes
Application fee	$60

Academics

The Kirksville College of Osteopathic Medicine is the founding school of osteopathic medicine and is distinguished by offering an education firmly based on holistic care, wellness, and academic excellence. Kirksville has a reputation for training physicians in primary care areas, as well as providing a strong clinical and basic science education for specialization. Though the first two years are reserved for basic science instruction, a clerkship with a primary care physician is included in the first-year curriculum. Traditional tenets of osteopathic medicine are coupled with the use of all modern technology, thus providing a well-rounded, comprehensive education. Problem solving and critical thinking are emphasized in both the basic science courses and clinical training. Clinical rotations currently take place in one of the following areas: Arizona, Michigan, Missouri, Ohio, Utah, Colorado, Pennsylvania/New Jersey, and Florida. Kirksville is a community of approximately 20,000 residents. With a 2005 class size of 172, the average age is 25 with a composite MCAT of 25 and an overall GPA of 3.50.

The osteopathic curriculum involves four years of academic study. Reflecting the osteopathic philosophy, the curriculum emphasizes preventive medicine and holistic patient care. Medical students learn to use osteopathic principles and techniques for the diagnosis and treatment of disease.

KCOM students spend the first two years studying the basic sciences and clinical introductions in a classroom setting. The Complete DOctor, a course specific to KCOM, incorporates early clinical experiences with didactic study in medical law and ethics, physical exam skills, cultural diversity and spirituality in medicine, and communication skills.

Third- and fourth-year students have the option of completing their clinical rotations in one of KCOM's National Rotation Regions. These regions currently include Arizona, Colorado, Florida, Michigan, Missouri, New Jersey, and Utah.

After completing osteopathic medical college, DOs serve a one-year internship, gaining hands-on experience in internal medicine, obstetrics/gynecology, general practice, pediatrics, and surgery. This experience ensures that osteopathic physicians are first trained as primary care physicians even if they plan to pursue a specialty. The internship provides every DO with the opportunity to see and treat every patient as a whole person.

After the one-year internship, DOs enroll in a residency program of their choice. A residency typically requires from two to six years of additional training, depending on their chosen area of medicine.

All physicians (both DOs and MDs) must pass a national medical board examination in order to obtain a license. DOs are eligible to take the Comprehensive Osteopathic Medical Licensing Examination (COMLEX-USA) and the United States Medical Licensing Exam (USMLE). There are three parts to each examination that are taken throughout the medical education experience. Additionally, all physicians must pass a state licensing exam. Each state board sets its own requirements and then issues the license for the physician to practice in that state.

Students

STUDENT LIFE

The Admissions program strives to recruit, select, and orientate intellectually and physically healthy applicants. They seek creative, compassionate, and motivated applicants that want to serve humanity. If an applicant is to choose ATSU or ASHS, they must fe safe and be able to secure housing in peaceful and friendly neighborhoods. A student's physiological needs of food, clothing, and protection are assured only if provided with financial assistance and the skills to manage debt.

Students can escape loneliness and alienation while receiving empathy, affection, and a sense of belonging by participating in student organizations, leadership development, and volunteer experiences encouraged and sponsored by Student Affairs.

ATSU students can experience a stable, firmly based level of self respect by being involved in the Still-Well wellness program or by being a member of individual and team sports and exercise programs at the Thompson Campus Center. Emotional and academic support is readily available through Counseling Services and the Learning Resources Office. The Registrar's Office verifies a lifelong record of course work, grades, and the granting of a diploma to recognize significant achievement.

Admissions and Enrollment Services, Counseling Services, Registrar, Financial Assistance, Thompson Campus Center, Learning Resources, and Student Housing are led by Student Affairs professionals enthusiastically dedicated to providing students with result-oriented and personal service. Each office is a high volume, high contact department determined to support the basic needs of students so that they can be competent and compassionate caregivers.

GRADUATES

Top postgraduate programs across the nation seek out our graduates each year. These include traditional and transitional internships as well as prestigious residency programs. Whether you are interested in primary care or a specialty, a KCOM education will ensure your future success!

Internship and residency placements for the class of 2005 include: Anesthesiology, dermatology, diagnostic radiology, emergency medicine, facial plastic surgery, family practice, internal medicine, ob/gyn, ophthalmology, orthopedic surgery, pathology, pediatrics, physical medicine and rehab, psychiatry, and surgery.

Admissions

REQUIREMENTS

As a private institution, no preference is given to Missouri residents, and almost all states are represented in the student body. Course requirements are biology (8 semester hours); chemistry (8 hours), organic chemistry (8 hours), physics (8 hours), and English (6 hours). To be considered for admission, applicants should have a minimum GPA of 2.5 in both the sciences and overall. The MCAT is required and scores must be no more than three years old. About 10 percent of AACOMAS applicants are interviewed, with interviews consisting of two sessions with faculty or administrators. Financial aid, both merit- and need-based, is available in the form of grants and loans.

PROCESS

The Kirksville College of Osteopathic Medicine participates with other osteopathic colleges in a centralized application processing service called the American Association of Colleges of Osteopathic Medicine Application Service (AACOMAS). An application may be submitted online at www.AACOM.org or obtained from AACOMAS, Suite 310, 5550 Friendship Boulevard, Chevy Chase, MD 20815-7231, 301-968-4190.

Applicants meeting the minimum 2.5 cumulative and science grade point average requirement will receive a KCOM Secondary Application. A nonrefundable application fee of $60 and letters of evaluation from the pre-professional college and a physician or employer are required at the time the additional information is submitted. Applications should be submitted no later than February 1 of the academic year prior to which admission is sought. Applicants are encouraged to apply far in advance of the February 1 deadline. As "The National College of Osteopathic Medicine," KCOM seeks students from all parts of the United States who are interested in a career in osteopathic medicine. The college also actively seeks and encourages underrepresented minority students to apply.

Admissions Requirements (Required)

MCAT scores, science GPA, letters of recommendation, interview, essays/personal statement, extracurricular activities, exposure to medical profession.

Admissions Requirements (Optional)

Exposure to osteopathic medicine.

COSTS AND AID

Tuition & Fees

Tuition	$33,255
Room and board (off campus)	$10,010
Cost of books	$2,672
Fees	$690

Financial Aid

% students receiving aid	94
Average grant	$12,740
Average loan	$40,450
Average debt	$151,160

DES MOINES UNIVERSITY
COLLEGE OF OSTEOPATHIC MEDICINE

3200 GRAND AVENUE, DES MOINES, IA 50312-4198 • ADMISSION: 515-271-1451 • FAX: 515-271-7163
E-MAIL: DOADMIT@DMU.EDU • WEBSITE: WWW.DMU.EDU

STUDENT BODY

Type	Private
Enrollment	819
% male/female	52/48
% underrepresented minorities	4
# applied (total/out)	2,387/2,227
# accepted (total/out)	435/359
# enrolled (total/out)	215/156
Average age	25

FACULTY

Total faculty (number)	62
% female	32
% minority	1
% part-time	35
Student-faculty ratio	13:1

ADMISSIONS

Average GPA and MCAT Scores

Overall GPA	3.56
MCAT Bio	8.7
MCAT Phys	8.3
MCAT Verbal	8.2
MCAT Essay	O

Application Information

Regular application	2/1
Regular notification	rolling
Are transfers accepted?	yes
Admissions may be deferred?	yes
Interview required?	yes
Application fee	$50

Academics

At the Des Moines University College of Osteopathic Medicine, students learn within a supportive environment. This includes a solid basic sciences education, extensive practical experience in the clinical setting, and one-on-one interaction with seasoned educators and clinicians. The curriculum emphasizes state-of-the-art standardized patient assessment laboratories and problem-based learning opportunities, which emphasize critical thinking and problem solving. The college is the second-oldest osteopathic school in the country. Located in a safe metropolitan setting, the campus offers proximity to affordable housing. A new 143,000-square-foot Student Education Center provides students with modern facilities and a location to exercise, relax, and learn. Other distinguishing features of DMU include the following: a wireless campus, laptops, hand-held computers for incoming students, and a dual master's degree program in health care administration or public health.

BASIC SCIENCES: The College of Osteopathic Medicine provides a flexible program that allows students to explore a range of professional goals. Students learn to consider the overall needs of the patient rather than an isolated medical problem. During the first two years, basic science lectures and laboratory studies are combined with experience in hospitals, clinics, and community-service agencies. This pre-clinical phase features a systems approach and the innovative use of simulated patients. The last two years of the four-year program involve clinical training. Third- and fourth-year rotations in hospitals and clinics may be selected from sites across the country.

Students

STUDENT LIFE

Each entering class has about 210 students. A wide variety of undergraduate majors are represented, ranging from biology to the humanities. Though the average age of incoming students is 25, student ages range from the early 20s to 50s. Beyond classes and labs, students have numerous opportunities to get involved and meet others through community service, clubs, and social events. From the beginning, first-year students are paired up with second-year students as part of Big Brother/Little Sister. DMU also offers peer tutoring. More than 30 professional clubs and organizations invite students to become part of a larger community of students and student concerns. Many students also get involved in community outreach. Through La Clinica they provide free medical care. The Literacy Army tutors reading and other subjects to elementary schools. At various local races and marathons DMU students have provided free OMM to the involved athletes.

GRADUATES

Graduates may enter residency programs in any specialty or subspecialty area. Des Moines University has over 8,600 alumni in virtually every state in the nation.

Admissions

REQUIREMENTS

Eight semester hours (with lab) each in biology, chemistry, organic chemistry, and physics are required. In addition, applicants must have taken six semester hours of English. We accept students without regard to legal state of residence. Usually 75 percent of students are from states other than Iowa. You can apply while working on your undergraduate degree, but you should have plans to receive it by the time you register with the college. The MCAT (taken within the last two years) is required. Those AACOMAS applicants who meet the minimum requirements for GPA and MCAT are sent secondary applications and about half of those who return secondary applications are invited for an interview. Notification occurs on a rolling basis.

Admissions Requirements (Required)

MCAT scores, science GPA, non-science GPA, letters of recommendation, interview, essays/personal statement, extracurricular activities, exposure to medical profession.

Admissions Requirements (Optional)

State residency.

Overlap Schools

A.T. Still University of Health Sciences, Kansas City University of Medicine and Biosciences, Michigan State University, Midwestern University, New York Institute of Technology.

COSTS AND AID

Tuition & Fees

Tuition	$30,210
Room and board (off campus)	$12,690
Cost of books	$3,050

Financial Aid

% students receiving aid	96
Average grant	$22,287
Average loan	$37,426
Average debt	$146,940

KANSAS CITY UNIVERSITY OF MEDICINE AND BIOSCIENCES
COLLEGE OF OSTEOPATHIC MEDICINE

OFFICE OF ADMISSIONS, 1750 INDEPENDENCE AVENUE, KANSAS CITY, MO 64106-1453 • ADMISSION: 800-234-4847
FAX: 816-460-0566 • E-MAIL: ADMISSIONS@KCUMB.EDU • WEBSITE: WWW.KCUMB.EDU

STUDENT BODY

Type	Private
Enrollment	887
% male/female	50/50
% underrepresented minorities	18
# applied (total/out)	2,400/1,926
# accepted (total/out)	487/433
# enrolled (total/out)	250/199
Average age	24

FACULTY

Total faculty (number)	54
% female	54
% minority	6
% part-time	100
Student-faculty ratio	8:1

ADMISSIONS

Average GPA and MCAT Scores

Overall GPA	3.45
MCAT Bio	8.64
MCAT Phys	8.13
MCAT Verbal	8.09
MCAT Essay	Q

Application Information

Regular application	2/6
Regular notification	rolling
Early application	Fall
Early notification	11/6
Are transfers accepted?	no
Admissions may be deferred?	yes
Interview required?	yes
Application fee	$50

Academics

Kansas City University of Medicine and Biosciences is both the largest medical school in the state of Missouri and the oldest in Kansas City, Missouri. Affordable and friendly, Kansas City's metropolitan area encompasses counties in both Kansas and Missouri. The university's core values are leadership, humility, faith and positivity, integrity, compassion, and service. These core values, coupled with exemplary basic sciences and clinical training, are at the heart of the KCUMB educational process from a student's first day on campus to the end of postdoctoral training and beyond. In 2006, 51 percent of the entering class was female, and the average age was 24. The age range of the class was 20–48 with a class size of 250. During their years at KCUMB, the university helps its students build on that foundation by offering a progressive and innovative twenty-first century curriculum that emphasizes early clinical experience and an integrated, patient-centered approach to medicine. An outstanding faculty who keep students' interests uppermost and state-of-the-art facilities provide unparalleled educational opportunities. High standards and educational excellence make KCUMB an award-winning academic institution, but it is the human dimension that makes KCUMB such a meaningful and special place.

CLINICAL TRAINING

KCUMB puts the patient at the center of the learning process with an innovative new curriculum. This curriculum eliminates the artificial separation of the basic and clinical sciences, integrating all essential concepts and information into a seamless continuum of clinical presentations. The foundations of anatomy, biochemistry, epidemiology, genetics, immunology, ob/gyn pathology, pharmacology, physiology, and the clinical disciplines of family medicine, internal medicine, pediatrics, surgery, and psychiatry are incorporated into clinical presentations. Topics such as health-care policy, medical informatics, and health and wellness are integrated into the curricular structure.

The case-based, patient-centered curriculum prepares students to begin analyzing and integrating medical information in a format used by medical practitioners. This approach integrates the basic and clinical sciences from the first day of medical school, rather than the traditional postponing of meaningful clinical interaction and decision-making until the third year of medical school.

A variety of teaching and learning methods are used in the first two years. These methods include classroom lectures, laboratory exercises, small-group discussions, computer-assisted instruction, specialized workshops, the use of standardized patients, and other simulated clinical activities.

Students

While the Kansas City area might be best known for its smooth jazz, beautiful fountains, and superior barbecue, the area has so much to offer, from upscale shopping districts and world-class entertainment, to ample recreational activities and thrilling professional sporting events. Located at the junction of the Missouri and Kansas rivers, Kansas City sits in the middle of the United States, about 1,900 miles from each coast. Approximately 1.8 million people live in the Kansas City metro area, which includes more than 135 cities in 11 counties on both sides of the state line.

In the historic northeast area of Kansas City, the KCUMB campus is just minutes from the Country Club Plaza, Arrowhead and Kauffman stadiums, the Nelson-Atkins Museum of Art, the Negro Leagues Baseball Museum, Worlds of Fun, Oceans of Fun, Union Station and the River Market. The city and its surrounding communities offer a combination of urban sophistication and small-town friendliness that is distinctly Kansas City.

Admissions

REQUIREMENTS

The minimum academic requirements for admission to the first-year class are as follows:

- The Medical College Admissions Test (MCAT). The MCAT is administered in April and August of every year. If applying for the 2006 entering class, only April 2003 through August 2005 scores will be accepted.

- A baccalaureate degree or commendable completion of at least 90 semester hours or 135 term credit hours of the required credits for a baccalaureate degree, from a regionally accredited college or university. The baccalaureate degree is preferred and preference is given to those candidates who will have earned the degree prior to matriculation in the medical school program.

- Satisfactory completion, with a grade of C or higher, of the following college courses, including laboratory work: Biological sciences (12 semester hours), biochemistry (3 hours in addition to chemistry hours), chemistry (13 semester hours), English composition/literature (six semester hours), genetics (3 semester hours in addition to biological sciences), physics (eight semester hours). Total number of semester hours equals 45.

SUGGESTIONS

Applicants are encouraged to begin the application process a year prior to matriculation. The following represents a monthly guide for application preparation:

- May: Contact all colleges and universities attended and have official transcripts forwarded directly from the educational institution to AACOMAS. Submit AACOMAS application. Supplemental application or materials are mailed to qualified applicants immediately upon receipt of the AACOMAS application in the Admissions Office.

- September: Personal interviews begin.

- February 1: Application deadline (AACOMAS). Supplemental applications are accepted and processed until all interview positions have been filled.

- February 15: Transcript deadline to AACOMAS.

PROCESS

AACOMAS online is available in early May 2006 for the 2007 entering class. All application materials, including detailed instructions, can be accessed through the AACOM website, http://www.aacom.org.

AACOMAS gathers all the necessary material about each applicant and transmits the information in a standardized format to the college(s) of osteopathic medicine selected by the applicant. AACOMAS has no participation in the selection process.

The applicant will receive a computer-generated applicant profile with a calculation of GPA and MCAT averages from AACOMAS. KCUMB will also receive the applicant profile, accompanied by a photocopy of the AACOMAS application and personal statement. KCUMB conducts an initial review of the transmitted AACOMAS application, MCAT scores, and academic record to determine which applications will be further processed.

Applicants meeting the initial review criteria will receive a KCUMB supplemental application. A supplemental application may be forwarded to an applicant under some circumstances when specific information is not available or will be submitted later. These circumstances generally relate to applicants who have not taken the MCAT and/or are registered to take the next scheduled MCAT exam. Applicants are encouraged to include the scheduled MCAT test dates on the AACOMAS application to indicate the intent of taking or retaking the exam.

Admissions Requirements (Required)

MCAT scores, science GPA, non-science GPA, letters of recommendation, interview, essays/personal statement, extracurricular activities, exposure to medical profession, community service/volunteer work.

Admissions Requirements (Optional)

State residency.

Overlap Schools

A.T. Still University of Health Sciences, Des Moines University.

COSTS AND AID

Tuition & Fees

Tuition	$35,055
Room and board (off campus)	$15,174
Cost of books	$2,300
Fees	$60

Financial Aid

% students receiving aid	96
Average grant	$1,500
Average loan	$40,000
Average debt	$154,000

LAKE ERIE COLLEGE OF OSTEOPATHIC MEDICINE

OFFICE OF ADMISSIONS, 1858 WEST GRANDVIEW BOULEVARD, ERIE, PA 16509 • ADMISSION: 814-866-6641
FAX: 814-866-8123 • EMAIL: ADMISSIONS@LECOM.EDU • WEBSITE: WWW.LECOM.EDU

STUDENT BODY

Type	Private
Enrollment	1206
% male/female	54/46
% underrepresented minorities	8
# applied (total/out)	4,251/2,681

FACULTY

Total faculty (number)	1,247
% part-time	93
Student-faculty ratio	1:1

ADMISSIONS

Application Information

Regular application	3/1
Regular notification	rolling
Are transfers accepted?	no
Admissions may be deferred?	no
Interview required?	yes
Application fee	$50

Academics

Lake Erie College of Osteopathic Medicine located in Erie, Pennsylvania with a branch campus in Bradenton, Florida, is the nation's second largest medical college. Its mission is to train physicians to meet the country's growing demand for health care professionals. The majority of LECOM graduates become primary care physicians. LECOM recognizes student-centered learning styles by offering three curriculum pathways. The traditional, lecture-discussion curriculum begins with core basic science and pre-clinical courses and progresses with a systems-based curriculum in year two. Problem-based learning offers small-group training following patient cases and Independent Study allows qualified students to use educational modules based on the core and systems curriculums.

BASIC SCIENCES: All students are required to complete 12 weeks of gross anatomy in the first semester. Microbiology, immunology, physiology, pharmacology, biochemistry, pathology, health care management, and spirituality, medicine, and ethics are the core of the Lecture-Discussion and Independent Study Pathways and integrated into the cases of the Problem-Based Learning Pathway.

CLINICAL TRAINING

Clinical training at LECOM begins in the first year as students spend time in local physician offices. LECOM has affiliations with more than 100 hospitals in a dozen states where third-year and fourth-year students complete their clinical rotations.

Admissions

REQUIREMENTS

LECOM is a private college and a majority of students come from out of state. Students are required to apply through AACOMAS, the central processor for osteopathic colleges. Applicants may download the LECOM Supplemental application from the college web site or one will be mailed upon receipt of the AACOMAS application. LECOM schedules interviews between October and March. Acceptance notification occurs on a rolling basis. The MCAT is required and must be no more than three years old. The mean MCAT score for successful candidates is 24 and their science GPA is a 3.2 or higher. The college requires two letters of recommendation and a letter from an osteopathic physician. Science course requirements are: 8 semester hours of biology, chemistry, organic chemistry, and physics. In addition, 6 semester hours of English and behavioral science are required.

SUGGESTIONS

LECOM encourages applicants to learn more about the profession by getting to know an osteopathic physician to enhance awareness of the osteopathic medical philosophy and prepare for the admissions interview. The college looks for students who exemplify the osteopathic philosophy of compassionate, total person health care.

Students

LECOM's main campus is located in Pennsylvania's fourth largest city and overlooks Lake Erie. The city is a resort community with a large number of tourist, entertainment, and recreational facilities. Erie County has five colleges and supports several professional minor league teams in baseball, football, and hockey. LECOM Bradenton is located in a master-planned community in one of the fastest growing regions of Florida.

STUDENT LIFE

LECOM encourages students to participate in community service and extracurricular activities. LECOM clubs offer social activities and opportunities to become involved in local events. LECOM students have organized mentoring programs for underserved children, Boy Scout and Girl Scout Troops, and provided health care screening and other related services to local citizens.

GRADUATES

While the majority of LECOM graduates become primary care physicians, many alumni have completed residencies and fellowships in other medical specialties. LECOM has developed postgraduate training at 26 hospitals. Graduates have matched for residencies at major hospitals around the country.

MICHIGAN STATE UNIVERSITY
COLLEGE OF OSTEOPATHIC MEDICINE

C110 EAST FEE HALL, MSUCOM, EAST LANSING, MI 48824-1316 • ADMISSION: 517-353-7740
FAX: 517-355-3296 • E-MAIL: COMADM@COM.MSU.EDU • WEBSITE: WWW.COM.MSU.EDU

STUDENT BODY

Type	Public
Enrollment	556
% male/female	54/46
% underrepresented minorities	6
# applied (total/out)	1,621/1,224
# accepted (total/out)	194/24
# enrolled (total/out)	124/5
Average age	25

FACULTY

Total faculty (number)	177
% female	37
% minority	19
% part-time	11
Student-faculty ratio	3:1

ADMISSIONS

Average GPA and MCAT Scores

Overall GPA	3.5
MCAT Bio	8.7
MCAT Phys	8.0
MCAT Verbal	8.2
MCAT Essay	O

Application Information

Regular application	12/1
Regular notification	rolling
Early application	8/15
Early notification	10/15
Are transfers accepted?	yes
Admissions may be deferred?	yes
Interview required?	yes
Application fee	$75

Academics

The Michigan State University College of Osteopathic Medicine (MSUCOM) was created by the Michigan legislature in 1971 to provide osteopathic physicians to meet the health care needs of the state's population. Educating primary care and specialty care osteopathic physicians occurs in a spectrum that includes premedical programs, osteopathic medical college, internships, residencies, and fellowships. The college has partnerships for clinical education with 20 osteopathic hospitals in Michigan in its Statewide Campus System, and it also occurs in private clinics and other environments. Medical research is a high priority of the college, and MSUCOM provides educational opportunities for physician/scientists, especially in its joint DO/PhD curriculum, the Medical Scientist Training Program. The curriculum, based on a study of the body's organ systems, emphasizes osteopathic principles and practices, early patient care, behavioral and diversity aspects of medicine, lifelong learning, and use of technology. The smallest college in university with nearly 45,000 students, MSUCOM is a close-knit community known for compassionate care and its volunteer work in the communities. For further information, see www.com.msu.edu.

The Michigan State University College of Osteopathic Medicine (MSUCOM) provides a full continuum of education—premedical programs, osteopathic medical school, internships, residencies, fellowships, and continuing medical education. The college has partnerships for clinical education with 25 hospitals in its Statewide Campus System and with nearly 2,000 clinical faculty practicing in communities.

Students learn from a faculty of top-flight educators in the heart of one of the premier scientific and research institutions in the nation. The curriculum emphasizes patient-centered care, osteopathic principles and practices, early exposure to the clinical setting, behavioral and diversity aspects of medicine, lifelong learning, and the use of technology.

The college offers the nation's first DO/PhD program; the MA in bioethics, humanities, and society; a joint DO/MPH; and the Osteopathic Medical Scholars Program for undergraduate students.

BASIC SCIENCES: Unit I is a four-semester sequence of basic science courses including anatomy, biochemistry, molecular biology/genetics, neuroscience, radiology, microbiology, histology, cell biology/physiology, pathology, and pharmacology. Students are introduced to physical examination, doctor-patient interactions, and the principles of osteopathic palpatory diagnosis and manipulative therapy.

Unit II is a three-semester sequence with an emphasis on body systems: integumentary, neuromusculoskeletal, hematopoietic, cardiovascular, respiratory, gastrointestinal, endocrine, genitourinary, reproductive, growth and development, and behavioral systems. These courses provide integrated presentations of basic and behavioral science and clinical aspects of each system. Students are required to master clinical skills associated with each system and to observe and selectively participate in patient care and office management under the direct supervision of a physician.

Unit III, the clerkship curriculum is a 76–84-week program designed to equip osteopathic physicians with skills necessary to enter primary care practice or pursue further specialty training. There is an emphasis on preparing for practice in ambulatory settings, with continuity in training and experience in working with allied health professionals in a team approach.

Students

Located on one of largest and most beautiful campuses in the nation, MSUCOM offers all the benefits of a fine university—from world-class arts and entertainment to Big Ten sports, from daily seminars and performances to research that spans hundreds of disciplines. Nearly 45,000 students from all over the world attend MSU, offering diversity and a rich cultural exposure.

STUDENT LIFE

Because academic life is so rigorous at MSUCOM, students must be highly motivated and organized to maintain a healthy life balance. The college maintains an active array of events, social options, extracurricular learning opportunities, and student support services. MSUCOM has a strong reputation as an institution that values the individual, cooperation, compassion, excellence, and community service.

GRADUATES

Wherever MSUCOM graduates live and work, their caring and commitment have made an impact on the communities they serve. Among our alumni are medical school deans, nationally recognized researchers in areas such as cardiovascular disease and genomics, a former surgeon general of the U.S. Coast Guard, the head of the largest U.S. study concerning women's health, the forensic psychiatrist who worked on the Jon Benet Ramsey, Columbine High School, and Kobe Bryant cases, and a physician who has received international attention for her decades of work with the poor in Mississippi.

Admissions Requirements

To satisfy the requirements, students must achieve a 2.0 grade in the required number of credit hours for each subject area. Students are required to have at least 8 credits of biology, but preferably 16–20 advanced level credits (biology, physiology, microbiology, anatomy, neuroscience, etc.)—AP credits are not accepted; 8 credits of physics; 6 credits of English; 6 credits of behavioral science, and a minimum total of 90 completed credit hours. There are prerequisite changes pending; please see the website for additional information.

The average for each entering class has consistently been 3.5. Most important are your grades in upper level science classes. The average MCAT for each entering class has ranged from 26–27. Community service is a heavily weighted factor. You must have experience in a clinical setting to be considered, but this can also include paid employment, shadowing, or other voluntarism. We require two recommendations (the individuals should know you well).

For additional information on other admission factors, see our website. We also suggest starting admissions counseling early in your admissions process: Call us at 517-353-7740 to schedule your appointment.

ADMISSIONS PROCESS

MSUCOM employs an aggressive rolling admission process with the goal of filling the class by early December.

* The AACOMAS Application Service website (www.aacom.org) begins taking applications May 15. For MSUCOM, December 1 is the last day AACOMAS accepts applications and December 15 is the last day AACOMAS accepts transcripts. However, September 1 is the last day you should be submitting your AACOMAS application if you are serious about applying to MSUCOM.

Admissions Requirements (Required)

MCAT scores, science GPA, non-science GPA, letters of recommendation, interview, essays/personal statement, extracurricular activities, exposure to medical profession.

Admissions Requirements (Optional)

State residency.

COSTS AND AID

Tuition & Fees

In-state Tuition	$21,951
Out-of-state Tuition	$47,751
Room and board (on campus)	$10,656
Cost of books	$2,605
Fees	$85

Financial Aid

% students receiving aid	93
Average grant	$2,720
Average loan	$25,455
Average debt	$117,220

MIDWESTERN UNIVERSITY
ARIZONA COLLEGE OF OSTEOPATHIC MEDICINE

OFFICE OF ADMISSIONS, 19555 NORTH 59TH AVENUE, GLENDALE, AZ 85308 • ADMISSION: 623-572-3275
FAX: 623-572-3229 • E-MAIL: ADMISSAZ@ARIZONA.MIDWESTERN.EDU • WEBSITE: WWW.MIDWESTERN.EDU

STUDENT BODY

Type	Private
Enrollment	558
% male/female	63/37
% underrepresented minorities	54
# applied (total/out)	2,359/2,233
# accepted (total/out)	340/297
# enrolled (total/out)	142/119
Average age	26

ADMISSIONS

Average GPA and MCAT Scores

Overall GPA	3.37
MCAT Bio	9.0
MCAT Phys	9.0
MCAT Verbal	8.7
MCAT Essay	0

Application Information

Regular application	1/2
Regular notification	3/1
Are transfers accepted?	yes
Admissions may be deferred?	yes
Interview required?	yes
Application fee	$50

Academics

The Arizona College of Osteopathic Medicine (AZCOM) was founded in 1995. The college, along with its sister college, the Chicago College of Osteopathic Medicine (CCOM), is part of Midwestern University. In addition to the Colleges of Osteopathic Medicine, Midwestern University also includes a college of pharmacy and a college of health sciences. The school is located on a 124-acre site in scenic Glendale, Arizona, a suburb of Phoenix. Facilities include three main academic centers housing lecture halls; conference rooms; a student services facility; numerous lecture and laboratory classrooms boasting the finest in educational equipment; cadavers for anatomy laboratories rather than plastic models; on-campus housing, which features one- and two-bedroom student apartments and a heated pool; a comprehensive library with computer resources and study rooms; a research facility; a clinic; and a student clubhouse. The mission of Arizona College of Osteopathic Medicine of Midewestern University responds to the contemporary societal need for physicians by emphasizing primary care and education experiences needed to serve in rural and underserved urban communities.

Admissions

REQUIREMENTS

As a private institution, the college attracts a national applicant pool, and out-of-state residents account for over 80 percent of the group. Only 145 positions are available in each class, and in recent years there have been over 3,000 applicants. The average GPA of successful applicants is about 3.4 in both sciences and overall. Minimum course work includes six semester hours in English and eight semester hours in each of the following: biology, inorganic chemistry, organic chemistry, and physics. The MCAT is required and must be no more than three years old. In addition to the AACOMAS application, applicants must submit a supplemental application (provided by the AZCOM after the AACOMAS application has been received and the student meets the GPA criteria of 2.75 in both science and overall).

PROCESS

To be considered for admission within our competitive selection process, one must possess:

1. To be competitive, an applicant should possess both a science and a total GPA over 3.00 on a 4.00 scale as well as a bachelor's degree. A minimum science and overall GPA of 2.75 on a 4.00 scale is required to receive a supplemental application.

2. Complete a bachelor's degree at an accredited college or university prior to matriculation. Applicants participating in special affiliated programs with the college and other exceptions to this policy will be considered on an individual basis.

3. Submit competitive scores on the Medical College Admissions Test (MCAT). Students who entered AZCOM in 2005 had an average MCAT score of 27. The MCAT test must have been taken no more than 3 years prior to application. To register for the exam contact the MCAT Program Office at 319-337-1357, or visit www.aamc.org/students/mcat. The exam is offered each April and August.

4. Two letters of recommendation are required. One must be from either the premedical advisory committee or science professor; the other must be from either a DO or an MD. Letters from osteopathic physicians are strongly recommended. Letters written by immediate family members will not be accepted. All letters of evaluation must be submitted by the evaluators. The Office of Admissions does not accept letters submitted by students.

5. Demonstrate a sincere understanding of and interest in osteopathic medicine.

6. Reflect a people/service orientation through community service or extracurricular activities.

7. Reflect proper motivation for and commitment to health care as demonstrated by previous work, volunteer, or other life experiences.

8. Possess the oral and written communication skills necessary to interact with patients and colleagues.

9. Pass a criminal background check.

Agree to abide by Midwestern University Drug-Free Workplace and Substance Abuse Policy.

Admissions Requirements (Required)

MCAT scores, science GPA, non-science GPA, letters of recommendation, interview, essays/personal statement, extracurricular activities, exposure to medical profession, letter from a DO or MD.

Admissions Requirements (Optional)

State residency.

Overlap Schools

Midwestern University.

COSTS AND AID

Tuition & Fees

Tuition	$34,099
Room and board (on campus)	$4,376
Cost of books	$2,060
Fees	$225

Financial Aid

% students receiving aid	90
Average grant	$1,910
Average loan	$23,500

MIDWESTERN UNIVERSITY
CHICAGO COLLEGE OF OSTEOPATHIC MEDICINE

OFFICE OF ADMISSIONS, 555 31ST STREET, DOWNERS GROVE, IL 60515 • ADMISSION: 800-458-6253
FAX: 630-971-6086 • E-MAIL: ADMISSIL@MIDWESTERN.EDU • WEBSITE: WWW.MIDWESTERN.EDU

STUDENT BODY

Type	Private
Enrollment	690
% male/female	47/53
% underrepresented minorities	28
# applied	3,200
# accepted	380
# enrolled	173
Average age	24

FACULTY

Total faculty (number)	294
% female	23
% minority	11
% part-time	50
Student-faculty ratio	2:1

ADMISSIONS

Average GPA and MCAT Scores

Overall GPA	3.5
MCAT Bio	9.0
MCAT Phys	8.3
MCAT Verbal	8.5
MCAT Essay	O

Application Information

Regular application	1/1
Regular notification	rolling
Are transfers accepted?	yes
Admissions may be deferred?	yes
Interview required?	yes
Application fee	$50

Academics

Midwestern University administers the Chicago College of Osteopathic Medicine (CCOM), the Chicago College of Pharmacy, and the College of Health Sciences, in addition to related programs in Glendale, Arizona. The MWU campus is located in Downers Grove, which is a western suburb of Chicago, Illinois. Clinical training takes place at various sites around the city and throughout the Midwest region. Students enjoy early clinical exposure through volunteering, preceptor programs, and formal patient contact in the second quarter of year one. Research is also important at CCOM, which offers a combined DO/PhD program and has summer research awards for medical students. The Downers Grove campus offers modern academic and recreational facilities, in addition to on-campus housing. In Fall 2005, the Downers Grove campus enrolled a total of 1,884 students in its various professional degree seeking programs.

BASIC SCIENCE: CCOM has developed and continues to refine a four-year curriculum that educates students in the biopsychosocial approach to patient care, as well as the basic medical arts and sciences. Within this curricular format, CCOM students spend their first two years both completing a rigorous basic science curriculum and preparing for their clinical studies. During their third and fourth years, students rotate through a variety of clinical training sites accruing an impressive 92 weeks of direct patient care experience

CLINICAL TRAINING

Students begin obtaining hands-on experience during their first year through the introduction to clinical medicine courses that are taught within the program. Students must complete and successfully pass required clinical rotations in the following disciplines: family medicine, internal medicine, surgery, pediatrics, psychiatry, osteopathic manipulative medicine, obstetrics/gynecology, and emergency medicine. These rotations cannot be done at out-of-system sites. Students must also complete elective rotations in recognized fields of medicine that include the following areas: anesthesiology, cardiology, family medicine (division of community medicine), osteopathic manipulative medicine (additional rotation), dermatology, emergency medicine (additional rotation), gastroenterology, hematology/oncology, infectious disease, nephrology, neurology, neurosurgery, nuclear medicine/endocrinology/metabolism, obstetrics/gynecology (clinical and/or elective at Olympia Fields), ophthalmology, orthopedic surgery, otorhinolaryngology, pathology, rheumatology/immunology, general surgery (additional rotation), cardiovascular/thoracic surgery, and urology. Students can pursue clinical rotations at other osteopathic, allopathic, or military institutions; however, they must plan their elective program with the Office of Clinical Education in order to obtain academic credit for these rotations. In the past, students have also had an opportunity to complete one international rotation as an elective rotation.

Student Life

Believing that well-rounded individuals make more caring health care professionals, we offer our students a variety of social, academic, and personal enrichment activities. Midwestern University offers a few different housing options for students through traditional style residence halls and one bedroom apartments. Most of the facilities are designed to be single occupancy. MWU provides a variety of student services outside of the classroom for students. Our website highlights the student organizations, intramural sports, wellness center, tutoring services, and counseling services that are available for students. Please refer to www.midwestern.edu for additional information.

GRADUATES

CCOM's class of 2004 matched into 72 programs in 19 states. The graduates' match rate was 87.8 percent into a first or second residency choice, far surpassing the national match rate of 61.9 percent.

Admissions

REQUIREMENTS

Minimum overall and science GPAs of 2.75 on 4.00 scale, MCAT scores, AACOMAS application, secondary application materials, letters of recommendation, and an interview are required. Additional admission requirements can be found on our website at www.midwestern.edu.

PROCESS

Students may begin the application process through AACOMAS and must submit the AACOMAS application with all required materials by January 1 of a given year. Midwestern University will distribute a secondary application to those applicants meeting the minimum GPA requirements. The secondary application must be submitted to the Office of Admissions with all required materials by March 1 of a given year. Midwestern University operates on a rolling admissions basis. As completed applications are submitted, they are reviewed and considered for admission into the program. Competitive applicants will be invited on campus to participate in the interview process. The admissions committee for the Chicago College of Osteopathic Medicine meets approximately once a month to make final admissions decisions.

Admissions Requirements (Required)

MCAT scores, science GPA, non-science GPA, letters of recommendation, interview, essays/personal statement, extracurricular activities, exposure to medical profession, oral and written communication skills.

Admissions Requirements (Optional)

State residency.

COSTS AND AID

Tuition & Fees

Tuition	$31,838
Room and board (on campus)	$9.400
Cost of books	$2,300
Fees	$412

Financial Aid

% students receiving aid	85
Average grant	$12,000
Average loan	$40,500
Average debt	$150,000

NEW YORK INSTITUTE OF TECHNOLOGY
NEW YORK COLLEGE OF OSTEOPATHIC MEDICINE

OFFICE OF ADMISSIONS, NYCOM/NYIT, PO BOX 8000, OLD WESTBURY, NY 11568 • ADMISSION: 516-686-3747
FAX: 516-686-3831 E-MAIL: ADMISSIONS@NYIT.EDU • WEBSITE: WWW.NYIT.EDU

STUDENT BODY

Type	Private
% male/female	60/40
% underrepresented minorities	16

ADMISSIONS

Application Information

Regular application	2/1
Are transfers accepted?	no
Admissions may be deferred?	no
Interview required?	yes

Academics

The New York College of Osteopathic Medicine is committed to educating primary care physicians and the focus is on the health care problems of the inner city and rural communities. NYCOM allows incoming students to select one of two educational tracks: The Lecture-Discussion Based (LDB) track integrates the biomedical and clinical sciences through a systems-based approach, while the Doctor Patient Continuum (DPC) employs a problem-based curriculum whose cornerstone is small-group, case-based learning. The two tracks converge after completion of the second year, when clerkships in the third and fourth years provide students with a variety of clinical experiences. In addition to the four-year DO degree, combined DO/MBA and DO/MS programs are also open to qualified students.

BASIC SCIENCES: Depending on the track they select, the first- and second-year curriculum in basic and clinical sciences will differ for students.

(LDB) track: Here, the courses in the first two years are organized in a systems-based format. The systems are preceded by a fundamentals course, and the fundamentals course is composed of three components (threads): The cellular and molecular basis of medicine; the structural and functional basis of medicine; and the practice of medicine. The cellular and molecular basis of medicine thread discusses the scientific principles specific to each organ system as it relates to wellness and disease and includes content material from the following disciplines: biochemistry, genetics, histology, microbiology, neuroscience, pathology, pharmacology, and physiology. The structural and functional basis of medicine thread uses a systems-specific approach to discuss the interrelationship between structure and function in wellness and disease, and incorporates extensive didactic and laboratory experiences in applied anatomy and osteopathic principles and practices. In year 2 students take the practice of medicine, a systems-based introduction to the essentials of clinical medicine. It presents the principles of patient-centered health care, emphasizing primary care in the pediatric, adult, and geriatric patient populations. It includes didactic and practical experiences in the doctor-patient relationship, as well as simulated clinical exercises.

(DPC) Track: This problem-based curriculum is founded on "continuum" education principles and instruction is set in the context of clinical-case scenarios. The cases function as an interface between the patient and the physician, in which the skills, knowledge, and attitudes of the practicing clinician will later be applied. The curricular content is rooted in evidence-based medicine and students are expected to explore aspects of health and disease pertinent to the clinical case at seven levels: molecular; cellular; tissue; organ; integrated organ system; whole person; and family, society, and environment. The DPC curriculum is highly student-centered and promotes the development of critical thinking and clinical problem-solving skills. Course work in the DPC curriculum during the first two years includes: Introduction to the fundamentals of osteopathic medicine; cellular and molecular; structure and function; the practice of medicine; and a series of courses in biomedical and clinical sciences. Second-year courses in the clinical sciences include didactic and laboratory experiences in osteopathic manipulative medicine and physical diagnosis, as well as experiences with standardized and simulated patients.

CLINICAL TRAINING

NYCOM students spend most of their third and fourth years doing clinical clerkships. An equitable lottery system determines how the students are assigned to clerkships. Required third-year clinical clerkships include: Family medicine (6 weeks); medicine (12 weeks); ob/gyn (6 weeks); pediatrics (6 weeks); psychiatry (6 weeks); and surgery (12 weeks). Fourth-year students complete a set of clinical clerkships including: two sub-internships in medicine, pediatrics, surgery, ob/gyn, psychiatry, or family medicine (4 weeks each); emergency medicine (4 weeks); radiology (4 weeks); a preceptorship with a board-certified DO (4 weeks); two selectives in medicine, pediatrics, surgery, or ob/gyn.(4 weeks each); and 3 electives (4 weeks each). Students often use the fourth-year clerkships to highlight their competencies to potential postgraduate training institutions. Students are encouraged to integrate structural evaluations and osteopathic manipulative medicine throughout all clerkships.

STUDENTS

NYCOM offers a great education in one of the world's largest cultural centers. New York City provides students with an exciting life outside of the classroom, from world-renowned arts and entertainment, to exciting sports teams, great dining, and an incredible colloquium of educational resources across all disciplines.

STUDENT LIFE

The numerous student associations on campus include the American Medical Woman's Association, the Christian Student Fellowship, and Project for Latino Health and provide an invaluable support network for student-physicians and their families.

GRADUATES

NYCOM graduates make an impact on the communities they serve. Historically, NYCOM students have matched well before graduation and are ready and able to meet professional challenges.

ADMISSIONS

REQUIREMENTS

Applicants for admission into the 4 year medical program must first meet the following academic requirements prior to matriculation: Obtained a baccalaureate degree from an accredited college or university; achieved a pre-professional science grade point average of at least 2.75/4.0 and an overall grade point average of at least 2.75/4.0; completed eight semester hours of biology, chemistry, organic chemistry, and physics, in addition to six semester hours of English. The MCAT is required and scores must not be more than 3 years old.

SUGGESTIONS

In assessing an applicant for admission, NYCOM evaluates the whole record, environment, initiative, and circumstances of each applicant. Applicants are encouraged to take additional courses such as calculus, comparative anatomy, genetics, physical chemistry, biochemistry, and behavioral and neurosciences. Volunteer or professional work is another way students can express their commitment to the healing profession. The educational process at NYCOM relies heavily on modern educational technologies as well as good study and organizational skills of the students. Therefore, all potential students are expected to prepare themselves well on these fronts.

PROCESS

The New York College of Osteopathic Medicine participates with other colleges of osteopathic medicine in the American Association of Colleges of Osteopathic Medicine Application Service (AACOMAS). About 20 percent of AACOMAS applicants are interviewed, with interviews taking place between November and May. The supplementary application is given to candidates at the time of the interview. Interviews are conducted with basic science faculty and/or osteopathic physicians from the community. Preference is given to New York residents and to residents of states in the northeastern United States.

Admissions Requirements (Required)

Science GPA, nonscience GPA, letters of recommendation, interview, state residency, extracurricular activities, exposure to medical profession.

Admissions Requirements (Optional)

MCAT scores, essays/personal statement.

COSTS AND AID

Tuition & Fees

Tuition	$34,984
Fee	$60

NOVA SOUTHEASTERN UNIVERSITY
COLLEGE OF OSTEOPATHIC MEDICINE

3200 SOUTH UNIVERSITY DRIVE, FORT LAUDERDALE, FL 33328 • ADMISSION: 954-262-1101 • FAX: 954-262-2282
E-MAIL: COM@NOVA.EDU • WEBSITE: WWW.MEDICINE.NOVA.EDU

STUDENT BODY

Type	Private
Enrollment	822
% male/female	50/50
% underrepresented minorities	32
# applied (total/out)	2,800/2,277
# accepted (total/out)	430/256
# enrolled (total/out)	236/112
Average age	25

FACULTY

Total faculty (number)	956
% female	19
% minority	26

ADMISSIONS

Average GPA and MCAT Scores

Overall GPA	3.4
MCAT Bio	8.56
MCAT Phys	8.00
MCAT Verbal	8.45
MCAT Essay	0

Application Information

Regular application	1/15
Regular notification	rolling
Are transfers accepted?	yes
Admissions may be deferred?	yes
Interview required?	yes
Application fee	$50

Academics

Our innovative curriculum is designed to fulfill our mission of training primary-care physicians. The design of the curriculum is based on successful academic models—carefully developed and integrated. It emphasizes interdisciplinary collaboration, guiding students to develop a holistic, and more importantly, an osteopathic approach to medicine. Basic scientific information is continually correlated with fundamental clinical application. Students are exposed to clinical settings in their first semester, which gives them an opportunity to prepare for the "real world" of medicine. This clinical exposure continues into the second year when students have increased opportunity to interact with standardized patients on campus as well as be involved, under physician supervision, with real patients in the office and hospital setting. A notable aspect of the clinical program is a required three month rotation in a rural practice setting. In rural clinics throughout Florida, our students provide health care to medically underserved and indigent patients. Our students learn to treat various patients whose lifestyles, practices, and attitudes toward healthcare differ from those in more traditional training sites. This enriching educational experience cannot be taught in the classroom.

BASIC SCIENCES: Basic Sciences are covered during the first two years of medical school. Courses such as medical histology, gross anatomy, medical biochemistry, medical physiology, neuroanatomy, medical microbiology, principles of pharmacology, and principles of pathology are completed.

CLINICAL TRAINING

The Interdisciplinary Generalist Curriculum (IGC) Program exposes medical students to primary care clinical settings from the beginning of their first year, with the long term goal of increasing the numbers of graduates who will pursue careers in family medicine, general internal medicine and general pediatrics. The premise of the program is that exposure to professional role models is a significant determinant of medical students' career choices, and that an early clinical experience is an essential learning component for medical students to begin to correlate classroom knowledge with actual patient encounters.

During the third and fourth year, students complete the core clinical rotations. These include psychiatry, geriatrics, family medicine, internal medicine, obstetrics/gynecology, pediatrics, general surgery, emergency medicine, and rural medicine. Students complete their electives in their fourth year.

Student Life

The College of Osteopathic Medicine Student Council is the official voice of all osteopathic medical students. Its meetings are open to all students of the college and it welcomes proposals and participation from the entire student body. A variety of student clubs and organizations that address various professional and practice-related interests are also open for student membership.

Admissions

REQUIREMENTS

Nova Southeastern University receives over 3,000 applications each year to fill a class of 230 students. All AACOMAS applicants receive a secondary application, but not everyone that applies is granted an interview. Interviews begin in August and consist of a session with a panel of health professionals including a DO. Science prerequisites must include 8 hours of each (with labs) in biology, chemistry, organic chemistry, and physics. In addition, three semester hours of English Literature and three hours of English composition are required. The MCAT is required and should be no more than three years old. The best set of scores will be used.

SUGGESTIONS

Because of the time it takes for AACOMAS to provide all of the student information, and the fact that NSU is on rolling admissions, making application early is advisable.

PROCESS

Preference will be given to students with a cumulative grade point average (GPA) of 3.0 or higher. However, the dean is empowered to evaluate the total qualifications of every student and to modify requirements in unusual circumstances.

The college participates in the American Association of Colleges of Osteopathic Medicine Application Service (AACOMAS) for the receipt and processing of all applications. AACOMAS takes no part in the selection of students.

Admissions Requirements (Required)

MCAT scores, science GPA, non-science GPA, letters of recommendation, interview, state residency, essays/personal statement, extracurricular activities, exposure to medical profession, DO recommendation.

Overlap Schools

Des Moines University, New York Medical College, Philadelphia College of Osteopathic Medicine.

COSTS AND AID

Tuition & Fees

Tuition	$25,785
Room and board (on campus)	NA
Room and board (off campus)	$12,040
Cost of books	$2,000
Fees	$925

Financial Aid

% students receiving aid	96
Average loan	$42,944
Average debt	$225,000

OHIO UNIVERSITY
COLLEGE OF OSTEOPATHIC MEDICINE

102 GROSVENOR HALL, ATHENS, OH 45701 • ADMISSION: 800-345-1560 • FAX: 740-593-2256
E-MAIL: ADMISSIONS@EXCHANGE.OUCOM.OHIOU.EDU • WEBSITE: WWW.OUCOM.OHIOU.EDU

STUDENT BODY

Type	Public
Enrollment	433
% male/female	44/56
% underrepresented minorities	30
# applied (total/out)	2,338/1,971
# accepted (total/out)	157/26
# enrolled (total/out)	108/14
Average age	24

FACULTY

Total faculty (number)	115
% female	30
% minority	15
% part-time	33
Student-faculty ratio	4:1

ADMISSIONS

Average GPA and MCAT Scores

Overall GPA	3.54
MCAT Bio	8.32
MCAT Phys	7.61
MCAT Verbal	8.03
MCAT Essay	P

Application Information

Regular application	2/6
Regular notification	rolling
Are transfers accepted?	yes
Admissions may be deferred?	yes
Interview required?	yes
Application fee	$155

Academics

The Ohio University College of Osteopathic Medicine (OU-COM) is dedicated to preparing well-rounded primary care and specialty physicians for service to the state of Ohio as well as the nation. Students begin their first two years of training in Athens while the final two years take place at one of 13 hospitals in our Centers for Osteopathic Research and Education (CORE). The learning environment at OU-COM and the CORE is constructed based on the principles of adult learning, which include student empowerment and clinical relevance. Students will enroll in one of two tracks—the Patient-Centered Continuum (PCC) curriculum or the Clinical Presentation Continuum (CPC) curriculum. Both curricula view medical education as an organized building process that extends from the first day of medical school through residency training and beyond. Students in both curricula begin interacting with real patients in the first weeks of their medical education. The PCC curriculum is a student-directed approach that uses a problem-based learning environment and places emphasis on small-group discussions, case analysis, collaborative learning, and problem solving as its primary educational tools. The CPC curriculum provides students with opportunities to learn the biomedical science fundamentals of medicine in an integrated, clinically relevant environment. This faculty-directed curriculum uses the most common and/or important symptoms that patients present to primary care providers as its organizing focus. Demographic information includes a first-year student body that is 59 percent female, 30 percent underrepresented minority, 87 percent Ohio residents, and ranges in age from 21–45.

CLINICAL TRAINING

To become a patient-centered osteopathic physician, it is extremely important to have patient contact from the very beginning of the undergraduate medical education. As part of the OU-COM curricula, students will receive patient contact within the first week of their first year through our Clinical and Community Experience (CCE) Program. Students are able to see firsthand the roles of other health care professionals and become aware of cultural, economic, and social issues that can affect health status and health care delivery. Through OU-COM's pioneering Simulated Patient Program, students begin to hone their history-taking, psychosocial, and physical examination skills. One of the first in the country, this program has been in place for more than 25 years and features patient actors who role play a variety of conditions. Whenever possible, patients with actual symptoms or illnesses such as diabetes or rheumatoid arthritis are used as part of the simulated patient experience. Students are also able to get involved in health care initiatives and community health service programs related to rural Southeastern Ohio. The Childhood Immunization Program and the Breast and Cervical Cancer Screening Clinic are both delivered through one of the college's two Mobile Health Units. Opportunities for clinical service also abound at University Medical Associates—an ambulatory health care facility in Athens—and in OU-COM's satellite clinics in the outlying rural areas. Clinical rotations at one of the 13 CORE hospitals will take place in the third and fourth years of study.

Students

Being part of a major university has its advantages! From cultural and athletic events to phenomenal student recreation opportunities, OU-COM students enjoy it all. Located within minutes of Strouds Run State Park, students can relax by hiking, swimming, or fishing or they can blade, walk, bike, or jog our 19-mile, paved fitness path that extends from Athens to Nelsonville. Even more outdoor adventure is available in nearby Wayne National Forest. Ohio University also provides a nine-hole golf course, a natatorium, ice arena as well as indoor and outdoor tennis courts all within walking distance of the OU-COM campus. Intramural sports are also very popular. OU-COM has produced championship teams in both basketball and broomball over the past two years.

STUDENT LIFE

While it is no surprise that most of a med student's day is spent studying, there is still time for fun. Students can enjoy the many amenities offered by the university or get involved in OU-COM student government or other medically related student organizations. The environment at OU-COM is one of collegiality and cooperativeness. Students are often seen studying together, having a meal together, or even living in close proximity to one another. The quality of life for an OU-COM student is high. Support from caring and dedicated faculty and staff alongside the beauty and history of Ohio University make OU-COM an extraordinary place to obtain a medical education.

GRADUATES

OU-COM was founded for the express purpose of providing outstanding primary care physicians for the state of Ohio. Since our first graduating class in 1980, the school has accomplished that and more. Sixty percent of graduates go on to specialize in family medicine, internal medicine, or pediatrics, with 50 percent going specifically into family medicine. The remaining 40 percent are pursuing specialties such as orthopedic surgery, neurology, nephrology, psychiatry, anesthesiology, and ophthalmology.

Admissions

REQUIREMENTS

Eight semester hours each in biology, chemistry, organic chemistry, and physics are required. In addition, applicants must have taken six semester hours of English and behavioral science. As a state-affiliated institution, the college gives preference to Ohio residents, who make up about 80 percent of the student body. About 80 percent of AACOMAS applicants are sent supplemental applications. About 16 percent of those who submit supplemental applications are invited to interview. Interviews take place from October through April, and consist of three 30-minute sessions with members of the faculty and administration. Approximately half of interviewees are accepted, with notification occurring on a rolling basis. In the past, successful candidates have had a mean GPA of 3.5 and an average of at least 8 on each section of the MCAT.

SUGGESTIONS

Additional course work in biochemistry, gross anatomy, histology, and immunology is recommended but not required.

PROCESS

Students may begin the application process through AACOMAS on May 1. Primary applications will be reviewed to determine the eligibility of a secondary application. If a secondary application is granted, students will need to supply letters of recommendation, a supplemental essay and, if from outside Ohio, a signed contract of admission. A letter from a DO is strongly encouraged. Application status notices are sent electronically so it is imperative that students provide AACOMAS with a valid e-mail address. Only complete files will go before the selection committee for review. Students are responsible for making sure their file is complete. Admission decisions are made on a rolling basis with accepted candidates being notified via e-mail the next business day after the interview.

Admissions Requirements (Required)

MCAT scores, science GPA, non-science GPA, letters of recommendation, interview, essays/personal statement, extracurricular activities, exposure to medical profession.

Admissions Requirements (Optional)

State residency, letter of recommendation from a DO.

Overlap Schools

Lake Erie College of Osteopathic Medicine, Medical College of Ohio, Philadelphia College of Osteopathic Medicine, The Ohio State University, University of Cincinnati, West Virginia School of Osteopathic Medicine, Wright State University.

COSTS AND AID

Tuition & Fees

In-state Tuition	$20,622
Out-of-state Tuition	$30,054
Room and board (off campus)	$16,520
Cost of books	$4,554
Fees	$2,223

Financial Aid

% students receiving aid	100
Average grant	$3,940
Average loan	$35,297
Average debt	$132,927

OKLAHOMA STATE UNIVERSITY
COLLEGE OF OSTEOPATHIC MEDICINE

1111 WEST 17TH STREET, OFFICE OF STUDENT AFFAIRS, TULSA, OK 74107 • ADMISSION: 918-561-8421
FAX: 918-561-8243 • E-MAIL: LDHAINES@CHS.OKSTATE.EDU • WEBSITE: WWW.HEALTHSCIENCES.OKSTATE.EDU

STUDENT BODY

Type	Public
Enrollment	352
% male/female	53/47
% underrepresented minorities	18
# applied (total/out)	422/224
# accepted (total/out)	116/23
# enrolled (total/out)	88/12
Average age	25

FACULTY

Total faculty (number)	491
% female	25
% minority	10
% part-time	86
Student-faculty ratio	6:1

ADMISSIONS

Average GPA and MCAT Scores

Overall GPA	3.59
MCAT Bio	9.0
MCAT Phys	8.0
MCAT Verbal	9.0
MCAT Essay	O

Application Information

Regular application	2/1
Regular notification	rolling
Are transfers accepted?	yes
Admissions may be deferred?	no
Interview required?	yes
Application fee	$25

Academics

The OSU College of Osteopathic Medicine curriculum includes simulated clinical experiences, opportunities for independent study, and frequent consultation with faculty members and community-based physicians. In a spiral curriculum, study matter is continuously reintroduced to the student in greater depth and complexity. This method serves to reinforce prior learning and promote meaningful retention. The curriculum integrates subject matter derived from the biological, clinical, and behavioral sciences to permit full comprehension of the clinician's work and to provide a foundation for a lifetime of learning by the student. The curriculum is designed to implement a 24 month clerkship program within the four-year program of professional education.

BASIC SCIENCE AND CLINICAL TRAINING

The OSU-COM spiral curriculum is student-centered with focus on hands-on experience, as well as problem-based and small group learning. Students receive training in all areas of medicine, with additional emphasis on osteopathic manipulation. The first year focuses on biomedical sciences, and the second year emphasizes case-based learning and problem solving as it relates to conditions seen in primary care environments. The third and fourth years are composed of clinical rotations, most of which take place at Tulsa Regional Medical Center, the country's largest osteopathic hospital, as well as St. Anthony's Hospital in Oklahoma City. Students also do rotations in adjacent rural areas, and they may fulfill requirements at various medical institutions across the country. Although 64 percent of graduates enter primary care, they are prepared to enter residencies in all medical specialty fields.

Students

Located on the west bank of the Arkansas River, minutes from downtown Tulsa, the OSU Center for Health Sciences campus is housed in a modern, four-building complex on sixteen acres. The complex consists of classrooms, basic and clinical science teaching laboratories, offices, research areas, lecture halls, break-out rooms, a medical bookstore and a medical library. The OSU Health Care Center, located on six acres one-half mile south of the main campus, serves as both a teaching clinic for students and a health care resource for the community. At this comprehensive clinic, faculty physicians, resident physicians, and osteopathic medical students treat a large and varied patient load. The Health Care Center provides essential health care includes 37 patient examining rooms, radiology lab, student learning center, physician offices, and offers services in general health care, osteopathic manipulative therapy, psychiatry and behavioral medicine, diabetes foot care, and a women's health center.

STUDENT LIFE

OSU-COM students are leaders and have a voice and an active role in campus life. Student Senate officers represent students' interests to the faculty and administration. Senate officers, along with representatives from each class, are elected by the student body each year. College-student communications are aided by student representatives serving on several college committees. OSU-COM students are also actively involved in over 21 student clubs and organizations. These organizations bring an added value to the educational experience by providing community service opportunities and bringing in guest speakers, who expose students to new developments in medicine. Students also enjoy intramural activities, including softball, volleyball, and flag-football.

Admissions

REQUIREMENTS AND ADMISSIONS PROCESS

Eighty-eight students are admitted each year to the OSU-COM entering class. Of the 88 positions available, 68 are reserved for Oklahoma residents. Prerequisites for application are 8–10 semester hours each of biology, physics, inorganic chemistry, and organic chemistry course work with labs, as well as 6–8 hours of English course work. In addition, at least one upper division (3000–4000 level) science course, including lab, is required. The minimum undergraduate GPA is 3.0, and an average MCAT score of 7.0 (21 total) is required. All qualified applicants are encouraged to submit a secondary application, but only about 10 percent of applicants are interviewed. Interviews begin in November and continue through April of each admissions year. Each invited applicant will meet simultaneously with two faculty members (a DO and a PhD) for a 35-minute interview. Admissions notification is made on a rolling basis.

Admissions Requirements (Required)

MCAT scores, science GPA, non-science GPA, letters of recommendation, interview, essays/personal statement, extracurricular activities, exposure to medical profession, familiarity with osteopathic physician.

Admissions Requirements (Optional)

State residency.

Overlap Schools

University of Oklahoma.

COSTS AND AID

Tuition & Fees

In-state Tuition	$16,045
Out-of-state Tuition	$31,265
Room and board (off campus)	$7,200
Cost of books	$3,500
Fees	$893

Financial Aid

% students receiving aid	95
Average grant	$2,500
Average loan	$30,000
Average debt	$130,000

PHILADELPHIA COLLEGE OF OSTEOPATHIC MEDICINE

OFFICE OF ADMISSIONS, 4170 CITY AVENUE, PHILADELPHIA, PA 19131 • ADMISSION: 800-999-6998
FAX: 215-871-6719 • E-MAIL: ADMISSIONS@PCOM.EDU • WEBSITE: WWW.PCOM.EDU

STUDENT BODY

Type	Private
Enrollment	1,041
% male/female	47/53
% underrepresented minorities	23
# applied (total/out)	2,765/2,281
# accepted (total/out)	415/157
# enrolled (total/out)	266/104
Average age	24

FACULTY

Total faculty (number)	1,073
% female	6
% part-time	93
Student-faculty ratio	1:1

ADMISSIONS

Average GPA and MCAT Scores

Overall GPA	3.34
MCAT Bio	8.42
MCAT Phys	7.87
MCAT Verbal	8.10
MCAT Essay	P

Application Information

Regular application	2/1
Regular notification	rolling
Are transfers accepted?	no
Admissions may be deferred?	no
Interview required?	yes
Application fee	$50

Academics

Established in 1899, Philadelphia College of Osteopathic Medicine (PCOM) is a private, not for profit institution built on an over 100 year tradition of excellence in medical education. Students find the educational program at PCOM is an optimal blend of classroom teaching, clinical experience, and research. From the first day of medical school, PCOM students begin learning the osteopathic approach to health care: treating the whole person, not just the symptoms. Early clinical exposure through community service activities and formal course work implement basic science instruction. The curriculum is interdisciplinary, and includes topics such as medical ethics and medical law, and emphasizes primary care and prevention. Clinical training takes place at 37 affiliated institutions in and around Philadelphia. In addition, students may arrange to fulfill elective requirements in other states or in other countries. Joint degree programs lead to the DO/MBA, DO/MPH and DO/PhD. PCOM is committed to helping each of its students choose a career that matches their specific talents and interests. The entering class of 2005 in Philadelphia included 266 students from 22 states. The male/female ratio was 50/50 and the average age was 26.

We are pleased to announce the creation of our new branch campus outside of Atlanta. This campus opened in August, 2005 with 86 students. The contact information is 625 Old Peachtree Road NW, Suwannee, GA 30024; the telephone number is 678-225-7500.

BASIC SCIENCES: The first two years lay the foundation with intense concentration on the basic sciences: anatomy, biochemistry, molecular biology, neuroscience, physiology, microbiology, pathology, and pharmacology. The classes are taught in integrated course units that emphasize clinical applications. In addition, research development at PCOM has a strong focus on interdisciplinary research programs. The plan is twofold: to incorporate more research into students' training, and to enhance faculty scholarly activity. There are a number of numerous and diverse projects being carried out at PCOM; these along with information on the Sigma XI International science society can be found on the Research and Scholarly Activity page on the PCOM website.

CLINICAL TRAINING

There are a total of 24 clerkship periods. Fifteen of these are assigned in a manner prescribed by the Curriculum Committee and the Dean to ensure that every student obtains the core experience needed to become a well-trained osteopathic generalist physician. Flexibility is provided by six months of elective time and two months of selective time to give the student ample opportunity to pursue his/her special interests. The assigned clerkship sites for the Philadelphia campus are predominantly in Pennsylvania. Affiliate lists and specialties can be found on the PCOM website under Clinical Education.

Students

PCOM students are involved in a variety of academic related opportunities, as well as community service, recreational programs, and social activities. Each year, more than 100 students are active in the PCOM Student Government Association, which represents the students in all academic programs. PCOM offers everything from research clubs to dancing clubs to keep students active and engaged. PCOM students show great enthusiasm for the activities of the college and external communities. Many find the spirit on campus extraordinary, and think collegiality is the obvious way to make academic life, professional pursuits and human relationships most enjoyable. The Student Affairs website has a complete listing of clubs and organizations at PCOM.

GRADUATES

Philadelphia College of Osteopathic Medicine has trained over 10,000 osteopathic physicians; they practice throughout the United States and several foreign countries. Our graduates practice in all areas of medicine, hold leadership positions in the medical community, teach in the country's top medical schools and serve in every branch of the military. Nearly 65 percent of our graduates have chosen careers in primary care, family practice, general internal medicine, obstetrics/gynecology, and pediatrics.

Admissions

As Philadelphia College of Osteopathic Medicine enters its second century, it calls upon the experience of the past 100 years plus to set the standard. When an applicant is accepted as a student, they become a part of a rich tradition of excellence in education and leadership. PCOM is dedicated to providing every student with the resources to become a competent and caring professional. Our medical students are taught the osteopathic approach to medicine; treating patients as a whole and helping them lead healthy lives. PCOM is challenging; our academic training rigorous. Because we challenge you to meet the highest goals, we pledge our full support in helping you reach them.

Admissions Requirements (Required)

MCAT scores, science GPA, non-science GPA, letters of recommendation, interview, essays/personal statement.

Admissions Requirements (Optional)

State residency, extracurricular activities, exposure to medical profession.

Overlap Schools

Temple University, University of Medicine and Dentistry of New Jersey.

COSTS AND AID

Tuition & Fees

Tuition	$28,500
Room and board (on campus)	$13,190
Cost of books	$1,950
Fees	$525

Financial Aid

% students receiving aid	93
Average grant	$2,500
Average loan	$42,250
Average debt	$149,800

PIKEVILLE COLLEGE
SCHOOL OF OSTEOPATHIC MEDICINE

147 SYCAMORE STREET, PIKEVILLE, KY 41501 • ADMISSION: 606-218-5406 • FAX: 606-218-5405
E-MAIL: AHAMILTO@PC.EDU • WEBSITE: WWW.PCSOM.EDU

STUDENT BODY

Type	Private
Enrollment	278
% male/female	57/43
% underrepresented minorities	5
# applied (total/out)	1,458/1,369
# accepted (total/out)	140/51
# enrolled (total/out)	80/43
Average age	26

FACULTY

Total faculty (number)	24
% female	29
Student-faculty ratio	6:1

ADMISSIONS

Average GPA and MCAT Scores

Overall GPA	3.31
MCAT Bio	7.5
MCAT Phys	6.9
MCAT Verbal	7.3
MCAT Essay	0

Application Information

Regular application	2/5
Regular notification	rolling
Are transfers accepted?	yes
Admissions may be deferred?	yes
Interview required?	yes
Application fee	$75

Academics

The Pikeville College School of Osteopathic Medicine (PCSOM) is the nineteenth school of osteopathic medicine in the country. PCSOM offers a four-year program that leads to the degree of Doctor of Osteopathic Medicine (DO). The first two years of the curriculum focus on basic sciences, and the third and fourth years emphasize clinical work. Osteopathic principles are integrated throughout the four-year curriculum and students learn osteopathic manipulative treatment for prevention, diagnosis, and treatment of disease. Pikeville College's Board of Trustees has decided that no student should be organizationally or academically disadvantaged because of a lack of adequate personal funding. To this end, PCSOM provides each student with a state-of-the art Pentium laptop computer; all required texts and workbooks; all anatomy dissection equipment; a new portable OP&P table; stethoscope; opthalmoscope; otoscope; lab coats; scrub suits; outside board review; and the cost of taking Part I and Part II of the NBOME certification exam once.

BASIC SCIENCES: During the first two years, students take lecture-based courses with labs covering the typical medical school disciplines with special emphasis in the following areas: Manual medicine; community and behavior medicine; and ambulatory care. Friday afternoons are spent in doctors' offices, where students learn to take patient histories and conduct physical exams. First-year courses include: Osteopathic principles and practice; gross anatomy; radiology; clinical skills; neuroscience; opthalmology; immunology; and medical ethics. Second-year courses include: pathology; pharmacology; pediatrics; community and behavioral medicine; and psychiatry. During the summer of their second year, students take medicine and surgery, two intensive, full-time courses that will prepare students to fully interact at the bedside or in an ambulatory care setting during the final two years of their medical school education.

CLINICAL TRAINING

During the third and fourth years students enter their clinical training, rotating through urban, suburban, and rural settings, while gaining exposure to all areas of medicine. Rotations occur on a monthly basis, starting on the first day of each calendar month and ending the last day of the month. The following rotations are required and assigned: Family medicine (2 months); emergency medicine (2 months); general internal medicine (2 months); pediatrics (2 months); general surgery (2 months); osteopathic principles and practice (1 month); women's health (1 month); psychiatry (1 month); radiology (2 weeks); anesthesiology (2 weeks); 2 selective rotations in a clinical subspecialty (1 month each). In addition, students complete elective rotations in medicine and surgery (1 month each) and an additional 2 months in the elective of their choice.

STUDENTS

The Admissions Office seeks to recruit students who will help Pikeville fulfill its mission to provide men and women with an osteopathic medical education that emphasizes primary care, and produce graduates who are committed to serving the health care needs of communities in the Appalachian regions.

STUDENT LIFE

PCSOM offers students a variety of professional and social clubs and organizations on campus. The PCSOM Emergency Medicine Student Club is a new organization that focuses on emergency medicine and aims to foster professional growth and interest in emergency medicine by providing relevant educational programs and service projects to the PCSOM community.

The Student Government Association (SGA) is the official voice for students, and is responsible for dispersing funds for student activities; acting as liaison for the student body; and working to improve the quality of life for all PCSOM students.

Other clubs of note include the Student Osteopathic Surgical Association (SOSA) for students who want to learn more about careers in surgery, and the Student Osteopathic Medical Association (SOMA) which works to improve the quality of health care delivery, contribute to the education of osteopathic medical students, and promote the ideals of osteopathic medicine. SOMA is recognized by the American Osteopathic Association (AOA) and the American Medical Association (AMA) as the National Professional Society of Osteopathic Medical Students. Membership in SOMA offers students a legitimate voice in shaping the future of their chosen profession. It also provides a means of communication among the students of the 19 colleges of osteopathic medicine. All students of osteopathic medicine are eligible for membership in SOMA, which comes with an extensive student benefits package, including discounts on books and equipment.

GRADUATES

After graduation, students complete one year of a rotating internship and 2–5 years of residency, depending upon which specialty is selected. PCSOM continues to form affiliations with hospitals in the Appalachian region to ensure that adequate postgraduate training sites are available for PCSOM graduates so that they can and will stay in the area.

ADMISSIONS

REQUIREMENTS

The minimum requirements for admission are: Completion of at least 90 semester hours of the required credits for a baccalaureate degree from a regionally accredited college or university; MCAT scores from an MCAT exam not taken more than three years ago; 12 semester hours of biology (with labs); 8 semester hours each of chemistry, organic chemistry, and physics (with labs); and 6 semester hours of English.

SUGGESTED

The baccalaureate degree is preferred, and preference is given to those candidates who will have earned the degree prior to starting the medical school program. The ability to use a personal or network computer is an important skill that will assist students with PCSOM course work. Therefore, each entering student should have a good working knowledge of common PC use and applications.

PROCESS

Pikeville participates in the AACOMAS application process.

Admissions Requirements (Required)

MCAT scores, science GPA, non-science GPA, letters of recommendation, interview, essays/personal statement, extracurricular activities, exposure to medical profession.

Admissions Requirements (Optional)

State residency.

Overlap Schools

Marshall University, Ohio University, University of Kentucky, University of Louisville, West Virginia School of Osteopathic Medicine.

COSTS AND AID

Tuition & Fees

Tuition	$27,000
Room and board (off campus)	$8,000

Financial Aid

% students receiving aid	96
Average grant	$11,110
Average loan	$28,000
Average debt	$106,000

TOURO UNIVERSITY—CALIFORNIA
COLLEGE OF OSTEOPATHIC MEDICINE

OFFICE OF ADMISSIONS, 1310 JOHNSON LANE, VALLEJO, CA 94592 • ADMISSION: 707-638-5270
FAX: 707-638-5250 • E-MAIL: SDAVIS@TOURO.EDU • WEBSITE: WWW.TU.EDU

STUDENT BODY	
Type	Private
Enrollment	525
% male/female	53/47
% underrepresented minorities	5
# applied	3,267
# accepted	135
# enrolled	135
Average age	26

ADMISSIONS

Average GPA and MCAT Scores

Overall GPA	3.3
MCAT Bio	9.07
MCAT Phys	8.99
MCAT Verbal	8.19

Application Information

Regular application	4/1
Regular notification	rolling
Early application	8/15
Early notification	9/15
Are transfers accepted?	yes
Admissions may be deferred?	yes
Interview required?	yes
Application fee	$100

Academics

The Touro University College of Osteopathic Medicine (TUCOM), San Francisco, is located in the northeast part of San Francisco Bay on Mare Island. Touro University is an international institution based in New York, with branches in Israel and the Russian Federation. The mission of the TUCOM is to train osteopathic, family practice physicians to help meet the need for primary care practitioners in California and throughout the country. Though preventative medicine and primary care are emphasized, graduates are also prepared to enter residency programs that train osteopathic specialists. Patient contact begins in the first year, and clinical training takes place at sites throughout the greater Bay Area including hospitals, clinics, and physicians' offices. Students have the opportunity to experience both urban and rural patient populations.

TUCOM prepares students to become outstanding osteopathic physicians who uphold the values, philosophy, and practice of osteopathic medicine and who are committed to primary care and the holistic approach to the patient. The college advances the profession and serves its students and society through innovative education, research, and community service.

BASIC SCIENCES: TUCOM students take courses in all of the subject areas one would expect any physician to master, including anatomy, pathology, histology, osteopathic principles and practices, pharmacology, clinical skills, etc. Our goal is to prepare students for the realities of medicine as it presently exists, as well as how it is likely to be in the future. Practice in problem-solving is part of the daily classroom clinic experience as we strive to deliver a curriculum consistent with emerging directions of health care.

Student Life

Touro University—California occupies a spectacular 44-acre site on Mare Island, located in the Northeastern part of the San Francisco Bay Area. In addition to the College of Osteopathic Medicine, the university is home to the College of Education, College of Health Sciences, and the College of Pharmacy. The campus enjoys wireless internet access, state of the art lecture halls, breakout rooms, and an anatomy lab.

TUCOM students participate in several organizations, including the Student Osteopathic Medical Association, and a variety of student organized clubs. With a campus that is centrally located in the San Francisco Bay Area, students are within an hour's drive of Napa Valley, Sacramento, and San Francisco.

Admissions

ADMISSIONS REQUIREMENTS

Candidates are required to obtain a Bachelors Degree prior to matriculating into the College of Osteopathic Medicine. A qualifying MCAT score is also required and must have been taken within the last three years. In addition, candidates are required to obtain 8 semester units (with lab) of the following: biology/zoology, general (inorganic) chemistry, organic chemistry, and physics. Successful candidates typically have cumulative and science GPAs of 3.0 or above and MCAT scores of 23 and higher.

PROCESS

What follows is a brief summary of the admissions procedures to apply to TUCOM. Further details should be reviewed by going to www.tu.edu, and clicking on Prospective Students, followed by College of Osteopathic Medicine.

- Complete the primary application with AACOMAS. This can be accomplished by clicking on the AACOMAS link on our website or by going to www.aacom.org. TUCOM's school number is 618.

- Qualified applicants will be invited to complete a supplemental application. This application is available online but should not be completed or submitted until eligibility is determined.

- If eligible for a supplemental application, submit an evaluation from a pre-professional advisory committee, or letters from two science faculty familiar with your work.

- Submit a physician (DO or MD) letter of recommendation.

- If invited to do so, schedule a formal interview with the Admissions and Standards Committee.

Admissions Requirements (Required)

MCAT scores, science GPA, non-science GPA, letters of recommendation, interview, essays/personal statement, extracurricular activities, exposure to medical profession.

Admissions Requirements (Optional)

State residency.

COSTS AND AID

Tuition & Fees

Tuition	$35,000
Cost of books	$1,694

Financial Aid

% students receiving aid	94

University of Medicine and Dentistry of New Jersey

School of Osteopathic Medicine

1 Medical Center Drive, Suite 210, Stratford, NJ 08084 • Admission: 856-566-7050 • Fax: 856-566-6895
E-mail: SOMADM@UMDNJ.EDU • Website: SOM.UMDNJ.EDU

STUDENT BODY

Type	Public
Enrollment	382
% male/female	43/57
% underrepresented minorities	53
# applied (total/out)	2,401/2,078
# accepted (total/out)	290/112
# enrolled (total/out)	100/2
Average age	24

FACULTY

Total faculty (number)	187
% female	39
% minority	18
% part-time	19

ADMISSIONS

Average GPA and MCAT Scores

Overall GPA	3.5
MCAT Bio	9.2
MCAT Phys	9.0
MCAT Verbal	8.5
MCAT Essay	Q

Application Information

Regular application	2/1
Regular notification	rolling
Are transfers accepted?	yes
Admissions may be deferred?	yes
Interview required?	yes
Application fee	$75

Academics

All applicants are processed and reviewed without regard to state of residence. The minimum course requirements are eight semester hours of biology, physics, chemistry and organic chemistry, all with associated labs and six semester hours each of English, math, and social sciences. Applicants should have at least a 3.0 GPA in both sciences and overall, as the average GPA of successful applicants is 3.4. The MCAT is required and must be no more than three years old. The average MCAT of successful applicants is in the 89 range. Just over 15 percent of approximately 2,000 applicants are interviewed, with interviews taking place between August and April. About half of interviewees are accepted. Wait list candidates may send supplementary information to update their files.

The instructional program at the UMDNJ—School of Osteopathic Medicine reflects the essence of the holistic philosophy of osteopathic medicine which regards the human body as an integrated whole. The curriculum provides comprehensive instruction in the basic and clinical sciences, emphasizing the primary care of the patient. The ultimate goal of the curriculum is to develop in students the lifelong learning skills of a physician.

The primary focus of the first year of medical school is the development of a solid foundation in the basic sciences. The study of the history and conceptual framework of osteopathic medicine, including the basic techniques of osteopathic manipulative therapy, is also included. The second year is devoted to the integration of the basic sciences and clinical medicine. Using a modularized design based on body system, the information is taught through a coordinated effort of basic science and clinical faculty. Instruction is provided by a combination of lectures, independent reading, and problem-oriented group discussions which enable students to acquire, assimilate, and analyze clinical knowledge. Additionally, students receive instruction and practice in the basic clinical skills of history taking and physical examination as well as in the more complex techniques of osteopathic manipulative therapy.

The third and fourth years are devoted to the development of clinical competence through directly supervised patient care activities. Through didactic instruction and "hands-on" education, students increase the scope and depth of their clinical knowledge and skills. These clinical experiences permit students to apply their skills to solving patient problems, as well as to develop strategies which promote wellness and the prevention of disease. A unique feature of the clinical curriculum is the participation in a longitudinal community-based health care program. A variety of settings are utilized for the clinical education, including the three Kennedy Memorial Hospital—University Medical Center site, Our Lady of Lourdes Hospital, Christ Hospital, Barnert Hospital, ambulatory health care centers, private offices, nursing homes, and community-based clinics.

THE PROBLEM BASED LEARNING CURRICULUM

The Problem Based Learning Curriculum (PBLC) is an alternative curricular track available to seven students. The PBLC was established to meet the needs of those applicants who find problem-based learning an attractive option. It is a two-year program, and with the start of the clerkships in the third year, PBLC students join the rest of their classmates.

Admissions

The Admissions Committee requires that every applicant submit results from the Medical College Admissions Test, as well as a pre-medical committee letter. All accepted students must have earned a baccalaureate degree upon matriculation at UMDNJ—SOM. Other requirements include eight hours of biology, eight hours of organic chemistry, eight hours of inorganic chemistry and eight hours of physics, all with laboratories. Additionally, three hours of English composition are required, as well as three hours from the English department; six hours of college level mathematics are required, three hours of which may be satisfied by computer science or statistics and six hours of behavioral science (psychology, sociology or cultural anthropology). UMDNJ—SOM strongly recommends that applicants take six additional semester hours of science courses. Biochemistry, genetics, physiology, and anatomy are strongly suggested.

Those applicants whose credentials are judged to be most competitive will be invited for an interview; interviews are not granted at an applicant's request. Applicants who are not considered for the first round of interviews will be held for further review. Candidates whose credentials are considered noncompetitive will receive a rejection notice at an early date.

Applicants may complete an online application through the American Association of Colleges of Osteopathic Medicine Application Service (AACOMAS) by logging onto their website: www.aacom.org. Applications are available in early May and may be completed and submitted between June 1 of that year and February 1 of the year of the desired admission. All applications are considered without regard to state of residence. Applicants must be U.S. citizens or permanent residents at the time the application is filed.

COMBINED DEGREE PROGRAMS
DO/PhD

The joint DO/PhD program is a unique interdepartmental program between the departments of Cell Biology and Molecular Biology intended to prepare future physicians anticipating careers in biomedical research or teaching. All DO/PhD candidates receive an annual stipend and a tuition waiver for each year of participation in the combined degree programs.

DO/MPA
The joint DO/MPA is offered in cooperation with Rutgers University—Camden Campus. The Master of Public Administration degree is designed to prepare future physicians with proficiency in administration and public policy.

DO/JD
The joint DO/JD program is offered in cooperation with Rutgers University—School of Law, Camden Campus. The program is designed to prepare future physicians for joint careers in medicine and law.

DO/MPH
The joint DO/MPH program is offered in cooperation with the UMDNJ—School of Public Health. The Masters in Public Health degree is designed to prepare future physicians to address a multitude of health issues within our society.

DO/MS
The Joint DO/MS program is offered in cooperation with the UMDNJ—Graduate School of Biomedical Sciences. The program is designed to prepare future physicians with strong research orientation in the Biomedical Sciences.

Admissions Requirements (Required)
MCAT scores, science GPA, non-science GPA, letters of recommendation, interview, essays/personal statement, extracurricular activities, exposure to medical profession.

Admissions Requirements (Optional)
State residency.

COSTS AND AID

Tuition & Fees

In-state Tuition	$21,390
Out-of-state Tuition	$33,472
Room and board (off campus)	$10,000
Cost of books	$8,536
Fees	$2,587

Financial Aid

% students receiving aid	92
Average grant	$2,690
Average loan	$32,759
Average debt	$104,005

UNIVERSITY OF NEW ENGLAND
COLLEGE OF OSTEOPATHIC MEDICINE

UNECOM RECRUITMENT, STUDENT & ALUMNI SERVICES, 11 HILLS BEACH ROAD, BIDDEFORD, ME 04005 ADMISSION: 207-602-2329
FAX: 207-602-5967 • E-MAIL: UNECOMADMISSIONS@UNE.EDU • WEBSITE: WWW.UNE.EDU/COM

STUDENT BODY

Type	Private
Enrollment	500
% male/female	48/52
% underrepresented minorities	10
# applied (total/out)	2,448/2,396
# accepted (total/out)	221/188
# enrolled (total/out)	121/93
Average age	25

FACULTY

Total faculty (number)	532
% female	5
% minority	1
% part-time	81
Student-faculty ratio	10:1

ADMISSIONS

Average GPA and MCAT Scores

Overall GPA	3.37
MCAT Bio	8.64
MCAT Phys	7.81
MCAT Verbal	8.52
MCAT Essay	Q

Application Information

Regular application	2/1
Regular notification	rolling
Are transfers accepted?	yes
Admissions may be deferred?	no
Interview required?	yes
Application fee	$55

Academics

The University of New England College of Osteopathic Medicine (UNECOM) is a private, nonprofit institution with a mission to provide for the education of osteopathic physicians and other health professionals for the people of New England and the nation. The curriculum focuses on the following three areas of excellence: Primary care, osteopathic principles and practice, and geriatrics. The academic environment is one of collaboration and support among the student body and with faculty members. The typical class size is 117–120 students, who come from a wide variety of educational and professional backgrounds. While approximately 60 percent of the class is from New England, there are students from around the country. Some come directly from undergraduate studies, while others have earned master's and professional degrees. The male/female ratio is about 48/52 and the average age of entering students is 25–27 years old.

BASIC SCIENCES: The modified systems-based curriculum begins with a focus on developing a solid preparation in the basic sciences and an exposure to the physician-patient relationship through early clinical experiences in the Foundations of Doctoring course. The gross anatomy course is one of the most comprehensive in the country, providing for the full dissection of a cadaver with just three other students and the incorporation of radiographic anatomy and live (palpatory) anatomy in the overall course. Building on the first year, the systems-based modules of the second year are taught by a cadre of practicing clinicians and basic scientists who bring the real world into the classroom. Students' clinical skills are enhanced in the Experiences in Doctoring course, with community placements and practice with standardized patients at the Clinical Skills Assessment Center, as well as in the differential diagnosis classes.

CLINICAL TRAINING

The third year is devoted to clerkships in core disciplines of internal medicine, pediatrics, surgery, psychiatry, obstetrics, and family medicine at Clinical Training Centers (CTCs) in the Northeast. Students are involved in patient care and didactic sessions in ambulatory, hospital, and rural settings. The third year concludes with a student colloquium for the assessment of acquired skills in the simulated patient program. Year 4 requires clerkships in Osteopathic Manipulative Treatment (OMT) and rural medicine while providing an opportunity for electives throughout the United States and overseas as the students complete their preparation for residency.

Students

The College of Osteopathic Medicine is one of three colleges of the University of New England. The College of Osteopathic Medicine and the College of Arts and Sciences are located on the waterfront campus in Biddeford, Maine; the Westbrook college campus in Portland is home to the College of Health Professions. Osteopathic medical students have access to a full range of student services on both campuses. Most students live less than 6 miles from campus in the cities of Biddeford (21,000) and Saco (17,000).

STUDENT LIFE

With an active student government, class officers, and more than 30 clubs and organizations, there are many opportunities for first- and second-year students to be involved on campus and assume leadership positions. First- and second-year students also serve the Biddeford community through various programs including the Biddeford Free Clinic, local soup kitchen, and mentoring program with one of the elementary schools. Students maintain a healthy balance in their lives by utilizing the Campus Center (including the fitness room, racquetball courts, gym, indoor track, pool and hydro-spa, and saunas) and participating in the university's intramural leagues. The campus sits at the mouth of the Saco River where it meets the Atlantic Ocean, and the southern coastal Maine area is ideal for jogging and running, cycling, mountain biking, kayaking, and canoeing. Hiking, backpacking, camping, climbing, skiing, and snowboarding opportunities are less than two hours away in the White Mountains. Portland, Maine's largest city, is only a 30-minute drive to the north, and Boston is 90 minutes to the south.

GRADUATES

With the class of 2006, UNECOM has more than 2,000 graduates working in primary care and specialty fields around the country. Approximately 60 percent of each class pursue these four areas of primary care: family practice, general internal medicine, pediatric, and obstetrics. Others choose to bring a patient-centered approach to a wide variety of specialties, including anesthesiology, emergency medicine, general and orthopedic surgery, physical medicine and rehabilitation, and sports medicine. Others will specialize in Neuromuscular Medicine (NMM). Graduates continue to serve the osteopathic community by serving in leadership positions in state societies and specialty colleges.

Admissions

REQUIREMENTS

Specific academic requirements include eight semester hours of biology, and six hours of English composition or literature. Four semesters of chemistry are also required, one of which must be biochemistry. Appropriate labs are required for all science courses with the exception of biochemistry. The minimum GPA is 2.7 in both the sciences and overall, while the class average is in the 3.3–3.6 range. The MCAT is required and must be no more than two years old at time of application. The minimum MCAT is 18 with M on the writing sample, but the class average is in the 24–27 range (8s and 9s in each of the 3 sections). In addition to the requirements noted above, the following non-academic achievements are important in the evaluation process: Leadership experience and organizational involvement; health care experience, whether volunteer or paid employment; community service, and volunteer experience. Passion and commitment to working with and serving others is important to the Admissions Committee. There is some preference for candidates from the six New England states, but approximately 40 percent of the class is from the rest of the country.

PROCESS

The primary application to the University of New England College of Osteopathic Medicine (UNECOM) is through the American Association of Colleges of Osteopathic Medicine Application Service (AACOMAS). Nearly 2,500 AACOMAS applications were received during the 2004–2005 application cycle. Applicants who meet all prerequisites are invited to submit a UNECOM-specific online supplemental application and letters of recommendation. A letter from an osteopathic physician is not required but strongly encouraged. Once all materials have been received, the applicant's files are reviewed for a possible interview. On-campus interviews are conducted from September through April; interview teams are often comprised of a basic science faculty member, practicing clinician, and a second-year student. Qualified candidates are offered acceptance on a modified rolling admissions basis.

Admissions Requirements (Required)

MCAT scores, science GPA, non-science GPA, letters of recommendation, interview, essays/personal statement, extracurricular activities, exposure to medical profession, volunteerism/community service.

Admissions Requirements (Optional)

State residency.

Overlap Schools

A.T. Still University of Health Sciences, Dartmouth College, New York Institute of Technology, Nova Southeastern University, Philadelphia College of Osteopathic Medicine, UMDNJ—School of Osteopathic Medicine, University of Vermont.

COSTS AND AID

Tuition & Fees

Tuition	$36,740
Room and board (off campus)	$11,000
Cost of books	$1,850
Fees	$590

Financial Aid

% students receiving aid	94
Average grant	$9,500
Average loan	$48,868
Average debt	$151,733

UNIVERSITY OF NORTH TEXAS HEALTH SCIENCE CENTER

TEXAS COLLEGE OF OSTEOPATHIC MEDICINE

OFFICE OF ADMISSIONS AND OUTREACH, EAD-248, 3500 CAMP BOWIE BOULEVARD, FORT WORTH, TX 76107-2699
ADMISSION: 817-735-2204 • FAX: 817-735-2225 • E-MAIL: TCOMADMISSIONS@HSC.UNT.EDU
WEBSITE: WWW.HSC.UNT.EDU/EDUCATION/TCOM/ADMISSIONS.CFM

STUDENT BODY

Type	Public
Enrollment	520
% male/female	47/53
% underrepresented minorities	10
# applied (total/out)	1,701/97
# accepted (total/out)	177/29
# enrolled (total/out)	135/13
Average age	25

FACULTY

Total faculty (number)	286
% female	32
% minority	10

ADMISSIONS

Average GPA and MCAT Scores

Overall GPA	3.5
MCAT Bio	9.6
MCAT Phys	8.9
MCAT Verbal	9.0
MCAT Essay	P

Application Information

Regular application	10/15
Regular notification	7/20
Early application	5/1
Early notification	10/15
Are transfers accepted?	yes
Admissions may be deferred?	yes
Interview required?	yes

Academics

The University of North Texas Health Science Center at Fort Worth trains osteopathic physicians, physician assistants, biomedical scientists, and public health professionals. Its academic components are the Texas College of Osteopathic Medicine, the Graduate School of Biomedical Sciences, the School of Public Health, and the School of Health Professions. Dual-degree programs combine medical training with research and public health. *U.S. News & World Report* and the Texas Academy of Family Physicians have both recognized TCOM's commitment to primary care.

BASIC SCIENCES: The first portion of the curriculum is designed to help students integrate the basic and clinical sciences, further develop their ability to diagnose illness, and increase their understanding of the context within which medicine is practiced. The integrated systems approach is built on the same strong foundation of scientific and clinical knowledge that has long characterized TCOM's outstanding academic program.

CLINICAL TRAINING

During the third and fourth years of study, students pursue a number of clinical training programs throughout the state at university sites, clinics, and affiliated teaching hospitals. A rural medicine track provides extensive preparation for those who wish to practice in small communities.

Students

UNT Health Science Center is located on a 17-acre, $107 million medical care complex in Fort Worth, Texas, in the city's beautiful Cultural District. Downtown Fort Worth, major thoroughfares, parks, museums, theaters, restaurants, shops, and affordable housing are all within minutes of campus.

STUDENT LIFE

The campus is located in the midst of a world-renowned cultural district, near parks and a variety of arts and entertainment facilities. The DFW Metroplex is home to several major and minor league sports teams, including the Dallas Cowboys, Texas Rangers, Dallas Mavericks, Fort Worth Cats, and Dallas Stars. A variety of student organizations bring a sense of community and camaraderie to campus. The health science center does not provide on-campus student housing, but a variety of affordable housing options are available in the area. Every student is responsible for making his or her own housing arrangements.

GRADUATES

Named as one of the nation's top 50 medical schools for primary care medicine by *U.S. News & World Report*, TCOM is a leader in training physicians skilled in comprehensive primary care. Approximately 65 percent of TCOM's graduates practice primary care medicine (family practice, general internal medicine, pediatrics, obstetrics, and gynecology). One of the distinct advantages of an osteopathic medical education is that it prepares students to enter all three of the nation's residency programs: Allopathic, military, and osteopathic. Our graduates have been placed in residency and internship positions throughout the United States. UNT Health Science Center offers residency programs through the Texas Osteopathic Postdoctoral Training Institutions (OPTI) in the following areas: Family medicine, internal medicine, obstetrics and gynecology, orthopedics, radiology, surgery, and manipulative medicine. The Health Science Center also offers fellowship programs in osteopathic manipulative therapy, geriatric medicine, sports medicine, and vascular surgery.

Admissions

REQUIREMENTS

At least 90 percent of the positions in each class of 150 are reserved for Texas residents. Traditional premedical science training at an accredited undergraduate institution is necessary to prepare for matriculation. In addition, applicants are required to submit MCAT scores and test results must be from within the past three years. Applications are accepted through the Texas Medical and Dental Schools Application Service (TMDSAS). Selected applicants are invited to interview between August and December. Initial offers of acceptance are sent on February 1 and continue until the incoming class is full. Applications are accepted through the Texas Medical and Dental Schools Application Service (TMDSAS). Selected applicants are invited to interview between August and December. Initial offers of acceptance are sent on February 1 and continue until the incoming class is full.

SUGGESTIONS

In addition to the required science course work, it is recommended that students take advanced course work in biochemistry and genetics to prepare for the rigors of medical education.

Admissions Requirements (Required)

MCAT scores, science GPA, non-science GPA, letters of recommendation, interview, essays/personal statement, exposure to medical profession, secondary application.

Admissions Requirements (Optional)

State residency, extracurricular activities.

Overlap Schools

Baylor College of Medicine, Texas A&M University—College Station, Texas Tech University, The University of Texas HSC at Houston, University of Texas Health Science Center at San Antonio, University of Texas Southwestern Medical Center, University of Texas Medical Branch—Galveston

COSTS AND AID

Tuition & Fees

In-state Tuition	$10,150
Out-of-state Tuition	$25,900
Room and board (off campus)	$10,857
Cost of books	$2,500
Fees	$600

Financial Aid

% students receiving aid	90
Average grant	$5,000
Average loan	$29,028
Average debt	$93,200

VIRGINIA COLLEGE OF OSTEOPATHIC MEDICINE (VCOM)
EDWARD VIA VIRGINIA COLLEGE OF OSTEOPATHIC MEDICINE

OFFICE OF ADMISSIONS, VCOM, 2265 KRAFT DRIVE, BLACKSBURG, VA 24060 • ADMISSION: 540-231-6138
FAX: 540-231-5252 • E-MAIL: ADMISSIONS@VCOM.VT.EDU • WEBSITE: WWW.VCOM.VT.EDU

STUDENT BODY

Type	Private
Enrollment	610
% male/female	51/49
% underrepresented minorities	13
# applied (total/out)	2,200/2,010
# accepted (total/out)	257/170
# enrolled (total/out)	160/90
Average age	25

FACULTY

Total faculty (number)	443
% female	51
% minority	10
% part-time	60
Student-faculty ratio	5:1

ADMISSIONS

Average GPA and MCAT Scores

Overall GPA	3.5
MCAT Bio	8.0
MCAT Phys	8.0
MCAT Verbal	8.0
MCAT Essay	P

Application Information

Regular application	2/7
Regular notification	12/6
Early application	9/6
Early notification	10/6
Are transfers accepted?	yes
Admissions may be deferred?	yes
Interview required?	yes
Application fee	$75

Academics

The curriculum for students enrolled in VCOM is modern and innovative. The basic science and clinical content are interwoven throughout the four years. In the first two years students learn about the normal state of homeostasis of the human body, the propensity for health, and ability of the human body to heal, the clinical conditions that most often affect the human body, and the presentations of those conditions. The curriculum is "patient-centered" and integrates patient cases throughout the four years that focus on physical health (the body), mental health (the mind), and spiritual health, and also emphasizes the community-centered approach to health care.

Based upon a learner-centered approach, students are given the opportunity to learn relevant material through clinical systems' organized approach. Students attend lectures and labs that are interwoven with small-group conferences, self-directed learning computer tutorials, and clinical experiences. Students are given patient-centered cases to integrate biomedical and clinical curriculum and must employ problem solving through third-year clinical based modules that require literature searches, group analysis, and collaboration. They develop lifelong learning skills that foster the team approach to medicine as well as independent study. The clinical and basic science integration throughout the four years provides an opportunity for a continuous curriculum. The same clinical faculty physicians providing instruction in the classroom will be the faculty who plan/provide instruction in the clinical setting.

BASIC SCIENCES: The first 11 weeks of the medical curriculum are designated for the foundations of medicine. Courses within this block include the following: Biochemistry; genetics, reproduction, and embryology; immunology; epidemiology; and primary care (including professionalism and ethics). Students must pass the foundations block to continue in school.

Following the foundations of medicine, first-year students enter a sequence of systems based-clinical based blocks. The curriculum in each block is presented by faculty from the disciplines of anatomy, histology, microbiology, physiology, and principles of primary care. Physical diagnosis and clinical case presentations are also part of the curriculum.

The second year includes foundations of clinical medicine where students learn introductory pharmacology, clinical pathology, microbiology, nutrition, psychiatry, radiology, and an evidence-based medicine approach to clinical medicine.

Third-year and fourth-year students train primarily in the clinical setting. Students return to campus or are connected via teleconference periodically during the third year core rotations for advanced clinical conferences. The conferences are taught in both the lecture format and through small-group assignments.

CLINICAL TRAINING

Clinical experiences are found throughout the four years at VCOM. Students begin with experiences in the first two years. In the third and fourth years, students spend five days per week in the clinical setting. Students returning to campus or educational sites for clinical case conferences in the third year and online modules provide curriculum to the student at their clinical site.

During primary care experiences, students train predominately in the rural and under served clinical settings where a relationship is developed with the physician, as both a teacher and mentor. Approved elective experiences during the fourth year include mor specialized clerkships where students may focus their experiences to improve self-perceived weaknesses. VCOM provides opportunities to continue with the curriculum into postgraduate training through the Appalachia Osteopathic Postdoctoral Training Institute Consortia (AOPTIC).

Students

VCOM sponsors social, fitness, spiritual, cultural, and vocational activities throughout the year. Via Wellness strives to promote balance in the busy lives of medical students and provides incentives for participation in a spectrum of activities. Information and a schedule of activities sponsored through Via Wellness are available from the VCOM Office of Student Services and are listed on the activities calendar on the school's website.

STUDENT LIFE

VCOM promotes an environment where students balance curricular, extracurricular, and personal experiences. Introductory meetings for student organizations occur during the first three months of the first year. Students are encouraged to learn about all organizations and participate in those that will advance career and personal interests. The Via Wellness promotes balance for VCOM students by offering social, spiritual, fitness, vocational and intellectual programs. VCOM also currently has interest groups in anesthesia, internal medicine/geriatrics, neurology/mental health and addiction medicine, obstetrics and gynecology, complementary and integrative medicine, radiology, and Spanish.

Admissions

REQUIREMENTS

Following are a list of requirements: (1) Obtain an undergraduate degree before matriculation. (2) Complete all required course work before matriculation. They include biology (8 hours) chemistry (8 hours), organic chemistry (8 hours), physics (6 hours), additional science (6 hours), and English (6 hours). (3) A recent MCAT score no earlier than April 2003. (4) Science GPA minimum is 2.75 (average 3.4). (5) Overall GPA minimum is 2.75 (average 3.5). (6) Letter of recommendation from premed/pre-health advisor (or science faculty member). (7) Letter of recommendation from an osteopathic physician.

PROCESS

Individuals applying to the Edward Via Virginia College of Osteopathic Medicine may begin the application process by submitting a primary application to the American Association of Colleges of Osteopathic Medicine Application Service (AACOMAS). AACOMAS will begin accepting primary applications for the Class of 2011, which will matriculate in Fall 2007, on May 1. Once VCOM receives the primary application, the document will be screened for three factors: Requirements, academic factors, and nonacademic factors. In addition to the academic requirements listed above, nonacademic factors include volunteer and work experience in the health care field, extracurricular activities, community service and outreach, and the personal statement.

Candidates who present a competitive primary application will be invited, in writing, to submit a secondary application. The secondary application, located on the school website, will be available by June 15. VCOM requires two letters of recommendation—one from your premedical/pre-health committee (or science faculty member) and one from an osteopathic physician. All letters of recommendation must be originals on professional or college/university letterhead, signed by the evaluator, and accompanied by the first page of the evaluation form. Letters on professional or college/university letterhead may be submitted in lieu of answering the questionnaire on the evaluation form provided.

A rolling admissions process is used; applications are reviewed and interview decisions are made at regular intervals during the admissions cycle. The Admissions Committee meets every 2–4 weeks during the admissions cycle. After an interview is conducted and the committee meets, a student will be notified of his/her status. To be competitive, students should apply early in the cycle. Your primary application must be submitted to AACOMAS by February 1 and all secondary application materials must be received in the Office of Admissions at VCOM by March 15.

Admissions Requirements (Required)

MCAT scores, science GPA, non-science GPA, letters of recommendation, interview, essays/personal statement, extracurricular activities, exposure to medical profession, letter of recommendation from an osteopathic physician.

Admissions Requirements (Optional)

State residency.

Overlap Schools

East Tennessee State University, Eastern Virginia Medical School, Lake Erie College of Osteopathic Medicine, Nova Southeastern University, Ohio University of Osteopathic Medicine, Philadelphia College of Osteopathic Medicine, Southeastern College of Osteopathic Medicine, University of Virginia, Virginia Commonwealth University, West Virginia School of Osteopathic Medicine.

COSTS AND AID

Tuition & Fees

Tuition	$29,950
Room and board (off campus)	$23,000
Cost of books	$2,500

Financial Aid

% students receiving aid	99
Average grant	$1,000
Average loan	$50,000

WEST VIRGINIA SCHOOL OF OSTEOPATHIC MEDICINE

DIRECTOR OF ADMISSIONS, 400 NORTH LEE STREET, LEWISBURG, WV 24901 • ADMISSION: 800-356-7836
FAX: 304-645-4859 • E-MAIL: ADMISSIONS@WVSOM.EDU • WEBSITE: WWW.WVSOM.EDU

STUDENT BODY

Type	Public
Enrollment	397
% male/female	53/47
% underrepresented minorities	11
# applied (total/out)	1,635/1,512
# accepted (total/out)	310/250
# enrolled (total/out)	104/61
Average age	29

FACULTY

Total faculty (number)	57
% female	35
% minority	2
% part-time	19
Student-faculty ratio	4:1

ADMISSIONS

Average GPA and MCAT Scores

Overall GPA	3.48
MCAT Bio	7.3
MCAT Phys	6.8
MCAT Verbal	7.8
MCAT Essay	N

Application Information

Regular application	2/15
Regular notification	rolling
Early application	11/1
Early notification	12/6
Are transfers accepted?	yes
Admissions may be deferred?	yes
Interview required?	yes
Application fee	$155

Academics

West Virginia School of Osteopathic Medicine is part of the West Virginia State System of Higher Education. As a state school located in rural Appalachia, it is geared toward meeting the primary care needs of West Virginia's significantly rural population. Nine other states have loose affiliations with the school and are also served by its programs. This curriculum includes a system-based and problem-based approach to learning basic sciences and clinical training at community sites. Among all students the average age is 26, and the male/female ratio is 63/48.

West Virginia School of Osteopathic Medicine's curriculum is both demanding and enriching. Students should be aware that full participation in required classroom, small group, laboratory, and clinical training experiences is essential. WVSOM's curriculum reflects the school's interrelated education, service, and research mission and is designed to produce osteopathic physicians who are confident in rural settings, while assuring they have the educational competence and legal status for licensure and practice in all states. This curriculum includes a system-based and problem-based approach to learning basic sciences and clinical training at community sites.

CLINICAL TRAINING

Introduction to the clinical aspects of pre-clinical sciences occurs early in the student's studies, in the correlated organ systems instruction. Clinical education is designed to accomplish four objectives: provide ambulatory care training; provide hospital-based training; consolidate clinical knowledge and skills and learn to use them in a family medicine setting; and allow students, through electives, to augment their training in areas of medicine that are of special interest. The majority of years 3 and 4 of a student's medical education take place in clinical settings including physician offices, health centers, medical center, hospitals, etc.

BASIC SCIENCES: In the first year the systems based learning curriculum takes courses in the basic and clinical sciences that provide the foundation for the study of the organ systems that follow. The problem-based curriculum is an innovative curriculum that relies heavily on small group and student-directed learning to provide the foundation. Throughout the second year, basic science and clinical instruction are focused on one organ system. Integration of osteopathic principles with organ systems is maintained throughout both years.

Students

WVSOM students come to Lewisburg with diverse academic and professional backgrounds. Each class is composed of individuals with different levels of previous exposure to sciences and humanities. Historically, residents of West Virginia accounted for 50 percent of the student body; however, with a recent expansion, more out-of-state students are matriculating to WVSOM.

GRADUATES

For those students who fulfill the degree requirements, graduation exercises are held the last Saturday in May.

STUDENT LIFE

There are numerous campus organizations available to the students. Many involve community service projects calling for student volunteers.

Admissions

WVSOM uses the American Association of Colleges of Osteopathic Medicine Application Service (AACOMAS) to process its applications. WVSOM makes admissions decisions on a rolling basis; we review applications, conduct interviews, and make decision throughout the admissions cycle.

REQUIREMENTS

The minimum course requirements are eight semester hours of biology, physics, general chemistry, and organic chemistry, all with associated labs, and six semester hours of English. The MCAT is required and the test must be taken no later than the fall prior to the entering class year. Average MCAT or successful applicants is in the 7–8 range. About 26 percent of approximately 1,635 applicants are interviewed, with interviews taking place between August and April. Evaluation letters are required from a physician (DO or MD) and a premed advisor, premed committee, or an approved science faculty member.

SUGGESTIONS

It is strongly recommended that prospective students take additional upper level science courses, shadow physicians, and volunteer in health related settings.

Admissions Requirements (Required)

MCAT scores, science GPA, letters of recommendation, interview, essays/personal statement, exposure to medical profession, minimum 90 semester hours.

Admissions Requirements (Optional)

Nonscience GPA, state residency, extracurricular activities.

COSTS AND AID

Tuition & Fees

In-state Tuition	$17,650
Out-of-state Tuition	$43,678
Room and board (off campus)	$11,760
Cost of books	$6,020

Financial Aid

% students receiving aid	96
Average grant	$1,000
Average loan	$43,000
Average debt	$137,825

WESTERN UNIVERSITY OF HEALTH SCIENCES
COLLEGE OF OSTEOPATHIC MEDICINE OF THE PACIFIC

OFFICE OF ADMISSIONS, POMONA, CA 91766-1854 • ADMISSION: 909-469-5335 • FAX: 909-469-5570
E-MAIL: ADMISSIONS@WESTERNU.EDU • WEBSITE: WWW.WESTERNU.EDU

STUDENT BODY

Type	Private
Enrollment	724
% male/female	50/50
% underrepresented minorities	46
# applied (total/out)	2,344/1,604
# accepted (total/out)	543/278
# enrolled (total/out)	219/84
Average age	27

FACULTY

Total faculty (number)	27
% female	19
% minority	33
% part-time	4
Student-faculty ratio	27:1

ADMISSIONS

Average GPA and MCAT Scores

Overall GPA	3.47
MCAT Bio	9.43
MCAT Phys	8.78
MCAT Verbal	8.32
MCAT Essay	0

Application Information

Regular application	3/1
Regular notification	rolling
Early application	N/A
Early notification	N/A
Are transfers accepted?	yes
Admissions may be deferred?	yes
Interview required?	yes
Application fee	$65

Academics

Founded in 1977, Western University of Health Sciences is a nonprofit, graduate university for the health professions located next to Southern California's historic downtown Pomona. With five colleges and 1,885 students studying towards advanced degrees in osteopathic medicine, pharmacy, graduate nursing, physical therapy, physician assistant studies, health professions education, and veterinary medicine, Western University is one of the largest graduate schools for the health professions in California.

BASIC SCIENCE: The educational program is centered on the basic concepts of osteopathic medicine. The College of Osteopathic Medicine of the Pacific identifies and develops the knowledge, cognitive and psychomotor skills, and the personal and professional behaviors required of an osteopathic physician in order to provide competent and comprehensive health care to all members of a family on a continuing basis.

The first semester of the first year is designed to introduce the students to the basic concepts of anatomy (gross, embryology and histology), biochemistry, microbiology, pathology, pharmacology, and physiology. Interwoven throughout the curriculum are osteopathic principles and practice.

The second phase begins in the second semester of the first year and continues throughout the second year. The basic and clinical sciences concerned with one particular organ system of the body are integrated in classroom instruction. This approach emphasizes the relevance of basic sciences to clinical practice. The osteopathic approach is continually emphasized by lecture and laboratory demonstration including manipulative techniques. Other courses not directly related to a system are also included as Family Medicine Core Courses.

CLINICAL TRAINING

Clinical training via rotation through each of the major medical disciplines (family practice, internal medicine, surgery, pediatrics, obstetrics/gynecology, pathology, psychiatry, emergency medicine, and radiology) is accomplished in the third and fourth years of training. Twenty-two rotations of four weeks each provide an opportunity for clinical skill development in primary care medicine. Several elective options are also offered during this two-year period. The goal of the clinical curriculum is to prepare each student with the knowledge, attitudes, and skills to excel in his or her chosen postdoctoral training program.

Student Life

The main campus of Western University is in Pomona, a city of approximately 150,000 residents, located about 35 miles east of Los Angeles near the foothills of the San Gabriel Mountains. It is an area with a high concentration of private and state colleges and universities. Mountain resorts are nearby, and Pacific Ocean beaches, Palm Springs, Hollywood, Pasadena, Los Angeles, arboretums, theme parks, museums, art galleries, libraries, theaters, and concert halls are all within about an hour's drive.

RECREATIONAL FACILITIES

Western University provides YMCA or designated fitness club individual memberships for students at a minimal cost. On the campus, the Health Professions Center Student Commons provides billiards, television, and ping pong; and the parks offer picnic tables, basketball, and volleyball. There are also numerous tennis courts, golf courses, ski slopes, and hiking trails in the immediate area.

STUDENT GOVERNMENT

Currently, 66 organizations have been established within the student body. Students are encouraged, individually and collectively, to express their views on issues and administrative policy on campus. Through the elected representatives of the student body and membership on various university committees, students have the opportunity to participate in the administrative activities of the university. This body represents the students in all matters of concern with regard to faculty and administration.

GRADUATES

The College of Osteopathic Medicine of the Pacific supports Western University of Health Sciences (Western U) in its mission to increase the availability of Physicians to serve the needs of the people living in the western region of the United States. The College of Osteopathic Medicine provides the educational basis for internship and residencies in all medical specialties. The academic environment fosters respect for the uniqueness of humanity. Students are provided with classroom and clinical experiences designed to prepare them to function as competent, caring, lifelong learners with a distinctive Osteopathic philosophy.

Admissions

REQUIREMENTS

Applicants applying for admission to the DO program must meet the following minimum academic requirements at the time of application: A minimum of 90 semester hours, from a regionally-accredited college or university. Application may be submitted prior to taking the MCAT. The Medical College Admission Test (MCAT) is a requirement. The MCAT exam must be taken prior to January of the entering year. All applicants must complete eight (8) semester units of: biology, inorganic chemistry (with lab), organic chemistry (with lab), physics, and six (6) semester units of: English and behavioral science.

ADMISSIONS PROCESS

Prospective applicants must submit a Primary Application through The American Association of Colleges of Osteopathic Medicine Application Service (AACOMAS DEADLINE: April 15).

Once the AACOMAS application is received, selected applicants are contacted by postcard or e-mail with instructions on how to submit the supplementary application. At this time, applicants are instructed to complete the supplementary application online in Acrobat Reader, print, and mail to the Admissions Office. The supplementary application and all supporting documents should be received by the Admissions Office within 30 days of the date we contact you regarding supplementary application.

The deadline for supplemental material is one month after contact date. Once the interview process begins, students are admitted to the program on a rolling basis; therefore, students are encouraged to apply early.

You are required to submit letters of recommendation from a Pre-Health Professions Committee (or the committee on your campus responsible for writing recommendations) and one physician. If such a committee does not exist at your college you are required to submit two evaluations from science professors (i.e., biology, chemistry, physics), one evaluation from a non-science professor and one evaluation from a physician, DO, or MD, with whom you have worked or whom you have observed in a clinical setting. A recommendation letter from a DO is preferred.

The science/non-science letters must be from professors who have instructed you and the recommender should specify the course(s). All recommendations must be on the Western University form provided or on college or professional letterhead.

Admissions Requirements (Required)

MCAT scores, science GPA, non-science GPA, letters of recommendation, interview, essays/personal statement, extracurricular activities, exposure to medical profession.

Admissions Requirements (Optional)

State residency.

Overlap Schools

Touro University—California.

COSTS AND AID

Tuition & Fees

Tuition	$35,220
Room and board (off campus)	$10,380
Cost of books	$2,800
Fees	$40

Financial Aid

% students receiving aid	93
Average grant	$20,427
Average loan	$40,837
Average debt	$149,504

10 Post-baccalaureate Premedical Programs

Colleges and universities offer organized post-baccalaureate premedical programs. Although this list is quite comprehensive, it may be incomplete because many schools have just recently adopted post-bacc programs. In addition, many undergraduate institutions that do not offer formal programs have flexible enrollment policies that facilitate post-bacc studies.

For further listings of post-bacc programs, Syracuse University Health Professions Advisory Program (315-443-2321) has an online compilation at: http://services.aamc.org/postbac/.

AGNES SCOTT COLLEGE: POST-BACCALAUREATE PREMEDICAL PROGRAM

Dr. Nancy Devino
Program Director
141 East College Avenue
Decatur, GA 30030
404-471-6361
E-mail: post-bacc@agnesscott.edu

ALBRIGHT COLLEGE: POST-BACCALAUREATE PREMEDICAL PROGRAM

Dr. Karen A. Campbell
Program Director
Biology Department
Albright College
Reading, PA 19612-5234
610-921-7720
Fax: 610-921-7728
E-mail: kcampbell@alb.edu

AMERICAN UNIVERSITY

Post-baccalaureate Premedical Certificate
Program
Dr. Frederick W. Carson, Premedical
Programs Coordinator
Department of Chemistry
American University
4400 Massachusetts Avenue Northwest
Washington, DC 20016-8014
202-885-1770
Fax: 202-885-1752
E-mail: fcarson@american.edu

ARMSTRONG ATLANTIC STATE UNIVERSITY: POST-BACCALAUREATE PREMEDICAL PROGRAM

Dr. W. C. Zipperer
Program Director
11935 Abercorn Street
Savannah, GA 31419
912-921-5660
Fax: 912-961-3226
E-mail: zipperwc@mail.armstrong.edu

ASSUMPTION COLLEGE

Steven Theroux, PhD
Biology Department, Assumption College
Program Director
500 Salisbury Street
Worcester, MA 01615-0005
508-767-7545
E-mail: stheroux@assumption.edu

AVILA COLLEGE: POST-BACCALAUREATE PREMEDICAL PROGRAM

Dr. C. Larry Sullivan, Premedical Advisor
11901 Wornall Road
Kansas City, MO 64145
816-501-3655
Fax: 816-501-2457
E-mail: Larry.Sullivanl@mail.avila.edu

BARRY UNIVERSITY: BIOMEDICAL SCIENCES

Dr. Ralph Lauden, Associate Dean and
Director
School of Natural & Health Sciences
11300 Northeast Second Avenue
Miami Shores, FL 33161-6695
305-899-3227 or 800-756-6000, ext. 3541
Fax: 305-899-3232
Program Contact: Ms. Jocelyn Goulet
E-mail: healthsciences@mail.barry.edu

BENNINGTON COLLEGE: POST-BACCALAUREATE PREMEDICAL PROGRAM

Dr. Janet Foley, Program Director
Office of Admissions
Bennington College
One College Drive
Bennington, VT 05201
800-833-6845
Fax: 802-440-4320
Program Contact: Althea Bryant
E-mail: abryant@bennington.edu

BOSTON UNIVERSITY

Post-baccalaureate Certificate in
Premedical Studies
PMC Program Coordinator
725 Commonwealth Avenue, Room 102
Boston, MA 02215
617-353-2980
617-353-4190
E-mail: metuss@bu.edu

BOSTON UNIVERSITY SCHOOL OF MEDICINE, MASTER OF ARTS IN MEDICAL SCIENCES PROGRAM

Susan Wilcox
GMS, Boston University
School of Medicine
715 Albany Street, Suite L-317
Boston, MA 02446
617-638-5120
Fax: 617-638-4842
Program Contact: Susan Wilcox
E-mail: wilcox@bu.edu

BRANDEIS UNIVERSITY

Post-baccalaureate Certificate Program
Kate Fukawa-Connelly, Program Director
Office of Undergraduate Academic
Affairs
Kutz 108/MS 001
Waltham, MA 02254-9110
781-736-3470
E-mail: Kfconnelly@brandeis.edu

BRYN MAWR COLLEGE

Post-baccalaureate Premedical Program
Bryn Mawr College Canwyll House
101 North Merion Ave.
Bryn Mawr, PA 19010-2899
610-526-7350
E-mail: postbac@brynmawr.edu

CARSON-NEWMAN COLLEGE

Dr. Frank Pinkerton
Program Director
Carson-Newman College
Box 71992, Russell Avenue
Jefferson City, TN 37760
865-471-3257
Fax: 865-471-3578
E-mail: fpinkerton@cn.edu

CHAPMAN UNIVERSITY

Dr. Virginia Carson, PhD
Post-baccalaureate Premedical Program
One University Drive
Orange, CA 92866
714-997-6696
Fax: 714-532-6048
E-mail: carson@chapman.edu

CITY UNIVERSITY OF NEW YORK—CITY COLLEGE

Dr. Robert Goode
J-529 Program in Premedical Studies
138th Street at Convent Avenue
New York, NY 10031
212-650-7843
Fax: 212-650-7816
Program Contacts: Mr. B. Jinadu and Ms. Y. Scott
E-mail: rosario@sci.ccny.cuny.edu

CLEVELAND STATE UNIVERSITY

Post-baccalaureate Program
Dr. Madeline M. Hall
BGES Department 2121 Euclid, SI 219
Cleveland, OH 44115
216-687-2418
Fax: 216-687-6972
E-mail: m.hall@csuohio.edu

COLUMBIA UNIVERSITY

Post-baccalaureate Premedical Program
Dr. Mary McGee
2970 Broadway
404 Lewissohn Hall, MC 4109
New York, NY 10027
212-854-0467
Fax: 212-854-7257
E-mail: gspostbacc@columbia.edu

CREIGHTON UNIVERSITY

Premedical Post-bacculaureate
Dr. Sade Kosoko-Lasaki
Program Director
2500 California Plaza
Omaha, NE 68178
402-280-3029
Program Contact: Channing Bunch
E-mail: cbunch@creighton.edu

DARTMOUTH MEDICAL SCHOOL: CENTER FOR THE EVALUATIVE CLINICAL SCIENCES

Hinman Box 7252
Karen A. Tombs, MEd
14 MML Building
Hanover, NH 03755
603-650-1782
Fax: 603-650-1900
Program Contact: Karen A. Tombs, M.Ed.
E-mail: karen.a.tombs@dartmouth.edu

DOMINICAN UNIVERSITY

Post-baccalaureate Premedical Program
Dr. Louis Seannichio, Program Director
7900 West Division Street
River Forest, IL 60305-1066
708-366-6901
E-mail: lseann@email.dom.edu

DOWLING COLLEGE

Certificate Program in the Pre-health Professions
Dr. Richard Wilkens, Program Director
Department of Biology
Oakdale, NY 11769
631-244-3491
Fax: 631-244-1033
E-mail: wilkensr@dowling.edu

DREXEL UNIVERSITY

Medical Science Preparatory Program
Drexel University College of Medicine
245 North Fifteenth Street, MS 344,
Room 4122 NCB
Philadelphia, PA 19102
215-762-4692
Fax: 215-762-7434
Program Contact: Yolanda Pressley
E-mail: imsinfo@drexel.edu

DREXEL UNIVERSITY
Drexel Pathway to Medical School
Drexel University College of Medicine
Dr. Loretta Walker, Program Director
45 North 15th Street,
MS 344, Room 4122 NC
Philadelphia, PA 19102
215-762-4692
E-mail: imsinfo@drexel.edu

DREXEL UNIVERSITY
Evening Post-baccalaureate Premedical
Program
Drexel University College of Medicine
Dr. Laura Mangano, Program Director
245 North 15th Street,
MS 344, Room 4122 NCB
Philadephia, PA 19102
215-762-4692
E-mail: imsinfo@drexel.edu

DREXEL UNIVERSITY
Interdepartmental Medical Science
Program
Drexel University College of Medicine
245 North 15th Street,
MS 344, Room 4122 NCB
Philadelphia, PA 19102
Program Contact: Dr. Laura Mangano
215-762-4692
E-mail: imsinfo@drexel.edu

DUQUESNE UNIVERSITY
Post-baccalaureate Premedical Program
Dr. Kyle Selcer, Program Director
B101 Bayer Learning Center
Pittsburgh, PA 15282
412-396-6335
Fax: 412-396-5587
Program Contact: Cathy Dvorak
MSW/LSW, Associate Director
E-mail: dvorak@dug.edu

EAST TENNESSEE STATE UNVERSITY
FasTrack Program
Dr. Lattie Collins, Program Director
PO Box 70592—ETSU
East Tennessee State University
Johnson City, TN 37614
423-439-6903
Fax: 423-439-4840
E-mail: collinsl@mail.etsu.edu

EASTERN VIRGINIA MEDICAL SCHOOL
Medical Master's Program
Toni Dorn, Administrator
700 West Olney Road
Norfolk, VA 23507
757-446-8424
Fax: 757-446-8449
dornma@evms.edu

FISK UNIVERSITY AND VANDERBILT UNIVERSITY MEDICAL CENTER
Mary Wech, PhD, Program Director
UNCF Premedical Summer Institute, Fisk
University
1000 Seventeenth Avenue, North
Nashville, TN 37208-3051
615-329-8796
Fax: 615-329-8636
mckelvey@fisk.edu

GEORGETOWN UNIVERSITY
Post-baccalaureate Premedical Certificate
Program
Dr. Mark Esrick, Program Director
37th O Street, Northwest,
Reiss Building, Room 506
Washington, DC 20057
202-687-6039
E-mail: esrickm@georgetown.edu

GEORGETOWN UNIVERSITY
Adam Myers, Program Director
Special Master's Program, Department of
Physiology
Georgetown University, Box 571460
Washington, DC 20057-1460
Program Contact: Ms. Aureller Cabiness
202-687-1179
Fax: 202-687-7407
E-mail: physio@georgetown

HARVARD UNIVERSITY
Health Careers Program
Dr. William Fixsen, Program Director
51 Brattle Street
Cambridge, MA 02138
617-495-2926
Program Contact: Owen Peterson
E-mail: hcp@dcemail.harvard.edu

HOFSTRA UNIVERSITY
Post-baccalaureate Premedical Program
Marion Flomenhaft, Program Director
Hofstra University, 250 University
College Hall
Hempstead, NY 11549
516-463-7600
Program Contact: Marion Flomenhaft
E-mail: marion.flomenhaft@hofstra.edu

HUNTER COLLEGE—CITY UNIVERSITY OF NEW YORK
Post-baccalaureate Pre-health Professions
Program
695 Park Avenue
New York, NY 10021
212-772-5244
Program Contact: Woldine Guerrier
E-mail: woldine.guerrier@hunter.cuny.edu

GOUCHER COLLEGE
Liza Thompson, Program Director
Post-baccalaureate Premedical Program
1201 Dulaney Valley Road
Baltimore, MD 21204-2794
800-414-3437
Fax: 410-337-6461
E-mail: pbpm@goucher.edu

IMMACULATA COLLEGE
Post-baccalaureate Pre-professional
Program
Dr. James Murray, Jr., Program Director
1145 King Road, Box 650
Immaculata, PA 19345-0650
610-647-4400, Ext. 3307
E-mail: jmurray@immaculata.edu

INDIANA UNIVERSITY SCHOOL OF MEDICINE
Master of Science in Medical Science
Program
Indiana University School of Medicine
Dr. William Agbor Baiyee, Program
Director
Medical Science Building 207
635 Barnhill Drive
Indianapolis, IN 46202
317-278-1724
317-278-5211
E-mail: msms@iupui.edu

INDIANA UNIVERSITY SCHOOL OF MEDICINE
Dr. Stephen Kempson, Program Director
MS in Health Sciences
635 Barnhill Drive
Physiology—MS 309
Indianapolis, IN 46202-5120
317-274-7772
Program Contact: Marlene Brown
E-mail: msphysio@iupui.edu

JOHNS HOPKINS UNIVERSITY
Post-baccalaureate Premedical Program
David Trabilsy, Program Director
3003 N. Charles Street
Wyman Park Building, Suite G1
Baltimore, MD 21218
410-516-7748
Fax: 410-516-6017
Program Contact: Kristin Schulze, Coordinator
E-mail: postbacc@jhu.edu

LA SALLE UNIVERSITY
Post-baccalaureate Premedical
Certificate Program
Dr. Geri Seitchik, Program Director
1900 West Olney
Philadelphia, PA 19141-1199
215-951-1248
E-mail: seichik@lasalle.edu

LAKE ERIE COLLEGE OF OSTEOPATHIC MEDICINE (LECOM)
Dr. R. Nassiri, Program Director
LECOM
1858 West Grandview Boulevard
Erie, PA 16509
814-866-8146
Fax: 814-886-8411
E-mail: rnassiri@lecom.edu

LAMAR UNIVERSITY
Dr. James Westgate, Program Director
College of Arts and Sciences
PO Box 10058
Beaumont, TX 77710
409-880-7972
Fax: 409-880-8007
E-mail: westgatejw@hal.lamar.edu

LOMA LINDA UNIVERSITY
Biomedical Sciences Certificate
Kenneth Wright, Program Director
Faculty of Graduate Studies
Nelson House
Loma Linda, CA 92350
909-558-7602
Fax: 909-558-0119
E-mail: kwright@llu.edu

LOYOLA MARYMOUNT UNIVERSITY
Post-baccalaureate Premedical Program
Dr. Rebecca Crawford, Program Director
1 LMU Drive
MS 8225
Los Angeles, CA 90045-2659
310-338-7350
Fax: 310-338-7339
E-mail: rcrawford@lmu.edu

LOYOLA UNIVERSITY OF CHICAGO
Post-baccalaureate Pre-health Program
Loyola University Chicago Graduate &
Professor Enrollment
820 North Michigan Avenue, LT 800
Chicago, IL 60611-2196
773-508-3636 or 312-915-8900

LOYOLA UNIVERSITY OF CHICAGO
Master of Arts in Medical Sciences
Dr. Diane Suter, Graduate
Program Director
Department of Biology
6525 North Sheridan Road
Chicago, IL 60626
773-508-3285
E-mail: dsuter@luc.edu

MANHATTANVILLE COLLEGE
Post-baccalaureate Pre-health Professions
Program
Academic Advising Office
2900 Purchase Street
Purchase, NY 10577
914-798-2755
Fax: 914-323-5338
Program Contact: Andrew Bodenrader
E-mail: bodenradera@mville.edu

MEDICAL UNIVERSITY OF OHIO
Post-baccalaureate Premedical Program
Carol Bennett-Clarke, PhD, Program
Director
3045 Arlington Avenue
Toledo, OH 43614-5805
419-383-4903
E-mail: cbclarke@meduohio.edu

MIDWESTERN UNIVERSITY
Master of Biomedical Services
Fred D. Romano, PhD
555 31st Street
Downers Grove, IL 60515
630-515-6392
Fax: 630-971-6414
E-mail: froman@midwestern.edu

MILLS COLLEGE
Post-baccalaureate Program
5000 MacArthur Boulevard
Oakland, CA 94613
510-430-2317
Fax: 510-430-3314
Program Contact: Jo Sullivan
E-mail: jscullio@mills.edu

MONTANA STATE UNIVERSITY
Post-baccalaureate Premedical Certificate
Program
MSU Division of Health Sciences, 308
Leon Johnson Hall
Bozeman, MT 59717-3080
406-994-1670
Program Contact: Jane Cary
E-mail:hpa@montana.edu

MOUNT HOLYOKE
Frances Perkins Post-baccalaureate
Studies Program
Kay Althoff
6 Safford Hall
50 College Street
South Hadley, MA 01075
413-538-2077
Fax: 413-538-3013
E-mail: frances-perkins@mtholyoke.edu

NATIONAL INSTITUTES OF HEALTH
NIH Post-bacc Research Training
Program
Building 1, Room 135
1 Center Drive MSC 0151
Bethesda, MD 20892
301-402-1907
Fax: 301-402-8975
Program Contact: Debbie Cohen
E-mail: cohend@od.nih.gov

NEW YORK MEDICAL COLLEGE
Graduate School of Basic Medical
Sciences
Basic Sciences Building, Room A-41
Valhalla, NY 10595
Program Contact: Marge Riley
914-594-4110
Fax: 914-594-4944
E-mail: marge_riley@nymc.edu

NEW YORK UNIVERSITY
Post-baccalaureate/Pre-health Studies
Ms. Soomie Han, Program Director
Silver Professional Center
100 Washington Square East, #901
New York, NY 10003-6699
212-998-8160
Fax: 212-995-4549
E-mail: prehealth@nyu.edu

NORTHWESTERN UNIVERSITY SCHOOL OF CONTINUING STUDIES
Premedical Professional Health Careers
Program
Admissions Coordinator
405 Church Street
Evanston, IL 60208-2650
847-491-0990
Fax: 491-3660
E-mail: scadmissions@northwestern.edu

OKLAHOMA STATE UNIVERSITY
OSU Center for Health Sciences College
of Osteopathic Medicine
Leah Haines, Program Director
1111 West 17th Street
Tulsa, OK 74107-1898
918-561-8468
Program Contact: Amanda Gutierrez
E-mail: gutiera@chs.okstate.edu

OLD DOMINION UNIVERSITY
Pre-health Individualized Program
Ms. Sharon Melone-Orme, Program
Director
College of Sciences
OCNPS 131
Norfolk, VA 23529-0163
757-683-5200
Fax: 757-683-3034
E-mail: smelone@odu.edu

PENNSYLVANIA STATE UNIVERSITY
Post-baccalaureate Premedical Certificate
Program
Dr. Rodriguez, Program Director
213 Whitmore Lab
University Park, PA 16802
814-865-7620
Fax: 814-865-7214
E-mail: mxr22@psu.edu

PHILADELPHIA COLLEGE OF OSTEOPATHIC MEDICINE
Biomedical Sciences Program
Office of Admissions
4170 City Avenue
Philadelphia, PA 19131
800-999-6998
Fax: 215-871-6719
E-mail: admissions@pcom.edu

RICHARD STOCKTON COLLEGE OF NEW JERSEY
Post-baccalaureate Certificate Program in
Health Professions
Dr. Ralph Werner, Program Director
Jim Leeds Road
Pomona, NJ 08240
609-652-4462
E-mail: ralph.werner@stockton.edu

RIDER UNIVERSITY
Premedical Studies Program
Dr. Julie Drawbridge, Program Director
2083 Lawrenceville Road
Lawrenceville, NJ 08648
609-895-5428
Fax: 609-895-5782
E-mail: drawbridge@rider.edu

ROCKHURST UNIVERSITY
Post-baccalaureate Premedical Program
Dr. James Wheeler, Program Director
Department of Chemistry
1100 Rockhurst Road
Kansas City, MO 64110
816-501-4068
Fax: 816-501-4169
E-mail: james.wheeler@rockhurst.edu

RUTGERS UNIVERSITY—NEWARK
Post-baccalaureate Pre-health Program
Dr. Victoria U. Kachukwu
35 College Avenue, Deans Office
New Brunswich, NJ 08903
732-932-7234
E-mail: vukachuck@andromeda.rutgers.edu

SAN DIEGO STATE UNIVERSITY
Pre-professional Health Advising Office
Barbara Huntington
5500 Campanile Drive
MC-1017
San Diego, CA 92182-1017
619-594-6638
Fax: 619-594-0244
E-mail: healthpr@sciences.sdsu.edu

SAN FRANCISCO STATE UNIVERSITY
Barry Rothman, Program Director
Department of Biology,
1600 Holloway Avenue
San Francisco, CA 94132
415-338-2418
E-mail: brothman@sfsu.edu

SAN FRANCISCO STATE UNIVERSITY
Health Professions Prep and
Re-applicant Program
Dr. Barry Rothman, Program Director
1600 Holloway Avenue
San Francisco, CA 94132
415-338-2410
Fax: 415-338-2295
E-mail: brothman@sfsu.edu

SAN JOSE STATE UNIVERSITY
Post-baccalaureate Premedical Program
Dr. Robert Fowler, Program Director
Department of Biological Sciences
San Jose, CA 95192
408-924-4900 or 408-924-4843
Fax: 408-924-4840
E-mail: rfowler@email.sjsu.edu

SCRIPPS COLLEGE
Post-baccalaureate Premedical Program
Ms. Jodi Olson, Program Director
W. M. Keck Science Center
925 North Mills Avenue
Claremont, CA 91711
909-621-8764
Fax: 909-8588
E-mail: Jolson@scrippscollege.edu

SEATTLE UNIVERSITY
Post-baccalaureate Premedical Program
Dr. Margaret Hudson, Program Director
Biology Department Seattle University
901 Twelfth Avenue, PO Box 22200
Seattle, WA 98122
206-296-5486
E-mail: mhudson@seattleu.edu

SOUTHERN ILLINOIS UNIVERSITY SCHOOL OF MEDICINE
Medical/Dental Education Preparatory
Program (MEDPREP)
Dr. Harold Bardo, Program Director
Wheeler Hall
Carbondale, IL 62901-4323
618-453-1554
Fax: 618-453-1919
Program Contact: Vera Felts
E-mail: MedPrepAdmissions@siumed.edu

SPRING HILL COLLEGE
Post-baccalaureate Premedical Studies
Dr. David Dean, Program Director
4000 Dauphin Street
Mobile, AL 36608
215-380-3067
Fax: 215-460-2190
Program Contact: Consheda Wallace
E-mail: cwallace@shc.edu

STATE UNIVERSITY OF NEW YORK— STONY BROOK UNIVERSITY
Post-baccalaureate Premedical Program
James Montren
Room E2360
Stony Brook, NY 11704-3353
631-632-7093
E-mail: prehealth@notes.cc.sunysb.edu

TEXAS CHRISTIAN UNIVERSITY
Ruth Eakin
Box 298800
Fort Worth, TX 76129
817-257-5337
Fax: 817-257-6177
E-mail: r.eakin@tcu.edu

TOWSON UNIVERSITY
Post-baccalaureate Premedical and Pre-dental Program
Katherine Denniston, Program Director
Dean's Office, Fisher College of Science & Math
8000 York Road
Towson, MD 21252-0002
410-704-3128
E-mail: kdenniston@towson.edu

TUFTS UNIVERSITY
Post-baccalaureate Premedical Program
Carol Baffi-Dugan, Program Director
419 Boston Avenue
Dowling Hall
Medford, MA 02155
Program Contact: Liz Regan
617-627-2321
Fax: 617-627-3907
E-mail: liz.regan@tufts.edu

TULANE UNIVERSITY
Hayward Genetics Center One-year
Master's Degree Program
Gayle Pullen
1430 Tulane Avenue
New Orleans, LA 70112
504-584-1981
Fax: 504-584-3684
E-mail: hgcedprg@tulane.edu

UNIVERSITY AT BUFFALO—ROSWELL PARK CANCER INSTITUTE

Interdisciplinary Biomed/Oncology MS
Program
Craig Johnson, Program Director
Roswell Park Cancer Institute
408 Research Studies Center
Buffalo, NY 14263-0001
716-845-8134
E-mail: craig.johnson@roswellpark.org

UNIVERSITY OF CALIFORNIA— DAVIS SCHOOL OF MEDICINE

Post-baccalaureate Re-applicant Program
Edward Dagang, Program Director
One Shields Avenue
Davis, CA 95616
Program Contact: Alan Blakely
503-754-6033
Fax: 503-754-6252
E-mail: awblakely@ucdavis.edu

UNIVERSITY OF CALIFORNIA— IRVINE COLLEGE OF MEDICINE

Premedical Post-baccalaureate
Enhancement Program
Ms. Emma Ledesma
Office of Admissions and Outreach
College of Medicine
Medical Education Building 802
Irvine, CA 92697-4089
800-824-5388
Fax: 949-824-2485
E-mail: ppep@uci.edu

UNIVERSITY OF CALIFORNIA— IRVINE COLLEGE OF MEDICINE

Post-baccalaureate Reapplicant Program
Ms. Ellen Munoz
Medical Education Building 802
PO Box 4089
Irvine, CA 92697-4089
949-824-8930
E-mail: pbreapp@uci.edu

UNIVERSITY OF CALIFORNIA— LOS ANGELES, DAVID GEFFEN SCHOOL OF MEDICINE

UCLA Premedical Predental
Enhancement Program
Elizabeth Guerrero-Yzquierdo, Program
Director
13-154 CHS
10833 Le Conte Avenue
Los Angeles, CA 90095
310-825-3575
Fax: 310-206-7180
E-mail: aeotemp2@mednet.ucla.edu

UNIVERSITY OF CALIFORNIA— SAN DIEGO SCHOOL OF MEDICINE

Re-applicant Post-baccalaureate Program
Saundra Kirk
Student Outreach Services
Date Building, Room 105
La Jolla, CA 92093-0655
858-534-4171
Fax: 858-534-5293
E-mail: sjkirk@ucsd.edu

UNIVERSITY OF CALIFORNIA— SAN FRANCISCO

UCSF Post-baccalaureate Programs
Valerie Margol, Program Director
1855 Folsom Street
Room 305, Box 0409
San Francisco, CA 94143-0409
Program Contact: Felicia Tripp
415-514-1390
Fax: 415-502-1680
E-mail: tripp@medsch.ucsf.edu

UNIVERSITY OF CINCINNATI

Master of Science in Physiology
(12 Month Premedical Program)
Dr. Robert Banks, Program Director
231 Albert B. Sabin Way
PO Box 670576
Cincinnati, OH 45267-0576
513-558-3104
Program Contact: Karen Coleman
E-mail: Karen.Coleman@uc.edu

UNIVERSITY OF CONNECTICUT SCHOOL OF MEDICINE

Post-baccalaureate Program
Keat Sanford, Program Director
Admissions Center
263 Farmington Avenue
Farmington, CT 06030-3906
Program Contact: Tricia Avolt
860-679-4306
Fax: 860-679-1899
E-mail: robertson@nso2.uchc.edu

UNIVERSITY OF MARYLAND— COLLEGE PARK

Science in the Evening
Dr. Joelle Presson, Program Director
1322 Symons Hall
University of Maryland
College Park, MD 20742
301-405-6892
E-mail: jpresson@umd.edu

UNIVERSITY OF MASSACHUSETTS— BOSTON

Post-baccalaureate Premedical Program
Grace McSorley
University Career Services
100 Morrissey Boulevard
Boston, MA 02125
617-287-5519
Fax: 617-287-5525
E-mail: grace.mcsorley@umb.edu

UMDNJ—GRADUATE SCHOOL OF BIOMEDICAL SCIENCES

Master's in Biomedical Sciences
Dr. Nicholas Ingoglia, Program Director
ADMC 1, Suite 110
Newark, NJ 07103
973-972-4776 or 973-972-4511
Fax: 973-972-5656
E-mail: ingoglia@umdnj.edu

UNIVERSITY OF MIAMI

Pre-medical Post-baccalaureate Program
Linette Aguiar, Program Director
205 Ashe Building
Coral Gables, FL 33124-4622
Program Contact: Mariana Dunham
305-284-5176
Fax: 305-284-4686
E-mail: premed@miami.edu

UNIVERSITY OF NORTH CAROLINA— GREENSBORO

Premedical Program
Robert E. Cannon, PhD
Post-Baccalaureate Premed Program,
UNC—Greensboro
Department of Biology, PO Box 26170
Greensboro, NC 27402-6170
336-256-0071
Fax: 336-334-5839
E-mail: Robert_Cannon@uncg.edu

UNIVERSITY OF NORTH FLORIDA

Post-baccalaureate Premedical Program
Dr. Michael Lentz, Program Director
4567 St. Johns Bluff Road South
Jacksonville, FL 32224
904-620-2608
E-mail: mlentz@unf.edu

UNIVERSITY OF NORTH TEXAS

Post-baccalaureate Pre-certification in
Medical Science
Carla Lee, Program Director
3500 Camp Bowie Boulevard,
Suite EAD-816
Fort Worth, TX 76107
817-735-2560 or 800-511-4723
Program Contact: Amanda Griffith
E-mail: gsbs@hsc.unt.edu

UNIVERSITY OF OREGON

Post-baccalaureate Premedical Program
Office of Academic Advising 5217
University of Oregon
Eugene, OR 97403-5217
541-346-3211
Fax: 541-346-6048
Program Contact: Karen Cooper
E-mail: karenc@darkwing.uoregon.edu

UNIVERSITY OF PENNSYLVANIA

Post-baccalaureate Pre-health Program
Dr. Lynne Hunter, Program Director
3440 Market Street, Suite 100
College of General Studies
Philadelphia, PA 19104-3335
215-898-3110
Fax: 215-573-2053
E-mail: lynneh@sas.upenn.edu

UNIVERSITY OF PITTSBURGH

Arts and Sciences Post-baccalaureate
Program
Donna Walker, Program Director
252 Thackeray Hall
University of Pittsburgh
Pittsburgh, PA 15260
412-624-6444
Fax: 412-624-3707
E-mail: dlw5@pitt.edu

UNIVERSITY OF SOUTH FLORIDA

Biomedical Sciences
4202 East Fowler Ave.
SCA 400
Tampa, FL 33620
813-974-2144
Fax: 813-974-5314
E-mail: chemadvising@cas.usf.edu

UNIVERSITY OF SOUTHERN CALIFORNIA

Post-baccalaureate Premedical Program
Admissions Coordinator
CAS 120, USC College
Los Angeles, CA 90089-0151
213-821-2354
Fax: 213-740-3664
E-mail: postbacc@usc.edu

UNIVERSITY OF UTAH SCHOOL OF MEDICINE

Summer MCAP Preparation &
Research/Clinical Training Program
Ms. Sunshine Nakae-Gibson, Program
Director
30 North 1900 East
Room 1C117
Salt Lake City, UT 84132-2101
801-585-2430
Fax: 801-585-3300
E-mail: sunny.gibson@hsc.utah.edu

UNIVERSITY OF VERMONT

Post-baccalaureate Premedical Program
Beth Taylor-Nolan
1322 South Prospect Street
Burlington, VT 05401
802-656-2085
Fax: 802-656-0306
E-mail: Beth.Taylor-Nolan@uvm.edu

VIRGINIA COMMONWEALTH UNIVERSITY
Premedical Basic Sciences
Dr. Jan Chlebowski, Program Director
Office of Graduate Education VCU
School of Medicine
1101 East Marshall Street Box 980565
Richmond, VA 23298-9565
804-828-8366
Fax: 804-828-6011
E-mail: jfchlebo@vcu.edu

WASHINGTON UNIVERSITY IN ST. LOUIS
Post-baccalaureate Premedical Program
Dr. Steven Ehrlich, Program Director
One Brookings Drive, Campus Box 1064
St. Louis, MO 63130-4899
314-935-4320
E-mail: ehrlich@wustl.edu

WAKE FOREST UNIVERSITY
SCHOOL OF MEDICINE
Post-baccalaureate Premedical Program
Brenda Latham-Sadler, Program Director
Medical Center Boulevard
Office of Student Services
Winston-Salem, NC 27157
Program Contact: Nicole Henry
336-716-4271
Fax: 336-716-4271
E-mail: nhenry@wfubmc.edu

WEST CHESTER UNIVERSITY
Premedical Program
Dr. Melissa Cichowicz, Program Director
117 Schmucker Science Center South
West Chester, PA 19383
610-436-2978
Fax: 610-436-3277
E-mail: pmed@wcupa.edu

WORCESTER STATE COLLEGE
Post-baccalaureate Premedical Program
Dr. Allan Cooper, Program Director
486 Chandler Street
Worcester, MA 01602
508-929-8600
E-mail: acooper@worcester.edu

SCHOOL SAYS

In this section you'll find schools with extended listings describing admissions, curriculum, internships, and much more. This is your chance to get in-depth information on programs that interest you. The Princeton Review charges each school a small fee to be listed, and the editorial responsibility is solely that of the university.

AMERICAN UNIVERSITY OF THE CARIBBEAN

BACKGROUND

American University of the Caribbean School of Medicine (AUC) has been providing quality education continuously since 1978. Originally founded in Montserrat, British West Indies, AUC relocated its medical science campus to St. Maarten due to volcanic eruptions on Montserrat. In 1998, AUC built a new basic sciences campus on the island of St. Maarten that encompasses modern facilities for comprehensive medical study. The new campus facilities include contemporary lecture halls enhanced with audio/visual technology, fully equipped biological science and anatomical dissection laboratories, clinical patient examination rooms, an extensive library with an up-to-date student computer center, and numerous common areas appropriate both for student study and relaxation. The size and location of AUC's basic science campus contributes to a special atmosphere where faculty and staff are able to concentrate on students acquiring the basic medical knowledge necessary for their clinical experience. Students find that the faculty and staff are accessible and are committed to their progress. Thousands of AUC medical students have graduated to become caring, responsible and compassionate doctors who are licensed and practicing medicine throughout the United States. They have entered all aspects of mainstream medicine, private practice, universities, government agencies and managed care facilities.

FINANCIAL AID

AUC is approved for the Federal Family Education Loan Program (FFELP). The Office of Financial Aid is available to assist students through the intricacies of the financial aid process and paperwork. For qualified citizens and permanent residents of the United States, funding is available from both federal and privately sponsored loan programs to fully meet the cost of attending AUC (tuition, books & supplies, accommodation and travel). A private loan program is available for Canadian citizens.

LICENSURE, ACCREDITATION AND RECOGNITION

American University of the Caribbean School of Medicine is approved by the California State Medical Board, New York State Board for Medicine, and Florida State Commission for Independent Education. AUC is fully accredited by the Accreditation Commission on Colleges of Medicine (ACCM). The National Committee on Foreign Medical Education and Accreditation of the U.S. Department of Education recognizes the ACCM as an accreditation body having standards comparable to LCME. AUC is listed in the World Directory of Medical Schools, published by the World Health Organization (WHO).

SCHOLARSHIP

The Chancellor's Scholarship targets candidates from across the United States who have demonstrated excellent academic achievement and attained strong scores on the Medical College Admissions Test (MCAT). All admitted applicants who meet the scholarship requirements are considered. A separate application is not required. Scholarships will be awarded approximately three months prior to the student's semester start date subject to availability of funds. Scholarships may not be deferred to another semester. Recipients will be notified by mail of the scholarship amount and terms. Each Chancellor's Scholarship recipient is awarded a 50 percent tuition rebate. The recipient must maintain honor level status of 90 percent or better in order to continue receiving the tuition rebate.

APPLICATION

Students may apply online at www.aucmed.edu or request an application by calling toll-free at 866-DR2B-AUC (866-372-2282).

CAMPUS VISIT

Prospective students and their families are welcome to visit the AUC campus for a tour of its facilities and student housing. Campus tours provide prospects an opportunity to speak to faculty, as well as current students, about AUC. Tours are conducted from Monday to Friday between 10:00 A.M.–11:00 A.M. and in the afternoon between 3:00 P.M.–4:00 P.M., excluding final exam periods and holidays. To arrange a tour, please visit www.aucmed.edu, or call toll-free at 866-DR2B-AUC.

PHILADELPHIA COLLEGE OF OSTEOPATHIC MEDICINE

Established in 1899, Philadelphia College of Osteopathic Medicine (PCOM) is a private, nonprofit institution built on an over 100 year tradition of excellence in medical education. Students find the educational program at PCOM is an optimal blend of classroom teaching, clinical experience and research. From the first day of medical school, PCOM students begin learning the osteopathic approach to health care: treating the whole person, not just the symptoms. Early clinical exposure through community service activities and formal course work implement basic science instruction. The curriculum is interdisciplinary, and includes topics such as medical ethics and medical law, and emphasizes primary care and prevention. Clinical training takes place at 37 affiliated institutions in and around Philadelphia. In addition, students may arrange to fulfill elective requirements in other states or in other countries. Joint degree programs lead to the DO/MBA, DO/MPH and DO/PhD. PCOM is committed to helping each of its students choose a career that matches their specific talents and interests. The entering class of 2005 in Philadelphia included 266 students from 22 states. The male/female ration was 50/50 and the average age was 26.

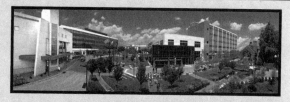

We are pleased to announce the creation of our new branch campus outside of Atlanta, Georgia. This campus opened in August, 2005 with 86 students. The contact information is 625 Old Peachtree Road NW, Suwannee, GA 30024; the telephone number is 678-225-7500.

As a private institution, PCOM accepts applicants from all over the country and does show preference for Pennsylvania residents. Science preparation must include eight semester hours (including lab) each in biology, inorganic chemistry, organic chemistry, and physics. In addition, six hours of English literature and composition are required. The MCAT is required and must be taken within three years of desired matriculation. All AACOMAS applicants receive secondary applications. Of the approximately 4,000 applicants returning secondaries, approximately 16 percent are invited (via e-mail) to interview on campus, with interviews beginning in September. The interview consists of one session with a panel which could include faculty, students, and administrators. Notification of committee decision occurs on a rolling basis until the class is filled.

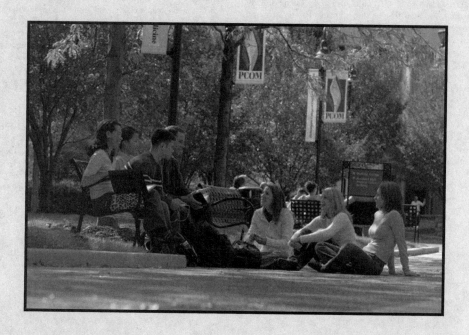

SPARTAN HEALTH SCIENCES UNIVERSITY, SCHOOL OF MEDICINE

AT A GLANCE

The primary objective of Spartan Health Sciences University, School of Medicine, is to provide qualified students an opportunity to fulfill their lifelong ambition of serving humanity with medical education and prolongation of human life through medical care and research. The university strives hard to attain a high standard of education with affordable tuition fees ever since its inception. This does not in anyway compromise the standard of medical education offered by this institution. The university is dedicated to train its graduates with an excellent medical knowledge and competent skills in order to assure the society and the medical profession to meet the health care demands of the societies to which they belong.

LOCATION AND ENVIRONMENT

Spartan Health Sciences University, School of Medicine, is located in the former British Colony of Saint Lucia. The people of Saint Lucia are English speaking, friendly, and very accommodating. The population of St. Lucia at the end of 2000 was 163,819. The local language is Creole (or Patois, an adulterated French) emerged as a result of British and French influences with English as the official language. Outside of the classroom, students are involved in various community health care events. Medical students take advantage of the fitness center, tennis courts on school premises, and cricket and soccer field behind the school. All students live off campus, within walking or biking distance of campus.

ACADEMICS

Spartan Health Sciences University, School of Medicine, offers a four academic year (36 calendar month) program leading to the Doctor of Medicine degree (M.D.), and is taught on a trimester (four months) schedule. The curriculum of the university's Doctor of Medicine degree program encompasses a comprehensive course of Basic Sciences (BS), Pre-clinical, and Clinical Sciences (CS) that lasts for four academic years. The trimester periods start in January, May, and September of each year. A student may elect to enter in any one of the three trimesters. To provide the best possible medical education to the students, the curriculum is under continuous review by the Deans of Basic and Clinical Sciences in conjunction with the faculty. All students are required to demonstrate competency in the basic medical sciences before being permitted to begin clinical rotations. Competency is assessed from the university administered and required Comprehensive Exit Examination at the end of Basic Sciences program. No student will be eligible for graduation until all academic requirements and financial obligations to the university have been fulfilled.

The initial four trimesters of the program represent an integrated course presentation of the Basic Sciences (BS) which include anatomy, physiology, pharmacology biochemistry, immunology, pathology, microbiology, behavioral sciences, neuroanatomy, general introduction to medicine, including physical diagnosis. Didactic lectures in internal medicine, pediatrics, psychiatry, obstetrics/gynecology, and surgery are offered. Clinical correlated conferences are conducted for related basic sciences to clinical medicine.

The final five trimesters are committed to broad clinical exposure in the major clinical disciplines of internal medicine (12 weeks), surgery and its sub-specialties (20 weeks), pediatrics (6 weeks), obstetrics and gynecology (8 weeks), psychiatry (6 weeks), family medicine (6 weeks), radiology (4 weeks), pathology (4 weeks), and clinical electives (14 weeks).

ADMISSIONS PROCESS

In evaluating individual applicant's credentials, the Admissions Committee looks for the applicant's capacity to do academic work for absorption of the material needed for sound foundation in the Basic Medical sciences. Evaluation is also carried out on Grade Point Average (GPA) from individual colleges and universities, and letters of recommendation. However, academic background is not the main criterion for selection; the individual's character and motivation to become a physician are essential determinants for admission.

The minimum requirement for admission is ninety (90) semester credit hours of college level work. Prerequisites are one year each of general chemistry, organic chemistry, biology, physics, English, and mathematics. The MCAT is recommended. Applicants from the United Kingdom, British Commonwealth of Nations and other countries with similar educational standards must possess a baccalaureate degree and have completed courses in biology, chemistry, mathematics, and physics. However, applicants with high grades in the General Certificate of Education (G.C.E.) advanced level with courses in the sciences may be considered. Prospective students from other countries with educational systems different from the British or U.S. will be evaluated on their own merits.

STUDENT LIFE

The University's student body is made up of multiracial backgrounds. Some of the students were professionals in their fields before they were admitted; some were pharmacists, biochemists, and researchers with postgraduate degrees. The university is a microcosm of the United Nations in the pursuit of eradication of diseases that plague the human race. Students come from different continents around the world (90 countries), North & South America, Africa, Europe, Asia, and Australia.

ALPHABETICAL INDEX

ABOUT THE AUTHOR

Malaika Stoll is a recent graduate of Stanford Medical School. She grew up in Berkeley, California, and graduated from Dartmouth College. After college she worked for two years as a Health Educator with the Peace Corps in Zaire. She earned a master's degree in public affairs from Princeton University, and went on to work in international health and development for the World Bank and the United States Agency for International Development. She completed her science requirements at Goucher College's Post-bacc Premedical Program. She is about to begin her family practice residency at Lehigh Valley Hospital in Pennsylvania.

NOTES

NOTES

More expert advice from 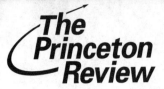The Princeton Review

I f you want to give yourself the best chance for getting into the medical school of your choice, we can help you get the highest test scores, make the most informed choices, and make the most of your experience once you get there. Whether you want to be an M.D., a nurse, or any other kind of health care professional, we can even help you ace the tests and make a career move that will let you use your skills and education to their best advantage.

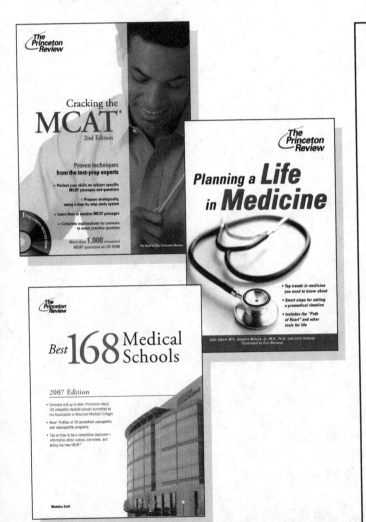

CRACKING THE MCAT CBT WITH CD-ROM
0-375-76597-2 • $59.95/C$77.00

PRACTICE MCATS
0-375-76456-9 • $22.95/C$32.95

CRACKING THE NCLEX-RN WITH SAMPLE TESTS ON CD-ROM
8TH EDITION
0-375-76542-5 • $34.95/C$44.00
WIN/MAC COMPATIBLE

ANATOMY COLORING WORKBOOK
2ND EDITION
0-375-76342-2 • $19.95/C$27.95

BIOLOGY COLORING WORKBOOK
0-679-77884-5 • $18.00/C$27.00

HUMAN BRAIN COLORING WORKBOOK
0-679-77885-3 • $17.00/C$25.00

PHYSIOLOGY COLORING WORKBOOK
0-679-77850-0 • $18.00/C$27.00

BEST 168 MEDICAL SCHOOLS
0-375-76566-2 • $22.95/C$29.95

PLANNING A LIFE IN MEDICINE
0-375-76460-7• $16.95/C$23.95

Available at Bookstores Everywhere.

www.PrincetonReview.com